Health & Medical Horizons

1991

MACMILLAN EDUCATIONAL COMPANY
A Division of Macmillan, Inc.
New York

MAXWELL MACMILLAN CANADA
Toronto

MAXWELL MACMILLAN INTERNATIONAL PUBLISHING GROUP
New York *Oxford* *Singapore* *Sydney*

Health & Medical Horizons 1991 is not intended as a substitute for the medical advice of physicians. Readers should regularly consult a physician in matters relating to their health and particularly regarding symptoms that may require diagnosis or medical attention.

Macmillan Educational Company
A Division of Macmillan, Inc.
A MAXWELL MACMILLAN COMMUNICATION GROUP COMPANY
881 Broadway, New York, N.Y. 10003

Maxwell Macmillan Canada, Inc.
1200 Eglinton Avenue East, Suite 200
Don Mills, Ontario M3C 3N1

ISBN 0-02-944091-2

Library of Congress Catalog Card Number 82-645223

Manufactured in the United States of America

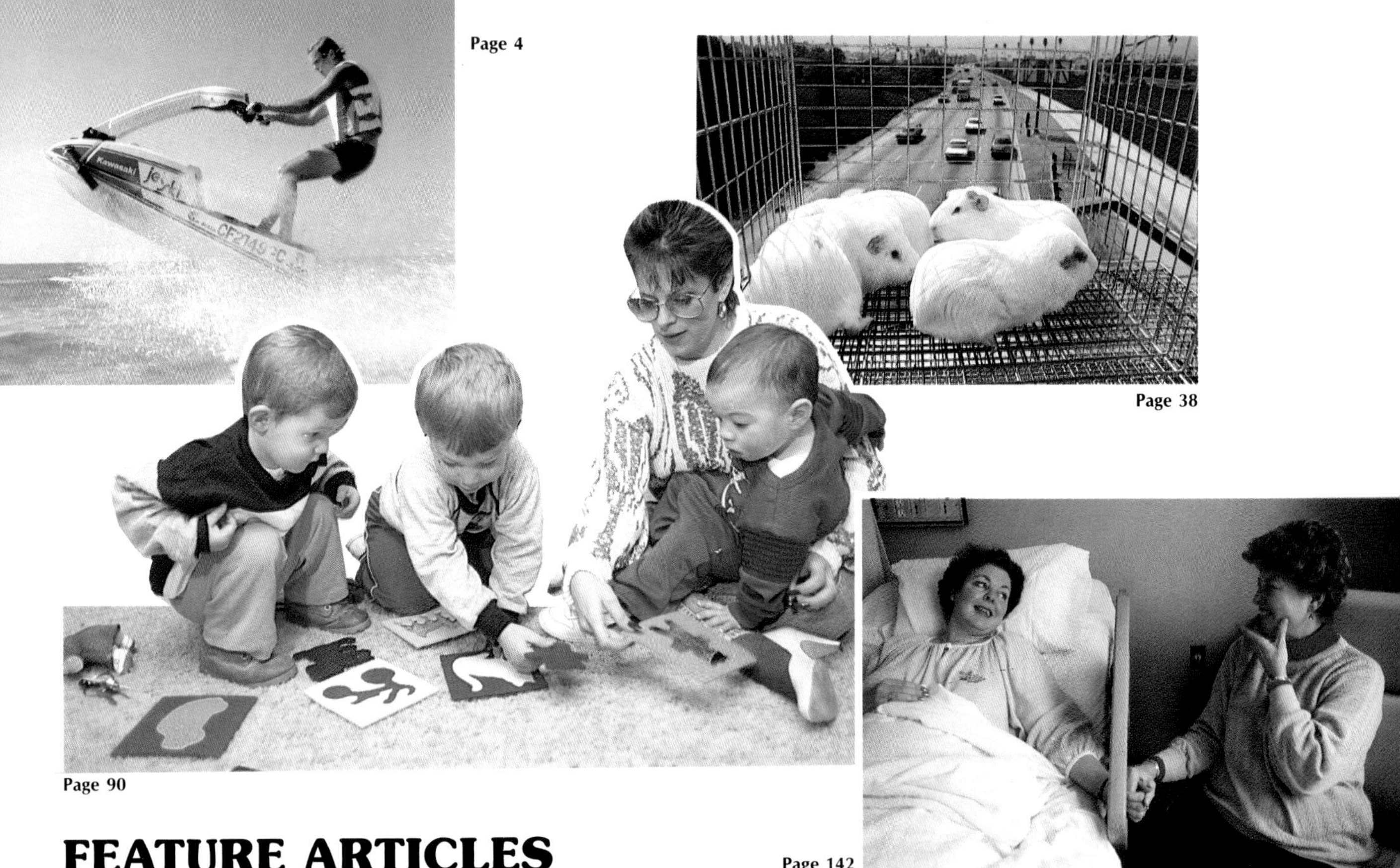

Page 4

Page 38

Page 90

Page 142

FEATURE ARTICLES

Contents Continues

SPOTLIGHT ON HEALTH

A series of concise reports on practical health topics.

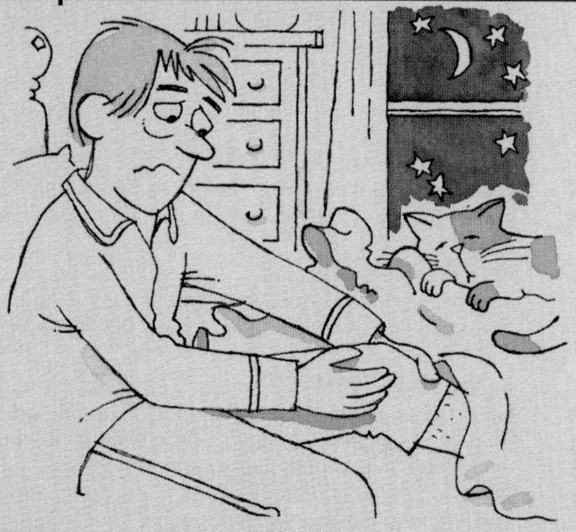

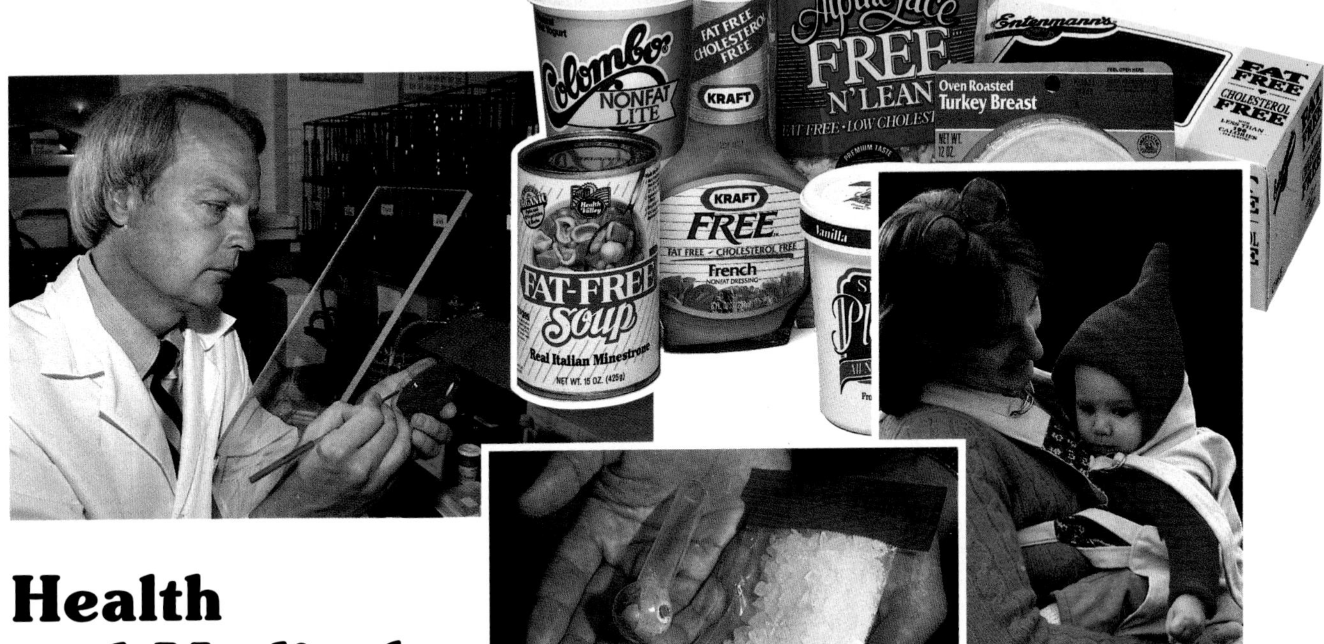

Health and Medical News

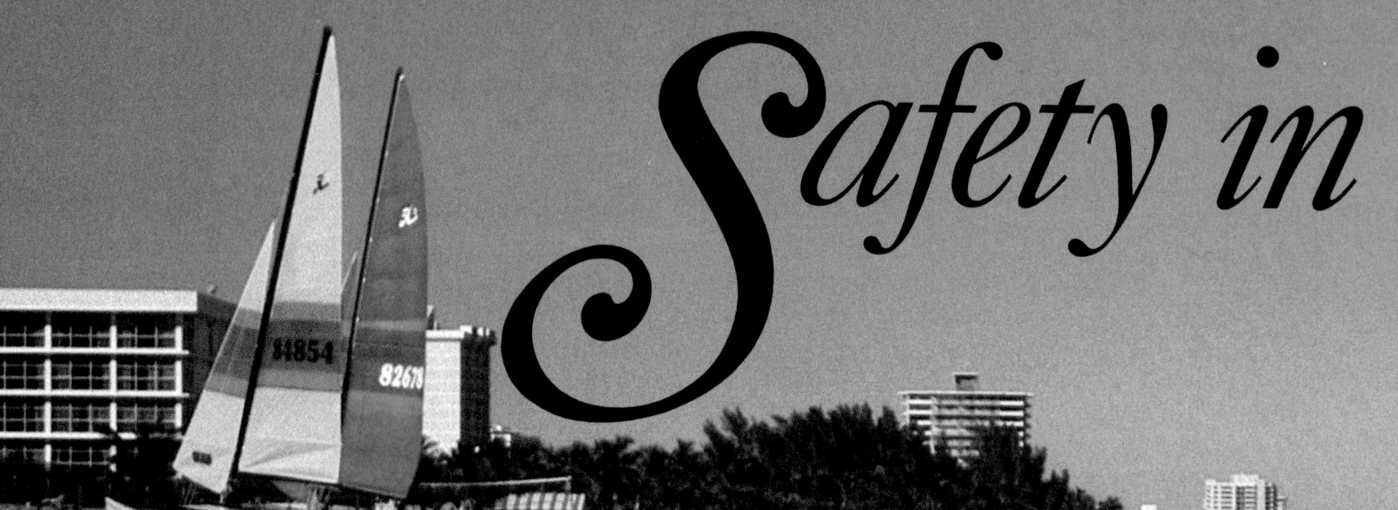

Safety in

A bracing sail across a windswept bay. A cool dip in a lake on a hot day. From windsurfing to scuba diving to waterskiing, water sports attract more and more people each year. Some are satisfying a sense of adventure by exploring the underwater world open only to the diver. Some are looking for the fitness benefits that vigorous swimming provides. Some are exhilarated by the never-ending challenge of wind and waves—allies to those who understand and respect them, hazards to those who do not. Some simply want to be in or on the water on a summer's day. And many are lured by the sheer sensual pleasure of it all and the sense of well-being that water sports can foster.

Unfortunately, many participants in water sports do not place enough emphasis on safety. According to the National Safety Council, drowning is the third

Water Sports

Renée Skelton

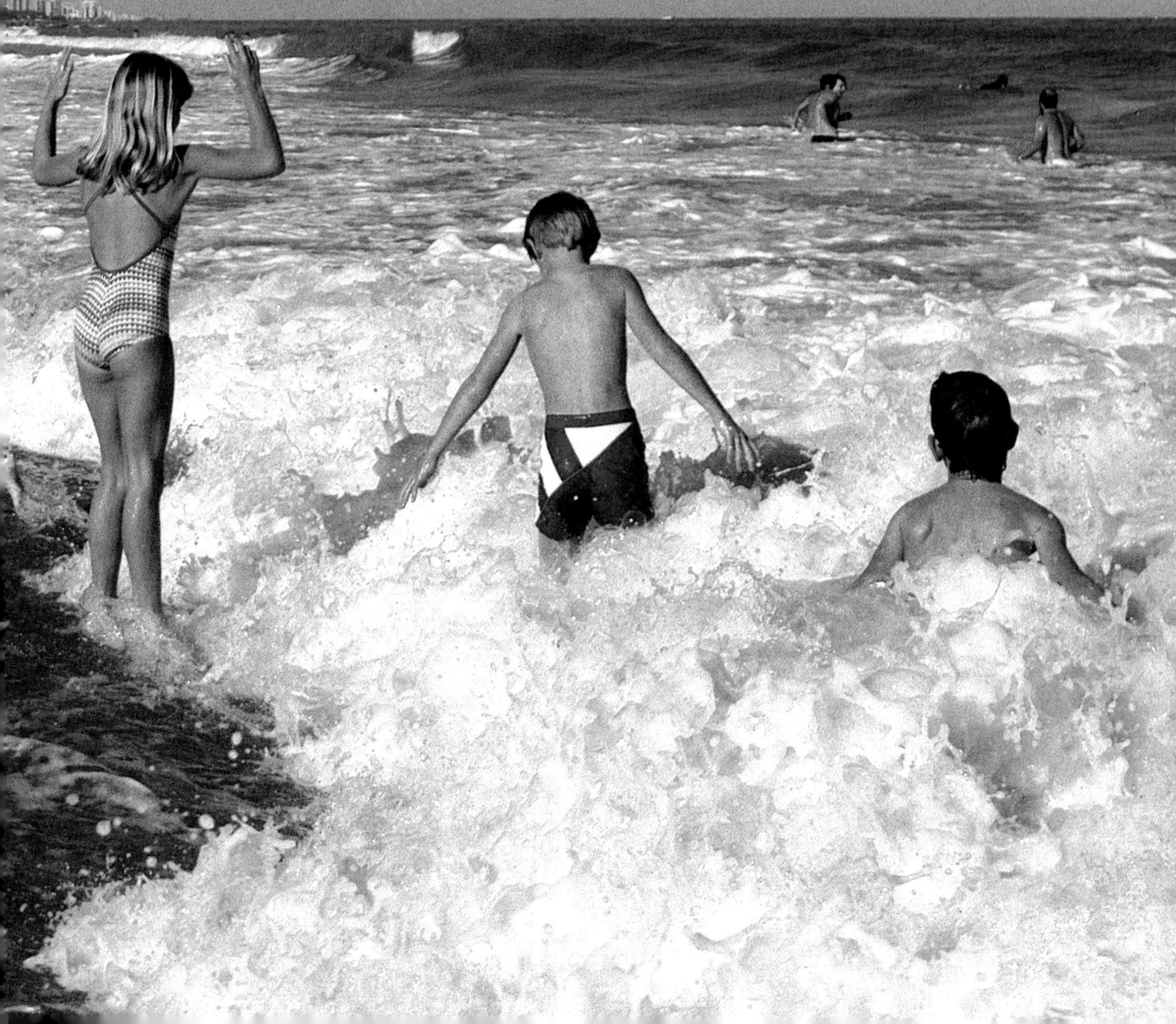

POOL SAFETY RULES FOR CHILDREN

Drowning is the third leading cause of accidental death for children under 15 and the second leading cause for those under 5. Many children do most of their swimming in pools. Taking a few safety precautions can help prevent mishaps.

- Enroll children in swimming and water safety courses.
- Never leave a small child alone in or near water.
- Do not allow children to swim right after they've eaten; they can get stomach cramps.
- Don't allow gum chewing or eating while swimming.
- Teach children to obey lifeguards and warning signs.
- Do not allow horseplay or jumping or diving from the sides of the pool.

In addition, if you have a pool at home:

- Keep rescue equipment nearby. Teach children to use it.
- Enclose an in-ground pool with fencing at least 5 feet high. Install a self-latching gate.
- If the pool has varying depths, mark them with numbers on the side.
- If the pool bottom drops off, mark the drop-off point with a floating line.
- Remove steps to an aboveground pool when it is not in use.
- Empty and remove inflatable pools when not in use.
- Do not leave floating objects in pools; they attract children, who can fall in.

leading cause of accidental death in the United States. This is not because the people involved don't know how to swim. Ironically, most drowning victims *are* capable swimmers. But swimming ability cannot make up for carelessness. Nor can it substitute for knowing one's limitations and the dangers that can lurk in the seemingly benign, sun-splashed waters of a lake or bay.

Each water sport has its own rules and standards. But a few such rules apply to all:

- Know how to swim.
- Get qualified training in whatever sport you choose.
- Know the laws for licensing or registering vehicles.
- Avoid alcohol and drugs while in or on the water.
- Wear a personal flotation device (PFD) on the water.
- Stay away from the water during thunderstorms.
- Know first aid, CPR (cardiopulmonary resuscitation), and how to perform a reaching rescue.
- Have someone with you at all times. If this is not possible—if you're sailing a one-person boat, for example—make sure someone knows your plans and is watching out for you.
- Obey lifeguards, warning flags, and signs.

In addition, here are some general guidelines for safe participation in some of the most popular water sports.

Swimming

Each summer day, as many as 46 million Americans go for a swim. Because swimming is such a common form of recreation, even for small children, people often assume that no special training is needed. This is a misconception. Instruction in swimming and water safety rules for both children and adults can go a long way toward ensuring that swimming fun does not turn into tragedy.

The first order of business should be swimming lessons. And that does *not* mean having Aunt Martha show you a few basic strokes in her backyard pool. Sign up for a swimming class taught by a trained instructor, where you will learn not only the basic strokes but also the "survival swim" techniques all those engaging in water sports should know. Many local chapters of the American Red Cross or the YMCA offer not only swimming classes but also instruction in lifesaving, water safety, first aid, and CPR. Local schools, community centers, and departments of parks and recreation often have organized swimming and water safety courses as well.

Even when you are sure of your swimming skills, you must always be aware of natural hazards. These include strong currents. Rely on lifeguards and warning signs to steer you away from the most dangerous areas. But if you're caught, knowing what to do to get yourself safely back to shore can head off panic.

A drift current can carry you down the beach parallel to shore. If

---

Renée Skelton writes on a variety of science, social studies, and consumer topics.

you are caught, keep swimming for shore. You *will* get there, although farther down the beach than where you went in. If you feel yourself being carried away from shore, you're probably in an undertow or rip current. Don't try to swim against it. You'll tire yourself, increasing the chances of being swept under. Instead, swim parallel to the shore until you're out of the current's flow. Then head for land.

Be aware of changing weather conditions, whether at the beach or pool. Thunder or lightning means get out of the water. Seek shelter in a large building or a car. Stay clear of large trees, poles, open fields, and metal objects such as fences or beach umbrella posts.

Become familiar with the presence and habits of any dangerous aquatic life, such as jellyfish, stingrays, and sea urchins, and know the first aid remedies if you are stung.

Become familiar also with other first aid and rescue techniques, including CPR. CPR, a rescue technique for someone whose heart or breathing has stopped, is often needed to revive victims of drowning accidents. Both teenagers and adults should know the technique. Many hospitals, employers, public health agencies, and community organizations (such as the American Red Cross and the American Heart Association) sponsor classes.

Know how to perform a reaching rescue in case you're in a place where there is no lifeguard. Avoid direct full contact when aiding someone in trouble in the water; the panicky, thrashing person can grab you and pull you under. Then there will be two people needing rescue instead of one. Brace yourself (for example, at the side of a pool or boat) and extend an arm or leg or an object (towel, rope, fishing pole) for the person to grab. Then pull the person in. If you're too far away, toss the person a throwable PFD or another floating object. Then get help.

Children learn how to swim at an organized class in a local California pool.

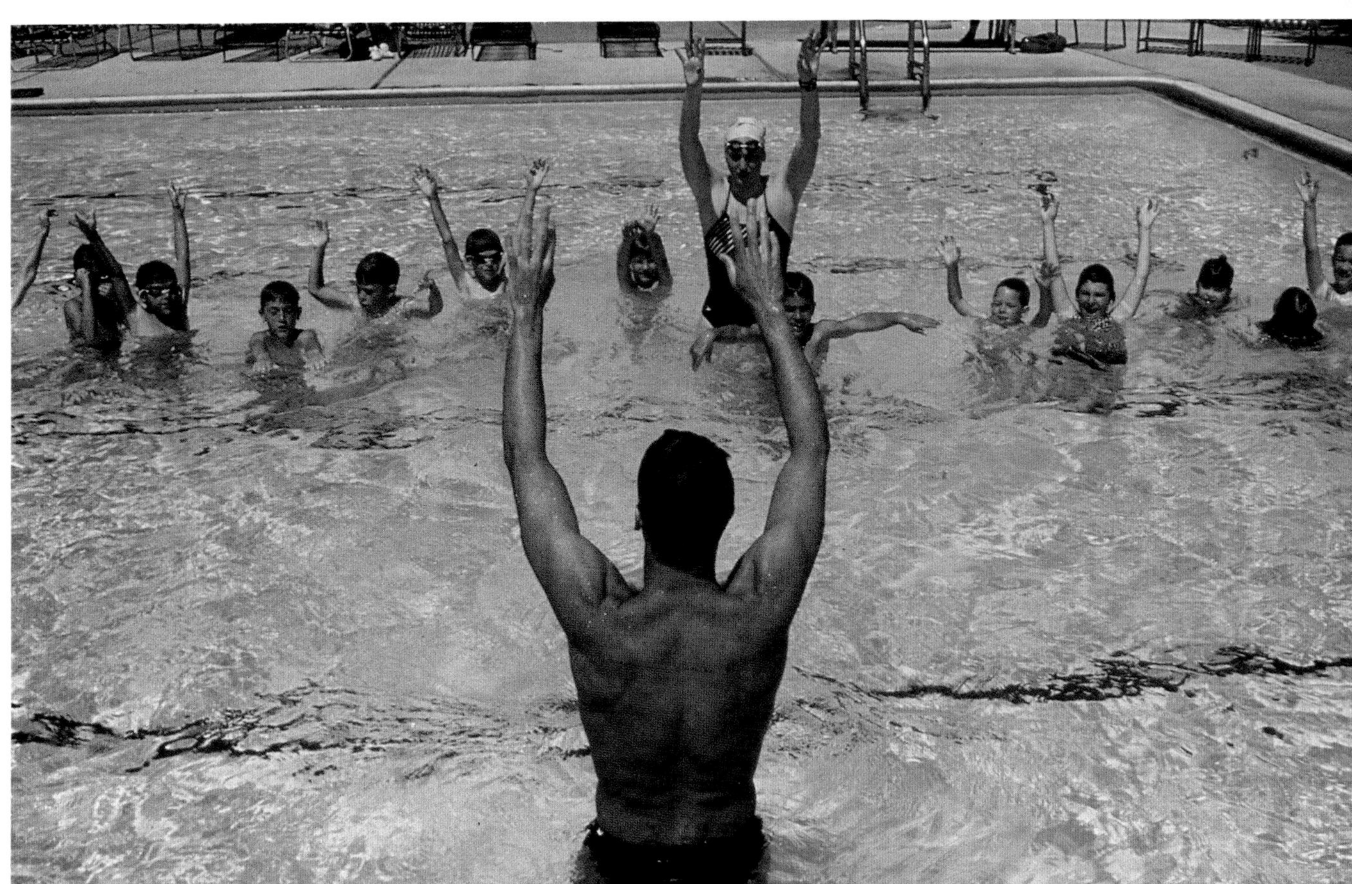

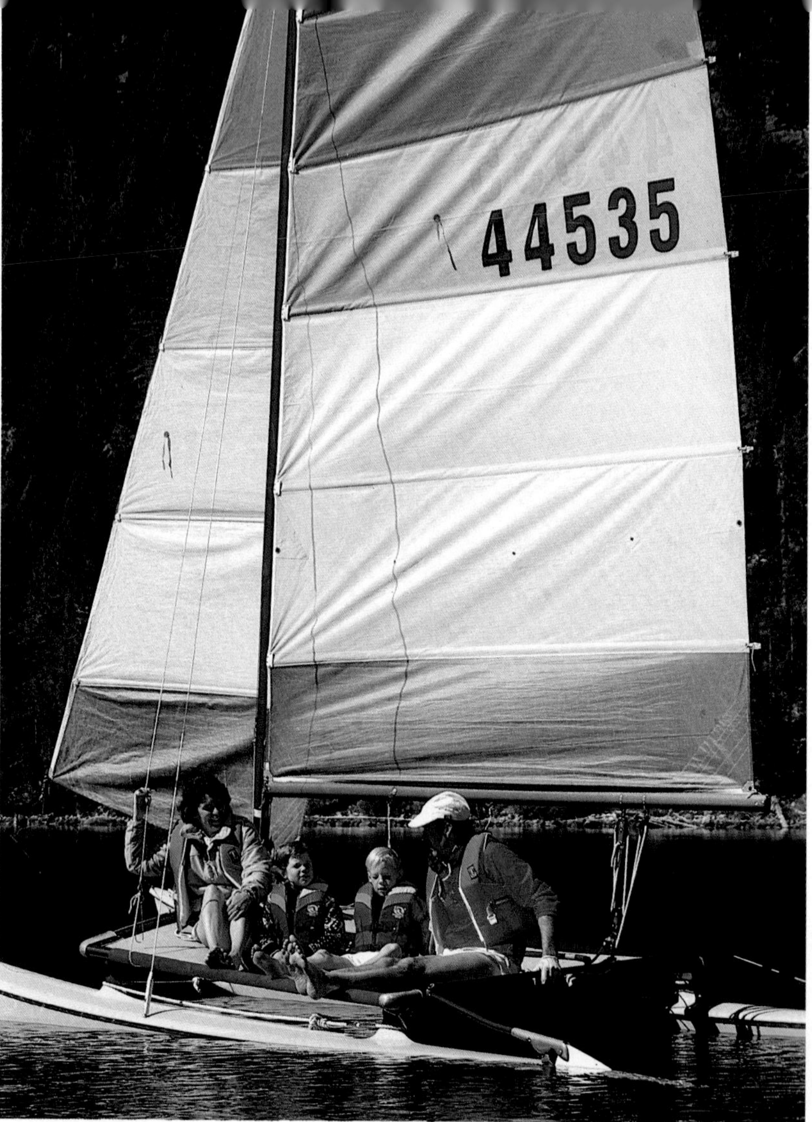

At a family outing in a small, sail-powered catamaran, Mom, Dad, and the kids are all wearing inflatable life jackets.

Also, be aware of the dangers of diving. Diving can be fun, but each year 13,000 people in the United States are injured seriously enough in diving mishaps to require emergency room treatment. Diving is also the leading cause of often-paralyzing spinal cord, head, and neck injuries. Follow these general diving rules:

- Learn from a qualified instructor.
- Never dive alone.
- Don't dive at the shallow end of a pool or in any body of water less than 8 feet deep.
- Don't dive into water where you are unfamiliar with depth or bottom contour.
- Never dive into an aboveground pool.
- Don't drink and dive.
- When using a diving board, be sure it has been properly installed.

Boating

Boaters 70 million strong take to America's waterways each year. Speed, wind, waves, and sun are pleasant parts of the experience. Unfortunately, tragedy can also play a part. Almost 1,000 Americans die each year in boating accidents, most by drowning. Sadly, many of these deaths were probably preventable with some attention to boating safety rules.

Most boating accidents are due to operator error. Beginning boaters, whether operating a sailboat, a motorboat, or a personal watercraft, are strongly advised to take a course that includes boat handling, safety, and navigation. The BOAT/U.S. Foundation provides information on where boating classes are offered throughout the United States.

One thing stressed in these courses is the importance of checking the weather *before* you go out. In the United States the National Weather Service provides marine forecasts (for ships on the oceans and the Great Lakes). Newspapers and radio stations often carry the information. In addition, most marinas and yacht clubs fly flags to signal dangerous conditions or approaching storms. It is also important to find out as much as possible about local currents, tides, and any other features of the area that might affect boaters.

Remember that any trip is only as safe as your boat. So check its seaworthiness. For instance, pump out any water that has accumulated in the bilge—the lowest point inside the boat—since your last trip. If the bilge seems overly full, look for leaks. Check that sails and lines are in order.

In the United States the Coast Guard can provide information about safety equipment requirements for different kinds of boats. (The Coast Guard is responsible for setting safety standards for recreational boats in the United States, whether they are to be used offshore or inland, and for enforcing federal safety laws and regulations affecting them.) Depending on the boat, required safety equipment ranges from a PFD for each passenger to fire extinguishers, visual distress signals (such as flares), noise devices (horns, bells, or whistles), running lights, and ventilators. It's good safety practice to carry also an anchor, a first aid kit, a flashlight, a bailing device, nautical charts, a compass, a radio, and if the boat has an engine, a tool kit and spare parts.

Before you leave the dock, it's a good idea to leave a float plan with some responsible person. It should detail who is on board, when and where you left port, your estimated time of arrival at any planned stops, and your ETA in port at day's end. If you don't arrive on time, the person with the float plan can notify authorities.

Boats should not be overloaded. Motorboats up to 20 feet long have a metal plate showing maximum weight capacity. By counting passengers and estimating their weights, you can figure your maximum safe load. If possible, have a backup pilot on board. And be sure that all passengers follow the safety rules.

Fueling a boat can be dangerous if not done properly, particularly if the boat has an inboard motor and is large enough to have a cabin. Gasoline vapors are explosive, and they settle in the low areas of the boat. During fueling, any doors, hatches, ports, and chests should be closed and any stoves, pilot lights, and electric circuits turned off. And positively no smoking. After fueling, ventilate any enclosed areas of the boat for at least one minute before starting up. Big boats (those over 26 feet long) should be ventilated longer, with blowers on and all ports open.

HYPOTHERMIA

Drowning is one of the leading causes of accidental death in the United States—and safety experts estimate that half of drowning victims die of hypothermia. Hypothermia is the condition that results when the body loses enough heat to drop its core temperature (in brain, lungs, heart, and spinal cord) dangerously low. The result is that the heart and lungs can't work properly, arms and legs become numb, and swimmers can lose consciousness. Drowning can result.

Body core tissues begin to lose heat quickly when a person enters cold water or is exposed to cool winds while wet. Under certain conditions, hypothermia can occur in 70°F water. Most heat is lost from the head, neck, sides of the chest, and groin. Extra protection in these areas is provided by PFDs or wet suits.

Symptoms of hypothermia include lack of coordination, weakness, confusion, shivering, semiconsciousness, and even unconsciousness. Victims of hypothermia need expert medical attention as soon as possible. Basic first aid treatment includes getting the victim out of the water, removing wet clothing, wrapping the victim in a blanket or sleeping bag, and giving warm fluids that contain no alcohol or caffeine (as long as there is no coughing or vomiting). Some victims may need CPR.

Once underway, follow the "rules of the road" that dictate how boats maneuver safely around each other when they meet. These rules are taught in boating classes.

Anticipate problems. Know what to do if someone falls overboard or the boat capsizes. (Again, this is taught in boating classes.) Most drownings occur after just such accidents. Make sure passengers wear PFDs at all times. Over 80 percent of boating accident drowning victims were not wearing PFDs. Chances are, many would still be alive if they had been.

Also, know your limitations. Research shows that under some circumstances just three hours of boating can tire your body and dull senses so much that your reaction time doubles. That's a big safety difference if you have to maneuver in an emergency. Alcohol also slows reaction times. According to the U.S. Coast Guard, 50 percent of boating accidents are alcohol-related.

Personal Watercraft. The small scooter-like vehicles that zip around lakes and bays, with names like Jet Ski and wet bike, are classified as boats by the Coast Guard and call for the same boating skills as traditional boats. The dealers who sell personal watercraft can provide information on their special operating features. Some dealers also provide riding lessons. Get familiar with your machine's operator's manual. It should contain a checklist of things to inspect before each day's riding.

Know how to swim. Falling off these machines is common—even expected. So part of your training should include how to safely retrieve and reboard your personal watercraft. Some have mechanisms that stop the engine when the driver falls off. Others are set to circle so they're easy to retrieve.

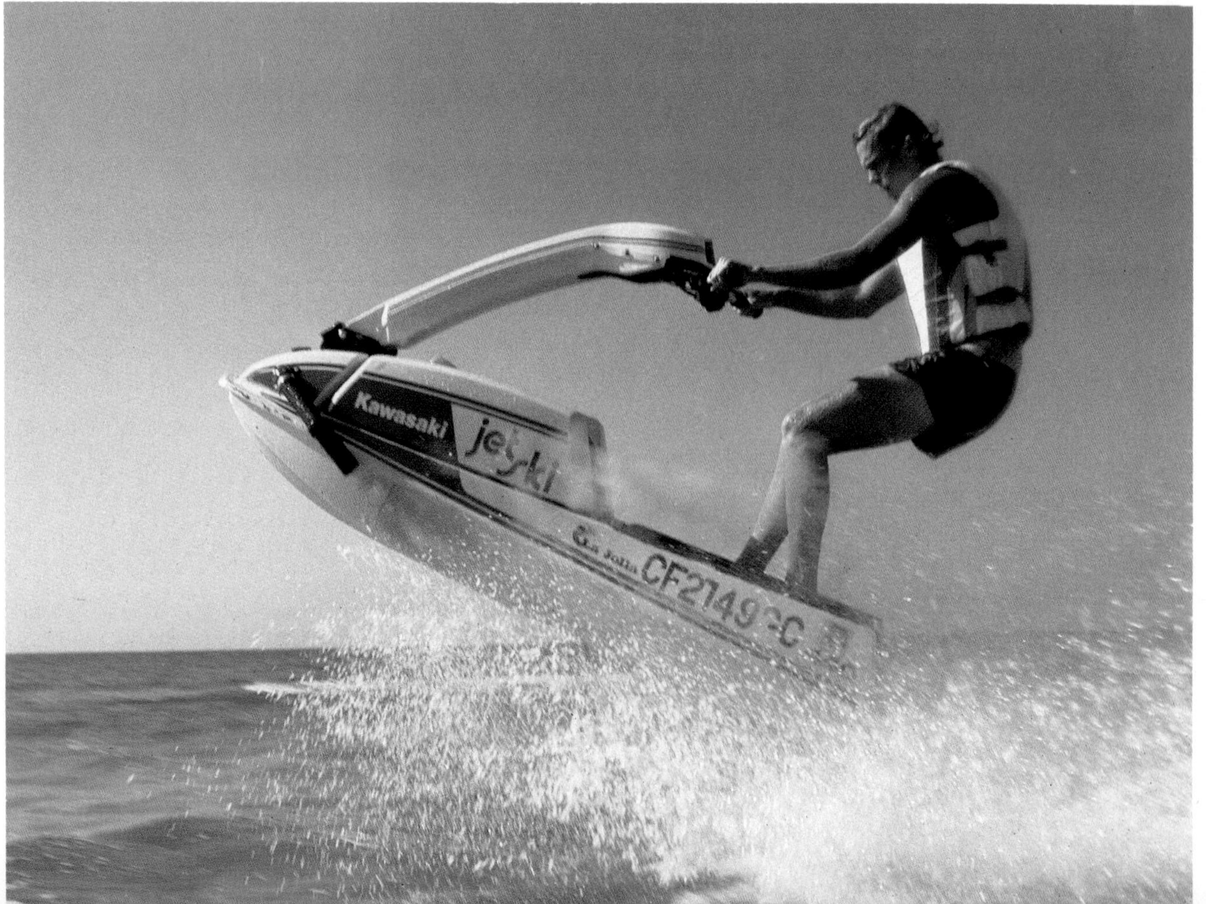

Personal watercraft are basically motor vehicles that require skill and care in handling.

Many personal watercraft are designed to get you wet. To avoid hypothermia, or dangerously low body temperature, you might want to wear a wet suit (a close-fitting suit, often made of foam rubber, that traps some water and warms it with body heat so that it acts as insulation against the cold). Deck shoes can protect against cuts and scrapes, and goggles block spray.

Also, remember that although personal watercraft look like toys, they are motor vehicles that require judgment and skill for safe operation. Some U.S. states have age restrictions for operating personal watercraft. The Personal Watercraft Industry Association suggests that no privately owned personal watercraft be operated by persons under 14 years of age.

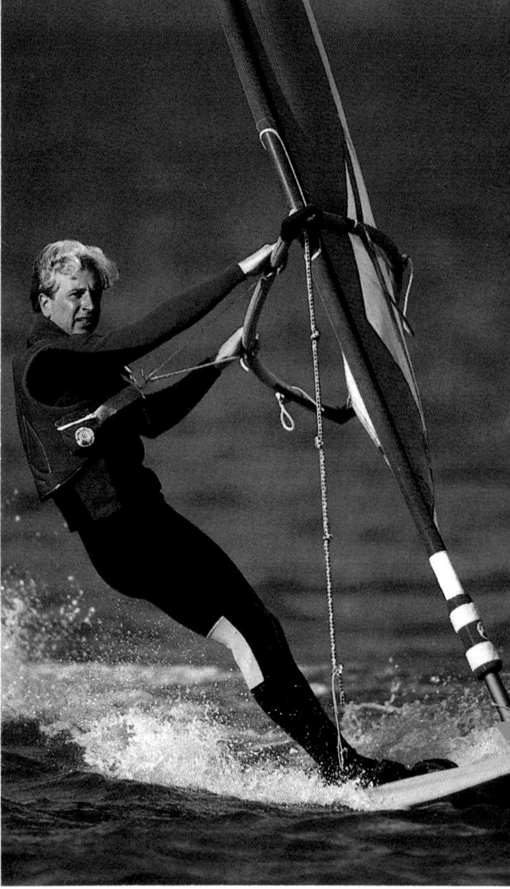

Windsurfing can be an exhilarating if strenuous sport; wearing a wet suit helps to keep away the chill from wind and water.

Windsurfing

Windsurfing solves an interesting problem: How do you surf when the waves are too small? Answer: Use wind to push the surfboard. A Windsurfer, or sailboard, is a movable sail rig mounted on a surfboard. When you windsurf, you use the sail and the position of your feet to steer. You can pick up windsurfing on your own, but you'll learn faster with lessons. Shops that sell windsurfing equipment can put you in touch with classes in your area.

Windsurfers will tell you that riding the board is only a small part of learning to windsurf safely. Knowing local weather and wind conditions is just as important, because the windsurfer is really at the mercy of the elements. Become familiar with wind and water patterns in the area. Know when the wind is too strong for you to handle. And if windsurfing in the ocean, never go out when the wind is offshore (blowing from the beach out to sea); you may have trouble getting back. Even if surfing on a river or bay, it's important to know local currents and tides. Some rivers have strong currents that can carry you farther than you want to go. In bays, tides can shift quickly, carrying you out to sea.

As in any water sport, check equipment before setting out. For instance, check the universal joint where the sail and mast are attached to the board. Check for fraying in the lines that attach the sail to the mast and boom. If something breaks far from shore, you will have to swim or paddle back.

Some people windsurf in bathing suits. If the water temperature is less than 70°F or if you might be out on the water for a while, wear a wet suit. Even if you don't fall in (unlikely), you'll get wet from spray. The evaporation of the water caused by wind hitting your skin will chill you. Hypothermia is then a threat. Wear a PFD as well. You can windsurf barefoot, but tennis shoes or specially designed nylon mesh slippers with rubber soles provide traction on the board. They also give warmth and protection against cuts and scrapes. In areas with heavy seas and high winds, wear a helmet made for water sports.

When you're on the water, follow the rules of the road observed by all sailing vessels. The U.S. Coast Guard provides copies of these rules.

If your sail rig and board get separated far from shore, swim to the board. It will keep you afloat. It's a good idea to have a safety line

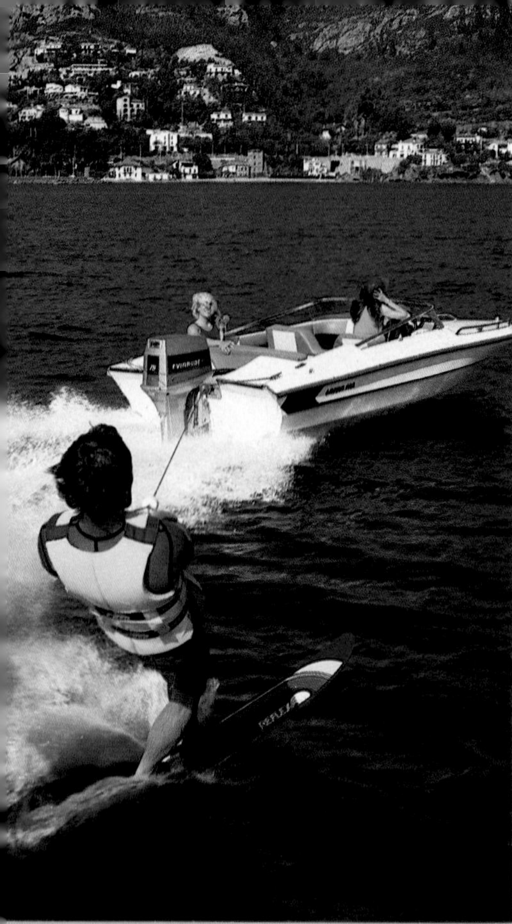

that connects the sail rig and the board so they can't drift apart if they separate.

Should you get stranded far from shore—because the wind is too strong or too weak—remove the mast and pull it out of the sail. Fold the sail and lay it on the board. Then use the mast to paddle to shore as you kneel on the board.

Make sure you know the international distress signal: Sit or kneel on the sailboard while raising and lowering your extended arms. Know how to tow and be towed. You should learn this in your training sessions.

Windsurfing puts many of your muscles under stress, so conditioning is important. Fingers and forearms can tire from holding onto the sail rig and twisting and turning. Thighs and calves are subject to tiring, too. Any exercises that strengthen forearm and leg muscles can be helpful. In the off-season, skiing, long distance running, or bicycling are useful.

Don't forget to spend a few minutes loosening up before you go windsurfing. Jump in place, do arm windmills, or crouch down and jump up to stretch yourself a bit.

Waterskiing

Waterskiing offers the exhilaration of speed on the open water. Although the sport looks like nothing more than a fun ride, it requires a great deal of skill—and attention to safety.

As with most other water sports, safe waterskiing starts with good instruction. The American Water Ski Association can provide a list of waterskiing instructors in a given area. Shops where equipment is purchased can also be helpful.

There are several kinds of waterskiing, each utilizing a different type of ski. They include standard recreational waterskiing, slalom, in which skiers use one specialized ski to do sharp twists and turns, and jump skiing. There are also various trick and novelty skis, including kneeboards, which you kneel on as you ski.

Standard skis come in three general price and performance groups: basic, for the recreational skier, intermediate, and tournament. Let the amount of skiing you intend to do, your skill level, and your budget dictate the type of equipment you buy.

Consider clothing as well. All water-skiers should know how to swim. But a Coast Guard-approved, Type III PFD should be worn. Wear a wet suit as well, especially when the water is cold. Some water-skiers also wear special helmets and gloves.

Keeping your equipment in good repair is essential. Inspect it before each use. Repair dents in skis with epoxy or have them repaired at a ski shop. Replace worn binders—the rubber "shoes" attached to the top of the skis. Replace ski vests that are torn or have broken straps and buckles. If your towrope is frayed, get rid of it and buy a new one.

It's important to have a towboat driver in whom you have confidence. Your towboat should also have an observer who sits facing the stern of the boat to keep an eye on you and relay your wishes to the

WATERSKIING SIGNALS

The skier, boat driver, and observer should know the following internationally recognized voice and hand signals for communication.

Voice Commands

- "In gear" or "take up slack"—tells boat driver to idle forward slowly.
- "Hit it"—tells driver you are ready to ski.

Hand Signals

- Thumbs up—speed up.
- Thumbs down—slow down.
- Okay sign—speed is fine.
- Slashing motion over neck—stop boat immediately.
- Circular motion with up-pointed finger, then point in wide arc to right—turn right.
- Circular motion with up-pointed finger, then point in wide arc to left—turn left.
- Pat top of head—want to return to shore.
- Clasp hands over head—indicates skier is okay after a fall.

boat driver. There are standard, internationally recognized voice commands and hand signals that water-skiers use to communicate with people in the towboat.

The towrope should be 75 feet long. Never wrap it around you or slip the rope handle over your head. Of course, there are general commonsense rules to observe, too. Don't water-ski during thunderstorms or in water that is less than 5 feet deep. Don't ski near beaches or marinas or in shipping channels. Also, stay away from fishing and other boats, and from other water-skiers. Be familiar with the area so you can avoid rocks, sandbars, and strong currents, and watch out for floating objects such as logs that can cause injury.

A water-skier must be in good shape. You are going to use muscles that are not used in everyday activities, and falls and twists are common. Muscle strains and sprained ligaments are a greater possibility in the out-of-shape. It is said that the best conditioning for waterskiing is waterskiing. But if you are only an occasional recreational skier, jogging and cycling are good conditioning exercises. In the off-season, ice skating and snow skiing can help keep your legs in shape and give your heart and lungs a healthy workout. Rowing machines are good for the arms, shoulders, and back. It is important to warm up before going out on the water. Stretch, run, and jump in place to get your muscles warmed up and your blood pumping. This is especially necessary when the water is cold.

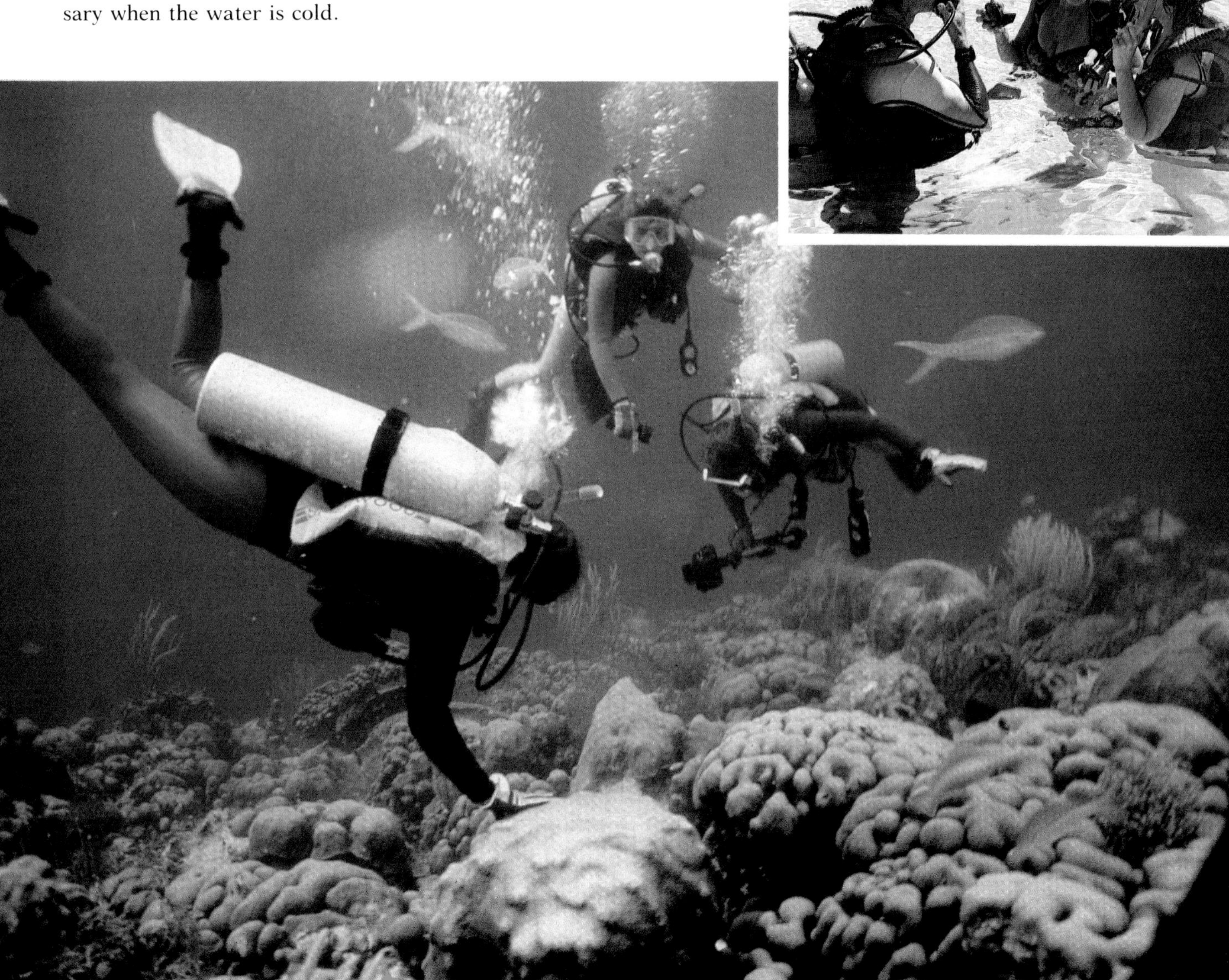

Lessons from qualified instructors are a must for scuba divers. Beginners learn the fundamentals in a pool or shallow water (inset). Even experienced divers do not venture below except with companions.

PERSONAL FLOTATION DEVICES (PFDs)

In a boating accident in which you are thrown into cold water, your ability to float is more important than your ability to swim. You might be too far from shore to swim to safety, or your body could be too chilled. A PFD will keep you afloat until help arrives. In the United States, federal law requires that all recreational boats carry a Coast Guard-approved PFD for each passenger. But that does no good unless the devices are worn. Four out of five people who die in boating accidents were *not* wearing PFDs. Here are the five main types:

TYPE I: Offshore Life Jacket

Best protection for open, rough, or remote waters.

Uses: Offshore cruising, racing, fishing.

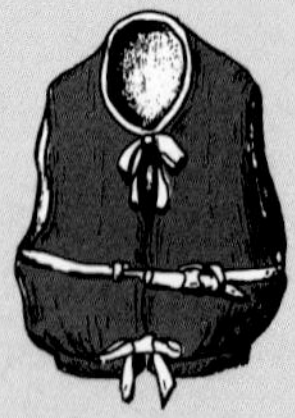

TYPE II: Near-shore Buoyant Vest

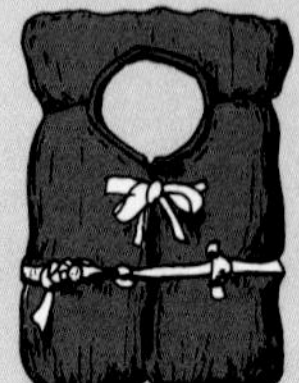

For protected water near shore. Not for extended time in rough water.

Uses: Inland cruising, dinghy sailing and racing.

TYPE III: Flotation Aid

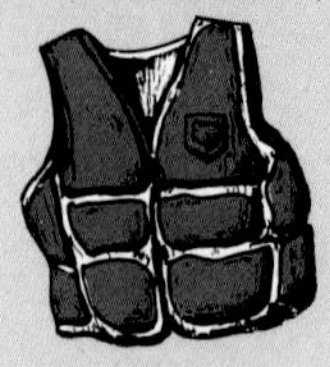

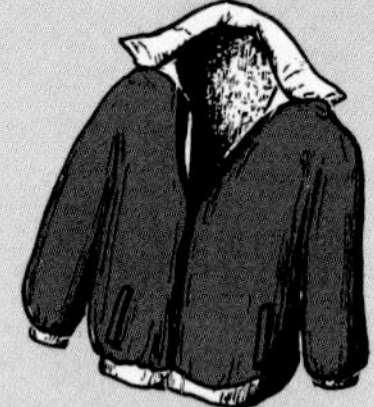

For protected water near shore. Not for extended time in rough water.

Uses: Waterskiing, sailing, personal watercraft.

TYPE IV: Throwable Devices

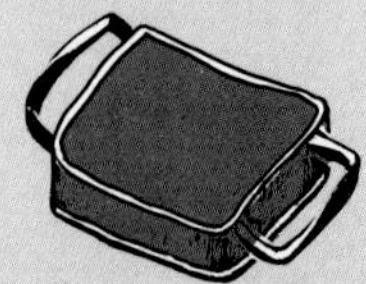

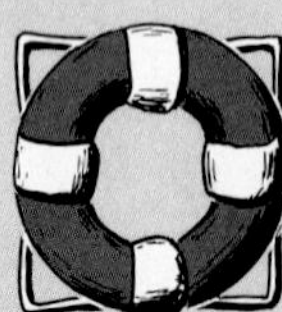

Cushions, rings, horseshoes. (Not to be worn.)

Uses: To be thrown to overboard victim.

TYPE V: Special Use Devices

White water vests, deck suits, and a variety of others.

Uses: Restricted to use for which each device is designed.

Snorkeling and Scuba Diving

People engage in snorkeling and scuba diving for the adventure and beauty of exploration underwater. But because scuba divers, especially, operate in a totally alien environment, safety is of supreme importance. Equipment failure or diver error many feet below the surface can quickly turn to tragedy. That is why it is imperative that anyone who wants to scuba dive take lessons from a qualified instructor. In the United States, the National Association of Underwater Instructors can direct people to scuba diving instructors in their area.

Snorkeling, unlike scuba diving, requires minimum equipment—only a face mask, a snorkel, and (optionally) fins. The snorkeler remains at or near the surface, breathing air through a snorkel that protrudes from the water's surface. Some snorkelers hold their breath to make short forays slightly deeper, then blow out the water from the snorkel. Sometimes snorkelers hyperventilate, or take a few deep, rapid breaths, before diving because they can then stay under water longer. But hyperventilation can cause snorkelers to misjudge when they really need another breath and to pass out under water.

Scuba divers go deep underwater wearing a mask, fins, and a *s*elf-*c*ontained *u*nderwater *b*reathing *a*pparatus (scuba)—basically a tank of compressed air connected to a tube and mouthpiece. Using the air supply properly is the foundation of the diver's safety. The further divers descend, the more the pressure on the body increases. As they ascend, the pressure decreases, and the compressed air in their lungs expands. If divers ascend too rapidly, the expanding air cannot leave the lungs fast enough. The pressure that builds up can damage the lungs or force bubbles known as gas or air embolisms from the lungs into blood vessels, causing intense pain and tissue damage—even death if the bubbles block the blood flow to the heart or brain. Embolisms can also form if divers hold their breath during the ascent (even if the ascent is only from a few feet down) or if they have respiratory problems. Anyone with problems of this kind should check with a doctor before diving.

Another danger facing divers is decompression sickness, or "the bends." Divers breathing compressed air breathe in more nitrogen than usual, and more of it ends up dissolved in the blood and tissues than is generally the case. The only way to get rid of excess nitrogen is to exhale it, but if the diver ascends too fast, the body can't eliminate it fast enough and the nitrogen forms bubbles in the blood and tissues. The bubbles cause local pain by stretching tissue. They can also put enough pressure on nerves to cause permanent paralysis. In rare cases, the circulatory system collapses, leading to death. To avoid medical problems, divers must learn how to use diving tables (or a dive computer), which tell them exactly how fast to ascend and how many stops to make along the way. Other equipment divers must be familiar with includes a depth gauge, an underwater compass, a submersible pressure gauge, a gas gauge that tells how much air is left in the tank, and some sort of timing device to keep track of how long they have been under water.

In order to scuba dive, you should be comfortable and proficient in the water—able to swim a certain distance nonstop on the surface or swim a certain distance underwater on one breath of air. If equipment fails, these skills could mean the difference between life and death.

Scuba classes are essential. Accompanied always by an intructor, beginners make practice dives in a swimming pool and then move on to progressively deeper dives in the ocean or other waterway. The certificate of proficiency given to those who successfully complete a scuba diving course is the key to further dives—without it no reputable outfit will take you diving or fill your air tanks for you.

Some general rules to remember include never to hold your breath while using scuba equipment because you may cause an embolism. Learn the local underwater conditions before diving. Know the signals divers use to communicate underwater. Never dive alone. Keep in mind that bodies of water above sea level require different decompression times than oceans, so the most common dive tables will need modifications. Also, don't fly within 24 hours of diving. Divers retain extra nitrogen in their blood for a number of hours. At high altitude, where pressure is low, it could form bubbles and cause illness.

Most scuba divers dive only during vacations. For such people, refresher courses to keep skills sharp are important.

Finally, divers should be alert for symptoms of decompression illness or embolisms. Victims of either condition may lose consciousness. Other symptoms of decompression illness include joint and limb pain, shortness of breath, pain on breathing, dizziness, and numbness. Divers with any of these symptoms need immediate medical attention, possibly in a decompression chamber. In a decompression chamber, the pressure is gradually adjusted to a level at which the air or nitrogen bubbles are compressed and redissolved. Pressure is then adjusted in stages until it is at the normal atmospheric level. Before you scuba dive, find out where the nearest decompression center or hospital is located and how to contact it if needed. □

SOURCES OF FURTHER INFORMATION

American Red Cross, YMCA (local chapters). Offer classes in swimming, water safety, lifesaving, first aid, and CPR.

American Water Ski Association, P.O. Box 191, 799 Overlook Drive SE, Winter Haven, FL 33884. Provides free pamphlets for beginning water-skiers. Offers a waterskiing school directory for a $2.00 fee.

BOAT/U.S. Foundation, 880 S. Pickett Street, Alexandria, VA 22304. Provides free booklet listing sources of services and information for boaters. Provides information about nearest location for boating classes at 800-336-BOAT, 800-245-BOAT (in VA). Will answer questions on boating in general at 703-823-9550.

National Association of Underwater Instructors, P.O. Box 14650, Montclair, CA 91763. Tel: 714-621-5801. Can provide locations of scuba diving schools with certified instructors.

U.S. Coast Guard Boating Safety Hotline. Tel: 800-368-5647. Will answer questions on boating safety, boating equipment, navigation, and the rules of the road.

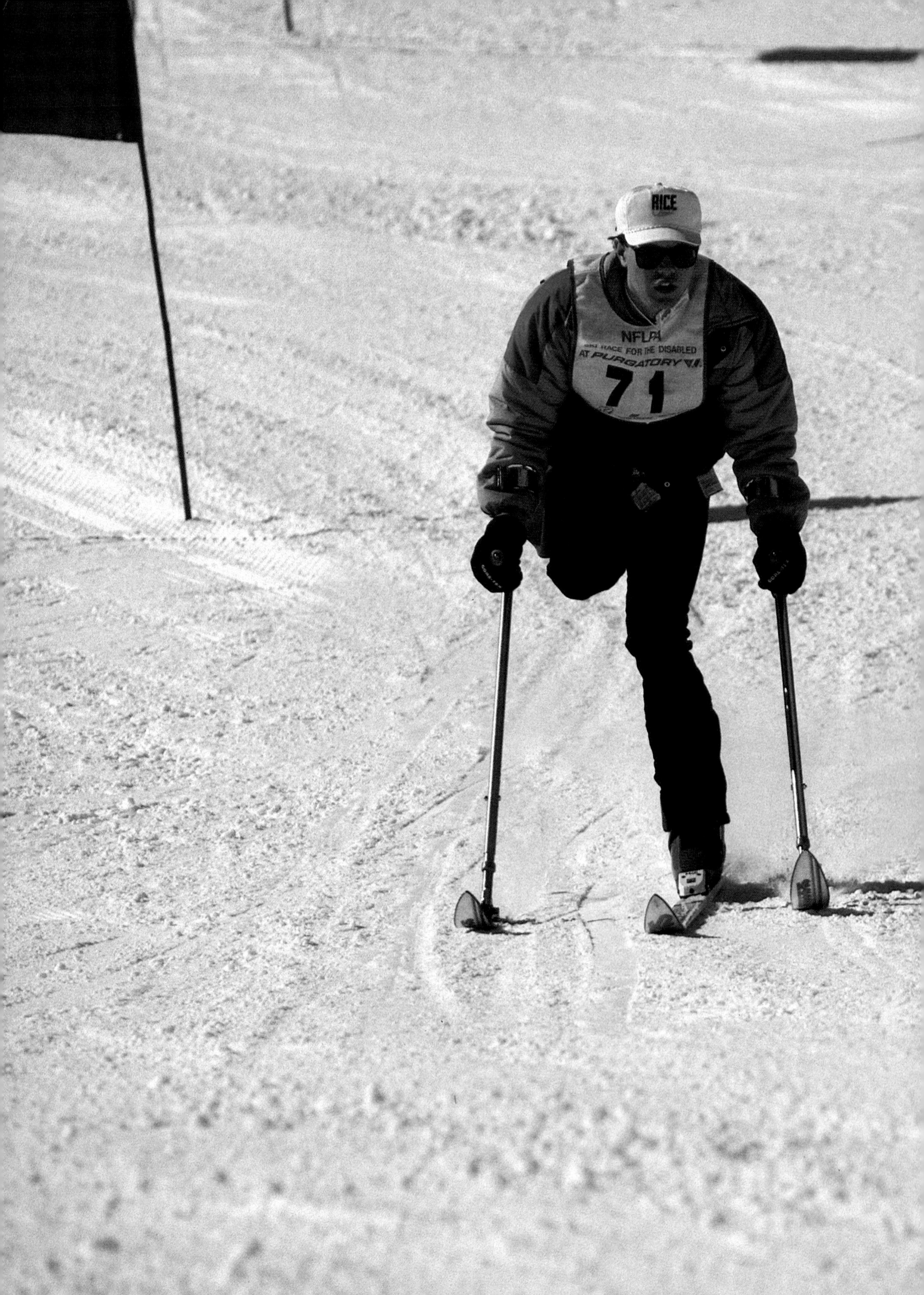
RICE
NFLPA
SKI RACE FOR THE DISABLED
AT PURGATORY
71

Sports for the Disabled

Herbert J. Kramer, Ph.D.

A blind athlete skiing down a steep mountain slope in Alpine competition? A runner with Down syndrome completing the Boston Marathon in under four hours? Ten basketball players in wheelchairs, all paralyzed below the waist, competing fiercely in international competition? A golfer whose legs have been amputated above the knee shooting under 80? An athlete with cerebral palsy competing in the long jump? Two teams of athletes all under 4 feet, 10 inches tall playing a hotly contested game of volleyball? Impossible? Incredible? No!

These athletes with physical and mental disabilities and many more like them are part of a 20th-century movement toward equality and full citizenship. Since the founding of the International Committee of Sports for the Deaf in 1924, millions of people with disabilities have used sports and athletic competition to prove to the rest of society that they are capable of playing a full role in the mainstream. They are ready, if society will only adapt some of its institutions to their particular limitations.

Sports, of course, have great curative, recreational, and psychological benefits for the individual with a disabling condition. But, as a poll taken among disabled athletes from 18 countries has clearly indicated, sport is used less for health and fitness than to create understanding and acceptance. Of those surveyed, 75 percent said that sports had improved their social contact with nondisabled people, and 92 percent said that they were taking full part in a normal social life.

Thus, sport for people with disabilities is more than just fun and games. According to the United States Cerebral Palsy Athletic Association, "For some individuals who have adjusted to their disability, sport is sport. For the majority of our athletes, sport is more than sport. It is a positive therapeutic activity that leads to the overall growth of the individual."

A Short History

Because it took so many years for people with disabilities to be accepted as true athletes and for their competitions to receive public acceptance, no description of the present, richly diversified landscape of sports for people with disabilities is complete without consideration of at least some past history.

In 1924 the International Committee of Sports for the Deaf was formed and the World Games for the Deaf were launched. U.S. athletes participated in the games for the first time in 1935, and a decade later the American Athletic Association of the Deaf was founded.

In 1944 wheelchair sports had been introduced at the Stoke Mandeville Hospital in England as part of the rehabilitation of war veterans with spinal cord injuries, and in 1945, U.S. war veterans at the Corona Naval Station in California played the first recorded game of wheelchair basketball in the United States. Four years later the first annual U.S. National Wheelchair Basketball Tournament was held, with six teams competing, and in 1957 the first U.S. National Wheelchair Games drew 63 competitors.

The year 1960 marked an important point in the movement for sports for the disabled. In that year, the first International Games for the Disabled were held, in conjunction with the Summer Olympics in Rome. Twenty-one countries were represented. This marked the beginning of the Paralympics, which are held every fourth year in the same country, if possible, as the Olympic Games. By the time of the eighth Paralympics, in 1988, participation had risen to 3,000 athletes from 60 countries competing in a wide range of sports. Among them were track and field, swimming, fencing, boccie, lawn bowling, archery, wheelchair basketball, volleyball, table tennis, bicycling, judo, weight lifting, and marksmanship. People with all disabilities were represented except the spinally paralyzed, deaf, and mentally retarded. The deaf, of course, had had their own world games since 1924. Individuals with mental retardation also had their own world games, the

---

Herbert J. Kramer is director of communications, the Joseph P. Kennedy, Jr., Foundation and special assistant to the chairman, Special Olympics.

Disabled but Not Handicapped

People with physical or mental disabilities generally want to be referred to just that way. Most do not want their conditions called "handicaps" or themselves called "the handicapped." They see these terms as being too suggestive of severe limitations, and putting too much emphasis on the disability and not enough on the individual.

Also gaining increased acceptance among people with physical disabilities is the term "physically challenged." And in the field of mental retardation, the term "the mentally retarded" or "mentally handicapped" is rapidly giving way to "people with mental retardation" or "individuals with mental disabilities." As Special Olympics athlete Michael Spencer replied when introduced as "one of our handicapped athletes," "I may be retarded, but I am certainly not handicapped."

International Special Olympics, founded in 1968. In that year 1,000 athletes with mental disabilities from 26 U.S. states and Canada took part in competitive events in track and field and swimming. Within 20 years around a million Special Olympics athletes from over 90 countries were taking part in 22 Olympic-type sports, from basketball to cross-country skiing.

In the years between the first and eighth Paralympics, the ever-increasing interest in and acceptance of sports for the disabled had been reflected in and helped along by the founding of new organizations, including the International Sports Organization for the Disabled, the International Blind Sports Association, the U.S. Association for Blind Athletes, the U.S. Amputee Athletic Association, and the U.S. Cerebral Palsy Athletic Association. A landmark statement by Unesco in 1976 that persons with disabilities have a "right to participate in physical education and sports" had led to the development of an international charter on physical education and sport and the creation of an international development fund to finance activities furthering that right. In the United States congressional legislation in 1978 had officially reaffirmed the U.S. Olympic Committee's commitment to serve *all* U.S. amateur athletes, including those with disabilities. In addition, a Committee on Sports for the Disabled had been formed, with representation from all the major U.S. organizations of sports for disabled athletes. In the 1984 Summer Olympics in Los Angeles two wheelchair races had been included as demonstration events, and in that year's Winter Olympics in Sarajevo, Yugoslavia, amputee skiers had displayed their skills in the giant slalom.

In 1989 the International Paralympic Committee was founded to parallel the efforts of its counterpart for able-bodied athletes, the International Olympic Committee.

The Third European Special Olympics Games, held in the summer of 1990 in Glasgow, Scotland, was only one of a number of international meets for athletes with disabilities held in that year. With 2,500 athletes representing 30 European and Middle Eastern countries, it was the largest sports event scheduled for Europe in 1990. Sports for those with disabilities had come a long way.

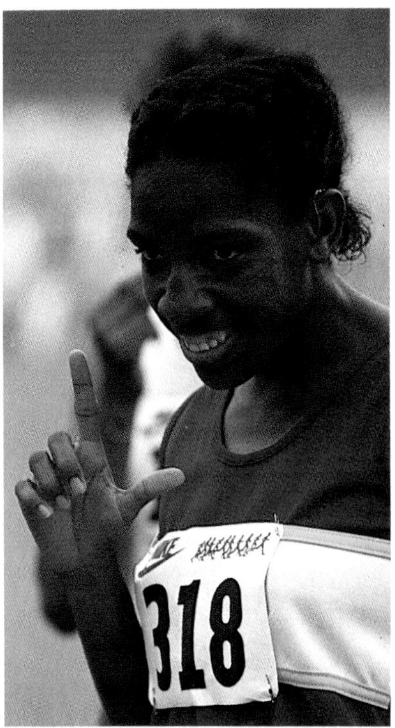

A deaf track and field athlete communicates in sign language.

Choices and Challenges

For persons with a disability, young or old, a wide variety of opportunities is now available in ongoing programs of fitness training and athletic competition. In the United States alone there are more than 30 associations—for sports ranging from archery to weight lifting—for people with physical disabilities.

For many years, parents and teachers tended to be overprotective of children with disabilities, fearing that failure to perform would frustrate them further or that participation in vigorous sports activity would damage them physically.

Increasingly, however, as the history of disabled sports clearly indicates, those with disabilities are no longer hearing, "You can't." Instead, it is recognized that there are very few limitations on their ability to participate in sports if three conditions are met: the will and desire must be there; opportunities must exist for sound training and expert coaching; and necessary adaptations to the disabling condition must be made.

Sports for the Deaf

Deaf athletes generally do not see themselves as disabled athletes. For most sports activities, their "handicap" is the least disabling, and so, historically, deaf sport has maintained a friendly separation from sports organizations for athletes with other disabilities.

The World Games for the Deaf (WGD), held every four years, are considered to be not only a sports competition but also "a source of leadership and cultural awareness for deaf communities throughout the world." In the World Games held in 1989 in New Zealand, more than 1,300 athletes from 31 countries took part. Children come to recognize early that the World Games for the Deaf are *their* Olympics, and many deaf children and deaf adults do not know them by any name other than "Deaf Olympics." To take part in these games becomes a goal of many young deaf athletes.

Disabilities need not stop people from participating in sports.

On the local level, sports programs for the deaf are available in the United States through schools, local sports associations of the deaf affiliated with the American Athletic Association of the Deaf (AAAD), and park and recreation departments. The ladder leading to participation in the WGD starts at this level, with training and competition in both team and individual sports, generally under the auspices of an AAAD affiliate. From the local level, athletes proceed to state competition, regional and national games, and finally, tryouts for the WGD. The AAAD is the national governing body.

Athletes With Cerebral Palsy

The U.S. Cerebral Palsy Athletic Association (USCPAA) offers competitive sports opportunities to persons of all ages in the United States with "cerebral palsy, strokes, or closed head injuries with motor dysfunction acquired congenitally or at any age." Participants range from beginners to athletes of international caliber. The USCPAA is a loosely knit confederation that administers a program of training and competition in 13 summer and winter sports ranging from archery to wheelchair team handball.

At the local level athletes with cerebral palsy can participate in activities organized not only by USCPAA-affiliated groups but also by schools, community park and recreation departments, and hospital sports and fitness programs. Throughout the year they can participate in local, state, and regional competitions and every second year in national games organized by the USCPAA. Internationally, there are the World CP Games and the Paralympics.

As is the case in most sports programs for persons with disabilities, participants are placed in divisions that permit them to compete against others with similar skills and functional abilities. There are four divisions for athletes who are in wheelchairs, four for those who are ambulatory.

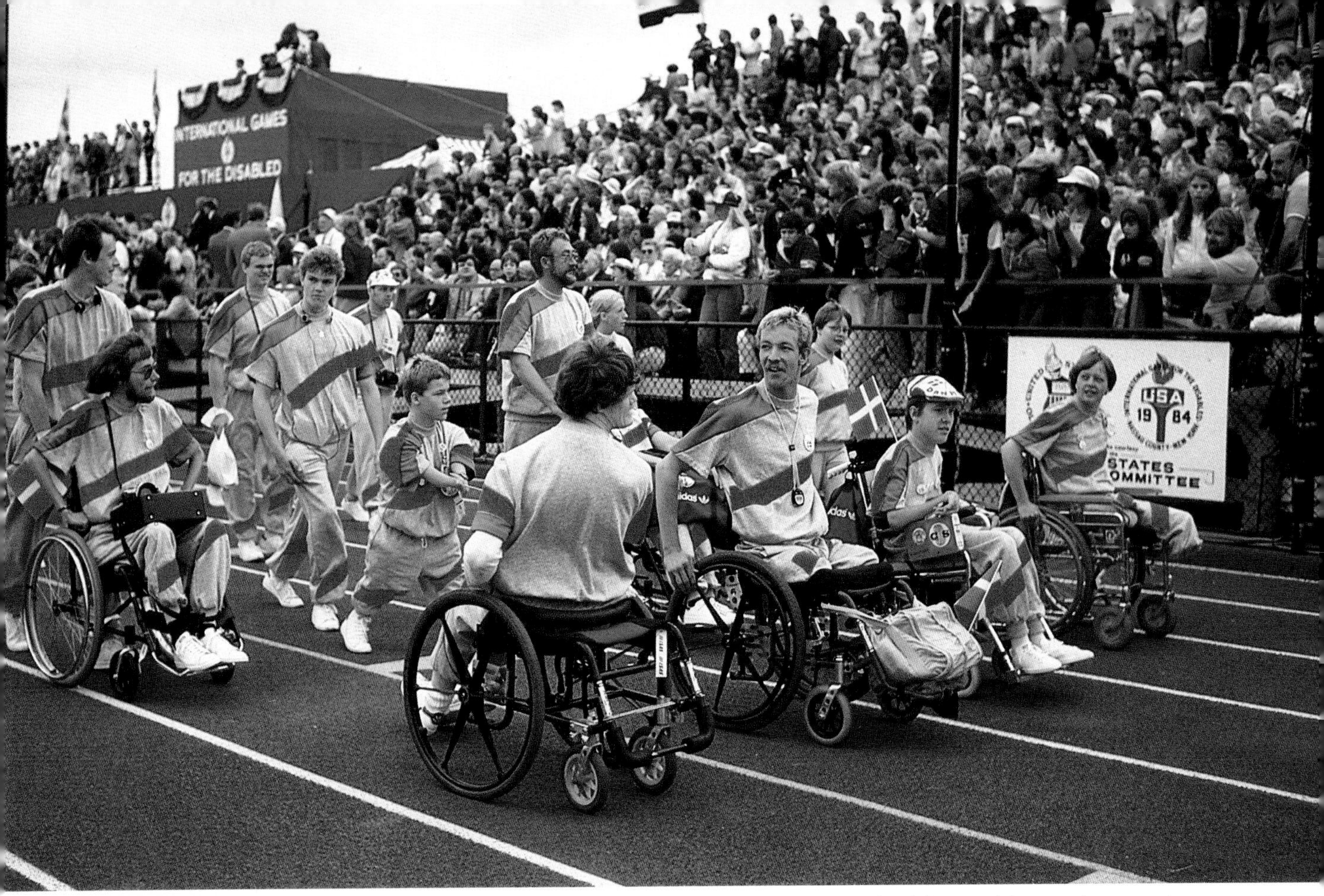

Sports for Wheelchair Athletes

Wheelchair athletes are those who, because of spinal cord disorders, amputations, polio, or other permanent neuromusculoskeletal disabilities of the lower extremities, use wheelchairs in their daily lives or to allow them to take part in sports not otherwise possible for them. Activities and competitions are available in almost every kind of sport.

The oldest sports association in North America for wheelchair athletes is the National Wheelchair Basketball Association. Started in 1947 by paralyzed World War II veterans, the NWBA has grown to a confederation of almost 200 member teams in the United States and Canada—each with 10 to 12 players.

Locally, wheelchair basketball is organized by recreational departments, rehabilitation centers, and individuals or groups interested in forming a team. Competitions take place on a local, regional, and sectional basis. At the national level there are annual Wheelchair Basketball Tournaments for men and women—single-elimination competitions between the winning teams of the Eastern, Midwestern, Southern, and Far Western sectional tournaments. Intercollegiate championships and world championships also take place.

The National Wheelchair Athletic Association sanctions regional events and national games in track and field, swimming, archery, table tennis, weight lifting, and shooting (with pistols and rifles). The offerings of other organizations include golf, bowling, tennis and other racquet sports, road racing, and softball.

(text continues on page 24)

Wheelchair athletes take part in a wide range of sports. Above, a group of men and boys wait for the qualifying rounds of wheelchair races. Below, a student athlete practices his tennis shots.

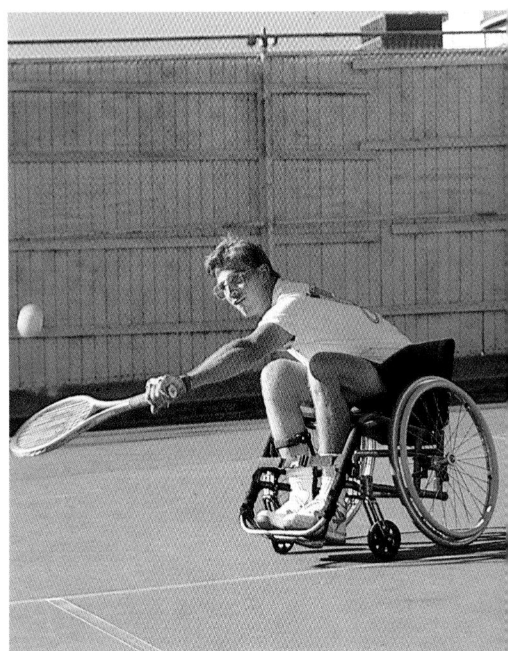

SOURCES OF FURTHER INFORMATION

ARCHERY

American Wheelchair Archers
Chuck Focht
R. D. #2, Box 2043
West Sunbury, PA 16061
(412) 735-4359

BASKETBALL

National Wheelchair Basketball Association
Stan Labanowich
110 Seaton Building
University of Kentucky
Lexington, KY 40506
(606) 257-1623

BASEBALL

National Beep Baseball Association
Dr. Ed Bradley
9623 Spencer Highway
LaPorte, TX 77571

BOWLING

American Wheelchair Bowling Association
Daryl Pfister
N54 W15858 Larkspur Lane
Menomonee Falls, WI 53051
(414) 781-6876

FLYING

International Wheelchair Aviators
Minday Desense, President
Bill Blackwood, Secretary
1117 Rising Hill Way
Escondido, CA 92029
(619) 746-5018

FOOTBALL

Blister Bowl
City Recreation Department
P.O. Box 1990
Santa Barbara, CA 93102-1990
(805) 962-1474

MULTISPORT

American Athletic Association of the Deaf
Shirley Platt, Executive Secretary
1052 Darling Street
Ogden, Utah 84403
TTD (801) 393-7916
Fax (801) 393-2263

Braille Sports Foundation
4601 Excelsior Boulevard
Minneapolis, MN 55416
(612) 920-9363

Canadian Federation of Sport Organizations for the Disabled
1600 James Naismith Drive
Suite 707A
Gloucester, Ont. K1B 5N4
Canada

Canadian Association for Disabled Skiing
P.O. Box 307
3860 Rotary Drive
Kimberley, V1A 2Y9
Canada
(604) 427-7112

Canadian Amputee Sports Association
Allan Dean, President
22 Moffet Crescent
Aurora, Ont. L4G 4Z6
(416) 727-5259

Canadian Blind Sports Association
1600 James Naismith Drive
Suite 707
Gloucester, Ont. K1B 5N4

Canadian Deaf Sports Association
1367 West Broadway
Suite 218
Vancouver, B.C., V6H 4A9
Canada
(604) 737-3041

Canadian Wheelchair Sports Association
1600 James Naismith Drive
Suite 212
Gloucester, Ont. K1B 5N4
Canada

Dwarf Athletic Association of America
Len Sawisch
3725 West Holmes
Lansing, MI 48911
(517) 393-3116

National Handicapped Sports
Kirk Bauer, Executive Director
1145 Nineteenth Street
Suite 717
Washington, D.C. 20036
(301) 652-7505

National Wheelchair Athletic Association
3595 East Fountain Boulevard
Suite L-10
Colorado Springs, CO 80910
(719) 574-1150

Special Olympics International
Tom Songster
Director of Sports and Recreation
1350 New York Avenue, NW
Suite 500
Washington, D.C. 20005

United States Association for Blind Athletes
Roger Neppl, Executive Director
33 North Institution Street
Brown Hall #O15
Colorado Springs, CO 80903
(719) 630-0422

United States Cerebral Palsy Athletic Association, Inc.
34518 Warren Road
Suite 264
Westland, MI 48185
(313) 425-8961

United States Les Autres Sports Association
David Stephenson
1101 Post Oak Boulevard
Suite 9-486
Houston, TX 77056
(713) 521-9007

QUAD SPORTS

United States Quad Rugby Association
Brad Mikelsen
2418 West Fallcreek Court
Grand Forks, ND 58201
(701) 772-1961

RACQUET SPORTS

International Foundation for Wheelchair Tennis
Sandy Hastings
2203 Timberloch Place
Suite 126
The Woodlands, TX 77380
(713) 363-4707

National Foundation of Wheelchair Tennis
Bradley Parks, Director
940 Calle Amanecer
Suite B
San Clemente, CA 92672
(714) 361-6811

RECREATION

National Association of Handicapped Outdoor Sportsmen
R.R. 6, Box 33
Centralia, IL 62801
(618) 532-4565

All Outdoors, Inc.
42 N.W. Grecley
Bend, Oregon 97701
(503) 388-8103

Breckenridge Outdoor Education Club Center
P.O. Box 697
Breckenridge, CO 80424
(303) 453-6422

C.W. HOG (Cooperative Wilderness Handicapped Outdoor Group)
Idaho State University Student Union
Box 8118
Pocatello, ID 83209
(208) 236-3912

National Handicap Motorcyclist Association
Bob Nevola, President
3534 84th Street #F8
Jackson Heights, NY 11372
(718) 565-1243

North American Riding for the Handicapped Association
P.O. Box 33150
Denver, CO 80233
(303) 452-1212

POINT (Paraplegics on Independent Nature Trips)
Shorty Powers, Director
3200 Mustang Drive
Grapevine, TX 76051
(817) 481-0119

Wheelchair Motorcycle Association
Dr. Eli Factor, President
101 Torrey Street
Brockton, MA 02401
(508) 583-8614

ROAD RACING

International Wheelchair Road Racers Club, Inc.
Joseph M. Dowling, President
30 Myano Lane
Stamford, CT 06902
(203) 967-2231

SKIING

Ski for Light, Inc.
Jeff Pagels, Mobility-impaired Coordinator
1400 Carole Lane
Green Bay, WI 54313
(414) 494-5572
Judy Dixon, contact for the blind
1455 West Lake Street
Minneapolis, MN 55408
(612) 827-3232

SOFTBALL

National Wheelchair Softball Association
Jon Speake, Commissioner
1616 Todd Court
Hastings, MN 55033
(612) 437-1792

TABLE TENNIS

American Wheelchair Table Tennis Association
Jennifer Johnson
23 Parker Street
Port Chester, NY 10573
(914) 937-3932

TRACK AND FIELD

Wheelchair Athletics of the USA
Judy Einbinder
1475 West Gray #161
Houston, TX 77019
(713) 522-9769

WATER SPORTS/RECREATION

American Canoe Association
Disabled Paddlers Committee
8580 Cinderbed Road
Suite 1900
P.O. Box 1190
Newington, VA 22122-1190
(703) 550-7523

American Water Ski Association
Elaine Bush, Chairwoman
Disabled Ski Committee
8920 Shortline Lane
Elk Grove, CA 95624
(916) 423-3377

Handicapped Scuba Association
Jim Gatacre, Program Director
116 West El Portal, Suite 104
San Clemente, CA 92672
(714) 498-6128

National Ocean Access Project
410 Severn Avenue
Suite 107
Annapolis, MD 721403
(301) 280-0464

Physically Challenged Swimmers of America
Joan Karpuk
22 William Street, #225
South Glastonbury, CT 06073
(203) 548-4500

U.S. Association of Disabled Sailors
Southern California Chapter
Mike Watson
P.O. Box 15245
Newport Beach, CA 92659
(714) 551-3641

U.S. Rowing Association
Adaptive Rowing Committee
201 South Capital Avenue
Suite 400
Indianapolis, IN 46225
(603) 778-0315

WEIGHTLIFTING

United States Wheelchair Weightlifting Federation
Bill Hens
39 Michael Place
Levittown, PA 19057
(215) 945-1964

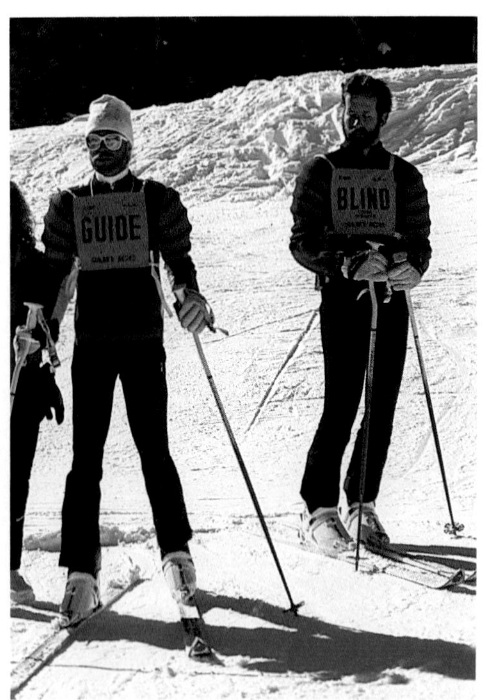

A sighted skier guides a blind athlete on the slopes.

Sports for Amputees

One of the most active of the U.S. sports organizations for athletes with disabilities is National Handicapped Sports (NHS), which was founded in 1967 by a group of Vietnam veterans to serve the rehabilitation needs of war-injured amputees. Today the organization provides year-round sports and recreational activities for over 36,000 persons in programs administered by a network of more than 60 chapters throughout the United States and in Puerto Rico. Although it is predominantly an organization for amputee winter sports, the NHS opens its annual ski championships to persons with orthopedic, spinal cord, neuromuscular, and visual impairments. The organization is extending its activities to include camping, hiking, biking, waterskiing, 10-kilometer runs, white-water rafting, mountain climbing, and horseback riding. It is also vigorously expanding its activities for disabled youths with programs like Ski/Learn to Race for young beginners.

The NHS has developed a Fitness for Everyone program with a national network of exercise classes for people with physical disabilities. It has conducted training and exercise classes nationwide and developed a series of videotapes on fitness.

Sports for Blind Athletes

Created in 1976, the U.S. Association for Blind Athletes provides opportunities for athletic participation and competition for children and adults who are blind or visually impaired. From its modest beginnings, with 27 athletes participating in three sports, the USABA today administers recreational and competitive programs for around 2,000 members who compete in eight summer and three winter sports on the local, regional, and national levels. Over 200 USABA athletes take part in various international championships. Sports offered by the USABA are track and field, swimming, Alpine and Nordic skiing, speed skating, gymnastics (women), judo, power lifting, wrestling (men), tandem cycling, and goal ball. Goal ball, played by three-player teams on an indoor court, is similar to soccer (although slower-paced); the ball, filled with bells, is rolled instead of kicked. The players wear blindfolds so that those with some sight do not have an unfair advantage.

Other sports successfully adapted for the blind include"beep baseball." In this game only the pitcher and catcher are sighted (and they are not allowed to field the ball); the other players wear blindfolds. The pitched ball beeps. If the batter hits it, the umpire, choosing randomly, activates another beeper on one of the game's two bases. If the batter reaches the beeping base before the ball is picked up by a fielder, a run is scored. In 1976 the National Beep Baseball Association (NBBA) was formed to serve as the national governing body for this sport. Today round-robin tournaments are held in many U.S. states to determine placements in the national championship tournaments culminating in the NBBA World Series.

The largest U.S. sports organization for the blind is the American Blind Bowling Association, which promotes tenpin bowling as a recreational activity for around 3,000 legally blind adults.

BEEP BASEBALL FOR THE BLIND

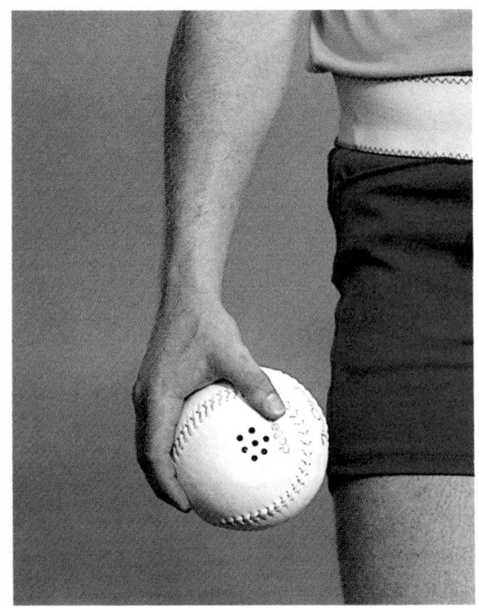

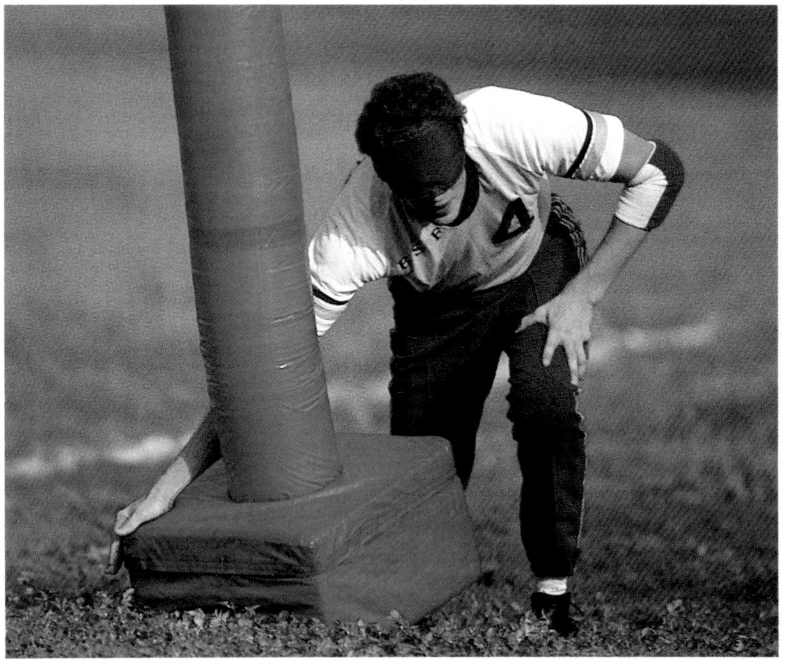

A beeper in the special ball (left) allows a blind batter to track its flight (below). After a hit the umpire activates a beeping base; a run is scored (above) when the batter gets to the base before the ball is picked up. Only the pitcher and catcher are sighted, and neither may field the ball.

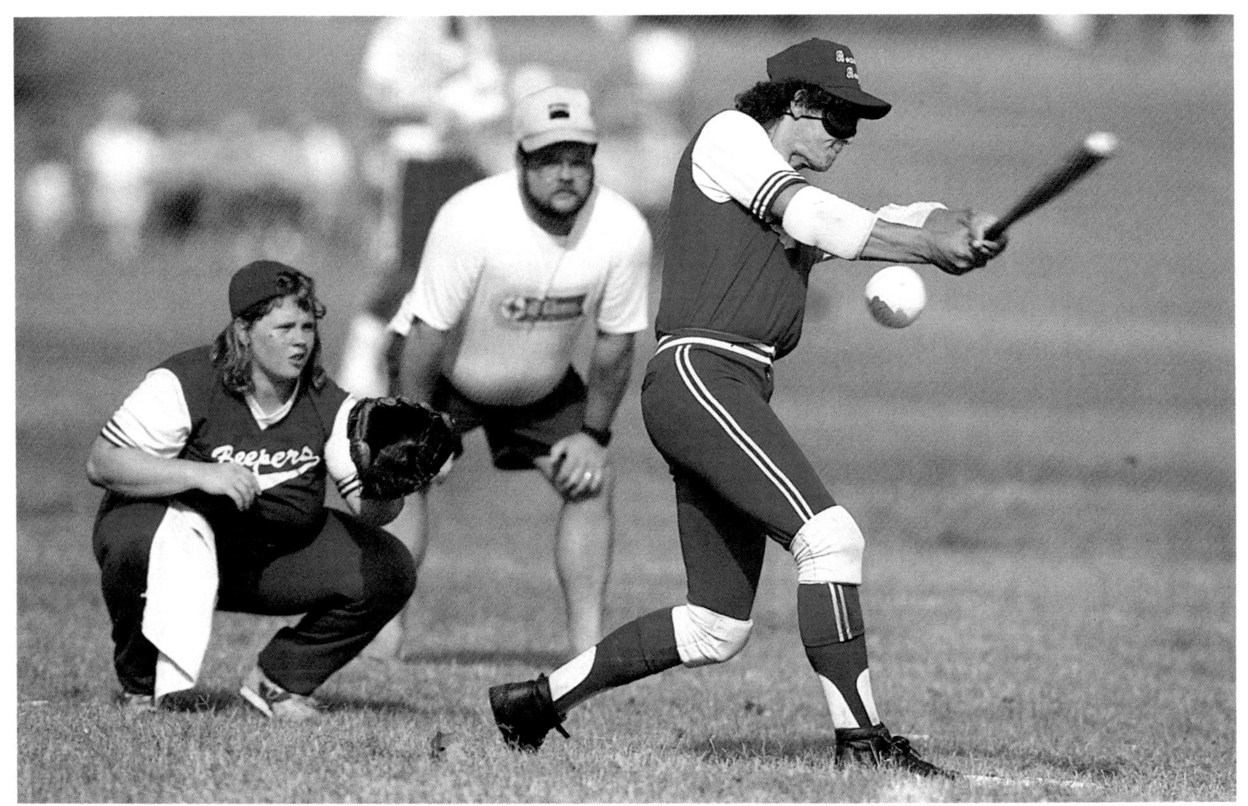

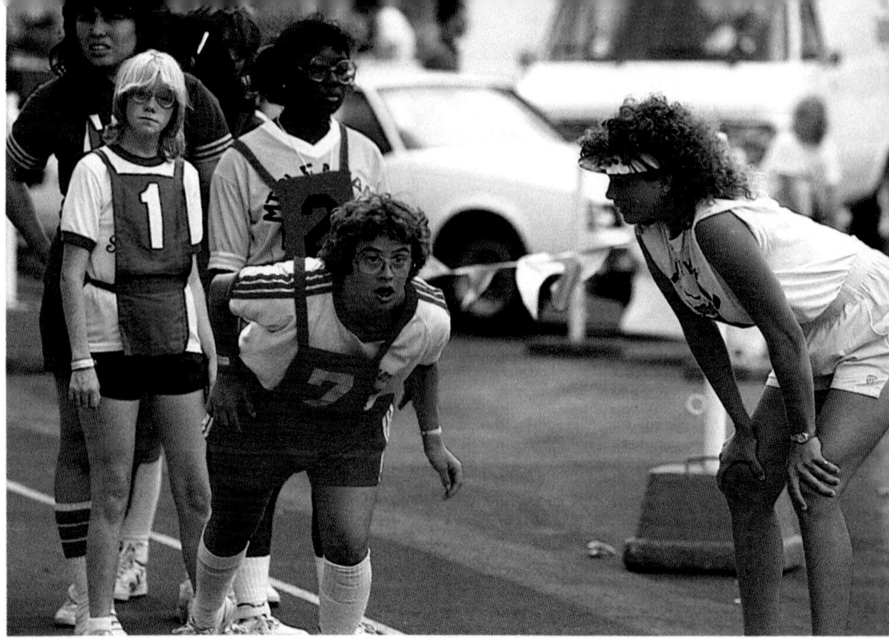

A Special Olympics athlete gets ready for the long jump.

Les Autres

The United States Les Autres Sports Association (from the French term meaning "the others") serves athletes with disabilities other than cerebral palsy, blindness, deafness, spinal cord injuries, mental retardation, or amputations. Included are a wide variety of disabilities that limit mobility, such as muscular dystrophy, multiple sclerosis, spina bifida, and arthritis.

Previously, many Les Autres athletes competed under the auspices of the U.S. Cerebral Palsy Athletic Association and the U.S. Amputee Athletic Association. Now they hold their own national games with events that include swimming, track and field, weight lifting, and table tennis. They also qualify for Paralympic competition. Eight Les Autres athletes were part of the contingent of American athletes with disabilities who participated in the 1988 Paralympics in Seoul, South Korea.

Sports for Dwarf Athletes

The Dwarf Athletic Association of America, founded in 1985, serves the recreational and sports needs of the estimated quarter-million dwarfs in the United States. Dwarfs are defined as individuals whose adult height is 4 feet, 10 inches or less as a result of chondrodystrophy—abnormal development of cartilage—or another medical condition. The DAAA provides a context in which sports for dwarf athletes can be challenging, fair, and rewarding.

With strong ties to the Little People of America organization, DAAA develops, promotes, and provides quality amateur-level athletic preparation, training, coaching, and competitive sports opportunities for the dwarf population in the United States. The DAAA offers competition in track and field, basketball, boccie, power lifting, swimming, skiing (Alpine and Nordic), table tennis, and volleyball. Except in basketball and volleyball, which are integrated, participants in all competitions sanctioned by the DAAA are placed in divisions based on age, sex, and functional ability.

DAAA athletes compete in their own national games every year. Internationally they compete in the Paralympics and the World Games for the Disabled, under the auspices of the International Sports Organization for the Disabled. (Nine dwarf athletes from the United States competed in the 1988 Paralympics in Seoul; in all, they won seven medals.) In 1993 the DAAA will host, on Long Island, New York, the first World Dwarf Games. It is hoped that this event will stimulate the formation of an international governing body for dwarf athletics.

Special Olympics

Founded in 1968 by Eunice Kennedy Shriver, sister of the late U.S. President John F. Kennedy, Special Olympics is the largest international organization devoted to sports training and athletic competition for athletes with mental retardation.

With chapters in every U.S. state and in over 90 other countries, Special Olympics offers year-round training and competition in 22 Olympic-type sports for around a million children and adults, ages 8 and up. The only criterion for eligibility is that the individual have an IQ of 75 or less or have "significantly subaverage intellectual functioning and marked impairment in adaptive behavior."

In local and regional games, meets, and competitions throughout the year and in international games that take place every two years, alternating summer and winter, Special Olympics pursues its goal of giving children and adults with mental retardation opportunities to develop physical fitness and competitive skills.

More than 200 schools in the United States include Special Olympics as part of their official sports program, honoring their Special Olympics athletes at school assemblies and awarding them varsity letters. One of only three sports organizations in the United States permitted by the U.S. Olympic Committee to use the word "Olympic," and officially recognized by the International Olympic Committee, Special Olympics provides coaching, training, competition, social and cultural events, and community-based mainstreaming activities to Special Olympics athletes and their families. Unlike most sports programs, it has very strong parent participation; many of its 150,000 coaches and 550,000 volunteers worldwide are the parents of its athletes.

Since 1968 more than 2 million children and adults have taken part in Special Olympics programs. Many of them have been able, through training and competition, to enter regular school or community sports programs. Mainstreaming of this kind is one of the major goals of the Special Olympics.

A relatively new Special Olympics program is Unified Sports, which integrates athletes with and without mental retardation on the same team. Unified Sports now includes basketball, bowling, distance running and walking, soccer, softball, and volleyball.

Special Olympics events are organized where appropriate in divisions based on age, sex, and performance level, so that every athlete has a fair chance to win. Participants in the International Special Olympics Games are selected in each country from among gold medal winners in the previous chapter or national games. □

Coach and athlete embrace after a race well run.

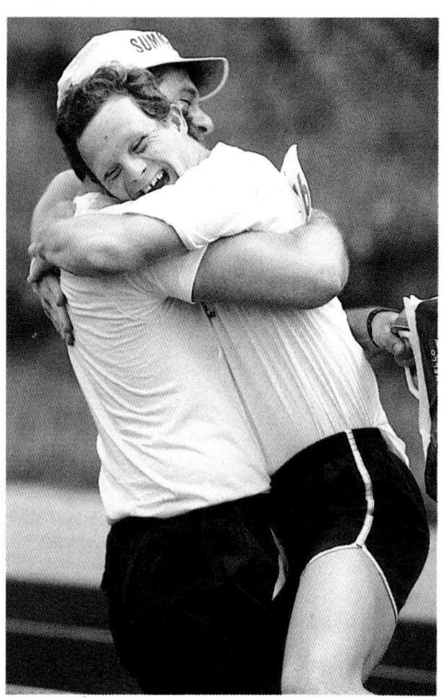

PRENATAL SCREENING

Thomas H. Maugh II, Ph.D.

Debbie Edwards was 26 years old and childless when she entered a fertility program at London's Hammersmith Hospital in an attempt to fulfill her long-cherished goal of having children. But a few months later she withdrew from the program in horror: she had learned that her nephew Simon, then 8, had developed adrenoleukodystrophy, a crippling genetic disorder that has since left him blind, incontinent, and helpless, and she feared that her own child might inherit the same disease. "I was convinced then that I would never have a family," she said.

Fortunately for her, however, geneticists Robert Winston and Alan Handyside of Hammersmith's Royal Postgraduate Medical School were launching a unique experimental program. They obtained eggs from prospective mothers, fertilized them in the laboratory, and grew them until they had divided into eight cells. They then removed one of the cells from each embryo and tested it to determine the embryo's sex. Because only males develop adrenoleukodystrophy, they selected two female embryos and implanted them in Debbie Edwards's womb. In July 1990 she gave birth to two healthy daughters, Natalie and Danielle—the first children to have been screened for genetic defects "in the test tube" before being implanted in their mother.

This breakthrough is one of the latest developments in the rapidly evolving field of genetic disease. Almost weekly, it seems, researchers are identifying another gene that causes one of the 3,000 or so disorders produced by a single genetic defect. Along with these discoveries,

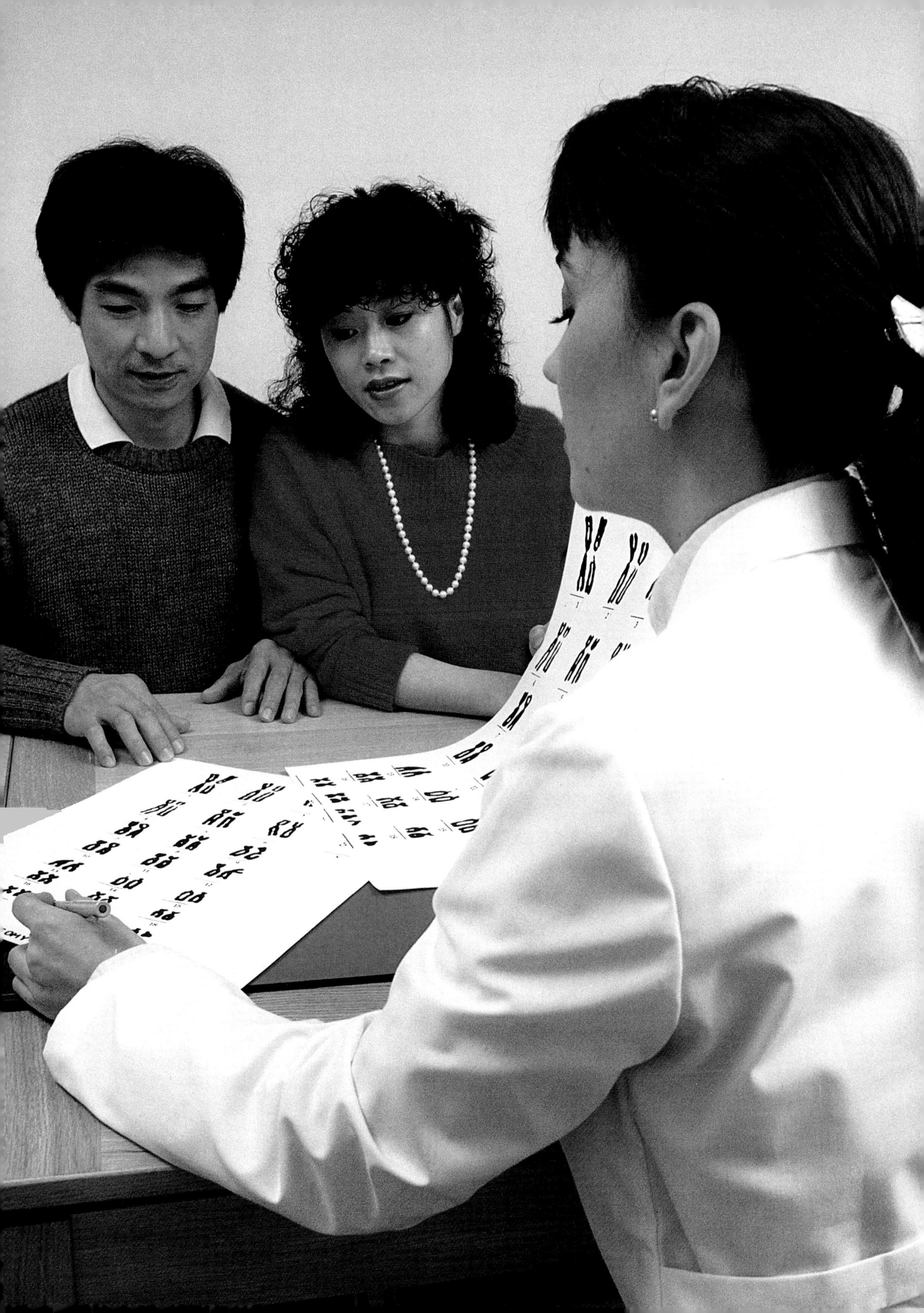

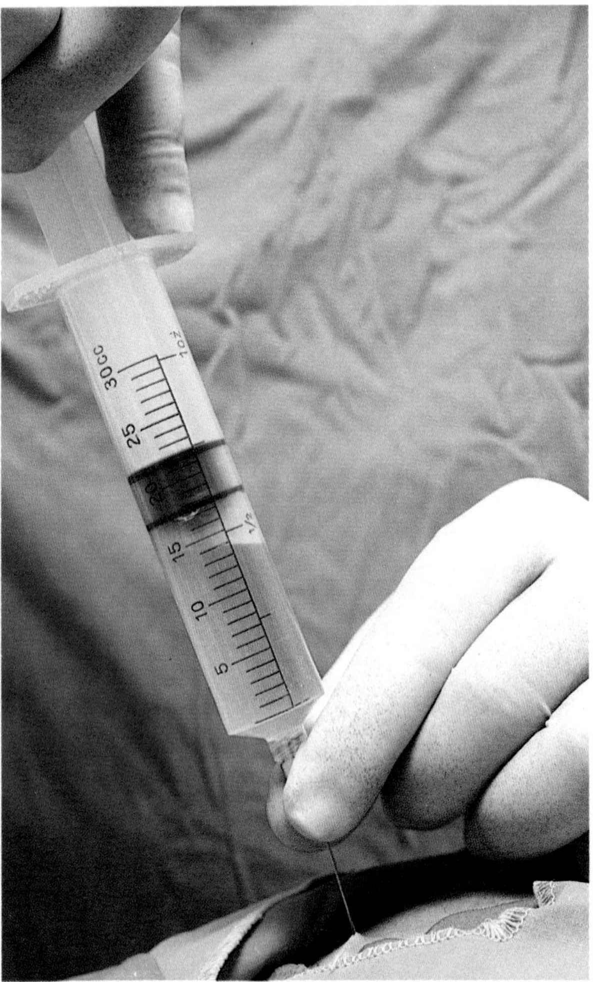

Amniocentesis, in which a needle is inserted into the mother's abdomen, was the first method of prenatal screening to be developed and is still the most commonly used.

researchers are developing new ways to screen for prenatal defects earlier and earlier in pregnancy. In certain cases, it is even possible to screen for defects before conception. These new developments promise to revolutionize the way physicians think about and handle congenital disorders.

A total of 20 million Americans, nearly one in every 12, carry a defective gene that could cause serious disease if passed on to any of their children or, in some cases, to any son; these genetic defects are either dominant or what is called sex-linked (see the accompanying box). In addition, everyone has an estimated seven to ten recessive genetic defects that can cause disease in offspring if the same defect is also inherited from the other parent. One in every 250 babies is born with a genetic disorder.

As recently as 20 years ago, physicians had only one test for prenatal diagnosis of birth defects—amniocentesis—and could detect only a handful of disorders. However, spurred by new discoveries in the rapidly growing field of genetic engineering, researchers have been developing a variety of more sophisticated techniques for identifying genetic defects, as well as expanding the number of diseases that can be tested for. In 1989, for example, researchers discovered the gene defect that causes most cases of cystic fibrosis and in 1990 the gene that causes neurofibromatosis, often known as Elephant Man's disease.

Researchers are closing in on the genes for a number of other disorders, including two progressive neurological disorders, Huntington's disease and Friedreich's ataxia. Within 15 years, furthermore, researchers hope to have completed the massive Human Genome Initiative, an unprecedented $3 billion project to identify and characterize each of the more than 100,000 genes that make up the entire genetic complement (the genome) in humans. When that is completed, geneticists will be well on their way to identifying the precise cause of each of the known 3,000 single-gene disorders.

But that research is raising a number of ethical and moral quandaries. Many people object to prenatal testing for birth defects because it often leads to abortion. Some ethicists fear that information about individuals' genetic makeup will be used against them, to keep them from purchasing insurance or obtaining certain types of jobs. Many scientists believe that these issues will take more time to resolve than will the scientific problems.

Physicians currently use two major techniques to check for genetic defects in fetuses—amniocentesis and chorionic villus sampling. But researchers are studying a variety of other techniques that may eventually supplement or supplant those two because of their increased safety. Because the risks of Down sydrome and neural tube defects, some of which are genetic, increase sharply when the mother reaches age 35, the American College of Obstetricians and Gynecologists recommends that all prospective mothers 35 or older be offered some sort of genetic screening to check for these defects in particular.

Thomas H. Maugh II is a science writer for the Los Angeles Times.

Down syndrome, which affects one in every 600 to 800 babies, is characterized by distinctive facial features, mental retardation, and a high risk of other disorders, including heart defects, leukemia, and Alzheimer's disease. About 250,000 Americans have Down syndrome. Spina bifida, a neural tube defect that affects one in 1,000 babies, varies in severity, but it can cause paralysis of the lower limbs and mental retardation. Another neural tube defect, anencephaly, also affects about one in 1,000 babies; it is marked by poor development of the brain and the spinal cord, and most infants with this disorder die shortly after birth.

Amniocentesis

Amniocentesis, developed more than 20 years ago for Rh monitoring of the fetus, was subsequently applied to prenatal screening and is still the most commonly used technique. It is based on the retrieval of fetal cells floating in the amniotic fluid, which surrounds and cushions the fetus while it is in the uterus. The procedure is usually carried out in the 14th or 15th week of pregnancy.

Physicians insert a needle through the skin of the mother's abdomen into the amniotic sac, from which some of the fluid is withdrawn. (An ultrasound image, or sonogram, of the uterus shows the physician precisely where to insert the needle.) Fetal cells found in the fluid are then grown in the laboratory to provide enough genetic material for analysis. Results are generally available about two to four weeks after the procedure is performed.

The primary drawback of amniocentesis is that it is performed in the second trimester of pregnancy, when the fetus has already started moving and when a woman is likely to have already announced that she is pregnant. These factors can make terminating the pregnancy more difficult, should that be the decision based on test results. Furthermore, abortion is riskier and more traumatic later in pregnancy. Amniocentesis itself has inherent risks, including infections and, most seriously, miscarriage, which occurs in 0.5 to 1 percent of the procedures.

Amniocentesis is considered highly accurate. A 1989 study conducted by the U.S. National Institute

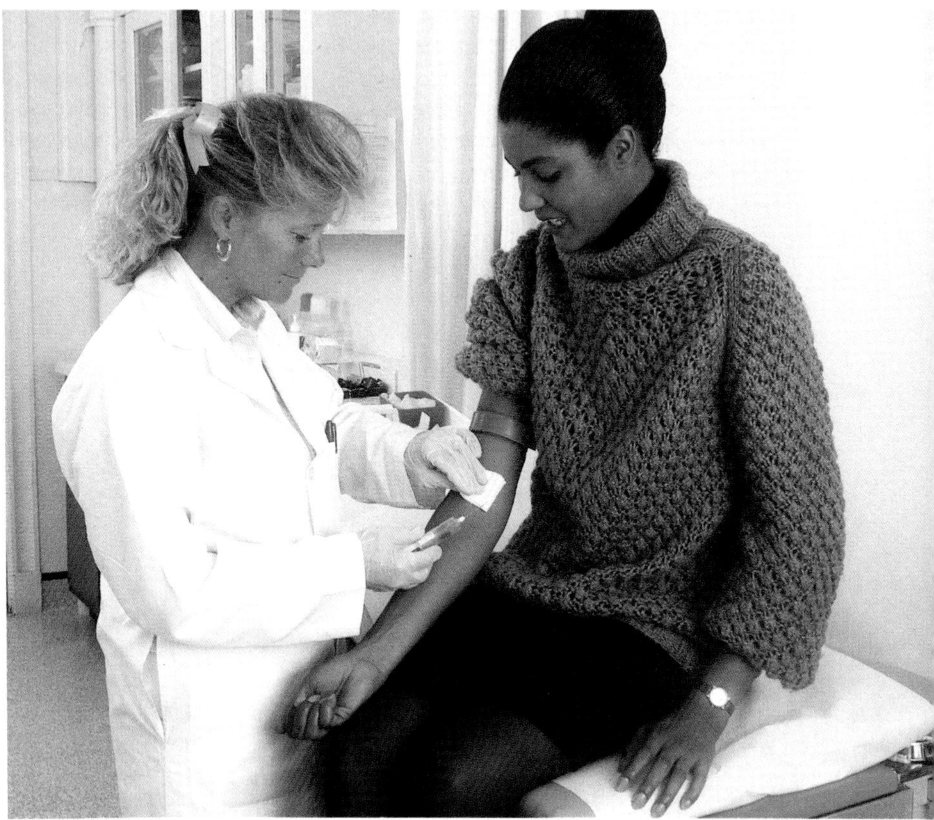

Blood tests are increasingly being used as a means of identifying genetic defects.

of Child Health and Human Development found that a correct diagnosis was obtained 99.4 percent of the time. The procedure generally takes 10 to 30 minutes and is uncomfortable but not painful.

Chorionic Villus Sampling

A newer technique called chorionic villus sampling (CVS) is being used by many doctors as a replacement for amniocentesis because it can be done as early as the eighth week of pregnancy. Chorionic villi are tiny hairlike projections on the surface of the chorionic plate, a membrane that grows around the embryo shortly after conception and later forms the placenta, which nourishes the fetus. The chorionic plate is made up of cells from the outer layer of the embryo and is thus genetically identical to the fetus.

To perform CVS, the physician inserts a flexible catheter through the vagina into the uterine cavity. (Ultrasonic imaging of the uterus shows the doctor where to manipulate the catheter.) The physician then removes a small sample of the chorionic villi. Because a larger quantity of cells is obtained than in amniocentesis, and because these cells grow faster, preliminary results are generally obtained in as little as two days, although confirmation may take longer.

CVS involves a greater risk of infection than amniocentesis because the catheter encounters bacteria as it passes through the vagina. In amniocentesis, in contrast, the skin into which the needle is inserted can be more thoroughly sterilized before the procedure begins. With CVS there is also a slightly higher risk of miscarriage, about 1 percentage point more, according to the 1989 study. That study also found CVS to be 97.8 percent accurate—slightly less reliable than amniocentesis. Furthermore, CVS does not detect defects, such as spina bifida, that become evident after the first trimester. Like amniocentesis, CVS takes 10 to 30 minutes and is considered merely uncomfortable; the most common side effects are cramping and spotting. The cost tends to be higher than for amniocentesis.

CVS is not for everyone. It is difficult to obtain results after the 12th week of pregnancy. If multiple births are involved, it is difficult to tell which fetus is being tested. If the mother has active genital herpes (or another venereal disease), the risk of exposing the baby is great. And fibroids or other benign growths in the uterus can make it impossible to sample the chorionic villi. In these cases, amniocentesis should be performed.

In a newer type of CVS called transabdominal, a needle is inserted through the abdomen, as in amniocentesis. This procedure is still experimental but shows potential. By dispensing with the vaginal catheter, it promises to lower the risk of infection that accompanies conventional CVS.

Alpha-fetoprotein Testing

A much less accurate but also less invasive test—the alpha-fetoprotein blood test—is being used increasingly to screen for Down syndrome and neural tube defects. Researchers have found that a protein called alpha-fetoprotein, or AFP, is produced by the fetus during development and released into the amniotic fluid and mother's blood, which can then be tested for AFP level. Unusually high concentrations of AFP can be a sign of an open neural tube defect, such as spina bifida or anencephaly, and unusually low concentrations have been associated with an increased risk of Down syndrome.

About 3 percent of the blood tests will show abnormally high levels of AFP, but only about 5 percent of these women will be found, after further evaluation, to actually have a fetus with a neural tube defect. Similarly, in the vast majority of women whose blood tests show low AFP levels, the fetus is normal. As a result, the AFP test results alone are not regarded as sufficient for a diagnosis, but they can indicate that more precise tests such as ultrasound or amniocentesis should be considered.

In spite of its imprecision, AFP testing is gaining popularity among older women, in large part because it does not increase the risk of miscarriage, as do amniocentesis and chorionic villus sampling. It is also being used by younger women considered at high risk of bearing a child with a neural tube defect because of a previous child with, or a family history of, such defects. Yet most babies with neural tube defects are born to couples assumed to be at low risk, and 80 percent of Down children are born to women under 35. For these reasons, some physicians recommend that *all* pregnant women take the AFP screening test.

The AFP test is usually done in the 16th or 17th week of pregnancy. If the test shows an abnormal elevation in AFP, a second blood sample is tested. In many cases the second test shows a normal level,

How Single-Gene Defects Are Inherited

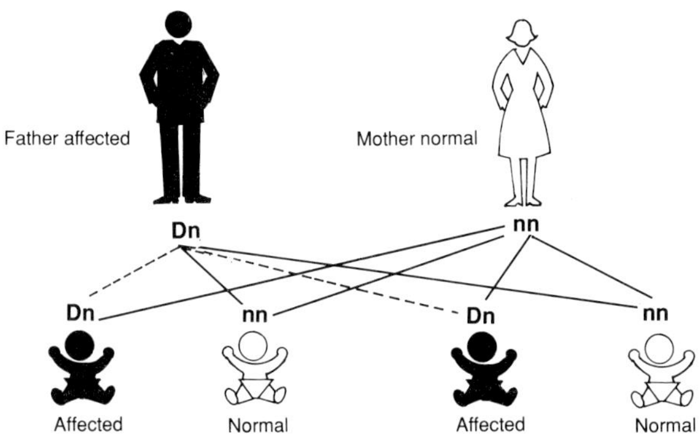

1. Dominant Inheritance

*One parent, who has the condition, has a faulty gene (**D**) that is dominant—it dominates the normal gene (**n**). The other parent has two normal genes. Each child has a 50 percent chance of inheriting the condition.*

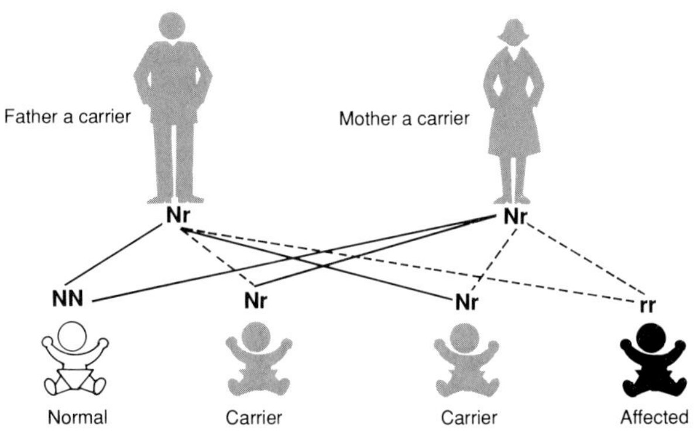

2. Recessive Inheritance

*Both parents are carriers of the condition: each has a normal dominant gene (**N**) and a faulty recessive gene (**r**). Each child has a 25 percent chance of inheriting the condition.*

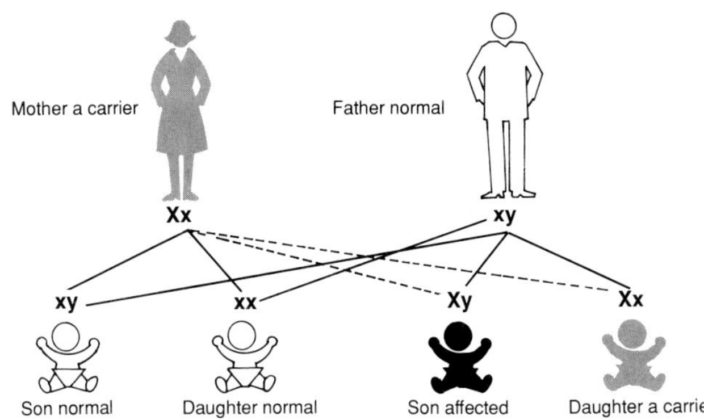

3. Sex-Linked Inheritance

*One of the mother's sex chromosomes carries a faulty gene (**X**) while her other sex chromosome is normal (**x**). The father's sex chromosomes (**x** and **y**) are both normal. Each male child has a 50 percent chance of inheriting the condition.*

Genes are the basic biochemical units of heredity. Each human being has 50,000 pairs of genes, which regulate the growth and functioning of cells, tissues, and organs. When a gene malfunctions or is defective in some way, the result may be a physical abnormality or disease.

Genes are contained in threadlike structures called chromosomes that are housed in the nuclei of cells. Humans cells have 23 pairs of chromosomes, or 46 in all. Two exceptions are the reproductive cells—the egg and sperm—which each contain only 23 chromosomes, one member of each pair. When an egg and sperm unite, the resulting cell contains the normal 46 chromosomes. In this way, children receive half of their genetic material from the mother and half from the father. That is why they resemble both but are identical to neither.

The inheritance of a genetic defect can take one of three forms, called dominant, recessive, and sex-linked inheritance.

Dominant Inheritance

Virtually everyone receives a few defective genes from their parents, but very few people get genetic diseases. This is because genes work in pairs, and usually a malfunctioning gene inherited from one parent is compensated for by a normally functioning gene inherited from the other. In such cases the malfunctioning gene is said to be recessive and the normal gene dominant. Sometimes, however, the defective gene is dominant. In these cases, every child who inherits the defective gene will suffer from the disorder it produces. (See Figure 1.) Huntington's disease is an example of such a disorder.

Recessive Inheritance

Inherited disorders can also result if both parents are carriers of a malfunctioning recessive gene. (See Figure 2.) Most recessive conditions are rare, since the chances are remote that a carrier of a defective gene will have children with another carrier of the same defective gene, but some disease-causing recessive genes occur more frequently among certain ethnic or racial groups—such as sickle-cell anemia in blacks. The likelihood of a recessive disorder also rises when two closely related people have children together.

Sex-linked Inheritance

In all but one of the 23 pairs of chromosomes, the two chromosomes always have the same number of genes, and the genes for a given trait are located at the same position on each chromosome. The one pair that may not match up this way is the pair that determines a person's sex. While females have two *X* chromosomes, males have an *X* and a *Y*. When the reproductive cells are formed, the sperm can have either an *X* or a *Y*, while the egg can have only an *X*.

The *X* chromosome contains some genes that have no corresponding gene on the *Y* chromosome. If one of these genes is defective, even if it is recessive every male child who inherits it will suffer from the disorder it causes, since he will have no dominant gene to compensate. (These diseases, such as hemophilia, are called sex-linked disorders.) A daughter, on the other hand, will most likely have a normal dominant gene on her other *X* chromosome and so will not develop the disease. But she may pass on the defective gene to her children. (See Figure 3.)

and no further tests are done. But if the second test also shows elevated AFP, ultrasound imaging is generally recommended. Ultrasound can often reveal an abnormality such as a malformed head or spine, or it may uncover a happier explanation, such as twins or a fetus that is older than previously estimated. If no explanation can be found by ultrasound, amniocentesis may be recommended. When a low AFP level is found, ultrasound and amniocentesis may be recommended to check for Down syndrome.

British and American researchers reported in 1988 that the accuracy of Down syndrome detection could be improved by combining the AFP test with tests for two other hormones, human chorionic gonadotropin (hCG) and estriol. In a healthy pregnancy the level of hCG rises steadily during the first 12 weeks; estriol levels rise throughout the pregnancy. The researchers found that if both estriol and AFP are low and hCG is high, the fetus is at high risk of having Down syndrome. Although this combination of tests is better than the AFP test alone, it still has a high rate of false positives (that is, test results indicate the defect is present when it is not). Thus, more accurate follow-up tests are necessary to confirm positive results.

Experimental Techniques

Other prenatal screening techniques are more experimental. Some make use of the fact that fetal red blood cells appear in the mother's blood in very small quantities, perhaps one cell for every billion of the mother's. Unlike adult red blood cells, these fetal red blood cells contain nuclei, which in turn contain chromosomes and thus can be used for prenatal diagnosis. Other experimental screening tests employ the techniques of in vitro fertilization (IVF) to examine the embryo before it implants itself in the uterus or even the egg before conception.

Fetal Blood Cells. Pediatrician Diana W. Bianchi of Harvard Medical School reported in 1989 that she had developed a way to isolate and study fetal cells in maternal blood. Bianchi withdrew a small sample of the mother's blood and added to it a special antibody that binds only to fetal cells. She then used a high-speed, automated, laser-based cell sorter that looks at the cells one at a time and separates those bound to an antibody from those that are not. The few cells obtained in this manner can then be analyzed. In her first studies, Bianchi was attempting to prove simply that the cells were, in fact, coming from the fetus. For that purpose, she identified in the cells the Y chromosome, which is found only in males.

Of the 19 women Bianchi studied initially, 8 had male and 11 had female babies. Bianchi was able to identify six of the eight males. She did not envision using the test simply for choosing the sex of babies but said it could be very useful in families with a history of sex-linked genetic disorders that affect males almost exclusively, such as certain types of mental retardation, hemophilia, adrenoleukodystrophy, Lesch-Nyhan syndrome, and the type of muscular dystrophy called Duchenne. As the sensitivity of the test is improved, she speculated, it should be possible to test the fetal cells directly for these and other defects.

A variation of this technique has been developed by James Wainscoat and Kenneth Flemming of the John Radcliffe Hospital in Oxford, England. They did not separate the fetal blood cells from the mother's but instead used highly sensitive techniques to examine the blood sample for the presence of DNA that is known to be located on the Y chromosome. They reported in late 1989 that they had tested blood from 19 pregnant women and found male genetic material in the blood of all 12 women who gave birth to boys, while none was found in the blood of the seven who had girls. Investigators predict that it will be several years before either variant of the test is used widely, particularly because both require highly skilled technicians.

Studying Embryos in Vitro. Even more ambitious is research aimed at detecting genetic defects shortly after conception and before the embryo has been implanted in the uterus. This approach has been pioneered by Handyside and Winston at Hammersmith Hospital. Their technique requires that the embryo be conceived in vitro—in the laboratory. It has so far been used primarily for sex selection in families with a history of sex-linked genetic disorders that affect only males.

Handyside and Winston's procedure begins with conventional IVF, in which eggs are removed from the mother and fertilized in the laboratory. The fertilized egg is then grown until it has divided into eight cells. The researchers carefully remove one of the cells and, using highly sensitive techniques, examine its DNA to determine the sex. If it is male, the fertilized egg is discarded. If it is female, the egg is implanted in the mother's womb, again by conventional techniques. Previous research with animals and with frozen human embryos has shown that removal of one cell does not impair development of the embryo.

In late 1989, Handyside and Winston performed the procedure for five couples who had a family history of sex-linked diseases. In each case the couple had previously terminated one or more pregnancies because the fetus had been found defective. The couples had found aborting the pregnancies very traumatic, Handyside said, and wanted to try the new in vitro procedure.

In the initial set of tests, five out of 17 implanted embryos "took," and three mothers became pregnant—a success rate that is about average for IVF. Conventional chorionic villus sampling at ten weeks showed that all five fetuses were female and apparently free from genetic defects. In the summer of 1990, the researchers received approval from their institutional bioethics committee to treat 50 more couples. Handyside predicted that, within a year, the technique would be refined so that they could screen for specific genetic defects and would thus be able to implant healthy embryos of either sex. By also eliminating carriers (individuals who carry a recessive gene but show no effects of it), Handyside said, the technology offers the promise of eliminating a genetic defect in particular families.

First Polar Body. Geneticist Yury Verlinsky of the Illinois Masonic Medical Center in Chicago has developed a technique to screen human eggs before conception. His technique analyzes the so-called first polar body, a packet of genes sloughed off by the eggs during development. Verlinsky collects eggs from the ovaries, detaches the first polar bodies, and uses genetic engineering technology to check them for genetic defects. The eggs that are found to be free of defects are then fertilized and implanted in the mother through conventional IVF techniques. Verlinsky revealed in the summer of 1990 that one of his patients was pregnant with a baby conceived after the screening was performed (the pregnancy subsequently ended in miscarriage).

There are two main problems with Verlinsky's technique—IVF has a low success rate, and the test does not screen for genetic defects contributed by the father. On the other hand, screening occurs before conception, so no abortion is involved. Anti-abortion activists, such as James Bopp, Jr., of the National Right to Life Committee, say they see no problem with the procedure because it does not involve "the taking of an innocent human life." The Roman Catholic Church and some fundamentalist religious groups, however, are opposed to IVF, viewing it as a threat to the sanctity of human life. The cost of both Handyside and Winston's procedure and Verlinsky's technique is greater than $6,000.

Thanks to a new test, Karen Sweeney (top left), who comes from a family afflicted by Huntington's disease, was able to learn that she almost certainly does not carry the defective disease-causing gene. With her are her husband Paul and their children (from left to right) Mellissa, Brenndan, Jessie, and Shawn.

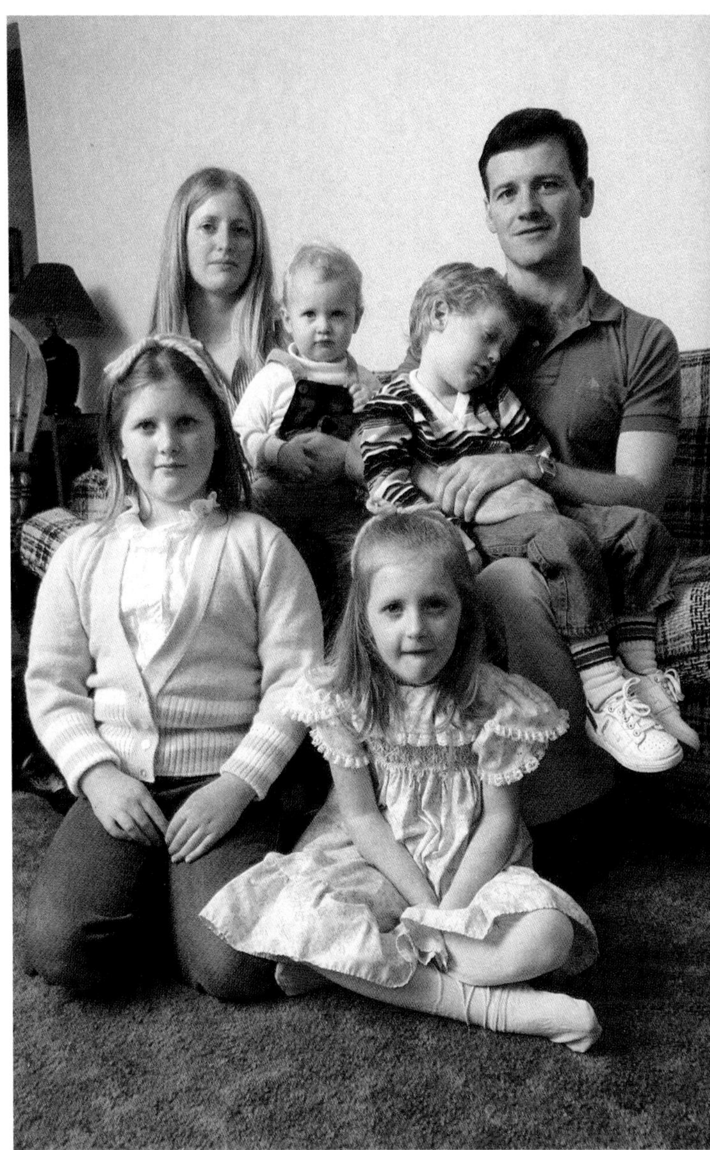

Genetic Counseling and Other Screening

Until very recently, genetic counselors could talk to prospective parents only in very general terms: If you have a family history of *X* defect, then you have an *x* percent risk of having a genetically defective baby. If you are both of a certain ethnic origin, then you have a *y* percent risk of this defect. If you are of a certain race, then you have a *z* percent risk of that defect. And so on.

But no longer. Today, researchers have identified the genes that cause two to three dozen specific genetic disorders and have found genetic markers—readily recognizable sequences of DNA—that serve as reliable indicators of literally hundreds more.

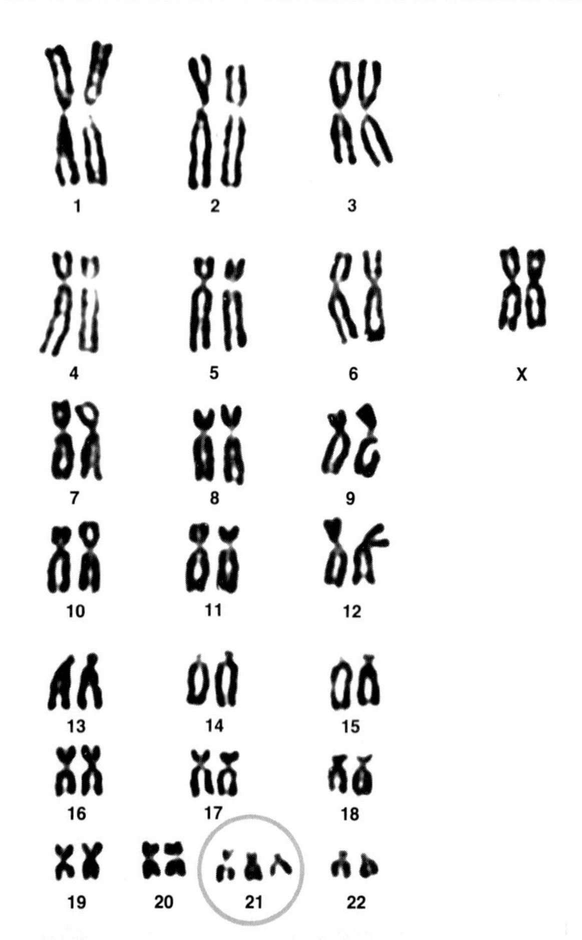

The presence of a third chromosome on pair number 21, which shows up clearly on the results of an amniocentesis test (left), indicates that the fetus has Down syndrome. Recent advances in care have enabled Down's children like little equestrian Elizabeth Lennard (below) to function at levels once thought impossible.

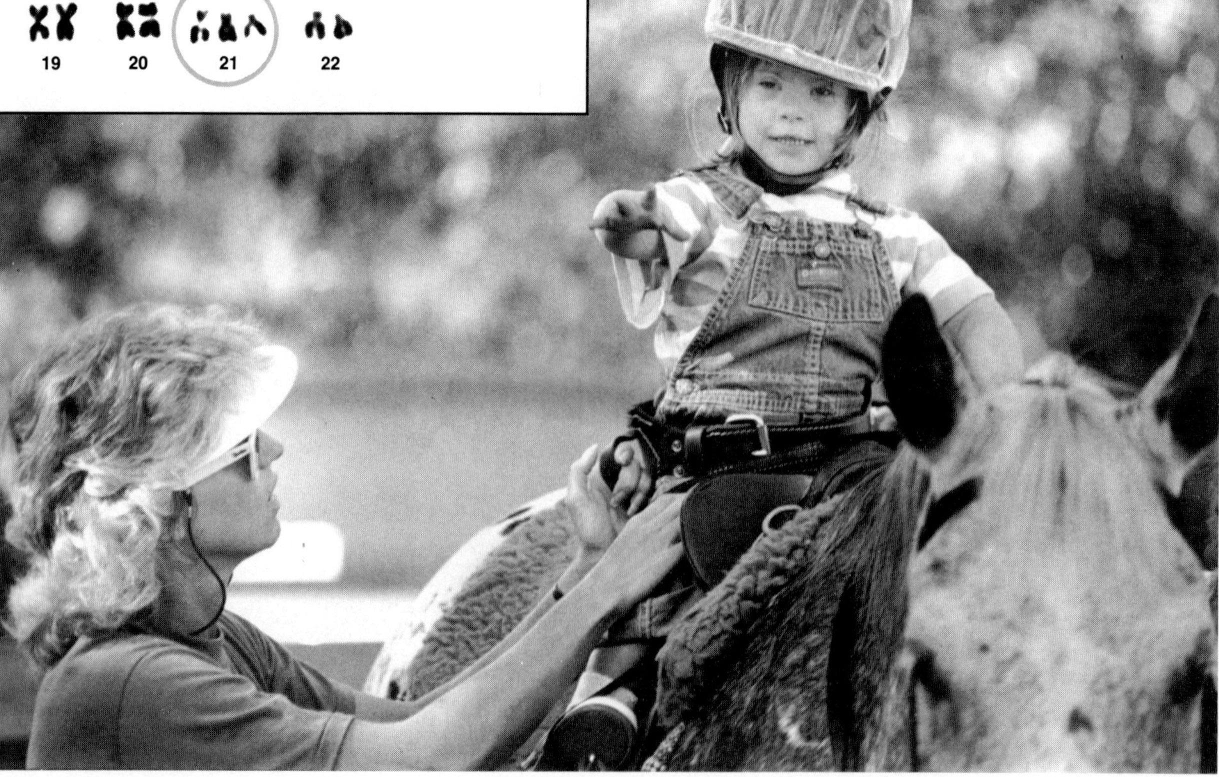

Diseases for which the responsible gene has been pinpointed include sickle-cell anemia, cystic fibrosis, Duchenne muscular dystrophy, and retinoblastoma (an eye cancer). While an individual is not normally screened for the whole spectrum of genetic diseases, it is becoming increasingly common to screen prospective parents for a disorder for which there is a family history or an ethnic predisposition.

Tests for these genetic disorders generally involve drawing a blood sample and examining the relevant genetic material for flaws. Because the test for Huntington's disease requires comparing the genetic material of close relatives, blood samples must be obtained from several family members. Although tests for recently isolated genes are becoming more widely available—a test for the cystic fibrosis gene was on the market literally days after the gene was discovered—many are still expensive and are conducted only at a few medical centers.

Many anti-abortionists are opposed to such prenatal screening because they believe detection of a defect most often leads to abortion of the fetus. But genetic counselors argue that screening actually has the opposite effect, showing concerned couples that their odds of a genetic disease-free child are higher than they expected. "Ninety-eight percent of all the prenatal diagnoses done in [the United States] lead to the birth of a child unafflicted with the genetic disorder for which the family was at risk," says pediatrician Michael M. Kaback of the University of California at San Diego. "It is a very pro-life technology."

Ethical Issues

Even thornier issues involve genetic analysis of children or adults. One commonly cited example is genetic analysis of individuals with a family history of Huntington's disease. The disorder, which generally develops between the ages of 30 and 45, destroys brain cells, leading to uncontrolled movements, an inability to talk, swallow, and remember, and, finally, death. If an individual inherits the gene for Huntington's, the disorder will develop, and no therapy exists to treat or delay it.

Although the gene responsible for Huntington's disease has not yet been isolated, researchers have found a genetic marker for it and have developed techniques to test for its presence before any symptoms appear. There are several arguments for advising people that they will develop the disorder: they can then decide whether to have children; they will have time to arrange for the future care of existing children or aging parents; they can set up a financial plan to pay for a possibly lengthy illness or prepare their home or workplace for the early stages of the disease when they may be clumsy but not totally disabled. On the other hand, such knowledge can bring on traumatic anxiety and despair.

Inevitably, genetic screening will move beyond the search for specific genetic defects and into broader areas. It may eventually become possible to remove a cell from an embryo and predict many things about the person-to-be's entire life: susceptibility to alcoholism or cancer, an increased risk of diabetes, or even blue eyes and blond hair. Then the question becomes where to draw the line. Is aborting a fetus because it will develop Huntington's disease or Duchenne muscular dystrophy morally different from aborting one because it has an above-normal risk of becoming an alcoholic? What is the morality of selecting for tallness if athletic ability is viewed as desirable? Or for other types of physical characteristics that do not affect health but that may influence life-style?

And assuming that such testing is done, who will have access to the results? Employers? Insurance companies? Will an individual be unable to get a blue-collar job because of an unusually high susceptibility to, say, a chemical that is found in the workplace? An executive job because of an increased risk of cancer?

Similarly, would an insurance company deny coverage to an individual because of an increased risk of cancer? Or, if the insurance company is denied access to the genetic screening results, would individuals who know they are likely to develop disorders that are expensive to treat purchase abnormally large amount of insurance, thereby taking advantage of the insurance company's ignorance? Similar issues have already been raised for individuals who are, for example, at risk for AIDS.

As of now, there are no answers to such questions. And in most cases, the questions are not immediately relevant because the technology still does not exist. But it is clear to all concerned that the continuing stream of discoveries is going to make the 1990s the decade of genetics and that those questions should be answered while there is still time to think about them in the abstract. □

YOUR AIR

Gary Legwold

Years ago, in one of his early experiments on the effects of air pollution on health, Ed Avol didn't think athletes would be part of the picture. After all, these types are resilient, hale and hardy hard-bodied folks in the pink of health. They are a far cry from the elderly, children, and people with heart disease or lung diseases like emphysema and asthma—the folks typically hit hardest by high levels of ozone, sulfur dioxide, and who knows what other kinds of industrial flatus that comes belching out of smokestacks or from the back ends of buses and cars.

Downtown Los Angeles cloaked in smog.

YOUR HEALTH

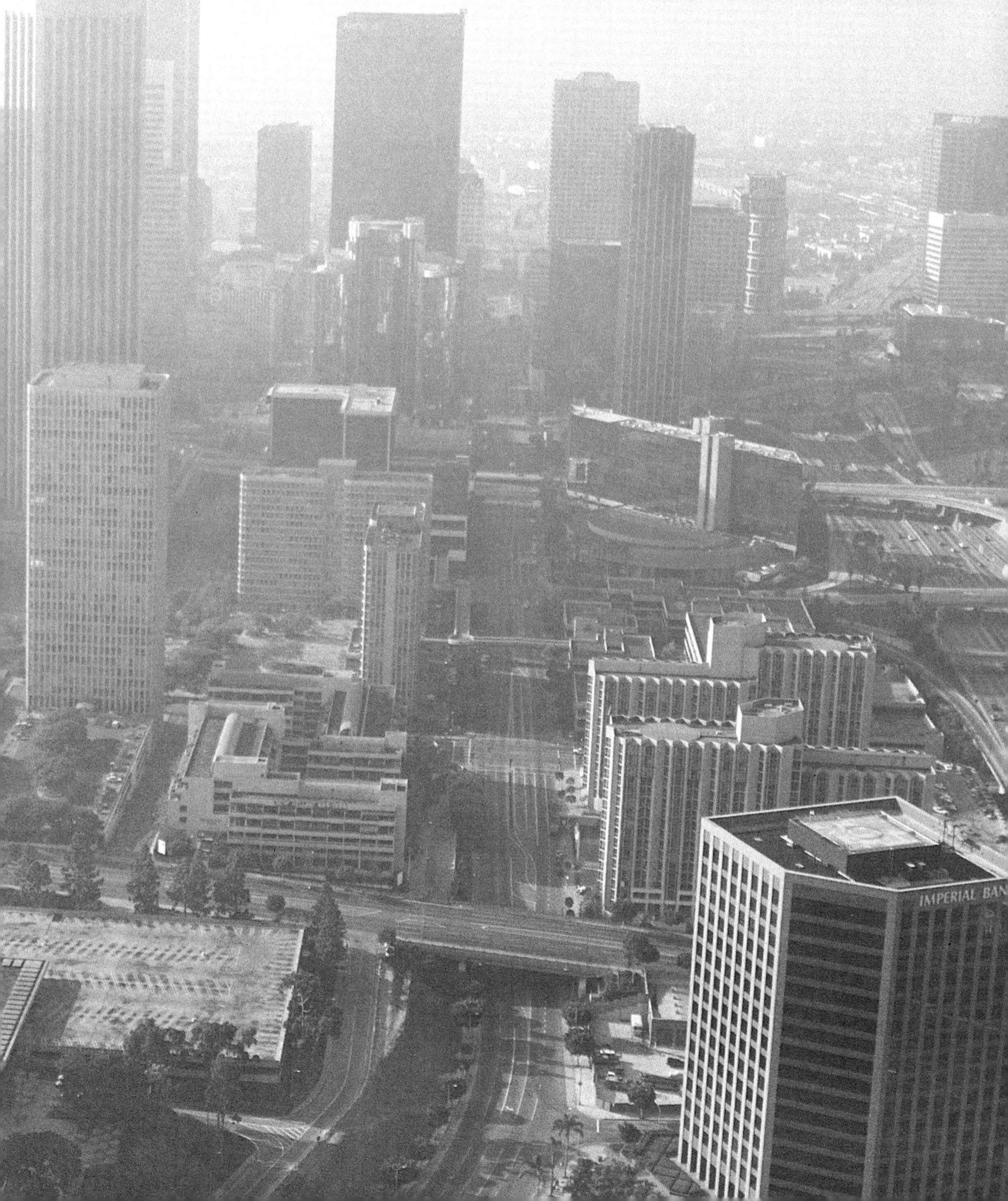

Then Avol, who is principal investigator of the Environmental Health Service at Rancho Los Amigos Medical Center in Los Angeles, gave the matter further consideration. "We thought that perhaps because they are outside exercising day-in, day-out, whether it's smoggy or not, that athletes may well be delivering large doses of air pollution to themselves," says Avol.

Indeed, that was the case. The lungs normally take in daily about 700 cubic feet of air—air, and all that's in the air. These pollutants are usually trapped by the lungs, in effect making the lungs a large vacuum cleaner, says Avol. During exercise, athletes process 10 to 20 times more air—and pollutants—than when they are at rest. Thus, their lungs are filtering out more pollutants, to the point where exercising athletes now can be considered a high-risk part of the population on particularly smoggy days.

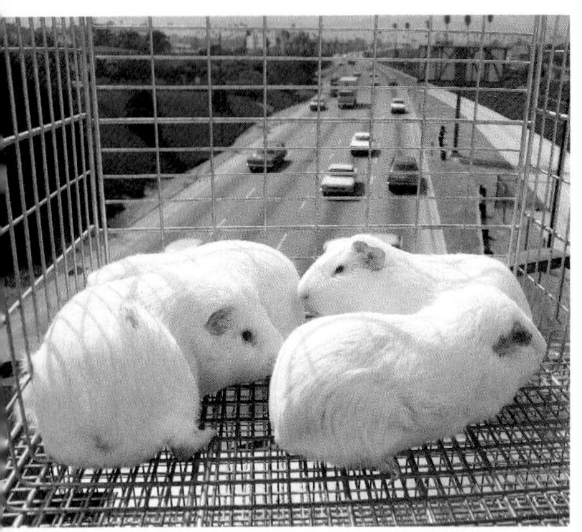

Guinea pigs suspended over a busy highway (above) provide one way of evaluating the cleanliness of the air. More sophisticated equipment is employed by a technician at the Desert Research Institute in Los Angeles (below).

Research on exercise and air pollution, which was stepped up around the time of the 1984 Summer Olympic Games in Los Angeles, is just one small area in a sprawling and, at times, confounding body of research on air pollution and health. But air pollution's effect on the health of exercisers is worth mentioning here because it reminds us—most of us have pooh-poohed air pollution, putting it out of mind repeatedly or blowing it off as someone else's problem—that air pollution can affect the health of us all, the firm and the infirm.

Killer Fogs

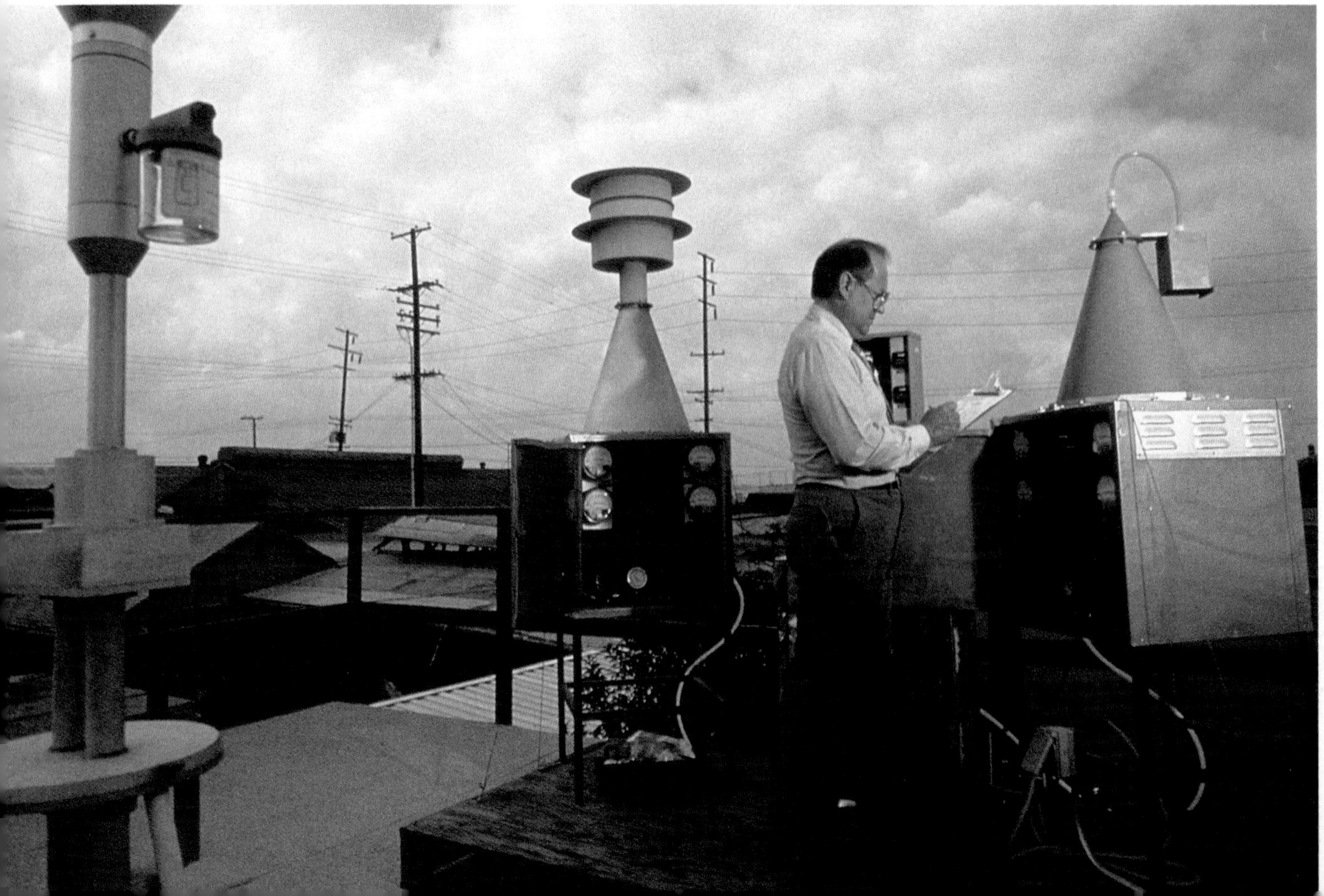

Many people remember vividly the bleak and grimy photos and news reports of the 1960s that showed the effects of air pollution. Those hazy days of summer that Nat King Cole sang of in the 1950s took on a more sinister association—smog—and psychedelic sunsets were seen by even the straightest urban dwellers witnessing the sun fighting through polluted skies. "Ecology" became a buzzword, and college students protesting pollution thought they were on to something new.

But they weren't. The first air pollution laws were passed in the 1880s. Chicago and Cleveland enacted legislation regulating smoke emissions, followed in the 1890s by Pittsburgh and New York. Also in the 1890s Ohio passed one of the first state air pollution laws, regulating smoke emissions from steam boilers. In 1952 Oregon became the first state to set up a state air pollution control agency.

There were several air pollution disasters recorded before the 1960s decade of discontent. The first that drew worldwide attention happened in 1930 in the heavily industrialized Meuse River valley in Belgium. For several days in December an inversion (a cool air layer trapped by a warm layer above) in the valley caused a buildup of pollutants. Thousands became ill and 60 people, most with preexisting heart and lung diseases, died.

The first air pollution laws were passed over a century ago.

In 1948 an inversion covering much of the northeastern United States caused a pollution tragedy. Twenty died and 6,000 of the 14,000 residents of Donora, Pa., fell ill from breathing polluted air trapped in the Monongahela River valley. Those who became ill complained of sore throats, chest tightness, headaches, breathlessness, burning and tearing eyes, vomiting, and nausea.

A five-day inversion in London in December 1952 led to 4,000 deaths attributed to air pollution. Applications for emergency hospitalization more than doubled that week to about 2,500. London, known for its smoke from soft coal and fog (the original smog), had had six similar incidents dating back to 1873, with air pollution deaths totaling 2,500. A 1962 inversion caused 750 Londoners to die.

In the 1960s, after similar incidents caused deaths related to air pollution in New York City and elsewhere, action was taken nationally in the United States. In 1963, Congress passed the Clean Air Act, empowering the U.S. Public Health Service to study air pollution, as well as funding research and training at the state and local levels. The Clean Air Act of 1970, and later of 1977, beefed up the previous legislation, making the U.S. Environmental Protection Agency (EPA) the center of federal anti-air pollution efforts.

The EPA became the link between the federal government and the state and local governments that, according to legislation, were primarily responsible for preventing and controlling pollution. The EPA oversaw these efforts in addition to doing research, providing technical and financial assistance to states, and administering programs involving such matters as solid waste disposal and clean air and water.

The EPA also set the National Ambient Air Quality Standards (NAAQS) for common pollutants that threaten health. These pollu-

---

Gary Legwold, a former editor of The Physician and Sportsmedicine, *is a free-lance writer in Minneapolis, Minn., and writes on a variety of health-related issues.*

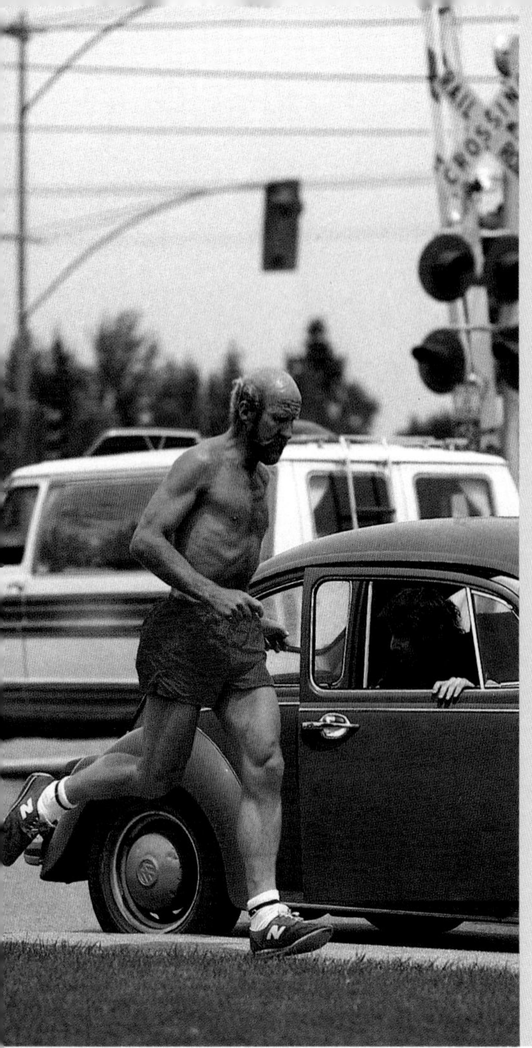

AIR POLLUTION AND EXERCISE

Nearly 150 million Americans live in areas where air pollutants reach unhealthy levels and exceed federal standards. Many of these people exercise, unaware that they are taking into their lungs 10 to 20 times more air than when at rest—and therefore much larger doses of pollutants than normal.

One solution, albeit drastic, is to stop exercising. But that is not necessary. A better solution is to exercise wisely. Be aware of air pollution and follow the guidelines below. More information on specific pollutants in different localities is available from local chapters of the American Lung Association.

1. **Know peak times.** Concentrations of pollutants like carbon monoxide and ozone vary in the course of the day. Carbon monoxide levels are highest at rush hours. The highest levels of ozone are found in the afternoon, since sunlight and time are necessary for ozone smog formation. So exercise in the early morning or late evening on smoggy days.
2. **Avoid congested highways.** Look at a map to see whether you can replace the heavily trafficked roads on your walk, run, or ride with back roads, access roads, paths, or bike routes. If you can't alter your route, at least make an effort to avoid high traffic times. If the shoulder of the road is wide enough, try to stay 30 to 50 feet away from vehicles.
3. **Altitude, heat, and humidity are factors.** If you live at a high altitude, where pollutants can be more potent, be especially careful about choosing days on which to exercise. And remember that heat and humidity compound the effects of pollutants.
4. **Take it easy.** If you must exercise on days with high levels of air pollution, try to do it inside in an air-conditioned environment where pollution levels can be half of what they are outside. If you must go outside, don't push yourself. Studies show that you simply can't perform at your best. If you go easy and do not huff and puff, you'll be taking in smaller amounts of pollutants. After exercising, go indoors and breathe clean air.
5. **Skip your workout.** Forget exercising on those extremely smoggy days when health officials issue health warnings. It's not worth the possible irritation and health risks.

tants, called criteria pollutants, include ozone, sulfur dioxide, particulate matter, carbon monoxide, nitrogen dioxide, and lead. Usually a primary standard is set to protect human health, and a secondary standard is established to protect livestock, crops, other vegetation, buildings, and visibility.

Many chemicals are less common than those covered by NAAQS and yet pose a serious threat to health. These less common pollutants, defined as those that contribute to an increase in mortality and serious illness, can cause cancers, birth defects, and genetic mutations. The EPA sets National Emission Standards for Hazardous Pollutants on some of these air pollutants, including asbestos, beryllium, mercury, vinyl chloride, arsenic, radionuclides, benzene, and coke oven emissions.

Health Effects of Common Pollutants

Hazardous pollutants are usually localized, according to industry in an area. They are not less of a concern to the EPA, but they are less widespread than criteria pollutants. Therefore, much of the EPA's clean-up efforts, now and especially in the early years of the EPA, have involved the six major criteria pollutants mentioned above. Let's take a closer look at these criteria pollutants and how they affect health.

Ozone. Ozone, a colorless, pungent gas that is the main ingredient of smog, is produced in the lower atmosphere when gases or vapors of organic chemicals called hydrocarbons combine with nitrogen compounds in the presence of sunlight. Major sources of hydrocarbons and/or nitrogen oxide are refineries, gas stations, automobile exhaust, chemical plants, paints, and solvents. Ozone was the main fear before the 1984 Summer Olympic Games in Los Angeles. This lower atmospheric pollutant is not to be confused with the "good ozone" in the upper atmosphere; this layer of stratospheric ozone protects us by screening potentially harmful ultraviolet rays.

The pollutant ozone irritates and constricts the airways, which can aggravate an asthma condition and can cause lung tissue to age prematurely. It can decrease the lungs' working ability and cause coughing, chest pain, shortness of breath, headache, nausea, dry mouth, eye irritation, nasal congestion, and reduced resistance to infection.

Ozone-related symptoms often go away after a few hours. After repeated exposure to high levels of ozone the body adapts. That's good for the now, but may be bad for the future, according to Dr. Henry Gong, professor of medicine in the pulmonary division of the UCLA Medical Center. Animal studies "certainly suggest that lungs that are recurrently exposed to ozone . . . may indeed have a faster decline in how the lungs function," he says. "You find evidence of fibrosis and emphysema."

Carbon Monoxide. Carbon monoxide is an odorless, colorless, poisonous gas. Its source is primarily automobile exhaust. Carbon mon-

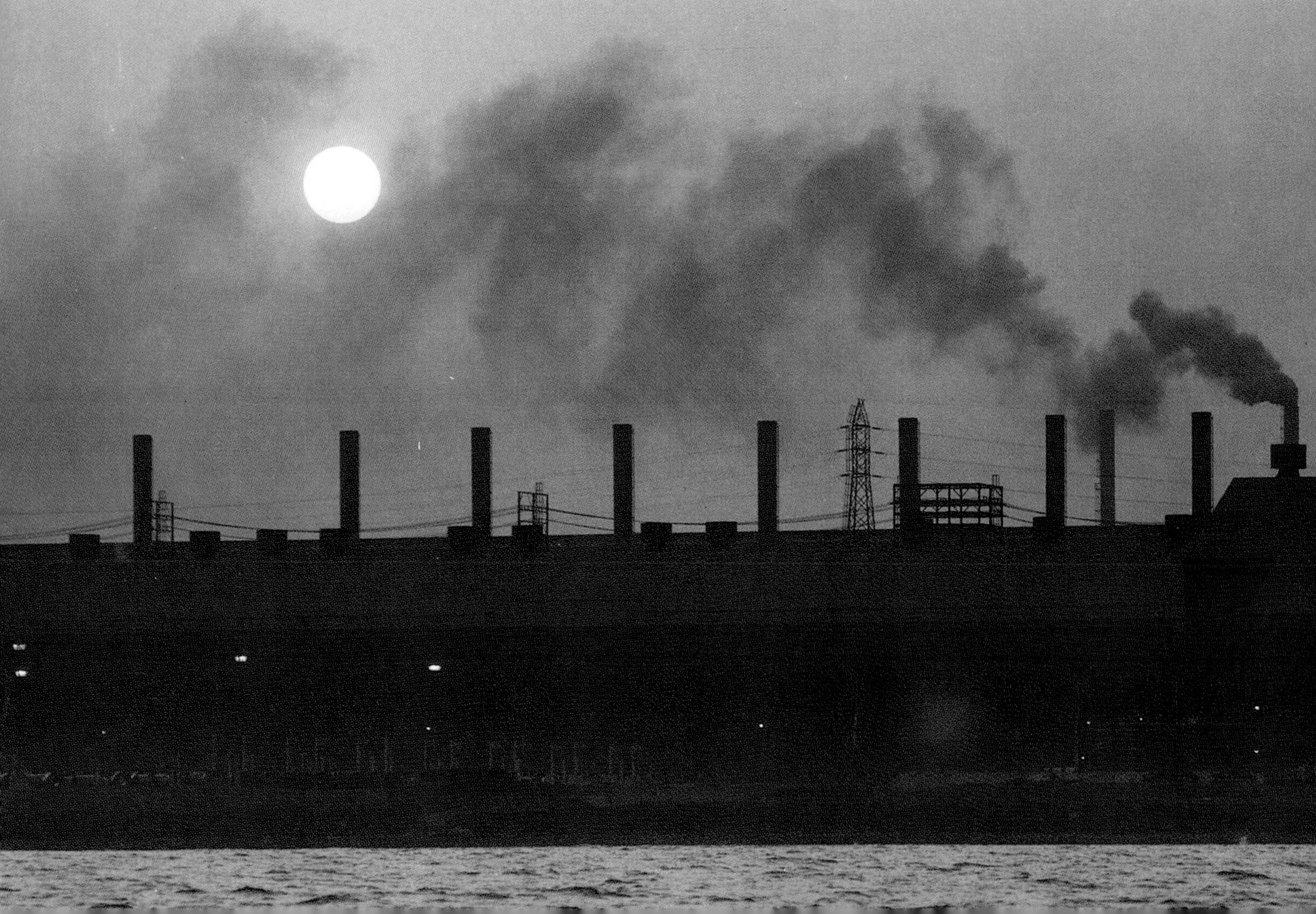

Heavy industries, such as this Indiana steel mill, are a major source of pollution. However, smaller sources, like backyard barbecues, are much harder to control.

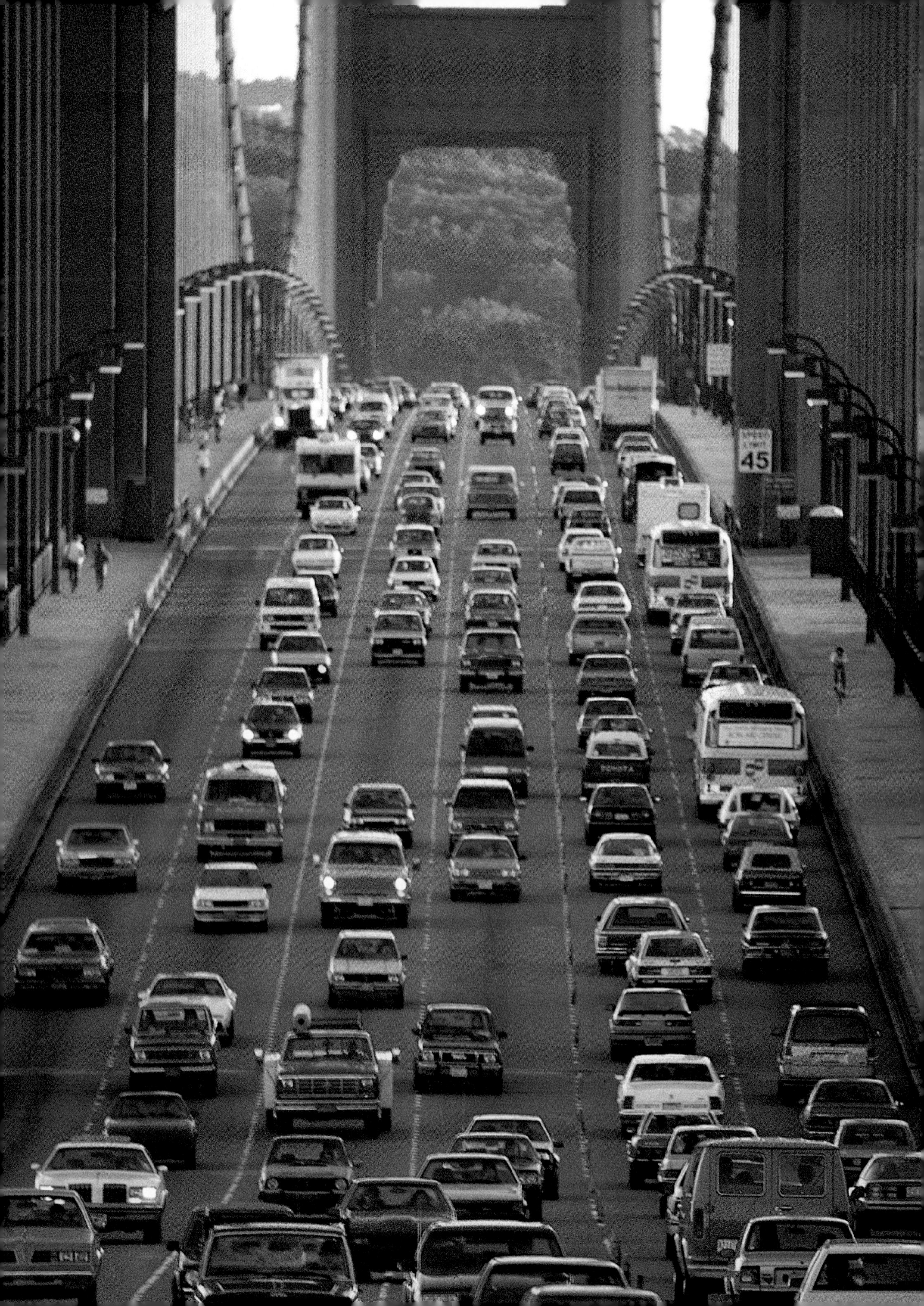
45

oxide binds with hemoglobin, the part of red blood cells responsible for carrying oxygen. Therefore, carbon monoxide impairs the blood's ability to supply oxygen to the brain, heart, and tissues throughout the body. High levels of carbon monoxide cause headache, nausea, dizziness, and visual disturbance. Carbon monoxide is especially dangerous for people with heart conditions and for pregnant women and their unborn children.

Nitrogen Dioxide. Again, fuels burned in automobiles and power plants are the main sources of this criteria pollutant. Nitrogen compounds contribute to smog formation, and nitrogen dioxide in the atmosphere forms nitric acid vapor. Nitrogen dioxide affects the body in ways similar to ozone and is considered by experts to be the fastest growing air pollutant.

Sulfur Dioxide. When sulfur-containing fuels are burned in power plants and diesel engines, sulfur dioxide is formed. In the atmosphere it can change into acidic particles and sulfuric acid droplets. Like ozone, sulfur dioxide constricts air passages and can be a major problem for people with asthma. It can also cause burning and tearing of the eyes, an irritated nose, dry coughing, and difficulty in breathing.

Particulate Matter. Particulate matter includes microscopic particles and droplets of liquid. Particles come from burning of fuels and from mining. Particulate matter can cause eye and throat irritation, bronchitis, and lung damage if the particles are small enough to escape the natural filters in the nose and airways.

Lead. Lead in the air comes mostly from older automobiles that use gasoline containing lead, which is added to gas to help prevent engine knocking. The shift to unleaded gasoline in the United States has resulted in a major drop in lead air pollution. Lead poisoning can reduce mental ability, especially in children, damage the blood, nerves, and organs, and raise blood pressure.

How Pollutants Hurt the Body

What we breathe is not always exactly what we want to breathe, and in the course of evolution our bodies have developed defense mechanisms to help filter out whatever may be harmful in the air. The body's first line of defense is the sticky mucus that coats the nasal passages and larger airways in the lungs and that traps large particles such as dust, pollen, and germs. Once trapped, these particles are swept up and out of the airways by tiny hairlike structures called cilia. When Avol first wondered whether athletes were taking in large doses of air pollutants while exercising in polluted areas, part of his suspicion was based on the practice athletes have of breathing primarily through the mouth. This mouth breathing bypasses a wonderful natural filter—the nose, with all its mucus and tiny hairs.

Many air pollutants, however, are small enough to flow by the mucus and cilia and go deep into the delicate lungs. Some of these small pollutants get trapped by mucus but can paralyze or destroy the cilia, allowing dirt and germs to build up in the mucus and sometimes leave the body more vulnerable to infection and disease. For example, air pollutants can paralyze the cilia and allow carcinogenic substances,

Automobile exhaust, such as spewed out during rush hour on San Francisco's Golden Gate Bridge, fouls the air with carbon monoxide and nitrogen dioxide. The shift to unleaded gasoline has led to a major drop in lead air pollution.

such as the hydrocarbon benzopyrene, to remain in contact with bronchial cells much longer than normal, which can lead to lung cancer.

Those pollutants making it deep into the lungs affect the alveoli, the tiny sacs making up the 600 to 900 square feet of surface area inside the lungs. It is at the alveoli where we actually breathe—that is, oxygen enters the bloodstream (to be circulated throughout the body) by passing through the walls of the tiny blood vessels called capillaries, and carbon dioxide moves from the capillaries to the alveoli to be exhaled. Pollution may cause some alveoli to enlarge and lose resilience, making breathing more difficult.

Pulmonary emphysema is the breakdown of the walls of these alveoli. In response to air pollutants or tobacco smoke, the alveoli walls become enlarged, lose resilience, and fall apart, causing an increasingly desperate shortness of breath as the disease progresses. Emphysema sufferers eventually suffocate because too many of these alveoli, the basic breathing units, disintegrate.

When air is bad, the body, in its wisdom, defends itself in another way—by trying to breathe less, thus taking in less of the polluted air. Air passages constrict and breathing becomes more labored. This can cause or aggravate asthma. In bronchial asthma attacks there is a temporary narrowing of the smaller airways called bronchioles, an increase in mucus secretions, and a swelling of the mucus membrane.

Even though air quality in the United States has improved in the past two decades, the health costs are still staggering.

The respiratory system is not the only system affected by air pollution. As we've seen, the circulatory system connects to the respiratory system at the alveoli. Therefore, when the alveoli are hampered by air pollutants—or, in the case of carbon monoxide, when the red blood cells are less efficient in carrying oxygen—the vital gas exchange process that occurs at the alveoli (oxygen for carbon dioxide) is not as efficient. This makes the heart work harder to maintain the same levels of oxygen in the blood at a time when less oxygen is being exchanged at the alveoli. Of course, making the heart work harder can be dangerous for someone with heart disease.

The Price of Air Pollution

To an individual whose health is affected by air pollution, no amount of money could make suffering with respiratory ailments or lung disease worth it. Therefore, there is no acceptable price of air pollution to that particular person. On a larger scale, no one has come up with a monetary figure representing all the health costs associated with human exposure to air pollution. The best science has done, in huge and complex studies, is to target specific populations and specific pollutants and try to link these to related health costs, including costs from illness, lost productivity, and premature death. The American Lung Association monograph "The Health Costs of Air Pollution" reviews 12 of these studies published between 1984 and 1989.

In this review the association found that health cost estimates ranged from $5.1 million annually for a local population near a polluting coal-fired power plant to a high of $93.49 billion annually for the American population exposed to automobile exhaust pollution. Most of the studies put the health cost range at $500 million to $15 billion per year. The pollutants covered in these 12 studies were four of the six criteria pollutants regulated by the Clean Air Act: ozone, lead, particulate matter, and sulfur dioxide.

Cleaner Air, But . . .

The health costs related to air pollution are staggering considering that the air in general has become cleaner in the United States in the past 20 years as a result of a variety of changes involving automobile exhaust and industrial emissions. One wonders what costs would be had the air become more polluted. "In many cases the air has gotten a lot cleaner," says Frederick W. Lipfert, Ph.D., a staff member in the Environmental Systems Analysis Group, Department of Applied Sciences, Brookhaven National Laboratory in Upton, N.Y. "For example, New York's air is about eight times as clean. Los Angeles started cleaning up before the 1970s, but they were clearly in very bad shape in the 1950s. Although it's been a struggle with L.A. because of the population growth, they've still made progress."

There are plenty of statistics to back up Lipfert's assessment. Examples: According to the EPA, between 1970 and 1988 particulate levels fell 63 percent, sulfur oxides (which include sulfur dioxide and sulfur trioxide) fell 27 percent, and carbon monoxide 40 percent. Nitrogen oxides (including nitrogen dioxide) increased 7 percent, but lead levels dropped an impressive 96 percent, primarily because of the efforts, starting in 1973, of the EPA and environmental groups to reduce average lead content in gasoline from 1.0 grams/gallon to 0.1 grams/gallon. About 70 percent of gas sold in the United States today is unleaded. Ozone levels have, in general, fallen as well—sometimes significantly, as in 1986 when winds were favorable and the weather cool and wet—despite an increase in vehicle miles traveled in the 1980s.

While there is no doubt that air quality has improved, the air is still polluted in much of the United States. The EPA estimates that 146 million Americans live in 487 counties that did not meet at least one air quality standard in 1988. That's about 60 percent of the U.S. population. Even though ozone levels have dropped since 1970, 112 million people (perhaps even more, according to experts) lived in some 340 counties that exceeded the ozone standard in 1988. That's more than the total for the other five criteria pollutants combined. Finally, approximately 60 percent of the higher risk population—the 5 to 10 percent of the entire U.S. population that includes pre-adolescent children, the elderly, people with asthma, and people with chronic bronchitis and emphysema—live in areas that did not meet one or more of NAAQS standards.

Clearly, there is work to be done. But Lipfert says from now on improvements in air quality and the accompanying rewards will be "subtle and hard to find, and they won't strike you in the face" like those of years ago. "A lot of the cleanup took place in the early to mid-1970s in major cities. Since then there has been a population growth, there are more vehicles, more backyard barbecues, more dry cleaning establishments [which use chemicals containing hydrocarbons that are vented in the cleaning process], more industry; it's kind of a

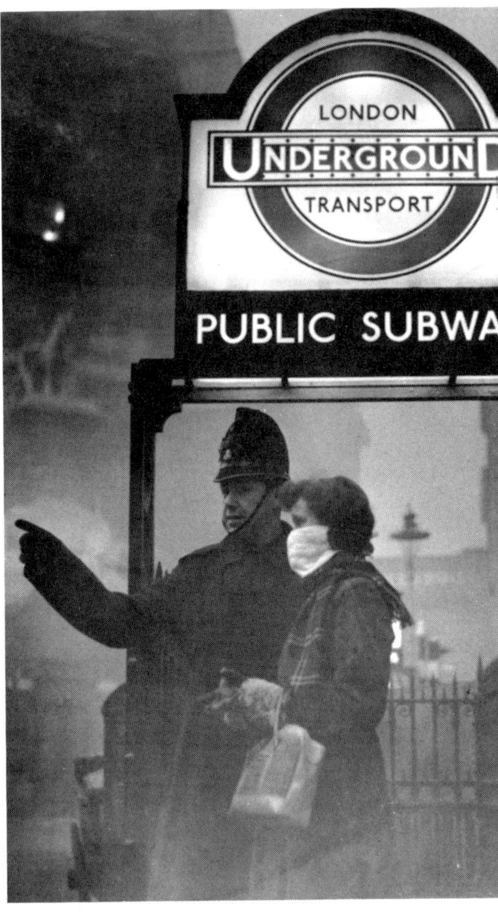

The air in London in the early 1950s was sometimes so harmful that people wore smog masks. One particularly bad pollution episode killed 4,000 people.

never-ending battle to keep up with it. Everything that we do has some sort of pollution consequences. The more people you put together in one place, as in Los Angeles for example, the more problems you'll have . . . Industry has installed what's called best available technology; so in many cases industry has done the best it can. If you still have a problem, then you have to go after the little sources. That's difficult to do because there are lots of little sources."

That's especially difficult when controversy exists about just how much blame, if any, can be placed on pollutants such as ozone for the variety of health problems related to bad air. Research trying to link air pollution to health problems can be confusing. The whole issue is much like the controversy around the claim that smoking causes lung cancer.

Several obstacles make it difficult to prove a link between pollutants and disease. First, research studies on human volunteers who inhale toxic gases in test chambers examine only healthy people; it would be dangerous to test sensitive subjects, such as people with asthma, the ones most affected by pollution. Animal studies, which have linked pollutants to disease, use higher concentrations of pollutants than found in the air; also, it is difficult to transfer data from one species to another—some animals are more sensitive than others. Epidemiological studies, which look at large numbers of people over time, are some-

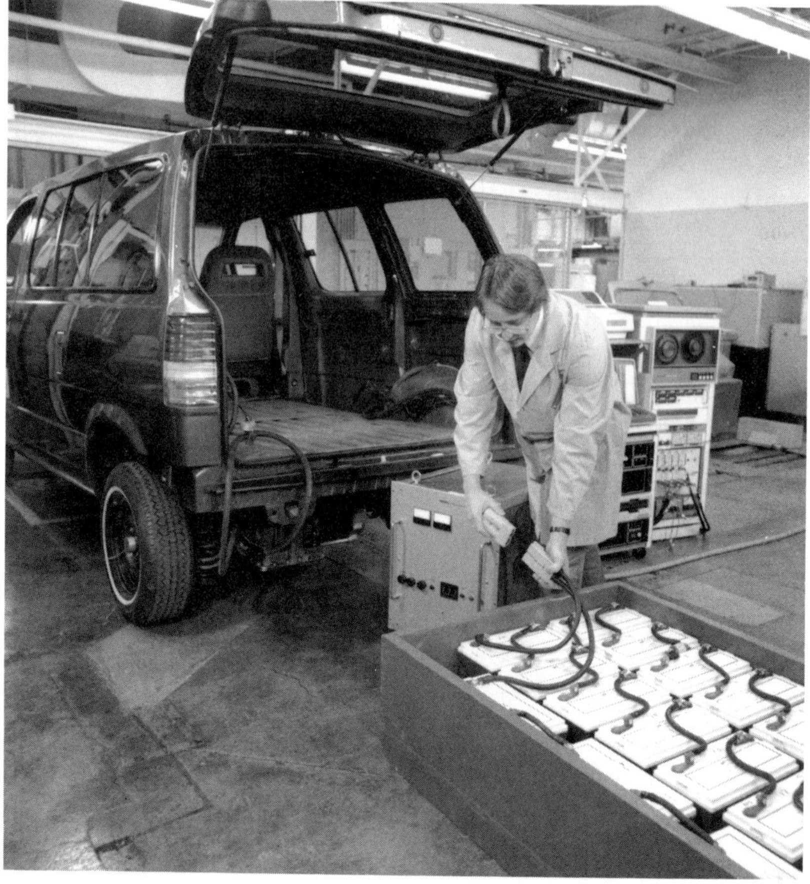

A technician charges a battery pack for an experimental electric vehicle. Nonpolluting electric cars promise to be major weapons in the battle against dirty air.

times revealing, but researchers are not exactly sure what pollutants people are exposed to. A researcher can measure air quality at a central location, but is is much harder to measure the quality in a person's house, car, and job site.

The Battle Continues

Research drawbacks aside, scientists and physicians must press on with the tools they have to study the connection between air pollution and health. Many Americans feel more should be done to reduce pollution levels, and in 1990 some encouraging actions were taken.

Polls show people overwhelmingly support environmental protection, even at a price.

Polls show people overwhelmingly have supported environmental protection, even if it costs them money. "I personally feel we could do better in cleaning up the air," says Lipfert. "The relative economic cost is not all that high, so we ought to do it even if it's difficult to prove to the last decimal point what the benefits are." Some environmentalists charge that as the EPA has grown, it has become bogged down with politics, image, and budgets. The National Clean Air Coalition (NCAC) in Washington, D.C., says that although the EPA is required to identify and regulate the dozens of known toxic air pollutants responsible for as many as 2,000 cases of cancer every year, in 20 years it has regulated only seven of them.

This apparent foot-dragging is in sharp contrast to the action taken in 1990 by the California Air Resources Board, which established strict rules and guidelines on less-polluting automobiles and fuels. The rules call for automobile makers to introduce models, starting in 1994, that emit no more than half the hydrocarbons allowed for 1993 models under present California regulations, already the strictest in the United States. By 1988, 2 percent of all cars sold in the state would have zero emissions (which means electric cars). By 2003 the zero-emissions cars would have to equal 10 percent, and most of the rest would have to meet emission standards 70 percent below the 1993 level. The rules also set standards on less-polluting gasoline. Ultimately, the board's plan is to reduce auto pollution by 50 to 84 percent.

The California action, impressive as it is, was overshadowed by passage in Congress of the Clean Air Act Amendments of 1990, the first amendments of the Clean Air Act of 1977. The 1990 act strengthened and expanded the 1977 statute and included provisions to reduce tailpipe emissions of hydrocarbons and nitrogen oxides by 35 to 60 percent, respectively, in many new cars starting with 1994 models and in all new cars by 1996. Also, most areas where smog is a problem would have to achieve 15 percent reductions in six years.

"The Clean Air Act gives us the first controlled program for acid rain pollutants, the first meaningful controlled program for toxic air pollutants, and it also regulates certain chemicals that deplete the earth's protective ozone layer," says the NCAC's Ed Barks. "Overall, we're happy with the act." He warns, however, that continued vigilance will be required from the president, the EPA, and congressional panels to monitor compliance with the act. "There's a lot more to be done," says Barks. "The Clean Air Act is 800 and some pages of paper. It alone is not going to get the job done." □

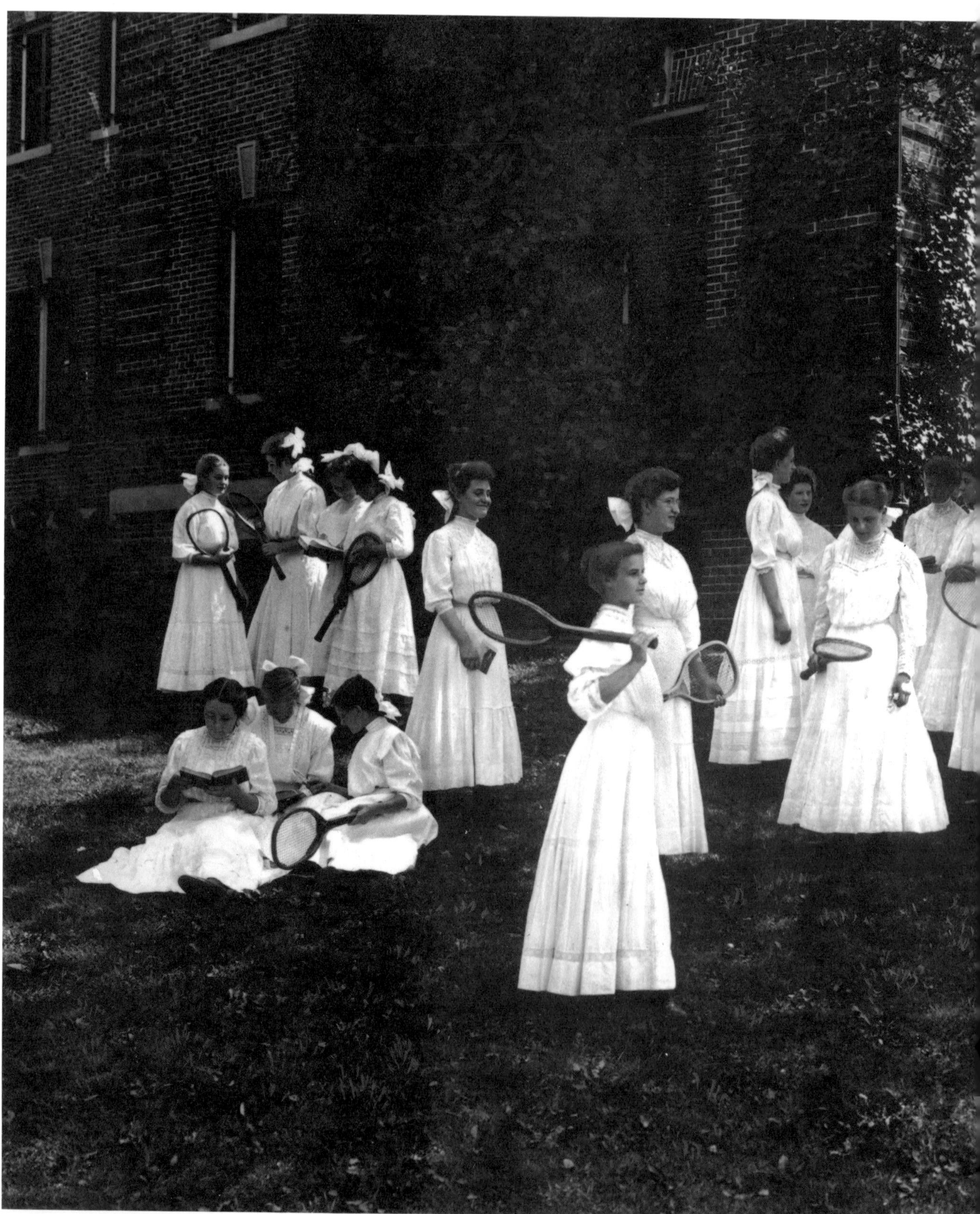

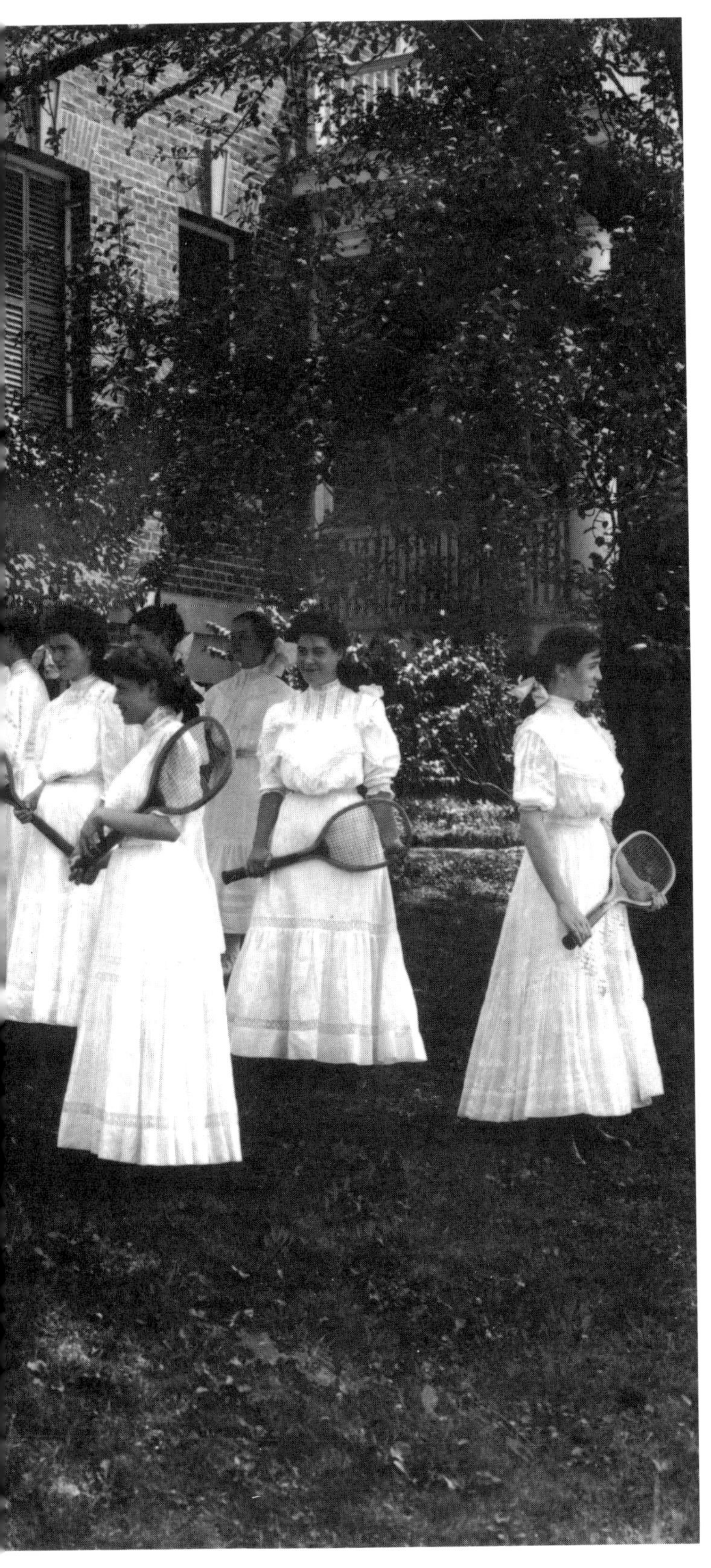

When America Discovered Fitness

Constance Urdang

From marathon runners, joggers in city parks, and mall walkers to the thousands enrolled in aerobics classes or dutifully following a solitary exercise routine in front of the television screen, Americans everywhere seem to be preoccupied with physical fitness. In the 1980s, sales of barbells, treadmills, trampolines, exercise bicycles, rowing machines, and jump ropes in the United States topped half a billion dollars. Over $300 million more was spent on running shorts, sweatshirts, warm-up suits, and specialized items like sports bras, not to mention sneakers, for which hundreds of brands were available in a staggering number of models. Thousands of companies provided fitness programs for their employees. Physicians prescribed individualized exercise regimens for their patients and sent them to cardiac rehabilitation clinics. *Jane Fonda's Workout Book* was No. 1 on the New York *Times* best-seller list for 51 weeks. In short, fitness became a major growth industry.

A picturesque group of tennis-playing college girls: circa 1905.

But this was not the first time that Americans sought a cure for the debilitating effects of sedentary urban living through physical education and exercise. When Hal Higdon of *Runner's World* magazine, wrote, "As a society we have become soft. We have succumbed to the blandishments of the Good Life. We . . . ride in automobiles, buses or trains instead of walking or bicycling . . . jam into elevators instead of climbing stairs . . . eat rich food . . . sit before television sets," he was only translating into contemporary terms the notion popular among 18th-century Americans that their long-lived forefathers were physically superior to their pampered selves. Even then, the simple sons of the soil were assumed to have been vigorous and healthy, while the "lewdness and luxury" of the city were thought to produce infirmity, devitalization, and disease.

Programs for improving the health, strength, endurance, and stamina of the populace have been a feature of American society since the early 1800s. They flourished particularly in times like the present—times of egalitarian ferment and social optimism, notably the Jacksonian 1830s and 1840s and the Progressive era of the early 20th century.

Health and Morality

The prevalence of tuberculosis in the United States in the first years of the 19th century, and especially the dreadful cholera epidemic of 1832, focused attention on the importance of hygiene. At the same time, traditional therapeutic methods were being perceived as useless in many

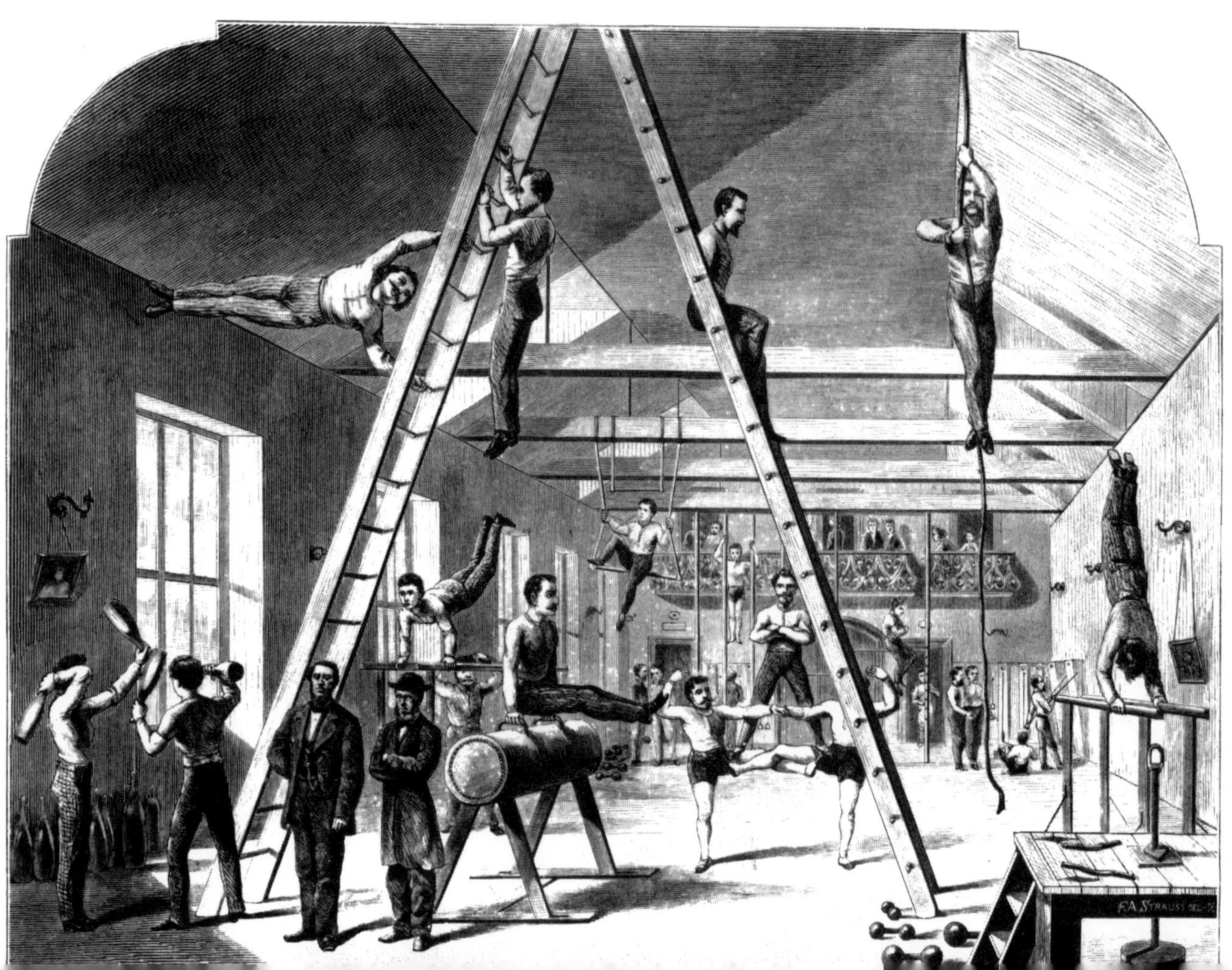

Gymnasiums, such as this early one in Boston, were hailed by reformers as a way of safeguarding young men from the wicked lures of city life.

cases and actually harmful in some. The result was popular mistrust of standard medical thought and practice. The average person became suspicious of intellectuals and book-learning and cynical about doctors. As one complained, "The application of some dashing, unmeaning, foreign, difficult name to a simple medicine, or to a simple, common disease, is calculated to strike an unlettered person speechless." Even the licensing of doctors was seen as interfering with individuals' freedom to select the kind of medical treatment they wanted.

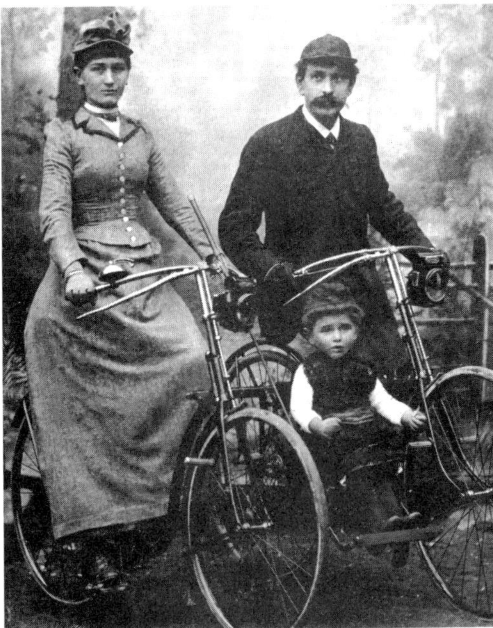

The advent of the bicycle introduced a sport that the whole family could enjoy together.

As a result, certain nontraditional health programs at the fringes of standard medicine became popular. Samuel Thomson's botanical self-treatment, the homeopathy of Samuel Hahnemann, and Vincent Priessnitz's hydropathy (the "water cure") won adherents through a combination of egalitarianism and the romanticism of trusting in a beneficent Nature. These systems were based on the notion that bodily health is achieved by following Nature, and they emphasized that each person is responsible for his or her own physical salvation and can earn it by adherence to certain laws of dress, exercise, and diet.

As early as 1823 systematic exercise classes were offered at the Round Hill School in Northampton, Mass., but it was not until the first German *Turners* emigrated to America toward the end of the 1820s that gymnastics attracted any attention. The *Turners* (from the German word meaning "gymnast") were men who followed a system of exercises designed in the first years of the century by Friedrich Jahn to promote physical education, hygiene, and patriotism in his native Germany. After the second wave of Germans arrived in America in the wake of the political upheavals of 1848, interest in physical fitness became widespread. Settling in Ohio, a group of Germans established the Cincinnati *Turngemeinde*, the first German *Turnverein* (gymnastics association) in the United States. By the end of the 1850s there were more than 70 such organizations throughout the East and the Midwest. More than simple gymnastics societies, they celebrated German culture with picnics, games, outings, and beer, along with an ideology of male physical perfectibility.

It did not take long for interest in physical fitness to spread through the larger population. Inexpensive and accessible in all seasons, the gymnasium, with its parallel and horizontal bars, horse, rings, weights, and climbing ropes offered a wide variety of exercises. Such manly exertions, with the positive feelings of health that they engendered, could not but benefit young men whose energy and daring might otherwise be diverted to gambling, licentiousness, and worse. The gymnasium was extolled as the innocent answer to the craving for excitement that tempts and endangers rootless youth in the city. At the same time healthful physical activity counteracted not only the drunkenness and debauchery of the slum dweller, but the nervous exhaustion that was diagnosed as the fundamental disorder of middle-class urban Americans.

The doctrine of fitness became so pervasive that by 1869 it was possible for Professor Moses Coit Tyler to state categorically, "Every vil-

---

Constance Urdang is a free-lance writer.

lage that has two churches now should . . . put both congregations . . . in one building and practice gymnastics in the other." Whether or not it was intended in that statement, the linking of physical culture with religion was not uncommon. "Muscular Christianity," an ideology that associated the robust physical life with a life of Christian morality, had become a popular ideal in England through the novels of the clergyman Charles Kingsley, Queen Victoria's chaplain. In *Tom Brown's Schooldays*, a popular novel by Thomas Hughes, the English found a hero who united physical fitness with moral probity and the tenets of Christianity.

These ideas became translated, both in England and in America, into a spiritual obligation to cultivate physical manliness and muscularity. It was assumed that not only would moral character be strengthened by disciplining the muscles and the will, but mental ability would be improved by the tension-relieving, mind-clearing effects of strenuous exercise. One of the most stalwart examples for 19th-century fitness fans was a certain Dr. George Windship, known as "The Roxbury Hercules." He had been the second smallest man in his Harvard class but through dedicated weight training became able to lift 1,000 pounds. Repeating his slogan, "Strength Is Health," he traveled around the country giving lectures in which he claimed for weight lifting such health-giving effects as relief from nervousness, headaches, and indigestion.

Amelia Bloomer, designer of the pantaloon outfit that carried her name, sought to free women from the restraints of 19th-century dress.

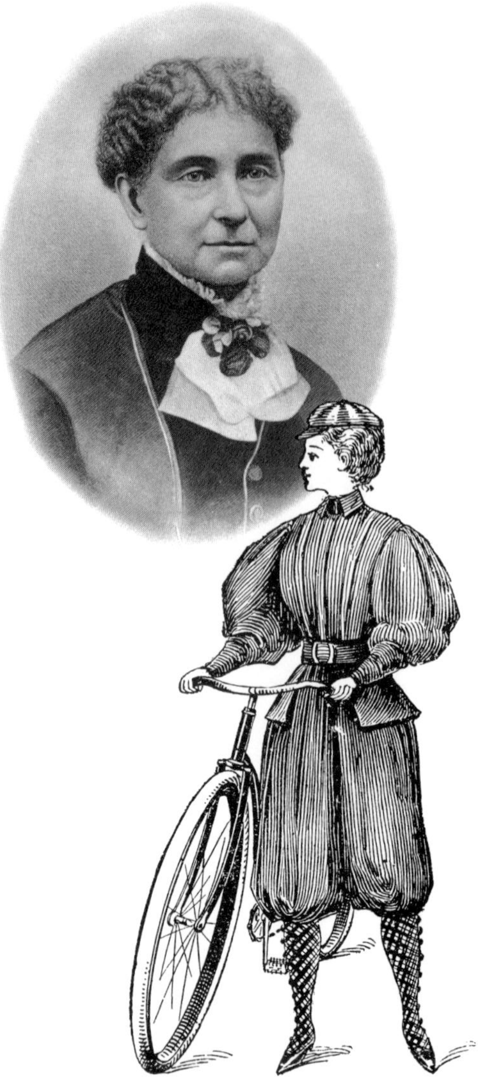

Including the Women

One of the chief limitations of Windship's regimen, like that of the German gymnasts, was that it was definitely not suited to that half of the population whose health was believed to be *most* in need of improvement. In their heavy, floor-length skirts and body-compressing corsets, women were unable to vault the horse or use the rings or trapeze. Of course, hoisting dumbbells was considered out of the question for the genteel ladies of the era.

This problem was addressed by Dioclesian Lewis of Boston, who studied gymnastics in Europe in the 1850s and became the promoter of the "New Gymnastics" of the 1860s. He built his exercise system on the premise that physical training was the foundation of all education and that it must be made available not only to young men but to women and children as well. Instead of stressing muscular strength and bodybuilding, Lewis emphasized exercises that increased whole body flexibility, coordination, agility, and grace. He pioneered the use of lightweight apparatus—beanbags, wooden rings and wands, dumbbells made of wood instead of iron, and Indian clubs (wooden clubs shaped somewhat like bowling pins)—along with dancing and marching, all usually to music. When he presented his system to the American Institute of Instruction in 1860, it was received with enthusiasm, and the delegates supported his proposal to set up a Normal Institute for Physical Education. This school turned out its first class of physical education teachers in 1861. Impressively, half of that first class were women. The Family School for Young Ladies, which Lewis opened in 1864, zeroed in on the health problems of young girls, whose

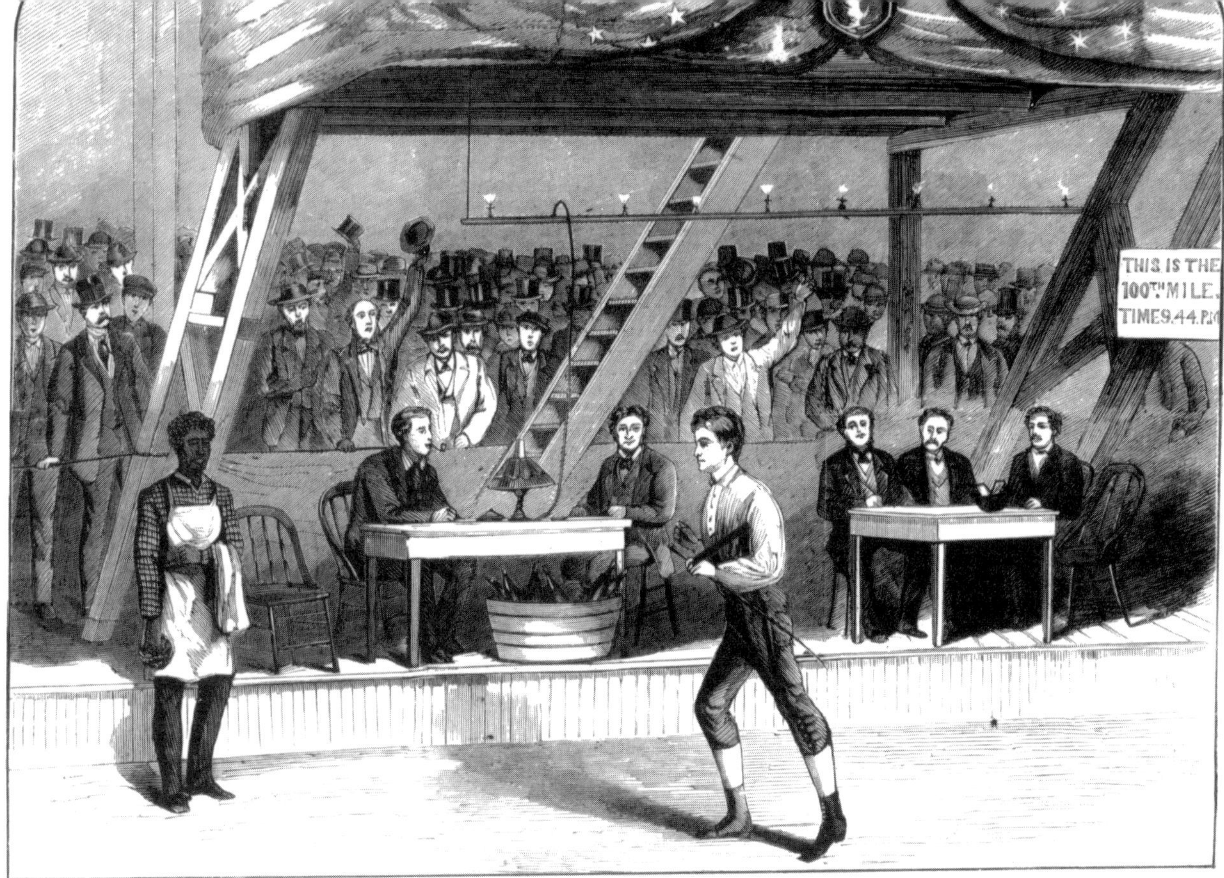

Endurance walking was popularized by "Weston the Pedestrian," shown here in New York City at the finish of a 100-mile, 22-hour hike.

bodies, he believed, were deformed by corsets and whose natural vitality was stifled by forced inactivity. Along with musical gymnastics Lewis prescribed fresh air, simple food, and loose clothing. The health thus acquired would not only make the young ladies more attractive to potential husbands, but would also make them better wives and mothers and be passed on to their children.

Body, Mind, and Spirit

"Improve the [physical] apparatus . . . and you facilitate and improve the work which the mind performs with it, precisely as you facilitate steam operation and enhance its product by improving the machinery," trumpeted S. D. Kehoe, one of the followers of the so-called Athletic Revival of the 1860s and booster of exercises with Indian clubs. Dr. Russell Trall, best known for his ardent espousal of hydropathy, maintained that even naturally stupid people might be made comparatively intelligent through gymnastic exercises.

As early as 1861, Edward Hitchcock, Jr., had introduced physical education at the college level at Amherst, and Dudley Allen Sargent's "mimetic exercises" at Harvard, designed so that students might imitate, using weight and pulley machines, the movements of various forms of physical labor and sports, were already being adopted by athletic clubs, schools, military bases, YMCAs, and the general public. For those who did not live in or near urban centers, home gymnasium equipment, forerunners of today's exercycles and stair-climbing machines, suitable for use in parlor, study, or bedroom, was available. The Patented Exercising Chair, with levers on both arms and a cushioned seat on a spring, was advertised as a substitute "for carriage and

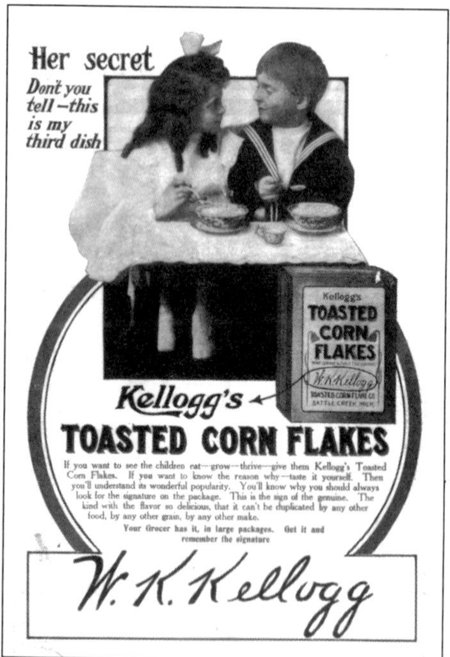

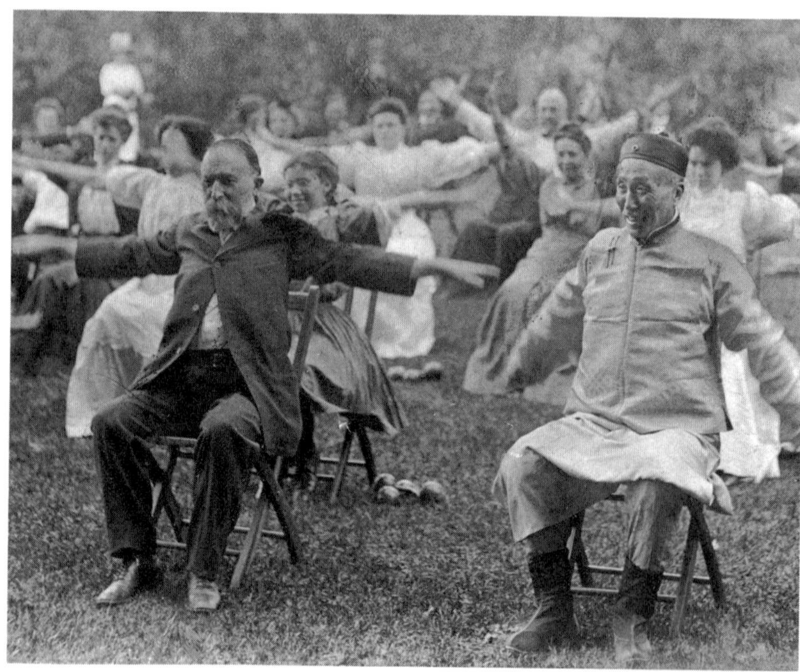

horse," and for many other forms of gymnastic exercise. The portable Parlor Gymnasium ("it can be carried in the pocket"), recommended for "every business or professional man . . . every teacher, clerk, and seamstress," consisted of a rubber cord with handles and with hooks that could be attached to the floor or wall. By pulling on the handles the sedentary worker could exercise shoulders, arms, legs, and back.

Following the Civil War, military drills became popular, as did walking and hiking, which required no equipment at all and were open to both men and women of all classes. Endurance walking, popularized by "Weston the Pedestrian," who walked from Portland, Maine, to Chicago in 26 days, became one of the newly fashionable spectator sports, along with rowing and sculling. A Parlor Rowing Machine that combined rocking with a sliding movement was promoted as an antidote for the nervousness that was identified as peculiarly women's. Bare-knuckle boxing, which had been a rough working-class sport, put gloves on, became "the manly art of self-defense," was taken up by the universities, and attracted a following, both as spectator and participatory activity.

It was Luther Gulick, who had been a student of Sargent's at Harvard nearly 30 years earlier, who transformed the Young Men's Christian Association into a sports and fitness organization for college graduates and disadvantaged slum-dwellers alike. His design of the triangle emblem of the YMCA symbolized Spirit upheld by Body and Mind, a graphic representation of the pervasive idea that physical training was the basis for moral training.

Between 1860 and 1920 belief in the importance of restoring the physical vigor that was seen to be sadly lacking in Americans continued to spread. By the last quarter of the 19th century the American frontier had all but disappeared, and with it an outlet for easing the

Fitness Through Food

The vegetarian cereal king John Harvey Kellogg, seen at left exercising with a Chinese colleague at Kellogg's famous Battle Creek, Mich., sanitarium, promoted his Corn Flakes as a wholesome countermeasure to the "vile" American diet. One of his most successful imitators was Charles W. Post of Grape-Nuts fame (right).

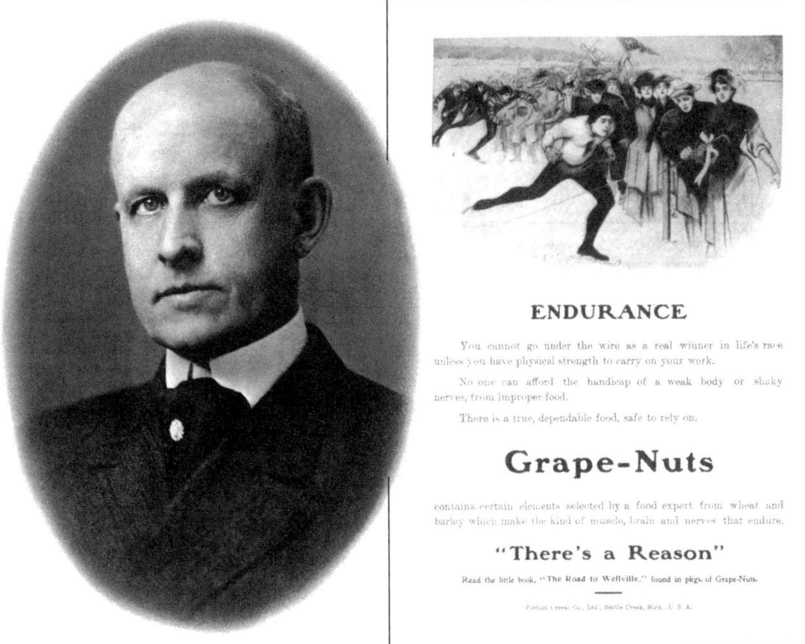

pressure of a population increasingly industrialized and urban. Increasingly, sports and physical training were seen as activities essential to the maintenance of social order. Duty to the country demanded hardy bodies and agile minds. Fears of a declining American stock demanded a new aristocracy—one of strength, health, and efficiency rather than noble birth.

By 1902, 270 colleges in the United States offered physical education programs, 300 city school systems required physical education, and there were 500 YMCA gymnasiums with a total of 80,000 members. Team sports— football, rowing, and baseball—were promoted as especially useful to prepare men for life in a democratic society. The team player must submit to certain rules and would thus learn to respect the law. He must learn to protect himself, while at the same time both attacking his opponent and controlling his aggression. While striving for victory, he must learn to anticipate defeat and meet it like a man.

In the post-Civil War years the most frequently diagnosed illness of the middle class was the condition known as "neurasthenia." At first it was considered a disease of the successful male urban "brain worker" (tacitly understood to be upper or middle class, white, and Protestant), whose status had been achieved because he had evolved into a form of human life more advanced than Catholics, blacks, and American Indians. But neurasthenia gradually became perceived as a malady of indolent women of leisure—the white, upper-class Protestant wives of those hardworking men. Its symptoms—sleeplessness, despondency, anxiety, neuralgia, and backache or headache—were treated with every remedy from the water cure to improved diets of varying degrees of strictness and the administering of mild electric shocks. Health spas on the European model, featuring the bathing in

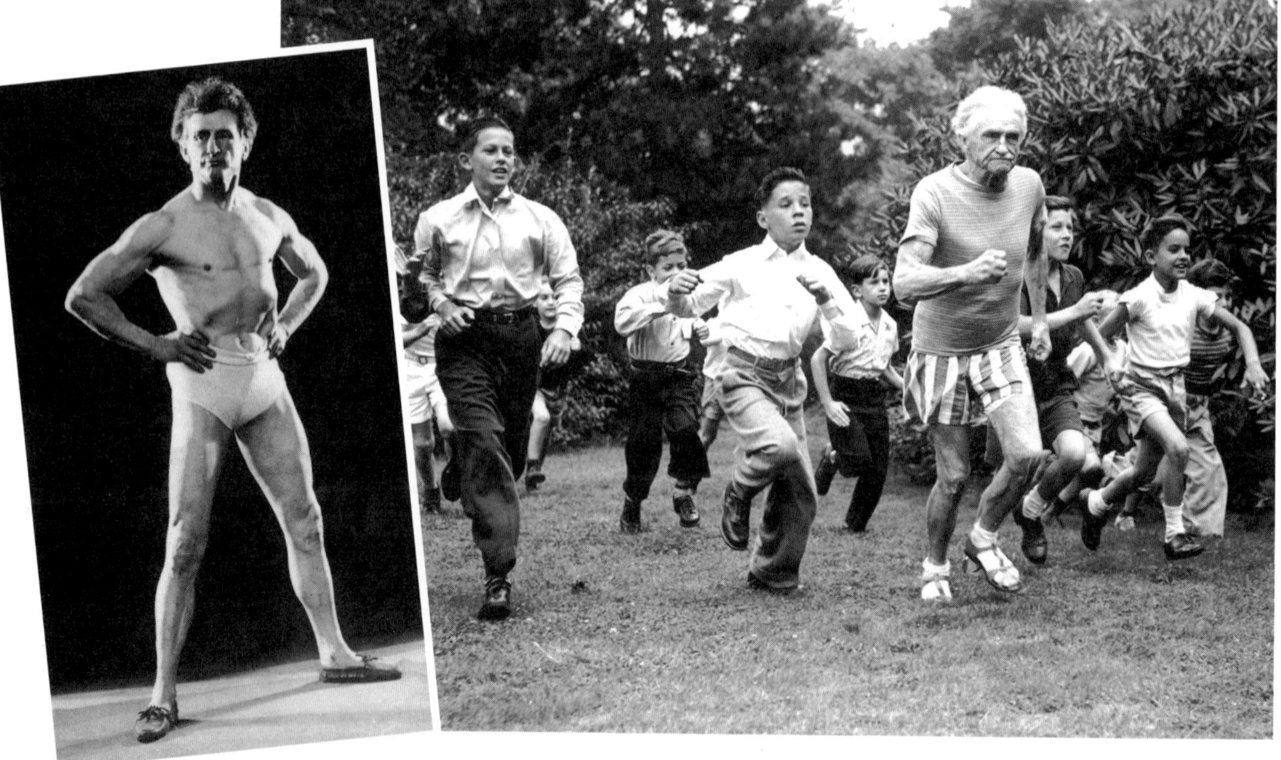

Indefatigable health advocate Bernarr Macfadden was in fine fettle at age 55 (above) and was still in front of the pack at 78 (above right). He was also a genius at self-promotion (below).

The Story of A Great American

Whose Amazing Success is a Monument to the Courage, Energy and Opportunity of America!

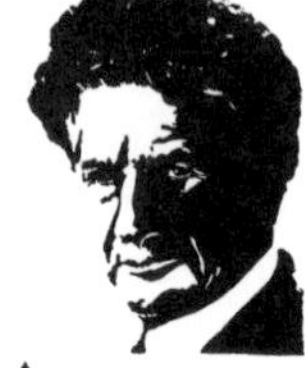

He overcame sickness and poverty to win strength and fortune!

He showed America the way to health!

He blazed the trail of clean living and rational sex education!

He defeated the forces of prudery and hypocrisy!

He created one of America's greatest business organizations!

Mr. Macfadden has consented to the writing and publishing of these books because we convinced him of their value as a guide to success to every earnest man and woman. His own life is a demonstration of the principles which he has fought for—and this revelation of his life is of incalculable value as a guide to you.

BERNARR MACFADDEN
A STUDY IN SUCCESS
by Clement Wood

The True Story of Bernarr Macfadden
by Fulton Oursler

The intimate biography of this great American—a life story revealing his amazing career from poverty-stricken boyhood to the wealth and power of his maturity. $2.50

Chats With The Macfadden Family
by Grace Perkins

Macfadden, the family man, is no longer a mystery. Here is the story of his family life from courtship to the present—the actual demonstration of the value of his principles of marriage and parenthood. $2.50

At All Bookstores or from

LEWIS COPELAND COMPANY
119 West 57th Street, New York, N. Y.

In This Man's Life We See Reflected the Vitality of America

No better example could be found of the courage, independence, and idealism of the American spirit—nor any more convincing demonstration of the rewards which America gives to those who fight and serve. Macfadden's life is an epic to inspire every ambitious man and woman struggling against great odds.

For the First Time a Brilliant, Successful Man Tells the Real Story Of How He Won Success

Now you may know the romance of his life and the secrets of his success, for every phase of the life of this extraordinary man and to profit by his personal counsel.

How He Built Mind, Body and Fortune

What is it worth to YOU to learn how this great genius has overcome sickness and won abounding health; has overcome poverty and gained great wealth; has practically with no schooling made himself one of America's most broadly educated men? What is it worth to YOU to have this mental, physical, and financial giant as YOUR PERSONAL COUNSELLOR? It is worth more than you can calculate, and yet that is what is offered you in these extraordinary books.

or drinking of mineral waters, had long been a feature of the American landscape, but these were only for the well-to-do. Exercise and improved nutrition, reformers pointed out, were within the reach of everyone.

Eating to Live

American eating habits had been the target of criticism by health reformers for years. Mountains of meats and starches dripping with lard or butter and the gluttonous haste with which this food was wolfed down were viewed with revulsion by such early temperance advocates as Sylvester Graham, now remembered chiefly as the inventor of the Graham cracker. Along with branding alcohol a tool of the devil, Graham crusaded against white flour. Motherless from an early age, he yearned for "the blessed days . . . when our good mothers used to make the family bread" of whole-grain flour instead of buying from a bakery an inferior product made with often adulterated white flour. Graham also fulminated against flesh-eating, praised "biologic living," and maintained that the only truly healthful diet consisted of eating nothing but what was available in the Garden of Eden, where Adam and Eve consumed no meat.

In 1876 the vegetarian movement acquired another powerful champion when John Harvey Kellogg was appointed physician-in-chief at the Battle Creek Sanitarium in Michigan, originally a Seventh-day Adventist institution. Starting with only a dozen patients, Kellogg soon attracted several thousand a year, including such people as President William Howard Taft, John D. Rockefeller, Jr., Alfred Du Pont, and J. C. Penney. His packaged cereals (corn flakes was one of the earliest) dominated the market. No amount of derision, no references to "Shredded Doormats" or "Eata-heapa-hay" discouraged Kellogg or imitators like Charles W. Post (of Grape-Nuts fame), a former patient at "the San." Along with vegetarianism, Kellogg stressed the importance of extremely thorough chewing, first promulgated by health reform activist Horace Fletcher. "Fletcherize!" commanded a large sign in the dining room in Battle Creek, and patients were entertained as well as instructed by a *Chewing Song* written by the chief. A certain Miss Palmer was held up for emulation; she reportedly devoted 20 minutes daily to the serving and enjoyment of a single cracker.

Physical Culture

Perhaps the chief guru of the physical culture movement at the end of the 19th century and the beginning of the 20th was Bernarr Macfadden, a tireless self-promoter and shrewd businessman whose "Healthatoriums" and book and magazine publishing empire publicized his fundamental, very American conviction that all individuals are responsible for themselves. "It lies with you," he wrote, "whether you shall be a strong virile animal or a miserable little crawling worm." Promoting a combination of muscular strength, self-actualization, preventive medicine, and sex proved to be a formula for success. Such magazines as *Physical Culture*, with its cover photographs or paintings of healthy, athletic young women in revealing costumes, attracted a wide readership, mostly among middle-class men. Macfadden himself posed nude in classical postures to display his own musculature, and the measurements of his wife, "waist, 25 in., bust, 38½, hips 39," were published to encourage the less well-endowed. In books like *The Virile Powers of Superb Manhood* and *The Power and Beauty of Superb Womanhood* he crusaded against masturbation and the curse of prudery and in favor of "health plus." Unfortunately, his ideas on improving the stamina and physique of Americans later turned into a form of racist eugenics. Victim, finally, of his own overdeveloped ego, Macfadden sought the nomination for governor of New York in 1928, and from 1932 until 1948, when he was 80 years old, he campaigned unsuccessfully for the Republican presidential nomination.

The Open Air

Indoor exercise had long been considered at best a substitute for activity in the open air, and walking, riding, rowing, swimming, fencing, and ice skating had been recognized as beneficial as far back as the 1830s. But horseback riding was only for the wealthy, and swimming was virtually impossible for women in the bulky and restrictive bathing dresses decreed by fashion as well as modesty. In fact, until late in the 19th century women's clothing had made it difficult for them to engage in any truly active sports. Loose clothing suspended from the shoulders continued to be recommended, but few wore it. The costume devised by Amelia Bloomer, with its full Turkish trousers under a short skirt, had never really caught on, and the corsets that created the much-admired wasp-waisted figure were more than confining. Hygienists and physicians alike denounced women's unnatural forms of dress, blaming corsets and tight-lacing for every female ill from prolapsed uterus to curvature of the spine, deformed thorax, personality changes, the excitation of amatory desires, and even diminished pelvic size that

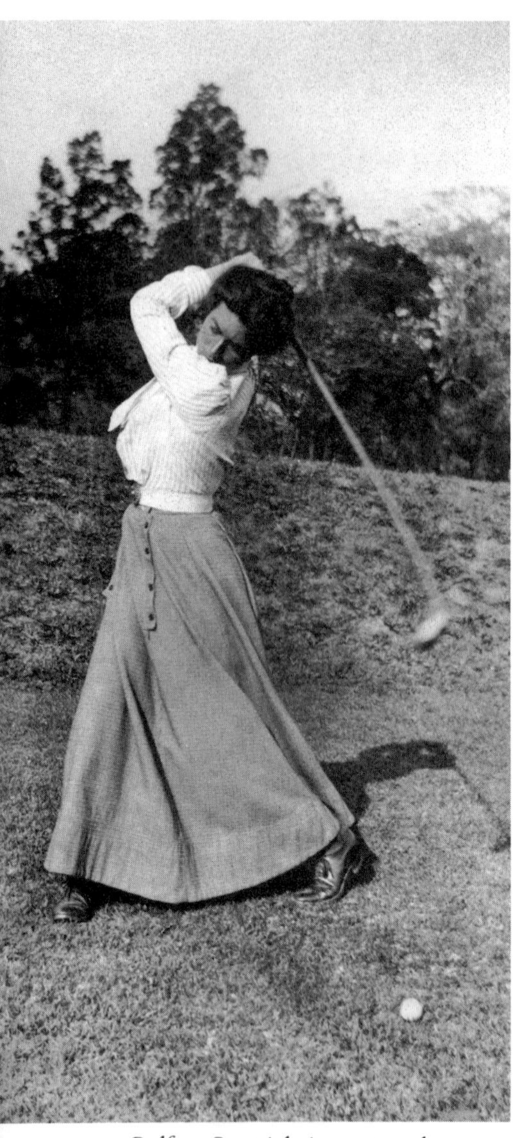

Golf, a Scottish import and a game for men, was soon taken up by women as well.

would be transmitted to daughters and result in the eventual enfeeblement of the race.

Croquet, a sport requiring skill but no strength, was open to women as soon as it was introduced in the 1860s, and roller-skating, with its potential for mixed socializing, quickly became popular. Nearly every town of any size had its hardwood-floored rink. Lawn tennis and archery also had their female adherents, particularly in the fashionable resorts. Golf, originally a man's game when it was imported from Scotland in the 1890s, was soon taken up by women as well. But it was the bicycle on which men, women, and children, rich and poor alike, saw themselves riding into a glorious era of health and freedom.

The earliest version of the bicycle, the celeripede, lacked both pedals and brakes and was too dangerous for all but the most daring. The crank-driven velocipede was too expensive. With the appearance of the "ordinary" bicycle in the 1870s, with its huge front wheel and tiny back wheel, more people took up the new sport, but the contrivance still had no brakes and was hard to control, while the design made it almost impossible for a decently clad woman to ride. Only after the production of the first "safety" bicycle with pneumatic tires in 1889 was the full potential of "The Wheel" realized. For the public in general it was exhilarating, but for women it promised true emancipation. Recognizing its potential threat, critics worried about how, when, where, and with whom women might ride. Indoor classes to initiate them in the mysteries of dominating the bicycle offered riding lessons in the morning, riding to music after lunch, and afternoon tea to follow. Women who dared to ride outdoors were expected to follow guidelines that prohibited solitary cycling and decreed that a lady never shared a tandem with another woman. The proper cycling costume consisted of a straight side-pleated skirt worn over an underskirt and flannel-lined trousers or knickerbockers. A lightly boned blouse, simple hat, and low shoes with spats completed the outfit.

By the mid-1890s the bicycle craze was in full swing. Millions were taking advantage of this new form of exercise that not only brought all the muscles of the body into play, advocates claimed, but stimulated the heart, lungs, and digestion and even invigorated the senses and improved the memory. An impressive list of ailments were allegedly cured by the new remedy: dyspepsia, anemia, curvature of the spine, asthma, varicose veins, alcoholism and morphine addiction, diabetes, and, of course, neurasthenia. The dark side of the "vehicle of healthy happiness" was revealed in the diagnosis of a list of new ailments, from bicycle heart to bicycle face and *kyphosis bicyclestarum* (cyclist's stoop), as well as inguinal hernia, appendicitis, impotence, and constipation.

Presiding at the very pinnacle of the crusade for health was the vigorous, grinning figure of Theodore Roosevelt, Rough Rider and champion of the strenuous life. Like many fitness advocates, Roosevelt achieved the physical development he admired by having had to overcome small stature and a sickly constitution. Coming to the presidency in the wake of McKinley's assassination in 1901, he became a kind of folk hero through his energetic espousal of athleticism and the outdoor life.

Run for Your Life

In the 1950s physicians jumped on the exercise bandwagon with, literally, both feet. The specific claim that exercise protects the heart from coronary artery disease was first advanced by Dr. Jeremy Morris in 1953 on the basis of a study, now considered questionable, of London transport workers. Twenty years later Dr. Thomas Bassler proposed the Marathon Hypothesis, claiming that marathon running, which now attracts thousands of Americans every year, actually guaranteed protection against death from coronary heart disease. The Road Runners Club, which started in 1958 with 42 members, had over 22,000 by the mid-1980s. Dr. Kenneth Cooper, who made "aerobics" a household word, identified five risk factors for heart disease and quantified exercise according to its cardiac benefits.

Running became transformed from a form of recreation to a veritable religion. It was credited by its more extreme advocates not only with reducing weight, blood pressure, and the risk of heart disease, but, like earlier fitness panaceas, with combating asthma, retarding the aging process, strengthening sexual prowess, easing pregnancy and labor, curing addiction to alcohol and nicotine, relieving stress and depression, and curing schizophrenia.

Profoundly American

Casting a dispassionate eye over the past century and a half, what seems clear is that the calisthenics, isometrics, "Callanetics," aerobics, yoga, jogging, running, walking, racquetball, squash, tennis, skiing, surfing, and other active pursuits of today's fitness boom are just the most recent manifestations of America's continuing effort in the direction of self-improvement. Repeatedly shocked and surprised to find out what bad shape they are in, Americans resolve to take themselves in hand and shape up.

In fact, exercise is beneficial (and if people need to buy equipment in order to become fit, the economy benefits too). Moreover, what is good for the country club member is also good for the inner-city youth. The pursuit of fitness is not only healthful, it is democratic. It is profoundly American. □

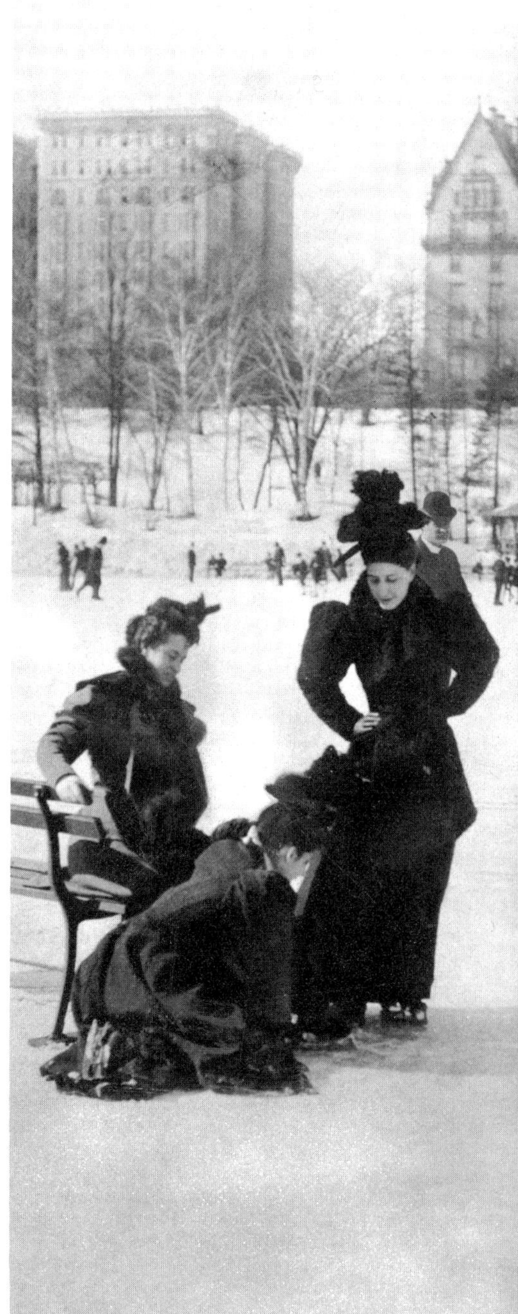

Properly clothed but daringly unaccompanied, women became enthusiastic skaters; here, a wintry scene in New York City's Central Park in 1893.

SUGGESTIONS FOR FURTHER READING

CERUTTY, PERCY. *Be Fit! Or Be Damned!* London, Pelham Books, 1967.

GREEN, HARVEY. *Fit for America: Health, Fitness, Sport, and American Society.* New York, Pantheon, 1986.

HIGDON, HAL. *Fitness After Forty.* Mountain View, Calif., Anderson World Publications, 1977.

SOLOMON, HENRY A. *The Exercise Myth.* San Diego, Harcourt Brace Jovanovich, 1984.

WHORTON, JAMES. *Crusaders for Fitness.* Princeton, N.J., Princeton University Press, 1982.

MEDICAL SPECIALISTS

A Look at the Increasingly Specialized World of Medicine

The world of medicine today is a far cry from the time when doctors paid house calls, took care of all members of the family, and ministered to whatever ailed them. Today, medicine is divided into specialties and subspecialties to such a degree that people sometimes have trouble figuring out who does what. This essay provides some of the answers. It looks at the world of medical specialists—from allergists to urologists and everything in between—and explains which area of medicine each of them deals with. It also describes what kind of training they receive that entitles them to call themselves specialists.

Reprinted from the February 1990 *Mayo Clinic Health Letter* with permission of the Mayo Foundation for Medical Education and Research, Rochester, Minn. 55905.

A

Allergist/Immunologist. An allergist/immunologist is a pediatrician or internist who has had additional training (usually two years) in allergy and immunology. This physician is an expert in the evaluation and management of disorders involving the immune system. Examples include asthma, eczema, hay fever, hives, food and drug allergies, and insect stings, as well as congenital or acquired immune deficiency conditions.

An allergist/immunologist performs tests to help identify offending agents that you should avoid or be immunized against. An allergist/immunologist also deals with the problems of organ transplantation or malignancies of the immune system.

Anesthesiologist. This physician administers anesthetics and monitors the anesthesia process before, during, and after surgery. After medical school, a physician spends four years of additional training to become an anesthesiologist. Training consists of studying the effects of various types of anesthetics on the human body. Developments in anesthesiology include new anesthetic agents and delivery techniques, new methods of reducing postoperative pain and new monitors to help ensure a favorable outcome from your operation.

Some anesthesiologists concentrate their efforts as members of the intensive care team treating critically ill patients. Others use their knowledge of drugs that control pain and the nervous system's conduction of impulses that the brain recognizes as pain to treat patients with chronic pain problems.

C

Cardiologist. A cardiologist spends a minimum of three years learning to manage abnormalities of your heart and blood vessels. This training provides experience in a wide range of activities including electrocardiography, echocardiography (non-X-ray imaging), cardiac catheterization (identifying the chambers of and blood supply to the heart), and pacemaker management. Once a cardiologist decides on an area of specific interest, such as cardiac catheterization, additional training focusing on the particular technique is necessary.

D

Dermatologist. A dermatologist specializes in the diagnosis and treatment of diseases of the skin—your body's largest organ. Dermatologists treat benign and some malignant conditions, ranging from eczema to squamous cell cancer. Dermatologists also treat disorders affecting your hair and nails. During three years of additional training, dermatologists gain expertise in areas such as the effects of ultraviolet light in treating skin diseases, as well as how the immune system influences the causes of skin disorders.

E

Emergency Medicine Specialist. A physician may elect to limit his or her practice to a trauma center. A three-year training program in trauma, medical, and pediatric emergencies qualifies a physician in this specialty. Some pediatricians and internists also concentrate their efforts in treating emergencies. But certification as an emergency medicine specialist is independent of certification in these specialties.

Endocrinologist. An endocrinologist spends three years after a residency in internal medicine learning to manage problems of hormone production. This could involve either overproduction or underproduction. In addition, he or she may spend time in a laboratory investigating the actions of one of the body's many hormones. The more common disorders that an endocrinologist manages include diabetes mellitus, problems of thyroid hormone production, and problems related to menstruation.

F

Family Physician. A physician may determine that his or her interest lies in the comprehensive care of the family. A three-year residency in family practice is the avenue to this specialty.

In training, a family practitioner gains experience in the various specialties of medicine. This enables a family practitioner to perform some minor surgical procedures or to manage uncomplicated pregnancies. This total, personal involvement with all members of a family, from the newborn to the grandparent, provides a challenging opportunity for an increasing number of medical school graduates.

G

Gastroenterologist. This internist diagnoses and treats disorders of the gastrointestinal (GI) tract and liver. A three-year training program teaches skills in examining the upper and lower gastrointestinal tract by means of a direct-viewing instrument called an endoscope.

Through this technology, small

How Physicians Become Physicians

With few exceptions, medical schools in the United States require prospective students to earn a bachelor's degree.

All medical schools require a minimum number of courses in biology, chemistry, physics, and mathematics. Medical schools encourage students to concentrate on the physical sciences. However, many medical schools also recognize the value of a "liberal education" that includes study of the humanities (such as literature and philosophy).

Curricula vary among medical schools. In most, the first two years cover basic sciences that deal with the workings of the human body. During this period, students examine the broad clinical areas of surgery, internal medicine, pediatrics, obstetrics, and psychiatry. Studies in these clinical sciences expand during the third and fourth years.

Medical school graduates earn the title Doctor of Medicine. By law, all physicians must be licensed by the state in which they practice.

Licensure follows the successful completion of an examination and, in most states, an additional year of training after medical school. To maintain a license, doctors must participate in programs of continuing medical education.

tumors within the gastrointestinal tract can be removed or, if too large, sampled for microscopic examination. A gastroenterologist also interprets X rays of the gastrointestinal tract.

Geneticist. Specialists in genetics evaluate individuals and families for the likelihood that inherited disorders, such as some forms of mental retardation, cystic fibrosis, muscular dystrophy, or hemophilia, might be passed to offspring.

A geneticist uses data from your medical and family history, as well as from a physical examination, to investigate the cause of the problem.

Genetic counseling can tell you how likely it is for a disease to occur in your family. A clinical geneticist receives training in a primary specialty, such as pediatrics or internal medicine, followed by two years of clinical genetics.

Gynecologist. See Obstetrician/Gynecologist.

H

Hematologist. Some physicians follow their internal medicine residency with a minimum of two years studying diseases of the blood and blood-forming organs. A hematologist diagnoses and treats anemias as well as malignant diseases of the blood such as leukemias and lymphomas. The most recent development in this field is bone marrow transplantation.

I

Infectious Disease Specialist. The two to three years of training in this subspecialty focus on the study of organisms that cause human infections, how they spread, and medications to treat them.

Prevention of infection through adequate immunization is a particular interest of this subspecialist. The AIDS epidemic and its infectious complications are within this field of expertise.

Internist. Internal medicine encompasses the diagnosis and nonsurgical treatment of disease in adults. An internist spends three to four years in training to gain an in-depth understanding of the various organ systems of your body, the diseases that can compromise them, and appropriate treatments.

After this residency, an internist may spend two or three more years developing expertise in a subspecialty of internal medicine. This additional training includes management of the patient's needs, as related to a particular group of diseases or area of internal medicine, and experience in laboratory research. The recognized subspecialists in internal medicine are cardiologists, endocrinologists, gastroenterologists, hematologists, infectious disease specialists, nephrologists, oncologists, rheumatologists, and thoracic disease specialists. See separate listings.

Medical Board Specialties That Doctors Most Commonly Choose

About 65 percent of all physicians have become certified in their specialty fields by taking an examination before their peers.

The largest number of board-certified physicians practice in the following 10 specialties*:

1. **Internal medicine**
2. **Family medicine**
3. **Pediatrics**
4. **Psychiatry and neurology**
5. **Obstetrics and gynecology**
6. **Surgery**
7. **Radiology**
8. **Anesthesiology**
9. **Emergency medicine**
10. **Pathology**

One value of specialty board certification is to help you identify physicians who have met a standard of training and experience above that required for licensure.

Licensure is not related to board certification. A physician may be a certified medical specialist, but he or she still needs a license to practice in a given state.

There are no legal requirements for a licensed physician to seek specialty board certification in order to practice his or her specialty. Physicians who choose to specialize may or may not elect to become board-certified.

*** Source: American Board of Medical Specialties.**

Primary Care: Your Gateway to the Healthcare System

The combination of a mobile society and increasing specialization within medicine has created a concern for many people: "How do I find the right physician for my problem?"

The answer: Start with a primary care physician.

A primary care physician is a doctor in family or internal medicine who has designed his or her practice to provide you with a point of entry into the healthcare system. To fulfill this role, a primary care physician must be:

- **Accessible. Your primary care physician is the doctor to contact initially when you have a medical problem.**
- **Comprehensive. Your primary care physician can care for the majority of your healthcare needs.**
- **A Coordinator. Your primary care physician coordinates your care, especially with regard to the selection and securing of specialty and subspecialty consultations. He or she is the "quarterback" on the healthcare team.**
- **Accountable. Your primary care physician accepts responsibility for the ongoing care and services that you receive.**

N

Nephrologist. A nephrologist is an expert in the function of the kidneys and the diseases that can affect them. During the three years of training in this subspecialty, a nephrologist may concentrate on the medical management of kidney disorders, the supervision of dialysis for patients whose kidneys have ceased to function, or the care of individuals who have received a kidney transplant.

Neurologist. Upon graduation from medical school, a physician may elect to specialize in the diagnosis and nonsurgical treatment of diseases of the brain, nerves, and muscles. Neurologists care for victims of stroke, Parkinson's disease, multiple sclerosis, and epilepsy, among other diseases. Three years of training follow a year of internal medicine residency. Expertise in interpreting brain wave recordings known as electroencephalograms (EEGs) or recordings of muscle function requires additional training.

Neurosurgeon. A neurosurgeon spends six to seven years in training to evaluate and surgically treat conditions such as brain tumors, abnormalities of the blood vessels that supply the brain, disorders affecting the spinal cord, and trauma to various parts of the nervous system. Advances in neurosurgery include microscope-aided and computer-aided surgery.

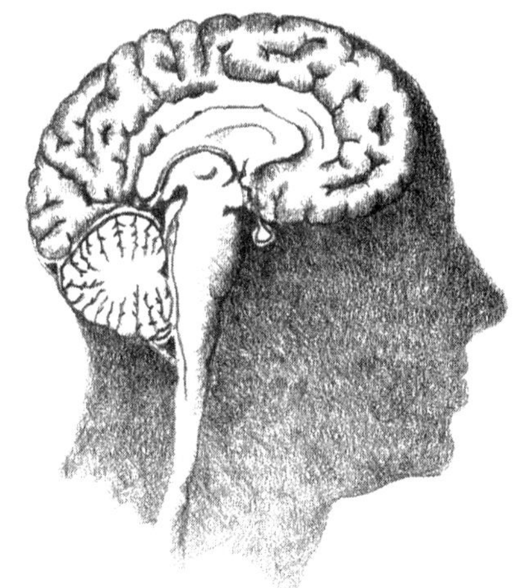

Obstetrician/Gynecologist. This physician specializes in the care of women during pregnancy and diseases that affect a woman's reproductive organs. During the four-year residency, a physician may elect to subspecialize in one of several facets of this discipline. For example, a gynecologist specializes in the surgical treatment of both benign and malignant diseases of the female reproductive organs. In other instances, the physician may choose to specialize in obstetrics. In addition to a residency, an obstetrician/gynecologist may take training in such areas as reproductive endocrinology—the body's mechanisms for fertility.

Oncologist. An oncologist specializes in the nonsurgical treatment of cancer. Today, the field of oncology encompasses a wide range of experimental and investigative techniques, as well as nonexperimental treatments. Among them are the investigation of the biochemical processes involved in cancer formation, study of abnormal genes associated with cancer, and analysis of the frequency and distribution of different types of cancer.

For this purpose, most large medical centers have an oncology record-keeping center called a "tumor registry." Groups of oncologists from various medical centers now combine their efforts in cancer treatment to include even greater numbers of patients in specific treatment programs.

Ophthalmologist. This physician specializes in care of the eyes. An ophthalmologist may limit his or her practice to diagnosing and treating eye disorders by nonsurgical means or to prescribing glasses and contact lenses that correct vision problems. Ophthalmologists surgically treat eye disorders such as cataracts, glaucoma, retinal detachment, or obstruction of tear ducts. After a four-year residency, this specialist may seek additional training in the diagnosis and treatment of specific eye-related diseases. (Optometrists and opticians, who also deal with eye care, are not physicians. Optometrists are trained to test eyes for focusing defects and to prescribe corrective lenses; opticians are trained to fill prescriptions for eyeglasses and lenses.)

Orthopedic Surgeon. This physician, upon completion of a five-year residency, specializes in diagnosing and treating disorders that affect bones and their supporting structures. An orthopedic surgeon treats a variety of conditions from setting fractures to implanting artificial joints.

After additional training, an orthopedic surgeon may limit his or her practice to an area such as the treatment of specific joint disorders, malignant diseases of the bones, or sports-related injuries. Microvascular surgery for reattaching limbs is a new development in the field.

Otorhinolaryngologist. An otorhinolaryngologist (oh'toe-rhye'know-lar'in-gol'o-jist) specializes in disorders of the ears, nose, throat, and related regions of the neck and base of the skull. For simplification, an otorhinolaryngologist frequently uses the title of ear, nose, and throat (ENT) specialist.

After a five-year residency, this physician is qualified to treat, both medically and surgically, a wide variety of disorders ranging from certain types of hearing impairment to cancer of the throat. Specialists in this field may concentrate their efforts in reconstructive and cosmetic plastic surgery of the head and neck region.

The Hippocratic Oath and Modern Medicine

Hippocrates is widely hailed as the "Father of Medicine." Yet we know almost nothing about the man himself. And contrary to popular belief, medical school graduates are not required to recite his oath.

According to tradition, Hippocrates was born near Asia Minor in about 460 B.C. He belonged to a guild of itinerant physicians.

The Hippocratic school rejected magical superstition as a way to understand illness. Hippocratic physicians emphasized careful observation and a reliance upon the healing power of nature.

Hippocratic writings give advice on the use of diet, medications, and "handwork" (surgery). Topics include ways to position the patient, proper illumination when giving treatment, and methods to treat burns, hemorrhoids, and fractures.

This practical approach, based upon reasoning and testing, has become the foundation of today's medical practice.

And while many modern doctors would hesitate to swear "by all the gods and goddesses," the Hippocratic commitment remains laudable. It states: "I will use treatment to help the sick according to my ability and judgment, but never with a view to injury and wrong-doing."

Pathologist. This physician specializes in the study of bodily fluids and tissues to determine the cause and status of disease. Pathologists may subspecialize to study anatomic structures, body chemistry or blood, and the effects of various diseases or microorganisms on them. Here are the subspecialists in this area:

- *Anatomic Pathologist.* After five years in specialty training, an anatomic pathologist is skilled in examining the various organs of the body, both in their intact state and under a microscope. This physician may be able to establish the nature of the disease affecting a specific organ and the extent to which the disease involves that organ and the body as a whole. An anatomic pathologist regularly uses a standard microscope to examine tissues but may also use an electron microscope and other technologies to examine each cell's individual components.
- *Laboratory Medicine Specialist.* This pathologist employs the latest in biomedical technology to identify and interpret abnormalities in the various tissues and fluids of the body. A laboratory medicine

specialist may concentrate on the study of chemical reactions within the body, measurement of hormones, or examination of the many cells that make up blood. After the standard five years of training, this specialist may embark on additional training to become an expert in areas such as "tissue typing" or "transfusion medicine." By studying blood samples, physicians in this evolving area of medicine can determine when a donated organ matches a potential recipient.

Pediatrician. Specialists in this field diagnose and treat acute and chronic childhood illness, as well as provide preventive care for infants, children, and adolescents. During a three-year residency, a pediatrician studies the normal function of the child's body as it develops from a newborn through the teenage years.

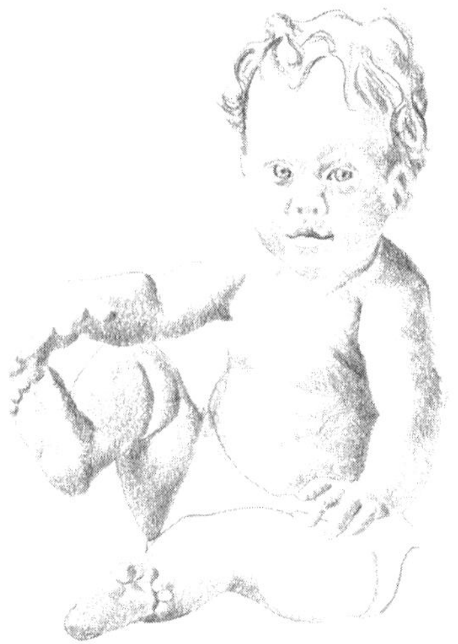

As in the case of the general internist, the general pediatrician may elect to extend his or her training for two to three years to study a particular organ system and the diseases that affect it. Pediatricians may subspecialize in an area such as cardiology or nephrology. Or, a pediatrician may select neonatology. In this field, a pediatrician develops expertise in dealing with the often life-threatening complications that can occur in the early hours and days following birth, whether full-term or premature.

Physiatrist. A physiatrist (fiz'e-ah-trist) nonsurgically treats acute and chronic disorders of the nervous and musculoskeletal systems. This specialist coordinates the rehabilitation of individuals who have sustained permanent injury to the nervous system, such as stroke or spinal cord injury, and related conditions in other organ systems.

A physiatrist trains for three years to competently evaluate how well patients can function in terms of their physical impairment. This expertise includes the use of techniques such as heat, cold, electrical stimulation, and biofeedback, as well as therapeutic exercises to manage chronic problems. Sometimes called a physical medicine and rehabilitation specialist, a physiatrist may practice in the area of prosthetics (artificial limbs, braces, and supports), sports medicine, or pediatric rehabilitation.

Preventive Medicine Specialist. The American Board of Preventive Medicine recognizes three related specialties: general preventive medicine and public health, occupational medicine, and aerospace medicine. After completion of medical school, a physician who is interested in preventive medicine pursues a two-year training program in one of these three specialty areas. In addition, specialists in these areas usually obtain a master's degree in public health or receive equivalent training.

Preventive medicine specialists focus on the prevention or early detection of disease. Occupational medicine specialists focus on the health and safety of employees in

Steps Toward Specialization

When you visit your doctor, you've no doubt noticed a number of certificates hanging on the wall of his or her office.

They represent different aspects of your physician's training. The medical profession has checkpoints that mark a doctor's professional growth—which can help you verify a practitioner's abilities.

Some physicians elect to specialize in a particular field of medicine. Specialization requires an additional period of training known as a residency. (Years ago, doctors actually lived at the hospital where they trained.)

Upon completion of the required number of years in residency, a physician undergoes a written and, in some specialities, an oral examination. A successful outcome results in certification by a board of examiners (such as the American Board of Internal Medicine). Each of the medical specialists described in this article are so tested.

Today, some doctors opt for subspecialty training within a specialty field: for example, plastic surgery. Upon completion of this postgraduate training, doctors take another examination. Some physicians are named to honorary societies, such as the American College of Chest Physicians. This recognition usually reflects a doctor's achievements during his or her career.

the workplace. Both of these areas also are concerned with the effects of the environment on an individual's health. Aerospace medicine specialists focus on the health and safety of people who travel by air—airline passengers, pilots, and astronauts.

Proctologist. See Surgeon—Colon and Rectal Surgeon.

Psychiatrist. A psychiatrist diagnoses and treats behavioral disorders. As physicians, psychiatrists can prescribe medications as well as use psychotherapy to treat these conditions. A psychiatrist's four years of training include aspects of both internal medicine and neurology. Psychiatry has many subspecialties including pediatric, geriatric, and forensic (legal) psychiatry.

(A psychiatrist may practice in concert with a psychologist. A psychologist attains, at minimum, a master's degree and usually a doctorate. This permits him or her to assess and manage problems of memory, behavior, and emotional function. A psychologist may specialize in chronic pain, substance abuse, or family conflict.)

R

Radiologist. A radiologist specializes in the use of multiple imaging technologies such as X rays, radioactive substances, ultrasound, and magnetic resonance imaging (MRI). Modern radiology provides images or scans of almost any organ or part of your body in a variety of ways, helping physicians diagnose diseases, and plan and monitor treatment. This often makes exploratory surgery unnecessary.

Radiologists now concentrate their five years of training to become one of the following specialists:

- *Diagnostic Radiologist.* These specialists use radiologic technology to diagnose medical conditions. Some radiologists use imaging techniques to biopsy tissue for microscopic examination and place catheters into blood vessels to define circulation.
- *Therapeutic Radiologist.* A therapeutic radiologist directs several forms of radiation to kill or slow the growth of cancer cells. This radiologist may use conventional X rays, radioactive isotopes, or high-energy particles like those generated by a linear accelerator.

Check the Yellow Pages

Where do you look to find a physician? More than one-third of American adults consult the Yellow Pages each month.

But if you let your fingers do the walking, step carefully.

To help you identify the 370,000 physicians recognized as specialists by the American Board of Medical Specialties (ABMS), this organization launched a national information program in 1990.

Many telephone directories throughout the country now list local physicians who are recognized as specialists by the ABMS, noting their specialty or subspecialty.

Not all specialists may be listed in this way, however. To verify whether a doctor is board-certified or not, call the ABMS toll-free at 1-800-776-CERT (1-800-776-2378).

Rheumatologist. A rheumatologist's main interest focuses on diseases of the joints and muscles caused by abnormalities in the immune system and degeneration of the joints, as well as inflammation of arteries (called vasculitis). Known as rheumatic diseases, these disorders are typified by rheumatoid arthritis.

This subspecialist spends three years training to diagnose and treat these diseases. A rheumatologist researches defects in the immune system that cause the system to fail to recognize your own musculoskeletal system and, therefore, turn against it.

S

Surgeon (General). A general surgeon spends five years after medical school studying the diagnosis and surgical treatment of diseases, ranging from breast cancer to gastrointestinal disorders to trauma. A general surgeon must have expertise in a variety of other specialties, including pathology and radiology, to diagnose and treat patients.

Following residency, a general surgeon may train an additional two to three years to specialize in treating specific diseases or diseases that affect a specific organ. The following are subspecialists:

- *Colon and Rectal Surgeon.* A two-year residency provides experience in treating diseases of the large bowel ranging from cancer to inflammatory bowel disease, such as ulcerative colitis. A colon-rectal surgeon also treats more common disorders such as hemorrhoids.
- *Pediatric Surgeon.* This general surgeon spends two years of ad-

ditional training to specialize in surgically treating childhood disorders. Examples include malignant tumors that occur only in children, trauma, and some forms of birth defects, as well as the more common problems of hernias and appendicitis.

- *Plastic Surgeon.* A plastic surgeon specializes in the areas of cosmetic and reconstructive surgery to enhance a patient's physical appearance or to restore normal appearance altered by tumors or injury. Examples of cosmetic surgery include liposuction (fat removal) and "face lifts." Reconstructive surgery involves correcting abnormalities brought about by disease, injury, or birth defect. A plastic surgeon spends two years after general surgical training to attain this degree of expertise.
- *Thoracic and Cardiovascular Surgeon.* This surgeon spends two to three years learning techniques necessary to correct structural abnormalities that can affect the heart, ranging from valve dysfunction to blockage of the arteries leading to the heart. Thoracic and cardiovascular surgeons also implant permanent cardiac pacemakers and perform surgery to treat diseases of the lungs and esophagus.
- *Transplantation Surgeon.* Physicians in this relatively new surgical subspecialty focus on organ transplantation and the use of medications that suppress the immune system. A surgeon's background determines the organs he or she will transplant. For example, a surgeon first must be an expert in cardiovascular surgery before being qualified to transplant hearts. Other surgeons specialize in liver, pancreas, or kidney transplantation.
- *Vascular Surgeon.* This surgical subspecialist corrects abnormalities that adversely affect arteries throughout the body, with the exception of the coronary arteries—the arteries that supply blood to your heart. A vascular surgeon clears clogged arteries by removing the material that causes the blockage or by using either a piece of vein or artificial material to bypass the area of obstruction. A vascular surgeon also repairs injured arteries.

T

Thoracic Disease Specialist. This internist specializes in diseases of the lungs. Examples include breathing abnormalities, infections, and cancer of the respiratory tract. Training encompasses two to three years and includes experience in measuring lung function and medically managing a variety of lung-related disorders. In addition, a thoracic disease specialist may develop the skills to use a direct-viewing instrument called a bronchoscope to examine and treat the airway system. Many thoracic specialists complete an additional year of training that deals with the care of critically ill patients.

Urologist. A urologist usually leaves the general surgery training course after two years and then completes three years of urological training. During this further training period, he or she studies how to diagnose and treat diseases and disorders of the urinary and urogenital tracts. Examples include benign and malignant diseases of the prostate gland (found in males), incontinence in both men and women, and male impotence.

SOURCES OF FURTHER INFORMATION

The following references can provide information about a physician's professional background. Look for them at your public library, local medical society, or libraries at a hospital or university medical school.

American Board of Medical Specialties (ABMS). *ABMS Compendium of Certified Medical Specialists.* Lists physicians who are certified by the examining boards of recognized specialty organizations. Provides information such as a doctor's medical school and internship training, type of practice and hospital affiliation, and address and telephone number.

American Medical Association. *American Medical Directory.* Lists physicians in the United States, Puerto Rico, the Virgin Islands, and certain Pacific Islands, and U.S. physicians temporarily located in foreign countries who belong to the AMA, whether board-certified or not. Provides such information as the physician's name, address, type of practice, and where he or she went to medical school.

Directory of Medical Specialties. Published by Marquis Who's Who. Provides information similar to that in the ABMS Compendium.

WHAT IS ENDOMETRIOSIS?

Linda Hughey Holt, M.D.

ILLUSTRATION BY KYE CARBONE

Endometriosis is a common condition, affecting some 5.5 million women in the United States and Canada. In endometriosis, tissue resembling the uterine lining (the endometrium) grows in other locations in the body, most commonly on the internal pelvic organs surrounding the uterus. This misplaced tissue usually responds to the hormones of the menstrual cycle as if it were true endometrial tissue, building up every month and then breaking down and bleeding.

Some women with endometriosis have no symptoms, but others experience pain such as very strong menstrual cramps and infertility. Endometriosis may cause regular internal bleeding and may result in extensive scar tissue in the abdomen. It is thought that the pain of severe endometriosis is caused by the monthly swelling and bleeding of the misplaced tissue, as well as by the resulting scar tissue and the large cysts that can develop in or on the ovaries. The scar tissue can also cause infertility by blocking off the fallopian tubes, which conduct fertilized eggs into the uterus, and by interfering with normal ovulation. It is less clear why mild endometriosis, in which only faint blue, brown, or reddish-blue blotches occur in the pelvis, can also seemingly cause both pain and infertility.

Endometriosis was once called "the career woman's disease" because it was commonly found in career-oriented working women in their 30s and 40s who had

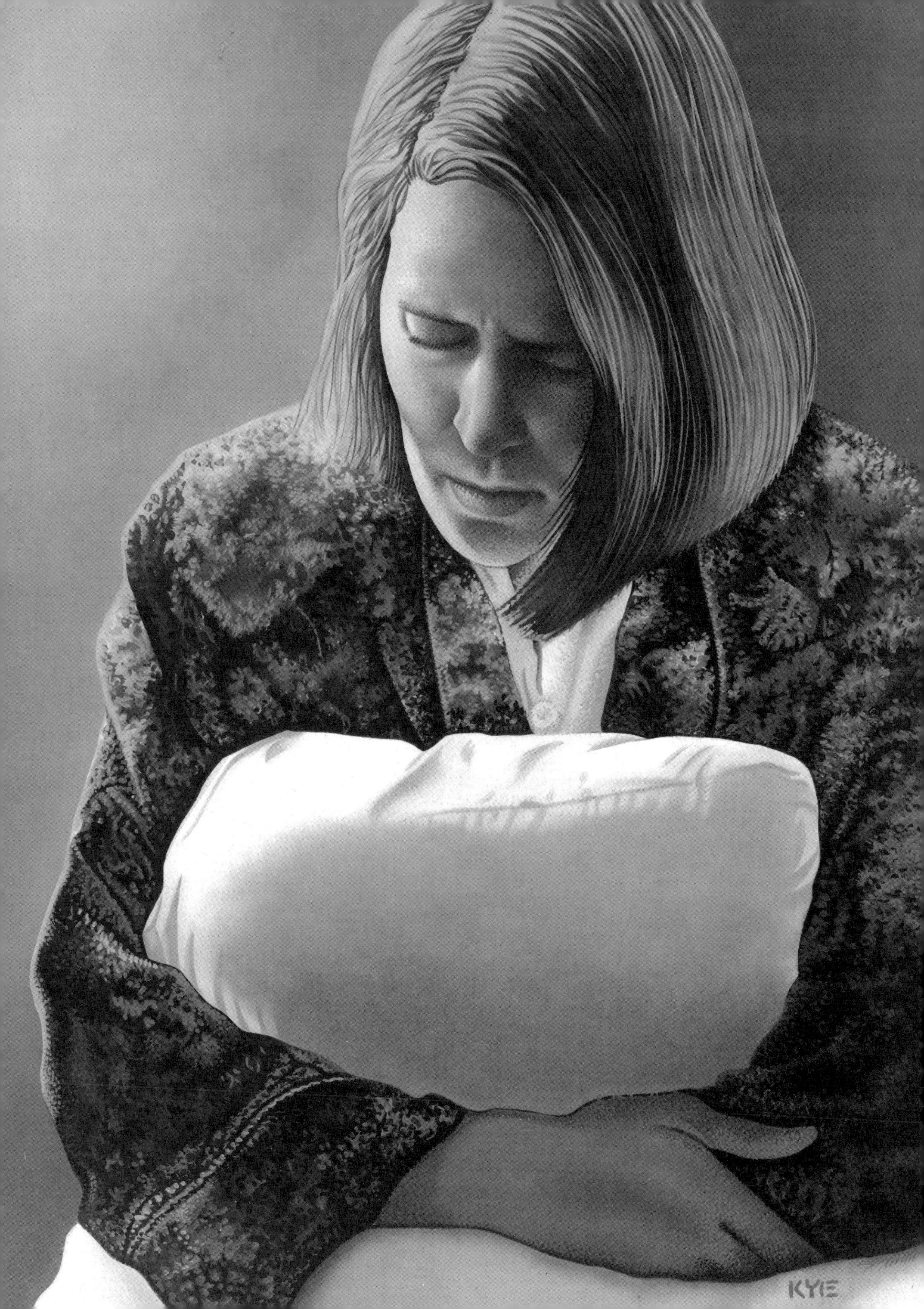
KYE

not had any children at the time of exploratory surgery for pain. It is now recognized that although delayed childbearing is a risk factor, the label is a misnomer. The increasingly widespread use of a minor surgical procedure called laparoscopy for the diagnosis of pelvic disorders has made it clear that endometriosis is not limited to any socioeconomic or occupational group. Most likely it was previously found primarily in middle-class, working women because they could better afford medical care and hesitated to miss work on account of menstrual pain. It does occur almost exclusively in women past puberty, and symptoms disappear or significantly improve after menopause.

Symptoms

Besides severe menstrual cramps, the symptoms of endometriosis include painful intercourse and irregular menstrual bleeding. When scar tissue occurs, the entire process of ovulating can become painful, with pain starting before ovulation and continuing until the menstrual period. Other symptoms may depend on where the misplaced endometrial tissue grows. The most commonly affected sites are the surfaces of the uterus, fallopian tubes, bladder, and rectum, but the endometrial implants can also occur on the surface of the colon, creating symptoms that mimic bowel disorders such as irritable bowel syndrome. Women with this type of endometriosis are often misdiagnosed as having primarily bowel problems, resulting in delays in obtaining appropriate diagnosis and treatment. Endometriosis on the bladder can result in such symptoms as frequent and painful urination. The appendix is also a common location for endometrial implants, and pain much like that of appendicitis can result.

STAGES OF ENDOMETRIOSIS

Endometriosis is described as minimal, mild, moderate, or severe, depending on the extent of implants and adhesions.

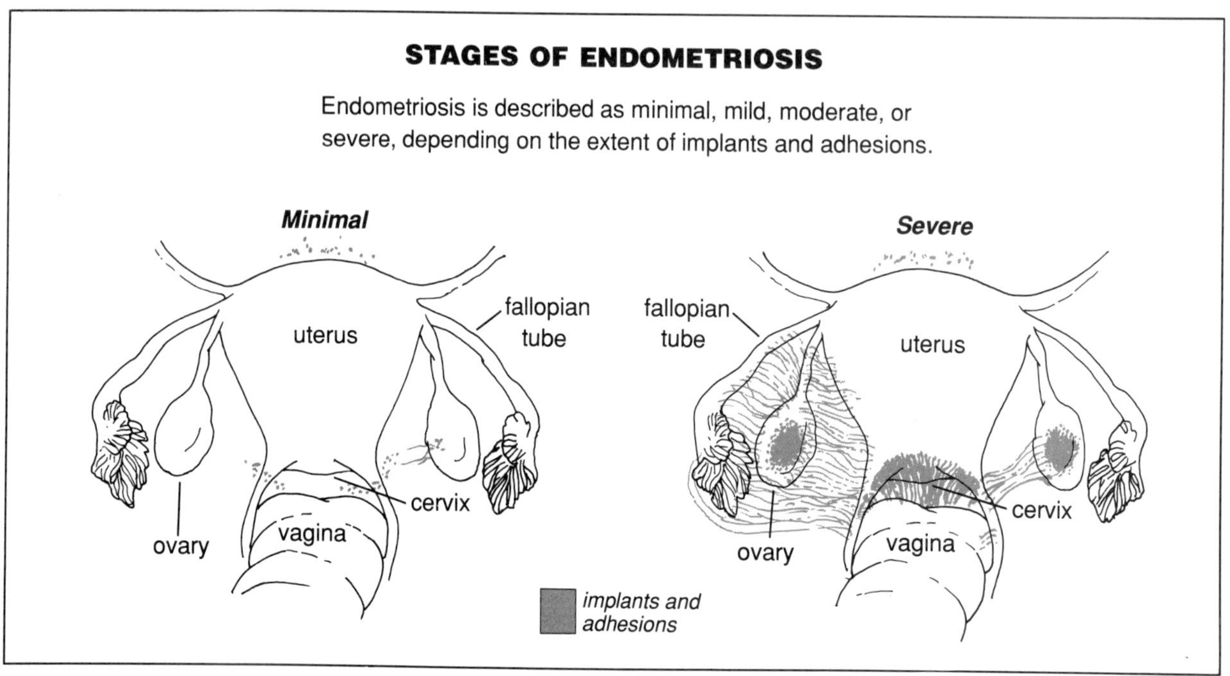

One of the most common sites for endometriosis is at the top of the vagina. Pressure on this area during intercourse can cause pain. When endometriosis occurs inside the ovaries, it creates large cysts, which usually require surgical removal because they can rupture. In addition, an enlarged ovary rouses suspicions of ovarian cancer, and a doctor may wish to remove the cyst to be sure it is not malignant. (Fortunately, endometrial implants rarely become malignant.)

Spotting, or small amounts of irregular bleeding, can occur during the menstrual cycle and is most likely caused by disruption of normal ovarian hormones by cysts or irritation of ovarian cells by the abnormal tissue. Most women with endometriosis have fairly regular periods, though, and women who frequently skip periods may have a reduced risk of endometriosis.

Endometriosis has been called "the great mimicker" because the symptoms can occur in many other conditions. Furthermore, endometriosis may cause no symptoms whatever, and the severity of symptoms does not always correlate with the extent of misplaced tissue growth. Endometriosis should be suspected in any woman with severe pelvic or bowel pain and in any woman with severe menstrual cramps that do not respond to over-the-counter medications.

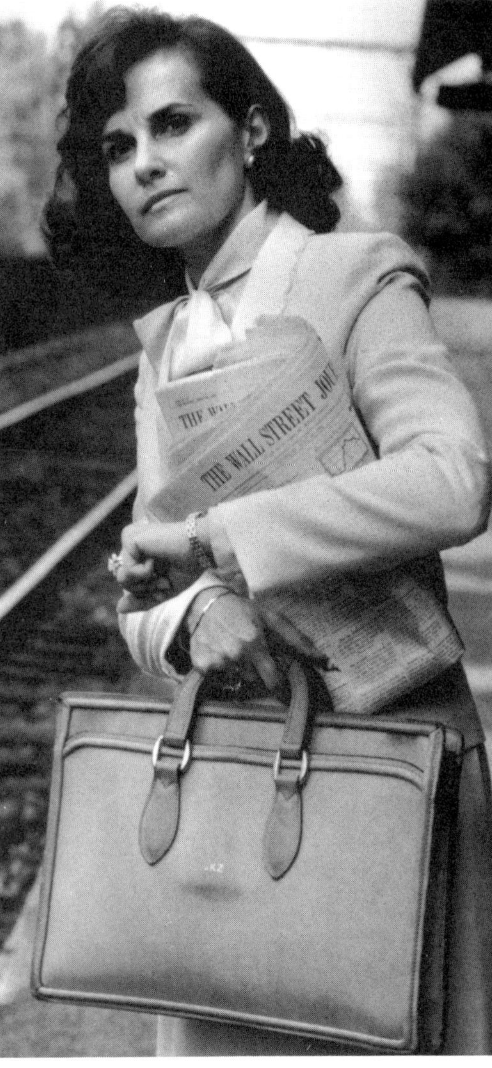

Career women were once thought to be the most likely to suffer from endometriosis, but it is now known to affect women in all socioeconomic and occupational groups.

Risk Factors

Risk factors for endometriosis include a family history of the disease and delayed childbearing. Also, the incidence of endometriosis is higher in women not using birth control pills. Endometriosis seems to be inherited in what is called a multifactorial mode—that is, several genes are involved. It was once thought that race played an important role, since in early studies black women showed less risk than white women. However, subsequent more sophisticated studies have shown a similar incidence in black and white women with similar socioeconomic backgrounds, access to healthcare, and childbearing patterns. Diet may play a role, since a high-fat diet increases a woman's estrogen levels, which may stimulate endometrial growth, and also leads to early puberty and therefore to more years of menstruation prior to childbearing.

The increased risk of endometriosis in women who delay having children stems from the fact that the hormonal changes of pregnancy can help prevent endometriosis. Birth control pills also exert a protective effect. Hence, women who delay childbearing and use nonhormonal forms of birth control are at increased risk for the disease.

Causes of Endometriosis

There are several theories regarding the cause of endometriosis. The most common route of endometrial tissue spread is probably spillage

---

Linda Hughey Holt is chairman of the Department of Obstetrics and Gynecology at Rush North Shore Medical Center in Skokie, Ill., and assistant professor at Rush-Presbyterian-St. Luke's Medical Center.

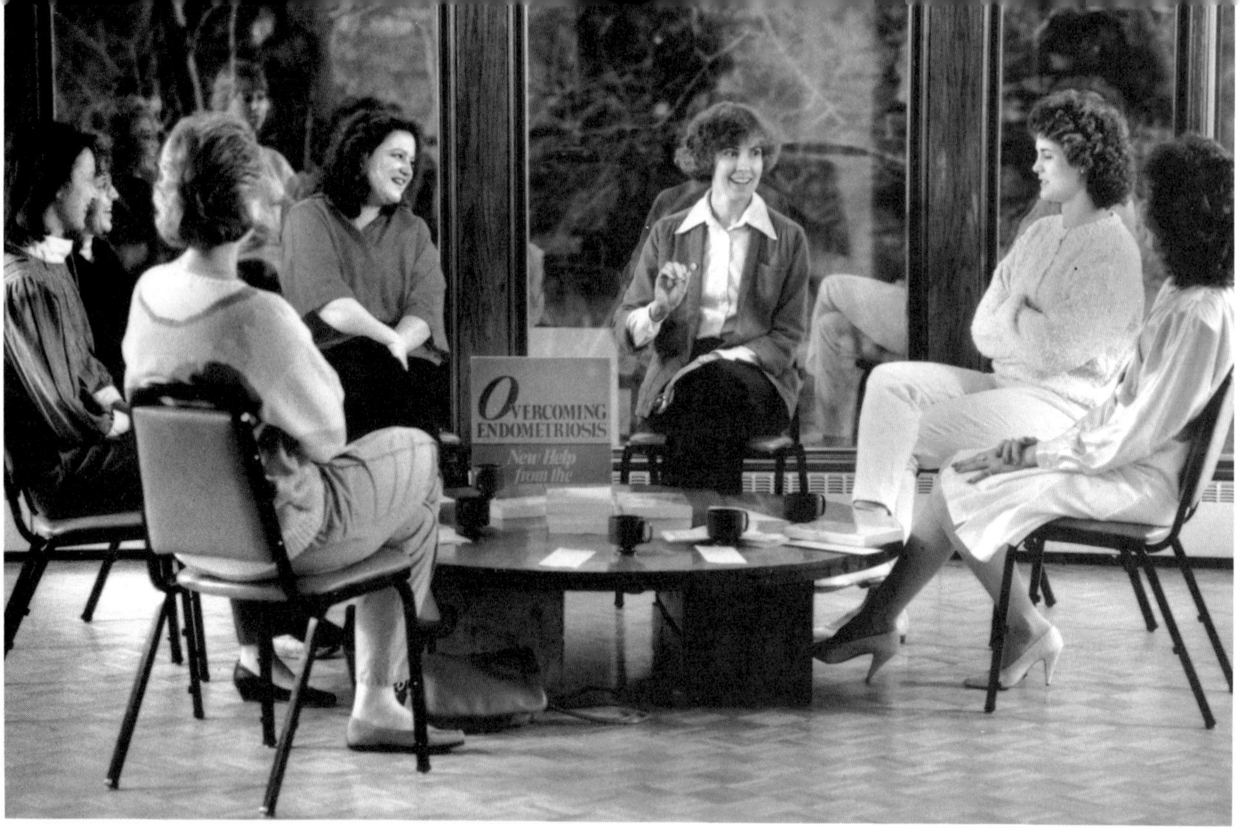

Support groups provide understanding listeners as well as opportunities to trade information about doctors, treatments, and ways of coping.

of remnants of endometrium through the fallopian tubes during menstrual periods, so-called retrograde menstruation. During a normal menstrual period, the uterine lining is shed mostly through the cervix, but many studies have confirmed that shreds of uterine lining and menstrual blood commonly spill through the fallopian tubes into the abdomen. Other studies showing that conditions in which the cervix is blocked off increase the risk of endometriosis and the fact that the most common locations for endometriosis are exactly where such spillage is likely to fall, support the retrograde menstruation theory. In addition, it has been observed that factors that cause a greater buildup of the uterine lining (including a high-fat diet, obesity, and early puberty) increase the risk of endometriosis, while factors that shrink it (such as use of birth control pills) or prevent menstruation (pregnancy or surgical or induced menopause) protect against endometriosis.

However, it is not clear why, if retrograde menstruation is a common event, only some women develop endometriosis—or why the condition is mild and nonprogressive in some cases and rapidly increases in severity in others. This puzzle has led investigators to postulate an immunologic component to endometriosis: Most women shed uterine lining onto the surfaces of the abdominal lining, the theory holds, but the normal female immune system will not allow it to grow; in some women the immune system fails in some way, allowing endometrial tissue to grow and sometimes spread.

The retrograde menstruation theory does not explain the occurrence of endometrial implants at distant sites such as the lungs. Therefore, a potential for spread by the blood stream or lymphatic system has been proposed. Endometriosis is also found in surgical incision sites and episiotomy scars (an episiotomy is an incision made below the vaginal opening to aid in childbirth), so spread via surgical instruments has been proposed.

These potential routes of spread of the disease still do not explain why endometriosis can occur in the lining of the abdomen in a woman who has had a hysterectomy (removal of the uterus). It has been theorized that the embryonic tissue that develops into the lining of the abdomen has some potential for spontaneously turning into the glandular tissue found in endometrial implants.

Whatever causes endometrial implants in the first place, once they have formed, the right hormonal environment is critical for successful growth. In simple terms, estrogen makes the implants grow, and a variety of other hormones (progesterone and some androgens, or male hormones) seem to either limit the growth of or actually shrink the implants.

Endometriosis and Infertility

Both mild and severe endometriosis have been linked with fertility problems.

Endometriosis is found in about 30 percent of women suffering from infertility and in only 2 to 5 percent of fertile women. When endometriosis is severe, the mechanism of infertility is well understood—scar tissue blocks off the fallopian tubes, and ovarian cysts interfere with normal ovulation. What is not clear is why so many women with mild endometriosis also have fertility problems.

Several possible reasons have been proposed: (1) Endometriosis may cause very subtle disruptions in ovulation and in the mobility of the fallopian tubes, which must transport fertilized eggs into the uterus. (2) Secretions from the endometrial implants may create a hostile environment for sperm and eggs. (3) Immunologic dysfunction may make eggs impenetrable to sperm. (4) Infertility from other causes may lead to endometriosis simply because, in the absence of pregnancy or use of oral contraceptives, more "unprotected" menstrual cycles take place.

Since endometriosis may not cause any symptoms, it is important for women who are having difficulty becoming pregnant to have a laparoscopy. The procedure should be done by a gynecologist or fertility specialist experienced in diagnosis and treatment of endometriosis, and it should be performed early in the course of an infertility evaluation—unless, of course, there is another obvious cause of infertility.

While it is clear, however, that treatment of severe or moderate endometriosis improves a woman's chance of becoming pregnant, many studies have indicated that pregnancy rates are similar in women with treated and untreated mild endometriosis.

Diagnosing the Problem

A woman and her doctor may suspect endometriosis on the basis of symptoms or otherwise unexplained infertility. Many women with endometriosis will have characteristic findings upon pelvic examination, including tender nodules behind the cervix or along the bladder, enlarged and tender ovaries, or a retroverted (backward tilted) uterus that does not move around easily. However, many other conditions can cause these problems.

There are no laboratory tests to diagnose endometriosis. Common blood tests are usually normal. Immunologic tests may show abnormalities, but none of these tests is specific for endometriosis. The only way to confirm the diagnosis is with a laparoscopy, in which a gynecological surgeon inserts a small viewing tube into the abdomen, inflates the abdomen with carbon dioxide (a harmless gas), and looks carefully at the pelvic structures. This procedure must be performed in a hospital or ambulatory surgery center. Although it is usually an outpatient procedure, it does require an anesthetic.

When performed by an experienced surgeon and anesthesiologist, laparoscopy is a very low-risk procedure, but there is one chance in a thousand of damage to the bowel or bladder, major bleeding, or major anesthetic complications. The risks are a bit higher in women who have had previous abdominal surgery, are very obese, or have heart or lung problems (which can make the anesthetic more dangerous). While the laparoscopy is an important step in diagnosis, it is nonetheless a surgical procedure and like any surgery should be done only when necessary. Many doctors recommend that a woman with suspected endometriosis simply be followed carefully with office visits and sonograms (painless, noninvasive procedures that use sound waves to produce an image of the pelvic organs) and reserve laparoscopy for situations in which severe pain or fertility problems merit the small risks of undergoing the surgery. Other doctors feel that any woman with significant pelvic pain should have a laparoscopy for diagnosis.

Combined surgical and medical treatment is common.

During laparoscopy, the severity, or stage, of endometriosis can be determined. Staging allows a woman's doctor to predict her chances of pregnancy, make better informed treatment decisions, and follow the course of her disease. It also allows researchers to assess the effectiveness of different treatments for different stages of the disease.

While laparoscopy is the mainstay of diagnosis, endometriosis may also be discovered during surgery for other reasons and is occasionally diagnosed by biopsy of endometrial implants of the bladder or bowel during diagnostic procedures on those organs.

Treatment

Treatment for endometriosis is a rapidly advancing area, although no treatment is perfect. Medical treatments alter the body's hormone levels to prevent or shrink tissue implants. The earliest medical treatments were based on the observation that pregnancy seemed to both prevent and alleviate endometriosis. Improving medical treatments have taken an increasingly sophisticated approach to changing the hormonal milieu that fosters the disease. Surgical treatments actually remove the implants; they also remove adhesions, fibrous tissues that develop as implants adhere to adjacent normal tissue, making pelvic organs stick together. Physicians have observed that simply removing chunks of diseased tissue often results in long-term symptom relief and improved pregnancy rates. Commonly, surgical and medical approaches are combined. It is important to recognize that the best treatment varies from woman to woman, taking into consideration the severity of the disease, her desire to bear children, the skills of the treating physician, and the availability of different equipment.

Medical Treatments. A number of medical treatments for endometriosis have been tried.

• *Pseudopregnancy.* One of the earliest forms of treatment was a high-dosage combination of estrogen and progesterone. Used together at high doses, these hormones mimic the hormonal changes of pregnancy, eliminating the menstrual cycle and therefore eliminating the cyclic internal bleeding that causes pain and tissue damage. Pseudopregnancy is rarely used at present because newer medications are more effective.

• *Androgens.* Androgens, such as testosterone, are male hormones that seem to be effective mainly by directly attaching to hormone receptors in the endometrial implants and causing them to shrink. They may also affect the immune system. They are rarely used now because of their side effects—including weight gain, acne, and abnormal facial hair—which make them less desirable than newer agents.

There is one androgen, however, that was specifically developed for endometriosis treatment. Danazol (brand name, Danocrine; in Canada, Cyclamen) is a weak androgen that is quite effective in shrinking small implants. At high doses, it also eliminates the menstrual cycle and may improve immunologic function as well. Although the potential side effects are the same as for other androgens, many women do not suffer from them. Usually, danazol is used for six months and followed by use of oral contraceptives or by attempts to conceive.

• *Oral contraceptives (OCPs).* The combination of estrogen and progesterone found in certain OCPs both prevents endometriosis and ameliorates symptoms in women who already have the disease. Such OCPs are the only agents used for long-term suppression. While their effects are not as dramatic as those of the agents listed below, they can when necessary be used for long periods of time and may be the treat-

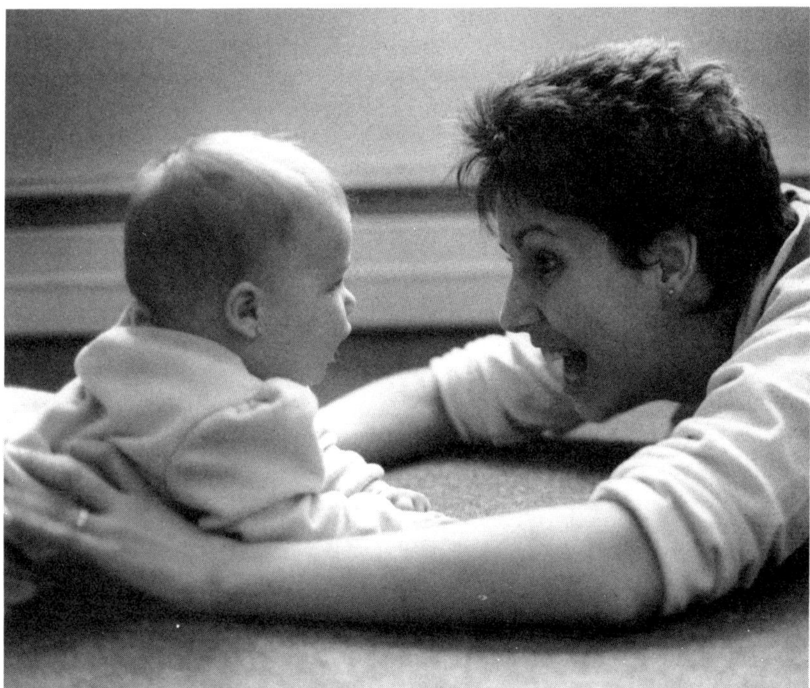

Pregnancy and breast feeding bring hormonal changes that can protect against endometriosis or improve its symptoms.

ment of choice for young women with known or strongly suspected endometriosis who may not be planning a pregnancy for many years but who may want to have children at some future date. Women who smoke should ideally quit smoking if they wish to use OCPs; women with a history of blood clots or breast cancer are also usually cautioned against OCP use.

• *Progesterone.* The hormone progesterone tends to shrink endometrial implants. It has commonly been given in long-acting injections or oral medication to be taken daily. Many women do very well on progesterone, but side effects such as weight gain, depression, and irregular bleeding are common. A new, long-acting progesterone implant, Norplant, was approved by the Food and Drug Administration at the end of 1990 for use in the United States as a contraceptive; if it helps keep endometriosis under control, it may be an excellent choice for women who do not wish to use OCPs.

Certain hormones can shrink endometrial implants.

• *Gonadotropin agonists.* Only recently approved for the treatment of endometriosis in the United States, these agents show great promise. They are chemically similar to the hormone called luteinizing hormone releasing hormone (LHRH), which is made in the brain and triggers the pituitary gland to initiate menstruation. "Pulses" of these agents can be used to bring about multiple ovulations, so they are widely used as fertility drugs. Continuous administration, however, shuts down stimulation of the ovaries, in effect creating a temporary menopause that relieves endometriosis. These agents are currently available in long-acting or daily injectable form and as a nasal spray. They are fairly expensive and not in widespread use, but they show great promise. Side effects are similar to menopause symptoms, which include hot flashes, vaginal dryness, and loss of bone mass.

Surgical Treatments. Surgical approaches to treatment include the following.

• *Laparoscopy.* During laparoscopy to treat (rather than just diagnose) endometriosis, small implants may be removed by either cautery (burning) or laser therapy. Adhesions can be lysed (cut apart), and pieces of affected abdominal lining can even be peeled off and removed. Since laparoscopy can be performed on an outpatient basis, it is rapidly becoming the surgical approach of choice for mild to moderate endometriosis. However, laparoscopic surgery does carry some risks of damage to other abdominal structures, such as the bowel or bladder, and its usefulness is directly related to the skill and experience of the surgeon.

At the present time, it is unclear whether laser treatment is any better than traditional cautery methods, or whether severe endometriosis is best dealt with by laparoscopy or by the more traditional open surgery. The ability of a laser to vaporize very small tissue implants without damaging surrounding tissues and to prevent bleeding while it cuts through scar tissue, however, makes this method a promising choice for the future, once the technology is widespread, the potential risks are minimized, and the necessary surgical skills have caught up with the technology.

• *"Conservative" surgery.* When large cysts or extensive scar tissue are present, "conservative" surgery may be the best treatment for women who wish to conserve the pelvic organs. Conservative surgery consists of removing visible implants, reconstructing blocked fallopian tubes if necessary, and at times suspending the uterus forward to prevent recurrent scarring. At times the nerves in back of the uterus may be partially cut for control of very severe pain; however, there are risks to this procedure, and it is not widely used.

• *Hysterectomy.* For women who do not wish to have children or have completed their families, a hysterectomy plus removal of the fallopian tubes and ovaries is often recommended. In the vast majority of cases, this will eliminate or at least relieve most of the symptoms of endometriosis. Women who have struggled with chronic pain for many years may welcome the relief afforded by this procedure. Rarely, the disease may continue in milder form, but any remaining symptoms can usually be controlled by one of the other treatments.

Pregnancy and Menopause

Pregnancy offers protection against the development of endometriosis. In women who already have endometriosis, symptoms usually improve; however, they can recur after the pregnancy. Breast feeding may also offer protection or lengthen the period of remission by suppressing the menstrual cycle and production of estrogen. Menopause almost always offers relief from symptoms of endometriosis.

When endometriosis has caused the fallopian tubes to become badly scarred and blocked, the best chance of pregnancy may be in vitro fertilization (IVF), a procedure that simply bypasses the fallopian tubes. Eggs are surgically retrieved from the ovaries, fertilized in the laboratory, and implanted into the uterus. Rates for successfully completed pregnancies are approximately 10 percent per egg retrieval cycle in good IVF programs.

Estrogen Replacement Therapy

Controversy exists over whether women with a history of endometriosis should be placed on estrogen replacement therapy after menopause (when production of estrogen by the ovaries drops sharply) or after a hysterectomy and removal of the fallopian tubes and ovaries. The benefits of replacement therapy include prevention of osteoporosis (thinning of the bones), prevention of heart disease, and relief from the hot flashes, vaginal dryness, and mood disorders such as depression that some women experience at the time of menopause. It was once felt that estrogen replacement therapy was absolutely out of the question for women with endometriosis, because of the chance that estrogen could reactivate endometrial implants even without functioning ovaries in place. The current thinking, however, is that it is unfair to automatically deny women with a history of endometriosis the benefits of replacement therapy. Not all women want or need to take hormones with menopause, but if a woman and her doctor decide replacement therapy is indicated, a low dose of estrogen may be used with enough progesterone to avoid stimulating endometrial implants. □

SOURCES OF FURTHER INFORMATION

American Fertility Society, 2131 Magnolia Avenue, Suite 201, Birmingham, AL 35256. Tel.: (205) 933-8494.

Endometriosis Association, 8585 North 76th Place, Milwaukee, WI 53223. Tel.: (800) 922-3636.

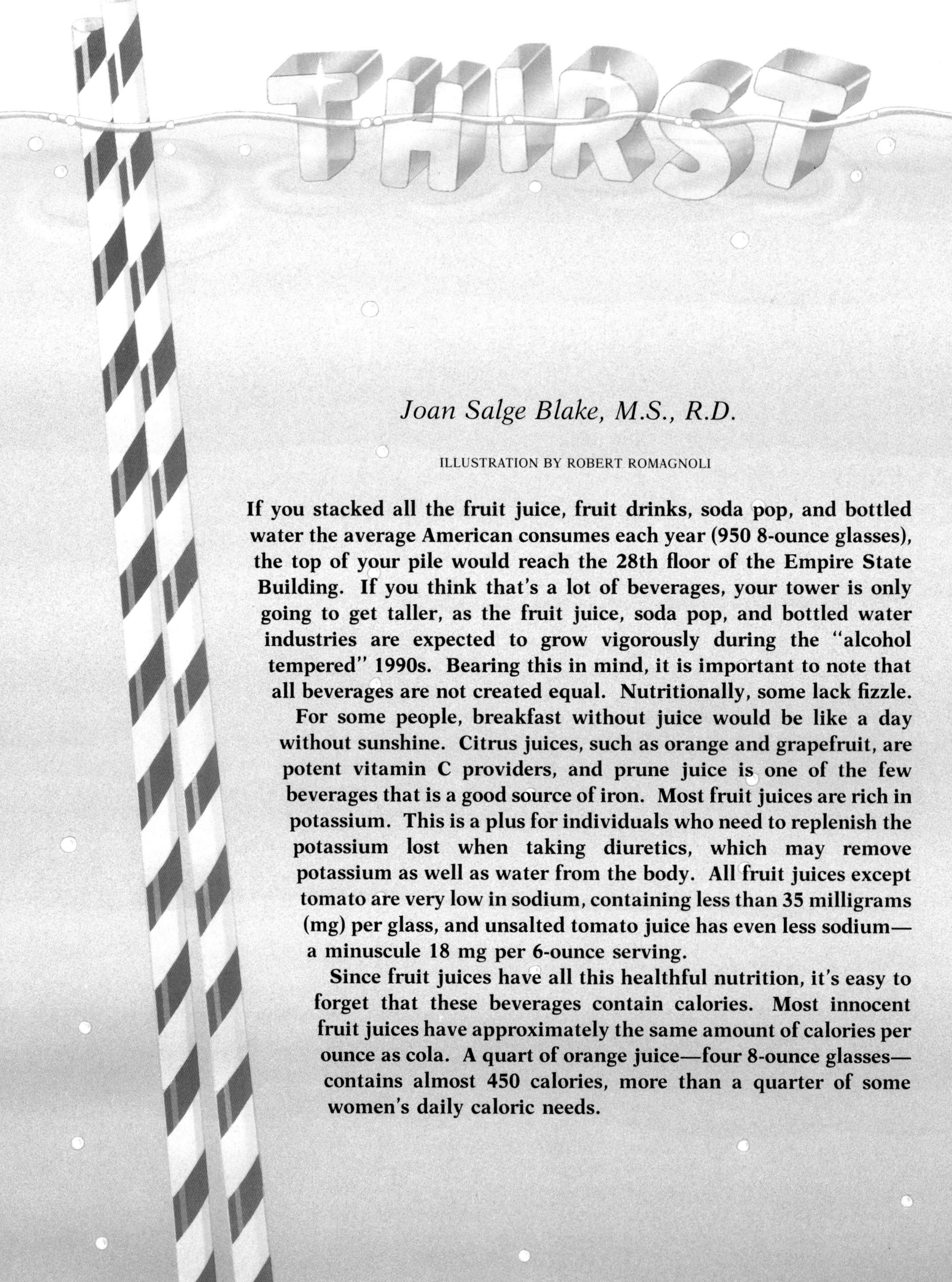

THIRST

Joan Salge Blake, M.S., R.D.

ILLUSTRATION BY ROBERT ROMAGNOLI

If you stacked all the fruit juice, fruit drinks, soda pop, and bottled water the average American consumes each year (950 8-ounce glasses), the top of your pile would reach the 28th floor of the Empire State Building. If you think that's a lot of beverages, your tower is only going to get taller, as the fruit juice, soda pop, and bottled water industries are expected to grow vigorously during the "alcohol tempered" 1990s. Bearing this in mind, it is important to note that all beverages are not created equal. Nutritionally, some lack fizzle.

For some people, breakfast without juice would be like a day without sunshine. Citrus juices, such as orange and grapefruit, are potent vitamin C providers, and prune juice is one of the few beverages that is a good source of iron. Most fruit juices are rich in potassium. This is a plus for individuals who need to replenish the potassium lost when taking diuretics, which may remove potassium as well as water from the body. All fruit juices except tomato are very low in sodium, containing less than 35 milligrams (mg) per glass, and unsalted tomato juice has even less sodium—a minuscule 18 mg per 6-ounce serving.

Since fruit juices have all this healthful nutrition, it's easy to forget that these beverages contain calories. Most innocent fruit juices have approximately the same amount of calories per ounce as cola. A quart of orange juice—four 8-ounce glasses—contains almost 450 calories, more than a quarter of some women's daily caloric needs.

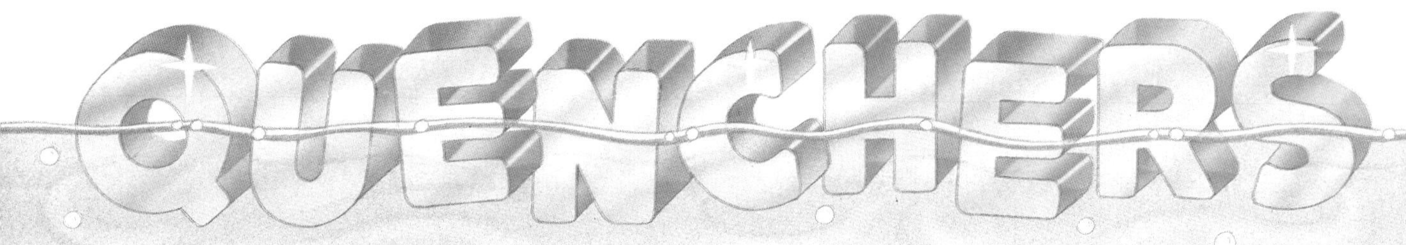

If calorie content makes you cut back on fruit juice, must your nutrition suffer? Not necessarily. For example, let's look at vitamin C. An adult's Recommended Dietary Allowance (RDA)—guidelines based on the dietary needs of healthy Americans—for vitamin C is 60 mg daily. (If you smoke, the amount jumps to 100 mg because smokers process and eliminate vitamin C more rapidly than nonsmokers.) A glass of vitamin C-rich orange juice in the morning will meet a nonsmoker's RDA before the person has left the breakfast table, but it's not the only natural source of this vitamin. In fact, it may not be the best source.

Juice has less of an important component of whole fruit—fiber, which can help regularize your elimination process. And some of the fiber in fruit is of the soluble type, which studies have shown may help lower your cholesterol. A navel orange not only meets a nonsmoker's RDA for vitamin C but also provides 2 grams of fiber with little more than half the calories of a glass of orange juice, which has less than half a gram of fiber. Other fiber-rich fruits, such as strawberries and cantaloupe, are also good sources of vitamin C for very few calories.

Since the current recommendation from the U.S. National Cancer Institute is to consume between 20 and 30 grams of fiber a day, which is far more than most Americans take in, you may want to limit the amount of juice you are drinking to a glass or two per day and eat more fruit instead.

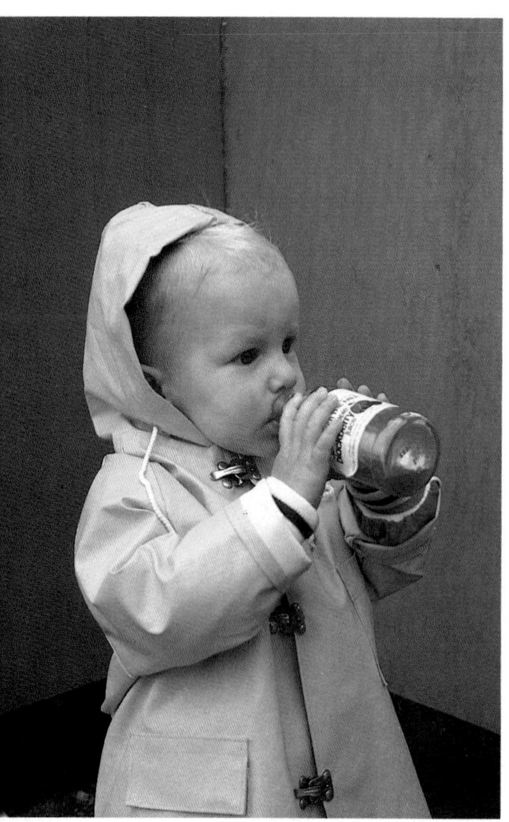

Children take naturally to the good taste of fruit juice. Fruit drinks and punches, however, may have added sugar.

Vitamin C and Colds

Back in the early 1970s, when the Nobel Prize-winning chemist Linus Pauling hypothesized that 1,000 mg of vitamin C a day would combat the common cold, people began clamoring for citrus juice at the first sign of a runny nose. Unfortunately, when scientists conducted studies to test Pauling's theory, vitamin C came up short. It has not been proved that large doses of this vitamin prevent colds. While some research has indicated that increased vitamin C intake may reduce the severity of cold symptoms, experts believe that the benefits are too small to justify recommending routinely taking large doses. This doesn't mean, however, that juices can't help when you suffer from a cold. These beverages, as well as other liquids, such as soup, decaffeinated tea or coffee, and water, can be used to replace the much-needed fluids that are lost from your body during the course of a cold or fever. Beverages containing caffeine are not recommended (since caffeine is a diuretic.)

What's in Fruit Drinks?

What does a glass of cranberry juice cocktail, fruit punch, or grape drink have in common with ten jelly beans? The answer is sugar: each can have about the same amount of sugar! The key word "cocktail," "drink," or "punch" on a label should be a warning that the beverage may contain added sugar. If any of the following words appear on the ingredients list, then a sweetener has been added:

- *Sucrose:* another name for table sugar.
- *Fructose:* the predominant sugar in fruit; sweeter than sucrose.
- *Corn Syrup:* a slurry made from cornstarch treated with acids, heat, and/or enzymes, producing a sweet syrup.
- *High Fructose Corn Syrup:* a sweetener made from the conversion of the glucose (a basic sugar found widely in plants) in cornstarch into fructose; high fructose corn syrup is the sweetener used most often in beverages.
- *Dextrose:* another name for glucose.

Since U.S. law requires that ingredients be listed in order of their predominance by weight, it is not uncommon for fruit drink labels to have one of these sugars near the top of the list, often second only to water. When a beverage has a label saying "10% Fruit Juice Added," that means only 10 percent of the drink (by volume) is fruit juice. For a 6-ounce serving, this translates into 0.6 ounces, an amount that equals a little over a tablespoon of fruit juice. The remainder is mostly water and sugar.

Since cranberries are known for their mouth-puckering qualities, it's no surprise that a lot of sugar is needed to make sweet-tasting cran-

---

Joan Salge Blake, a registered dietitian, writes on food and nutrition and is a nutrition counselor at Longfellow Health Center in Wayland, Mass.

berry juice cocktail. A 6-ounce serving may have only 30 percent cranberry juice—a little more than 1.5 ounces.

Other fruit drinks may boast that "7 Natural Fruit Juices" were added but neglect to tell you exactly how much of these juices were used and that sugar was also indtroduced. Words such as "100% Natural" on the label are not a guarantee that sugar isn't added; they can mean only that artificial colors or flavorings were not used.

One way to get a refreshing low-calorie beverage is to make it yourself. You can create your own "fruit drink" by combining an ounce of fruit juice with sparkling water or club soda for a sweet beverage without the added sugar.

The concern for "truth in juice labeling" is not new. In the early 1970s the U.S. Food and Drug Administration (FDA) proposed regulations requiring that the percentage of juice contained in diluted fruit or vegetable juice beverages be stated on the label, but with one exception—drinks with orange juice—the regulations never became final. With the passage of the Nutrition Labeling and Education Act in October 1990, however, labeling practices in the United States are due for a change. After the FDA completes Congress's directive to rewrite the labeling rules in accordance with the new law (which may happen before the end of 1991), manufacturers will be required to indicate the percentage of juice in all fruit and vegetable juice beverages.

Orange juice is a potent source of vitamin C, but it lacks most of the fiber that a whole orange would supply.

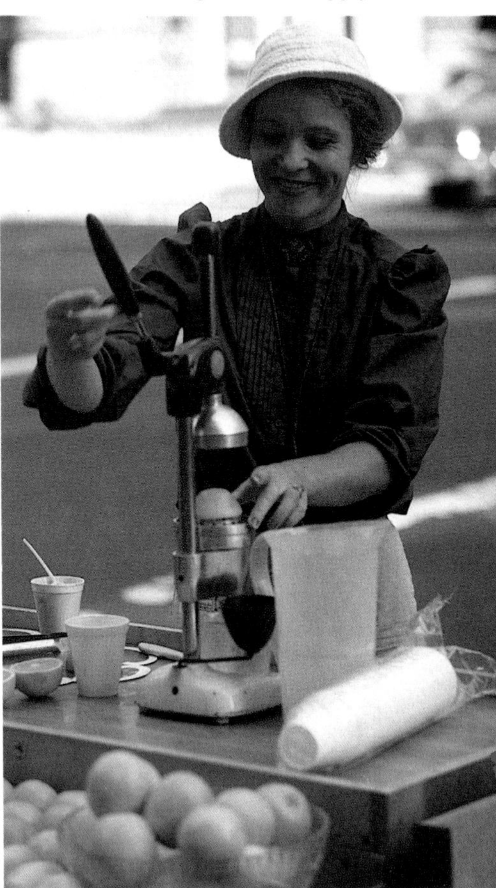

Soda Pop

When you mix carbonated water, caffeine, coloring and flavoring, and approximately ten teaspoons of sugar and pour it into a flip-top aluminum can, you have created every kid's delight and every parent's dilemma. Years ago, soda pop was usually saved for birthday parties and special occasions, but to the sorrow of most nutritionists, it now often appears daily at the dining table. All you get from these popular beverages are the "three C's": calories, cavities, and caffeine.

Counting Calories. Before you start flipping open your next can of soda pop, you may want to consider that one can of cola has about the same number of calories as 2½ slices of high-fiber, vitamin-rich whole wheat bread. Considering that all the calories in the soda pop come from its sugar, that's a lot of calories for so little nutrition. Soda pop with added fruit juice is not much more nutritious because as little as 2 percent fruit juice is added to these beverages—not exactly enough to make them health foods.

Soda pop not only contains a lot of calories, but the even more serious health issue is that for many people it takes the place of more nutritious drinks, such as calcium-rich milk. A survey conducted by the United States Department of Agriculture found that 42 percent of the population—in particular females over 11 years of age and males 35 and older—consumed less than 70 percent of their RDA for calcium. Since, on average, half the calcium Americans consume comes from milk products, the substitution of a two-liter bottle of soda pop for a quart of milk may rob a person's bones of a vital nutrient.

A diet deficient in calcium can set the stage for osteoporosis—a potentially crippling thinning of the bones that usually afflicts older people. In most people, the body is increasing its bone mass until around age 30. Later in life some loss of bone inevitably begins to occur. Since calcium gives bones strength and structure, it's important to have a diet adequate in calcium during childhood and early adulthood to help build up as much bone mass as possible. A study conducted at the University of Pittsburgh found that women who drank milk with every meal up to age 35 had significantly higher bone density than those who drank milk less frequently. After age 30 or so, a diet adequate in calcium is important to help keep bone loss to a minimum. If the prospect of high calories is turning you away from milk, try low-fat or skim milk. An 8-ounce glass of skim milk has approximately 80 calories and 300 mg of calcium—close to half of an adult's RDA of 800. The same amount of cola supplies 96 calories and no calcium at all.

In order to attract calorie-counting consumers, soft drink manufacturers sell diet soda with less than 2 calories per 12-ounce can. While this may have solved the calorie problem for many soda pop lovers, it may have caused another problem, at least for some people.

When cyclamate, a noncaloric sweetener, was taken off the market in the United States in 1970 for its apparent association with bladder cancer in laboratory animals, saccharin, another noncaloric sweetener, was all that remained to provide the sweetness of sugar without the calories. Unfortunately, saccharin not only has a slight aftertaste, but it too was reported to have an association with bladder cancer in rats.

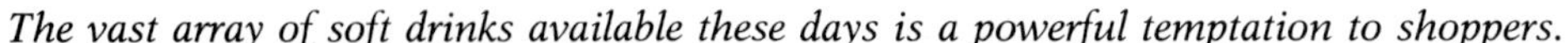

The vast array of soft drinks available these days is a powerful temptation to shoppers.

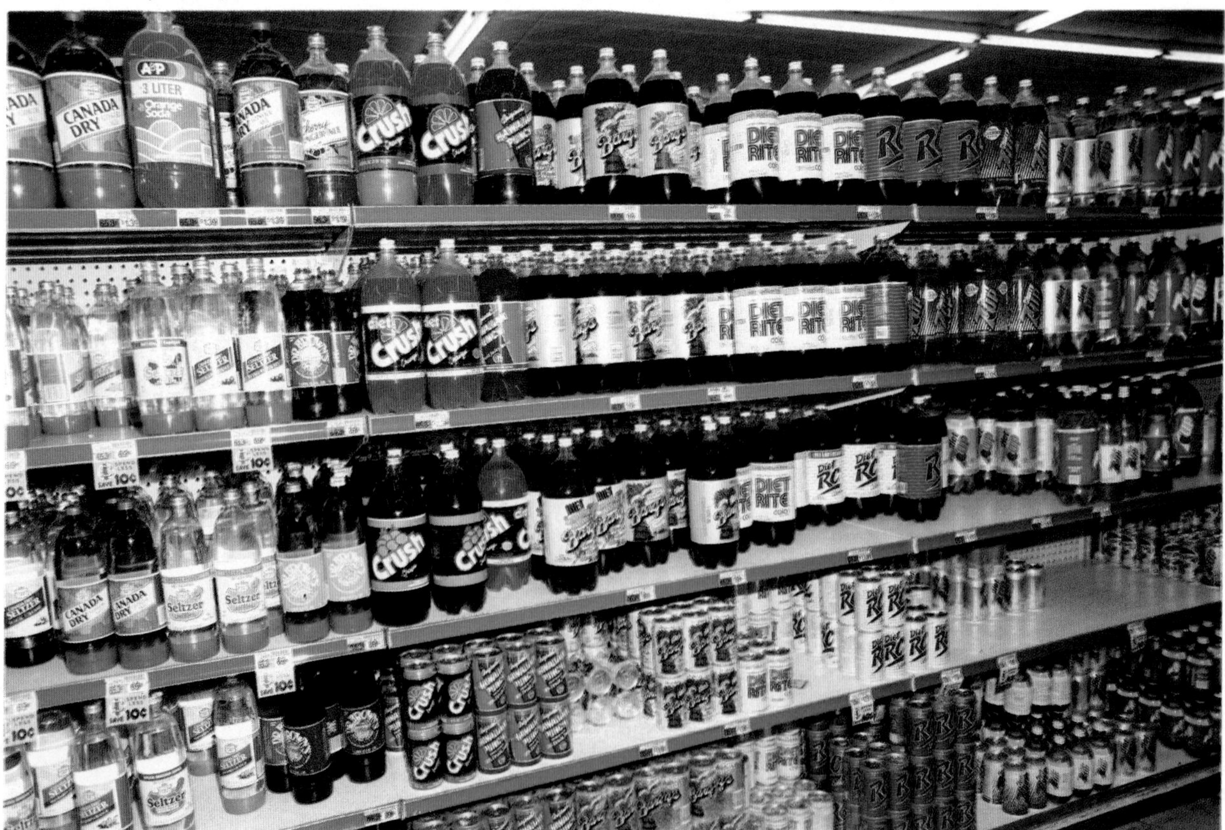

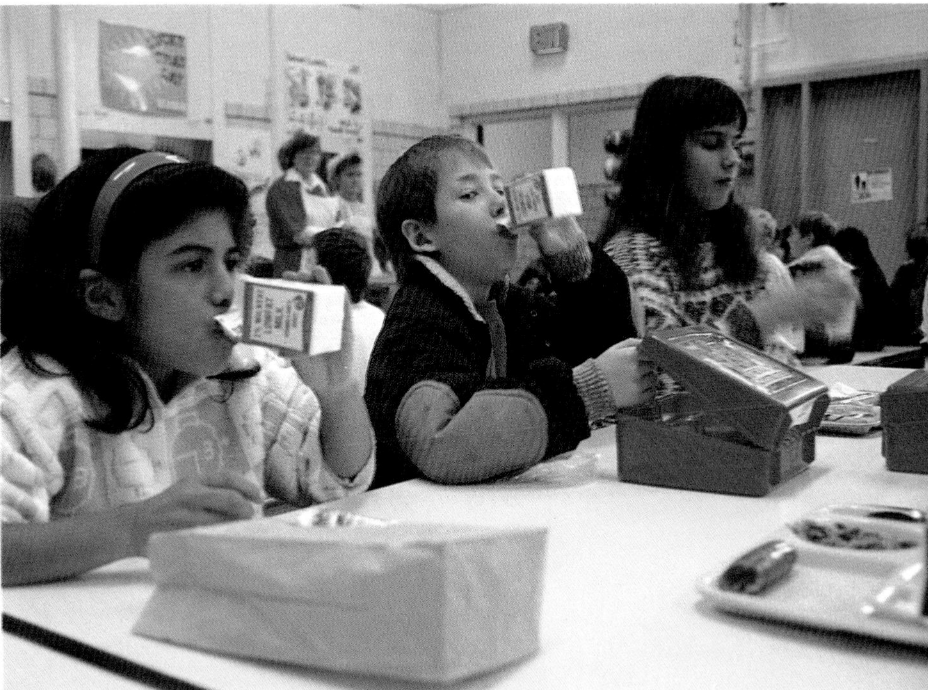

To get enough calcium, children usually need to drink milk. On average, half the calcium Americans consume comes from milk products.

In 1989 the U.S. National Academy of Sciences' Committee on Diet and Health concluded, after reviewing the scientific evidence, that the amount of saccharin and cyclamate (which is available in Canada) consumed by most people does not carry an increased risk of bladder cancer. Nevertheless, experts remain cautious about giving either substance a clean bill of health.

Meanwhile, a third sweetener came along. It was discovered when a research scientist working with proteins in a laboratory happened to lick his finger—and tasted the sweetness of aspartame. Better known by its trade name, NutraSweet, aspartame is made up of two amino acids, the building blocks of proteins. NutraSweet has almost 200 times the sweetening power of sugar. Since the amino acids in aspartame are found naturally in over half of the foods we eat, NutraSweet looked like a sure, safe bet as a good-tasting, low-calorie sweetener.

Unfortunately, large amounts of one of the amino acids, phenylalanine, is a potential danger to individuals with a disorder called phenylketonuria (PKU). These individuals are unable to metabolize phenylalanine, which can lead to brain damage and mental retardation. Such people need to avoid all foods containing phenylalanine, including products containing NutraSweet. Since NutraSweet is currently being used in over 1,200 products, from soft drinks to laxatives, in the United States products containing it must bear a warning label.

Courting Cavities. In defense of sugary soda pop, it does not have any unique cavity-causing property not found in other carbohydrate-rich foods. Soda pop, fruit juices and drinks, candy, bread, or crackers all can be broken down in the mouth into the perfect sugar feast for

(text continues on page 88)

THE BEVERAGE COUNTER

FRUIT JUICES *(6 ounces)*	CALORIES	VITAMIN C *(milligrams)*	POTASSIUM *(milligrams)*	SODIUM *(milligrams)*	CAFFEINE *(milligrams)*	COMMENTS
Apple Juice	87	2	222	3	0	
Carrot Juice	73	16	538	54	0	
Grapefruit Juice	72	71	300	2	0	
Orange Juice	83	93	372	2	0	
Pineapple Juice	104	11	251	2	0	
Prune Juice	136	8	530	9	0	Especially good source of iron.
Tomato Juice	32	33	400	658	0	Unsalted tomato juice has only 18 milligrams of sodium.
SPECIALTY JUICES *(6 ounces)*						
Apple & Eve Cranberry Grape Juice	94	<1	142	5	0	100% fruit juice.
Campbell's V-8 Juice	35	30	383	600	0	100% vegetable juice. Vitamin C added.
Campbell's V-8 Juice No Salt Added	40	30	439	45	0	
Citrus Hill Plus Lite Premium	60	72	210	10	0	60% orange juice. Contains aspartame.
Dole Pineapple-Orange Juice	100	60	59	8	0	100% fruit juice.
Dole Pure & Light Raspberry Juice	87	6	114	15	0	Made with 100% fruit juice. The light in "Pure & Light" refers to the "lighter" texture. All of the pulp has been removed.
Libby's Juicy Juice, Apple-Grape	90	n/a	170	10	0	100% fruit juice.
Minute Maid Pineapple Orange Juice	98	28	274	19	0	100% fruit juice.
Mott's Apple Cranberry Juice	83	0	189	17	0	100% fruit juice.
Tropicana Orange Strawberry Banana Juice	106	60	337	2	0	100% fruit juice.
Welch's Purple Grape Juice	120	27	230	10	0	100% fruit juice.
FRUIT DRINKS *(6 ounces)*						
Five Alive Citrus Beverage	87	51	209	23	0	Sweetened with high fructose corn syrup.
Hi-C Wild Fruit Punch	96	60	33	17	0	10% fruit juice. Sweetened with high fructose corn syrup.

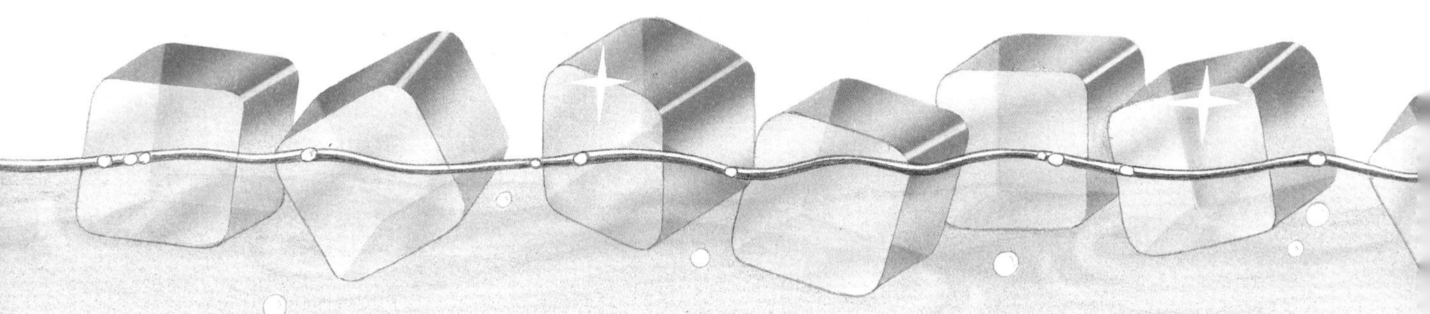

FRUIT DRINKS *(6 ounces)*	CALORIES	VITAMIN C *(milligrams)*	POTASSIUM *(milligrams)*	SODIUM *(milligrams)*	CAFFEINE *(milligrams)*	COMMENTS
Minute Maid Citrus Punch	93	trace	33	18	0	Sweetened with high fructose corn syrup.
Minute Maid Light & Juicy Fruit Beverage	14	1	125	17	0	Contains aspartame.
Mott's Apple Raspberry Drink	95	0	33	10	0	Contains added sugar.
Ocean Spray Cranberry Juice Cocktail	110	60	33	10	0	30% fruit juice. Sweetened with high fructose corn syrup.
Ocean Spray Low Calorie Cranberry Juice Cocktail	40	60	36	10	0	Contains aspartame.
Tropicana Orange Strawberry Banana Twister	71	23	64	<1	0	Sweetened with high fructose corn syrup.
Welch's Orchard Harvest Blend	110	13	70	20	0	50% fruit juice. Sweetened with sugar and corn syrup.

SODA POP *(6 ounces)*	CALORIES	VITAMIN C *(milligrams)*	POTASSIUM *(milligrams)*	SODIUM *(milligrams)*	CAFFEINE *(milligrams)*	COMMENTS
A & W Root Beer	82	n/a	4	22	0	
A & W Root Beer, Diet	1	n/a	17	25	0	Contains aspartame.
Coca-Cola Classic	72	n/a	trace	<18	23	
Coca-Cola Classic, Caffeine-Free	72	n/a	trace	<18	0	
Coca-Cola, Diet Coke	<1	n/a	9	<18	23	Contains aspartame.
Coca-Cola, Diet Coke, Caffeine-Free	<1	n/a	9	<18	0	Contains aspartame.
Jolt Cola	80	n/a	trace	10	36	
Mountain Dew	89	n/a	5	16	20	
Mountain Dew, Diet	<2	n/a	20	<1	27	Contains aspartame.
Pepsi-Cola	79	n/a	3	5	19	
Pepsi-Cola, Diet	<1	n/a	6	27	18	Contains aspartame.
Slice	76	n/a	50	5	0	
Slice, Diet	13	n/a	50	5	0	Contains aspartame.
Sunkist Orange	106	6	0	14	0	
Sunkist Orange With Caffeine	106	6	0	14	20	

n/a = not available
< = less than
Note: amounts may vary slightly.

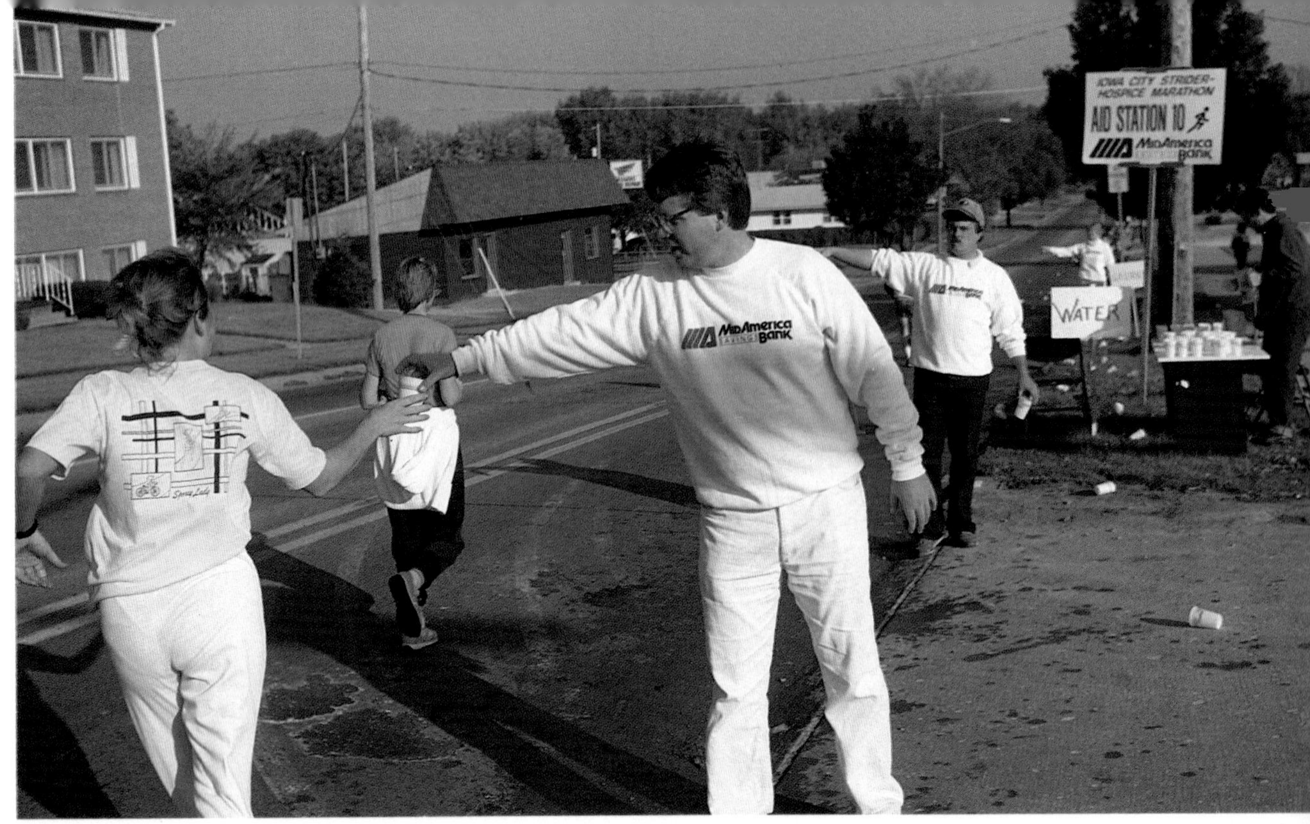

the bacteria that bathe the teeth. As the bacteria consume the sugar, an acid by-product develops that can erode teeth and cause cavities. Ironically, sweetened beverages may have *less* potential for causing cavities because they leave the mouth more quickly than the sticky candies, breads, and crackers that can adhere to and get caught between the teeth, providing a leisurely meal for the bacteria. This doesn't mean that it's a good idea to be sipping on soda pop all day long. The more often your teeth are exposed to carbohydrates, the more potential for developing cavities. If you drink beverages containing sugar, it's best to consume them with a meal. Food will help dilute the sugar and stimulate saliva, the natural mouth rinse that helps to clean teeth.

Getting a Kick Out of Soda Pop. If you get jittery after drinking a few cans of cola, you're not imagining things. A 12-ounce serving of cola provides as much as 46 mg of caffeine, an amount large enough to cause you to start feeling the effects of this central nervous system stimulant. A dose of caffeine larger than 200 mg—about four cans of cola or 1½ cups of brewed coffee—is considered a pharmacologically active amount and may cause headaches, tremors, nervousness, and irritability.

Caffeine is added to soda pop to provide a bitter edge to balance the sweetness of the sugar. Cola is not the only type of soda pop that contains caffeine. Orange and lemon-lime sodas can have it, too.

The stimulating potential of caffeinated soft drinks has some soda pop manufacturers trying to compete with the coffee producers. Jolt, a soft drink that is caffeine dynamite, provides almost twice the amount of caffeine as regular cola. With a little over 70 mg of caffeine per 12 ounces, Jolt is popular among college students cramming for exams. (To appeal to soda drinkers who want no such effect, some cola manufacturers now also offer caffeine-free colas.)

Sports Quencher

The drink of choice for athletes is water, which is now obtainable in a great number of varieties. Left: water is handed out to participants in an Iowa marathon. Right: a bicycle racer protects himself against dehydration.

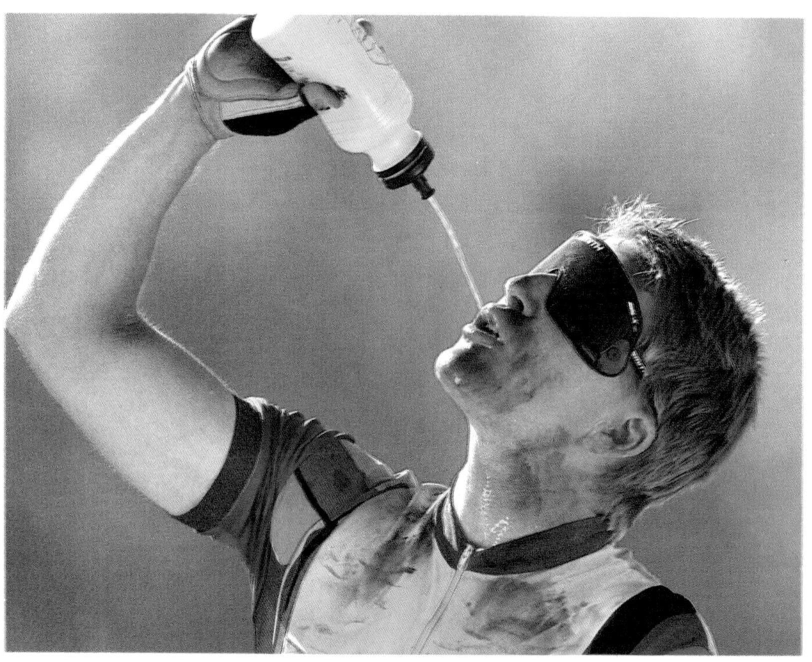

If you use caffeinated beverages to quench your thirst after that long, hot softball game or tennis match, the effect can be the same as reaching for an empty glass. Since caffeine is a diuretic, it causes the body to lose water. Drinking caffeinated soda to replenish the water loss after exercise is like pouring water into a bucket with a hole in the bottom. So what's the best fluid replacer? What else but water!

A Little Sparkle in Your Water

Water is the "in" drink. Over 600 different brands of bottled water are now available for Americans, who drink approximately 1.5 billion gallons of it each year.

While bottled water cannot claim to be better for you than tap water (assuming the latter has no impurities), true water connoisseurs would scorn filling a glass from the faucet. Bottled drinking water is obtained from a natural underground source—a spring, a well, or an artesian well (one in which natural underground pressure pushes the water up like a fountain). Mineral water—which is not legally defined by the FDA—also comes from these sources and is generally considered in the bottled water industry to contain an amount of total dissolved solids no less than 500 parts per million. Carbonated water—better known as sparkling water—can be naturally carbonated or have carbonation added.

All these bottled waters have no calories or sugar and are very low in sodium. Many varieties of sparkling water have a touch of added flavor, such as lemon, lime, or raspberry essence. But there are some brands with added fruit juice and sweetener, which put them close to fruit drinks and soda pop in calories per serving. To compete with soda pop, bottled waters are now being packaged in flip-top cans and plastic bottles. Drinking water has never been so easy. □

How to Choose CHILD CARE

Barbara Scherr Trenk

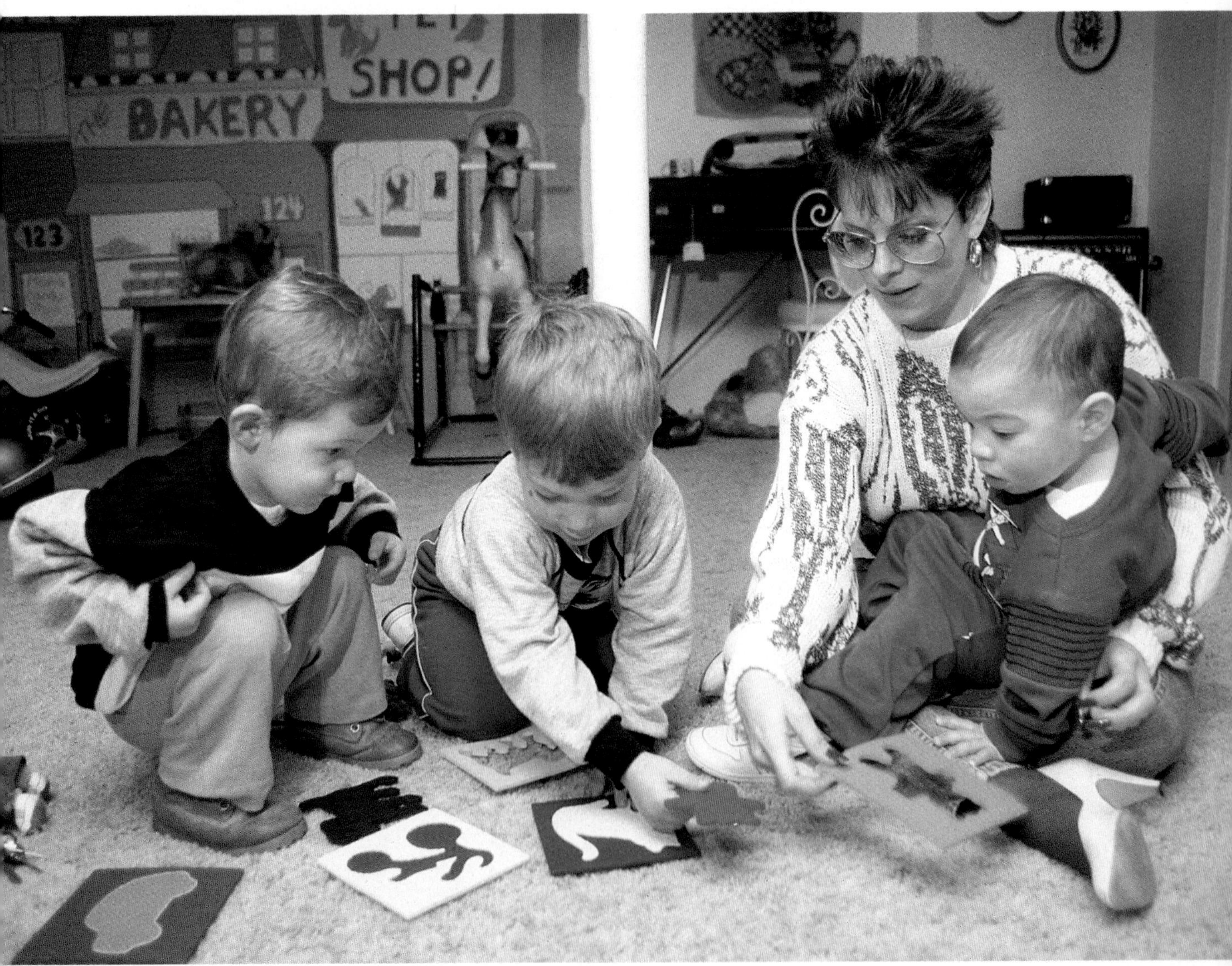

Mothers who work outside the home have become the rule rather than the exception in the United States. According to the National PTA (Parent Teachers Association), 50 percent of American women with children under the age of one year are working, 60 percent with children under age six.

Whether these women are the sole support of their families or are providing a second income, they have a common need: quality child care that is also convenient and affordable. Although women more often than men are responsible for arranging child care, they are not alone in their concern for children's welfare during the work day. One survey of 5,000 employees in five companies found that among workers who had children under age six, 57 percent of women and 33 percent of men reported spending unproductive time on the job because of child care concerns.

While some may argue that there is no shortage of child care, most professionals in the field say that in many communities reliable, high-quality, affordable care is in such limited supply as to prevent some women from entering the work force.

Child Care Options

The care that is available can take a variety of forms.

Family Members. Nearly half of all working parents with children under age five manage to arrange work hours so that one parent is always at home, or rely on a relative, older sibling, or very close friend—or on a combination of these arrangements. This usually eliminates the need to pay for child care, and many parents are more comfortable relying on relatives than they would be leaving a child with a paid caretaker.

In-home Care. This type of care is provided in the child's home by a paid caretaker. The labels vary—babysitter, nanny, housekeeper, or au pair—and the job descriptions may include some housework or other chores. Parents don't have to worry about dressing a child to go out to the caregiver, and needn't make an extra stop on the way to and from work. If a child is ill, there's less worry about making alternate care arrangements.

The National Association for the Education of Young Children says that in-home care is the easiest for a baby to adjust to, since the child remains in familiar surroundings. For somewhat older children, however, this type of care may be less desirable. Toddlers and preschoolers should have playmates and a change in environment for at least part of the week; sometimes these youngsters will spend part of the day at home with a caregiver and part at a nursery school or organized play group. About 6 percent of children whose parents work receive in-home care.

Family Day Care. The care of a small group of children in the provider's home, family day care is the most common form of paid child care in the United States. About half the providers have preschool children of their own. Many parents feel the family environment, the opportunity for their children to interact with other youngsters, and the flexible hours of family day care make it an ideal form of care. The Child Care Action Campaign estimates that 24 percent of children of working parents are in family day care; some experts say that the percentage would be higher if informal arrangements with friends and neighbors were counted as well.

This form of child care is very much in demand, and parents will want to choose a caretaker who resists the temptation to accept more children than can safely be handled. Sometimes a family day care provider will expand the operation into a group child care home by hiring an assistant and accepting more children.

Child Care Centers. Child care centers may be nonprofit or profit-making, and the number of children they serve may range from a dozen to hundreds. The facilities and quality of care vary widely, and good programs that are not too expensive tend to fill up very quickly. Some centers will accept infants; others insist that children be out of diapers before they can be enrolled.

The (nonprofit) YMCA operates the largest child care program in the United States, with more than 1,500 centers serving over 200,000 children. Many churches, synagogues, nursery schools, and public and private elementary schools also sponsor child care programs. In addition, day care centers may be operated as private businesses. Some of these are individually owned and operated; others are part of chains that can range in size from Kids First, Inc., with three locations in the Washington, D.C., area to the giant Kinder-Care, which operates close to 1,250 centers throughout the United States

---

Barbara Scherr Trenk is a writer specializing in healthcare issues.

and in two Canadian provinces. In 1987 roughly 16 percent of children of working single parents or dual-earner couples were placed in child care centers; about half as many attended nursery school or preschool while their parents were at work.

Cost of Child Care

A U.S. Census Bureau survey released in 1990 showed that families with employed mothers had spent $15.5 billion on child care in 1987, with an average weekly bill of $49 per family. For many families child care expenses are a severe financial burden; according to the survey they consumed an average of 25 percent of poor working parents' income. (In France, by contrast, child care is heavily supported by national and local governments alike, with the result that an average of 10 percent of parental income is spent on child care.)

In-home care from a qualified nanny gives a child the reassurance of familiar surroundings but is often very expensive.

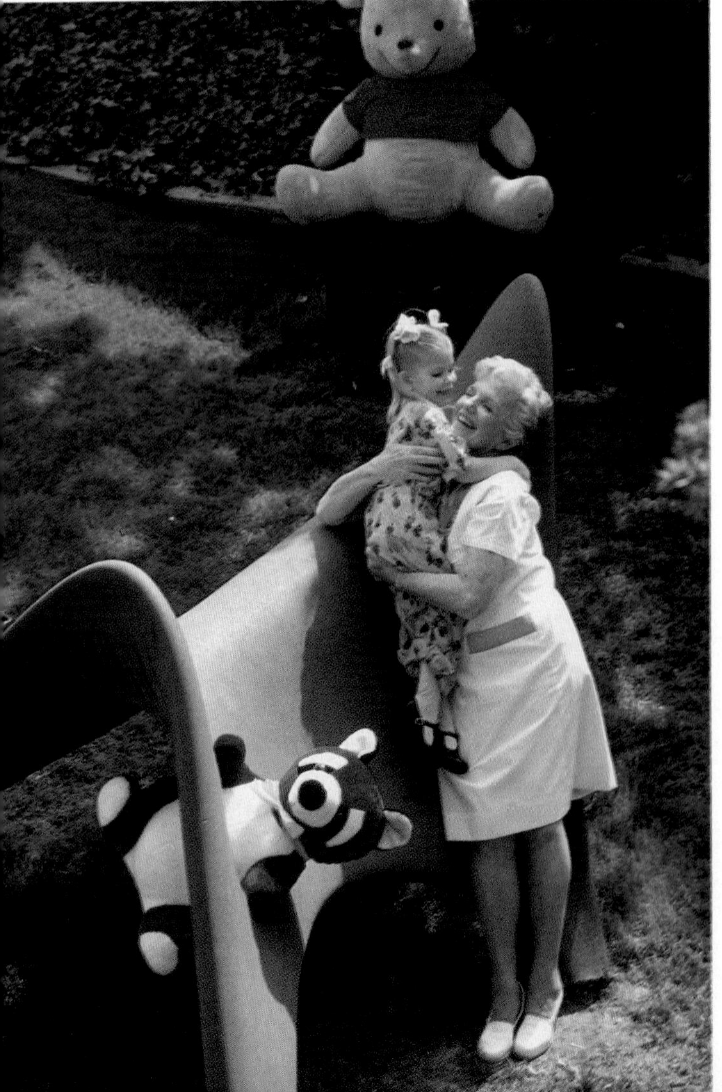

In 1990, Congress passed the first comprehensive federal child care legislation since World War II. A Child Care and Development Block Grant was established, to provide $2.5 billion over three years to subsidize the child care expenses of working parents. The money is to go to the states, which must give priority to low-income children and those with special needs; states can distribute the money to day care facilities or issue child care vouchers to families. The 1990 legislation also gave low-income families additional federal tax credits for child care, estimated to be worth $12 billion over five years. But this legislation does not alter the fact that cost is a critical factor for most families seeking child care.

In-home care is often the most expensive form of care, and reliable caregivers are hard to find. In-home caregivers are considered employees, and U.S. federal law requires that they receive at least the minimum wage and that the family pay employer Social Security taxes. Forty hours of care at just the minimum wage (effective January 1, 1991) of $4 an hour would run $160 per week, bringing the cost of a full year's care to over $8,000 (before Social Security taxes). Using an agency to locate the caregiver adds the agency's fee to the cost.

Live-in nannies may be paid $400 a week or more, plus room and board, in such high-cost areas as New York City; in Cleveland salaries range from $200 to $300 per week.

The annual cost of quality group child care can range from $3,000 to $10,000, depending upon form of care and geographic area, according to the Child Care Action Campaign. Parents in affluent Fairfax County, Va., outside Washington, pay about $100 a week, on average, for child care centers; infant care is more expensive because of the need for a higher staff to child ratio. It averages $125 a week in this community, more in some others.

YMCAs and some other nonprofit child care centers adjust fees according to family income, but many centers do not. Care in government-subsidized facilities is available for only a limited number of children.

Licensed and Unlicensed Care

In the United States the licensing of family day care homes and child care centers is a state responsibility, and license requirements vary greatly from state to state. All states have some form of licensing procedures; however, the regulations are minimal in some states, and many family day care providers essentially ignore state law by not seeking licenses, even though they may meet all the requirements. Unlicensed family day care facilities far outnumber licensed providers.

The Child Care Action Campaign says that licensing usually means a facility has met certain safety standards but may not guarantee that staff members are knowledgeable about child development or that the program is well organized. While some states limit the size of groups according to age, a Children's Defense Fund survey found that 22 states allowed five or more babies to be cared for by one person (picture being responsible for quintuplets all day!). And 31 states did not require any training for family day care providers.

Dr. Susan Aronson, a Philadelphia pediatrician who has studied child care extensively, points out that even where facilities are licensed, inspection may be lax or the inspectors poorly trained. Unlicensed family day care homes may in fact be as good as or better than licensed ones. Nevertheless, most child care experts advocate the licensing of child care facilities—and have urged the federal government to set national standards. (The 1990 child care legislation required only compliance with state and local standards.) The American Academy of Pediatrics and American Public Health Association have developed a set of standards for child care centers that health professionals hope will become the eventual basis for licensing.

What Do Children Need?

A low child-to-caretaker ratio reduces the likelihood of accidental injury while allowing caregivers time to respond to children's emotional and developmental needs. The youngest children do best when they have a steady caregiver who can nurture and care for them. A ratio of one adult for three children under 18 months is the proportion recommended by most experts. If this seems restrictive, consider the need to change diapers, to hold babies while they have a bottle of milk or juice without resorting to bottle-propping, and to watch over babies who need to spend some part of each day crawling and exploring. A caregiver should be able to do all this and still have time and energy to play individually with each child.

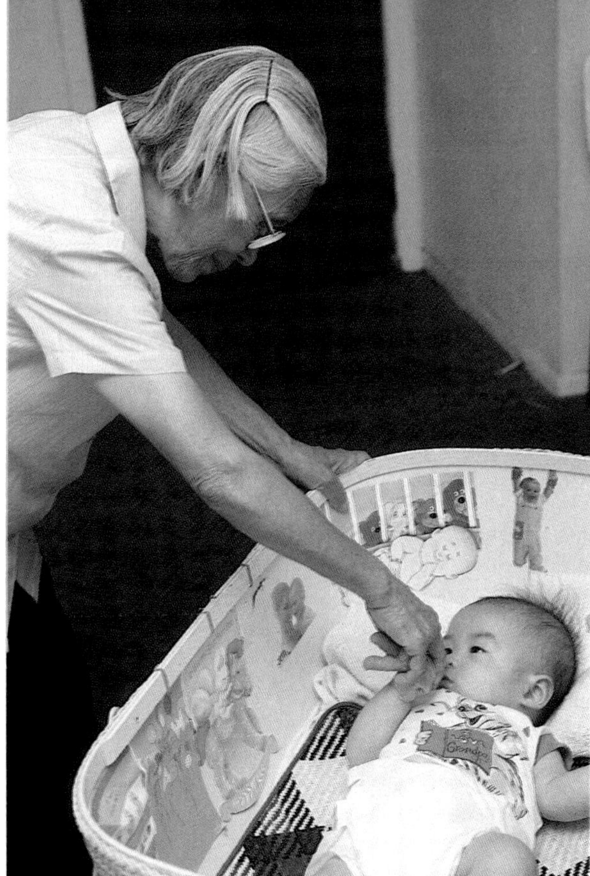

While this baby's parents are at work, his grandmother provides safe, affordable care at home.

Toddlers—children aged 18 months to three years—may still be in the diaper set, but they are more active and independent than infants. They should be in groups of four to five toddlers for each caregiver, suggests the American Academy of Pediatrics. Children in this age range need close supervision as they learn to play with their peers and express their growing independence. An adult who takes the time to tell these children the names of objects can help them to learn language skills. Most children are learning to use the toilet during this period, and parents will want to choose a caregiver who will encourage bathroom habits similar to those being taught at home.

Some experts believe that preschool children (three to five years old) can be adequately supervised in groups of eight children to one caregiver. But T. Berry Brazelton, the noted pediatrician and author of *Working and Caring*, suggests that no more than five children under age five should be looked after by one adult. These youngsters need a balance of active and quiet play. Preschoolers are starting to make friends and should be helped in developing social skills (like learning to take turns and share toys). They should also be learning to do things by themselves—using the bathroom, dressing, washing their hands, eating—and need caregivers who will encourage independence yet be ready to provide assistance when needed. Preschoolers should be learning to recognize colors, shapes, and letters of the alphabet, and a good child care setting should foster development of these skills.

Finding the Right Care

Parents who must look beyond their families for child care often start by asking everyone they know about suitable caregivers. Besides friends and relatives, members of the clergy and pediatricians are often good sources, as are teachers and school secretaries in local elementary schools.

Some communities have referral services for child care providers; these may be independent nonprofit agencies, or they might work through the United Way, Red Cross, YMCA, or state or local department of social services. Departments of education or early childhood development at local colleges and community colleges might provide names of caregivers who are sufficiently interested in their work to enroll for courses. Specialized employment agencies will help find in-home caregivers, for a fee. (They may be listed under Child Care Services, Home Health Services, or Sitting Services in the Yellow Pages.) Parents using such agencies should still screen potential caregivers themselves.

What to Look for

Parents will want to visit a family day care home or child care center at least once before contracting for services, and they should interview a prospective in-home caretaker. They should ask questions about a caregiver's experience and training. Has the individual worked previously with children the same age as theirs? How long has she or he been working with young children?

It's important to know whether the caregiver understands children's developmental stages, so that expectations of behavior and achievement will be realistic. Many child care workers take courses in child development or early childhood education. Nannies often take training courses lasting from three to six months, and some have degrees in early childhood education. Day care centers may have child development and pediatric consultants available to them.

Watch the way a caregiver interacts with the children being cared for, or with your own child during an interview. Is the person involved with the youngsters, or aloof? Annoyed by their attempts to get attention, or responsive? Try to visit the home or center soon after day care begins. Is the caregiver open and informative about the child's day?

Ask about a child care center's policy on discipline. Family Service America suggests that a provider should avoid negative methods of discipline such as spanking, threatening, shouting, or shaming the children. Appropriate discipline might include restricting playtime or directing the child to a new activity, but never withdrawing food.

Though there's never any guarantee that a single caregiver will be available to care for a child for several years, consistency is best for the child, experts say, and puts less strain on parents as well. Child care centers whose staff is well paid have lower rates of turnover. In general, however, child care workers receive very low wages, and centers in the United States have an average staff turnover rate of some 40 percent a year. (Often wages are higher at nonprofit centers than at profit-making facilities.) Family day care providers who have been in business for a few years may be less likely to change occupations than those just starting out.

It's important to ask caregivers for references—the names of former employers in the case of in-home sitters or nannies, and current clients for family day care providers or child care centers. When these people are contacted, questions calling for more than a "yes" or "no" response will usually elicit the most information. Instead of asking "Were you satisfied with the care?" try "How is discipline handled?"

Healthful, Safe Child Care

Some parents are reluctant to send their children to group child care because they fear a child may become ill more often. Pediatrician Dr. Aronson says that children are exposed to each other's germs when they come together in groups and may become mildly ill somewhat more often, but she does not advocate keeping children out of group care for this reason. Youngsters who are properly immunized are protected from many serious diseases, and Dr. Aronson recommends that providers of group child care require proof that children have had all immunizations appropriate for their age.

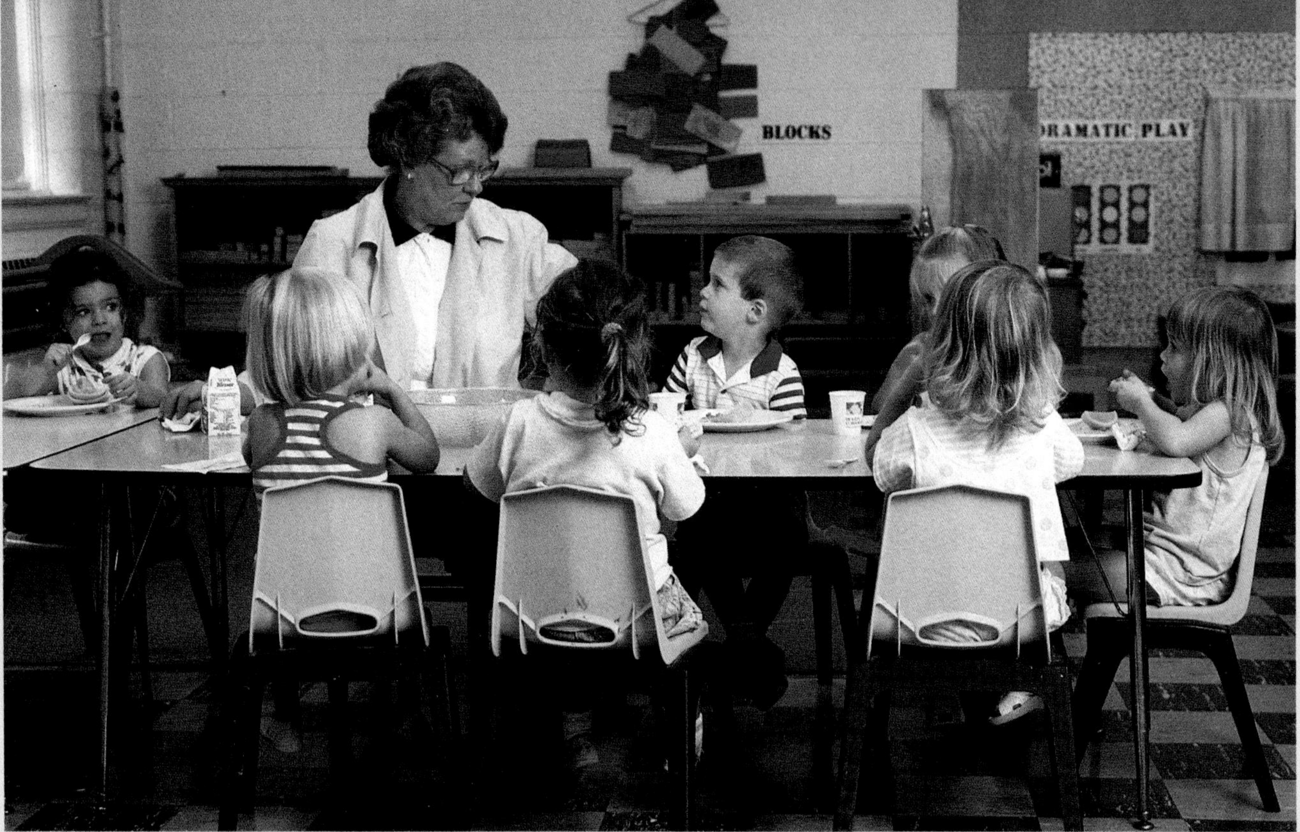

Mealtime at Gramma's Daycare Center in Memphis, Tenn.

DAY CARE CHECKLIST

Listed below are some key questions parents should ask of potential day care providers and some things to look for when touring child care facilities.

DAY CARE CENTERS

Ask:

Who owns and runs the center? Is it licensed?

Will the center supply references?

What is the ratio of children to staff members for infants? toddlers? preschoolers?

What educational qualifications and experience does the center require of its staff? How does it screen applicants?

What was the center's staff turnover rate for the preceding year?

What are the center's hygiene regulations?

How does it handle medical emergencies? illnesses that emerge during the day?

What is the center's policy on allowing sick children to attend? Does the center require proof of immunizations?

Can parents visit any time?

What is the center's discipline policy?

Look for:

Are all facilities clean and well maintained? Are they sufficient for the number of children?

Is child safety equipment fitted on heating and electrical installations?

Are all windows secured?

Are the food service area and the diapering area separated from other activities? Is there a sink near the diapering area? Is handwashing adequate?

Do the children seem happy and well looked after?

FAMILY DAY CARE

Ask:

How many children is the caregiver looking after?

If the caregiver has assistants, what is the ratio of children to care providers?

Is the home licensed for family day care?

Has the caregiver any educational background in child development?

What references can the caregiver supply?

How will a sudden illness or emergency be handled?

What is the caregiver's policy on discipline?

What is the caregiver's policy on TV?

Look for:

Does the home have smoke detectors? fire extinguishers?

Are there sufficient age-appropriate toys available?

If the caregiver's car may be used to transport the children, are there enough child seats?

How does the caregiver respond to your child?

AGENCIES FOR IN-HOME CARE

Ask:

What is the agency's screening procedure? Does it check qualifications and employment references supplied by applicants? Must applicants give their medical history? Does the agency check the driving records of each applicant? check for criminal records?

Under what circumstances is the agency's fee refundable?

Under what circumstances will the agency supply a replacement caregiver without an additional fee?

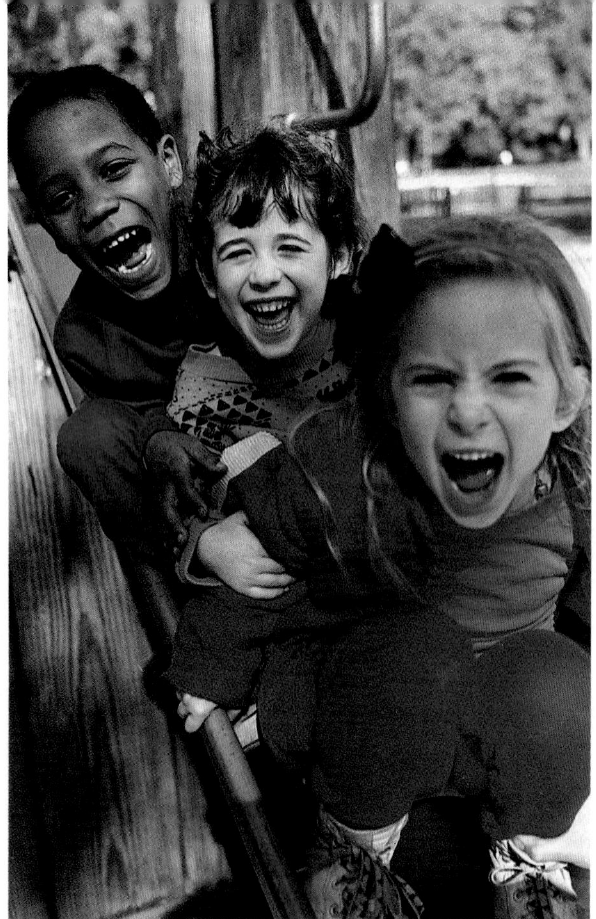

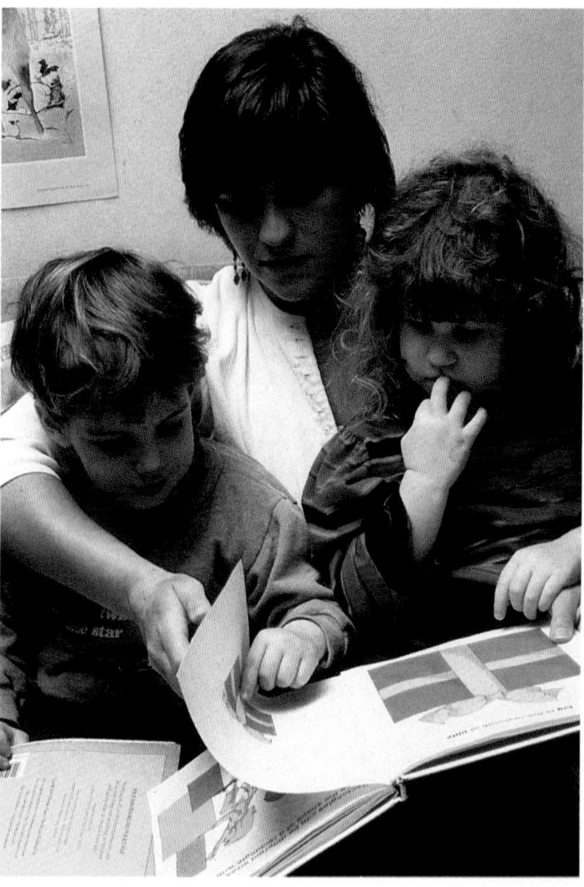

Good day care centers can foster social skills like sharing and cooperative play, as well as stimulation through story-telling and games. Preschoolers should have a balanced range of active and quiet pursuits.

Handwashing. Handwashing by staff members is an important way to cut down on the spread of infections associated with child care, particularly because of the ease with which infection can be transmitted through fecal matter.

There should be a sink near the diapering area, so that caregivers can wash their hands with soap after every diaper change. It's important that they wash after finishing the diapering of one child and before beginning to change another, and after disposing of used diapers. The changing area should be cleaned after each use. A disposable paper sheet should be used to cover the changing table.

Children should learn to wash their hands after using the bathroom and before eating, and staff should practice the same habits. Soap should always be available in bathrooms. Caregivers should also wash their hands after wiping a child's runny nose, and youngsters should learn to wash their hands after wiping their noses or covering coughs. To be sure that this good health practice doesn't become a hazard for the children, the hot water temperature should not exceed 120 degrees Fahrenheit.

Emergency Precautions. Caregivers should be prepared to handle potential health and safety emergencies, as well as less serious medical problems that may come up during the day. A health manual should be readily available and caregivers should be trained in CPR. The telephone numbers of the nearest emergency room, poison information center, and police and fire departments should be posted near the telephone. The names and phone numbers of each child's parents and pediatrician should be easily accessible.

Smoke detectors should be installed and in working order, or the building should be equipped with a sprinkler system. The home or center should also have easily accessible fire extinguishers. It's especially important for parents to look for these safety devices if the caregiver being considered is not licensed (and therefore not inspected). Caregivers should have a fire evacuation plan, and fire drills should be held regularly.

Injury Prevention. If children are transported in buses or automobiles during field trips, safety restraints should be used. A sitter or family child care provider who takes infants or toddlers on outings should have appropriate child seats in the car.

Unused electrical outlets should be covered with safety caps, and lamp and appliance cords should be well away from children's play areas. Space heaters should not be used. The American Academy of Pediatrics suggests that windows above the ground floor should have devices that keep them from being opened more than 6 inches.

Play Facilities

It's important for children to have age-appropriate toys and equipment at a child care center or family day care home. If children of several ages are cared for in the same home or center, the caregiver must see to it that youngsters are not attempting to handle toys that will be unsafe or inappropriate. For example, jigsaw puzzles provide constructive entertainment for preschoolers but would be a safety hazard if left where a curious infant could place small pieces in the mouth.

Toys that infants put in their mouths should be washable and kept clean. Slides and swings should be well maintained, with a soft surface underneath to provide a safe landing spot for active youngsters. Climbing apparatus should be less than 6 feet high, with 8-12 inches of loose impact-absorbing material below.

Meals and Snacks

Since child care providers will be responsible for feeding an infant several times during the day, or serving at least one meal to a child plus snacks every day, parents will want to know about mealtime arrangements. If an infant is on formula, parents should ask in advance whether they or the caregiver will be responsible for having an adequate amount on hand. A nursing mother who wants to leave bottles of expressed milk every day will want to be sure the caretaker is receptive to this arrangement.

Meals should be prepared and served under sanitary conditions. If the same table is used for lunch and craft projects, is it scrubbed and covered before mealtimes? If youngsters bring bag lunches from home, are they properly refrigerated?

If a child has food allergies, the parents should be sure that the caregiver will be attentive to the child's special needs. Parents who feel strongly about limiting sugary snacks will probably want to choose a caregiver who shares this view or will at least be cooperative. Styrofoam cups and plastic tableware should not be used by young children, according to the American Academy of Pediatrics, because they break easily and a child could choke on the pieces.

TV or Not TV?

If a child is cared for at home or in someone else's home, there will undoubtedly be a television set available, and probably a VCR too. Many parents will want the TV to be used as a source of quiet entertainment for short periods only, so that watching television does not become the child's major daily activity. Parents who want to limit their child's viewing to appropriate programs should let it be known that they don't want their child watching soaps. Some parents ask caregivers to limit the use of videotapes as entertainment to days when the weather doesn't permit outdoor play.

Guarding Against Child Abuse

Experts agree that children should not be left with a caregiver who discourages parents from dropping in during the day. Not only should parents be allowed to visit, says the American Academy of Pediatrics, but they should be admitted without delay to the area where their child is resting or at play.

Dr. Brazelton suggests that good training makes caregivers better able to handle the demands of the job and thus less likely to become abusive or neglectful. He also recommends that children as young as ages three or four can learn that their genitals are private parts that should not be touched by anyone without permission.

Employers and Child Care

There was a time when employers would refuse to hire a worker if they felt that lack of appropriate care for the prospective employee's young children would interfere with job performance. Today, however, some employers are dealing with their workers' difficulties in making child care arrangements in a different way: by helping them. Assisting par-

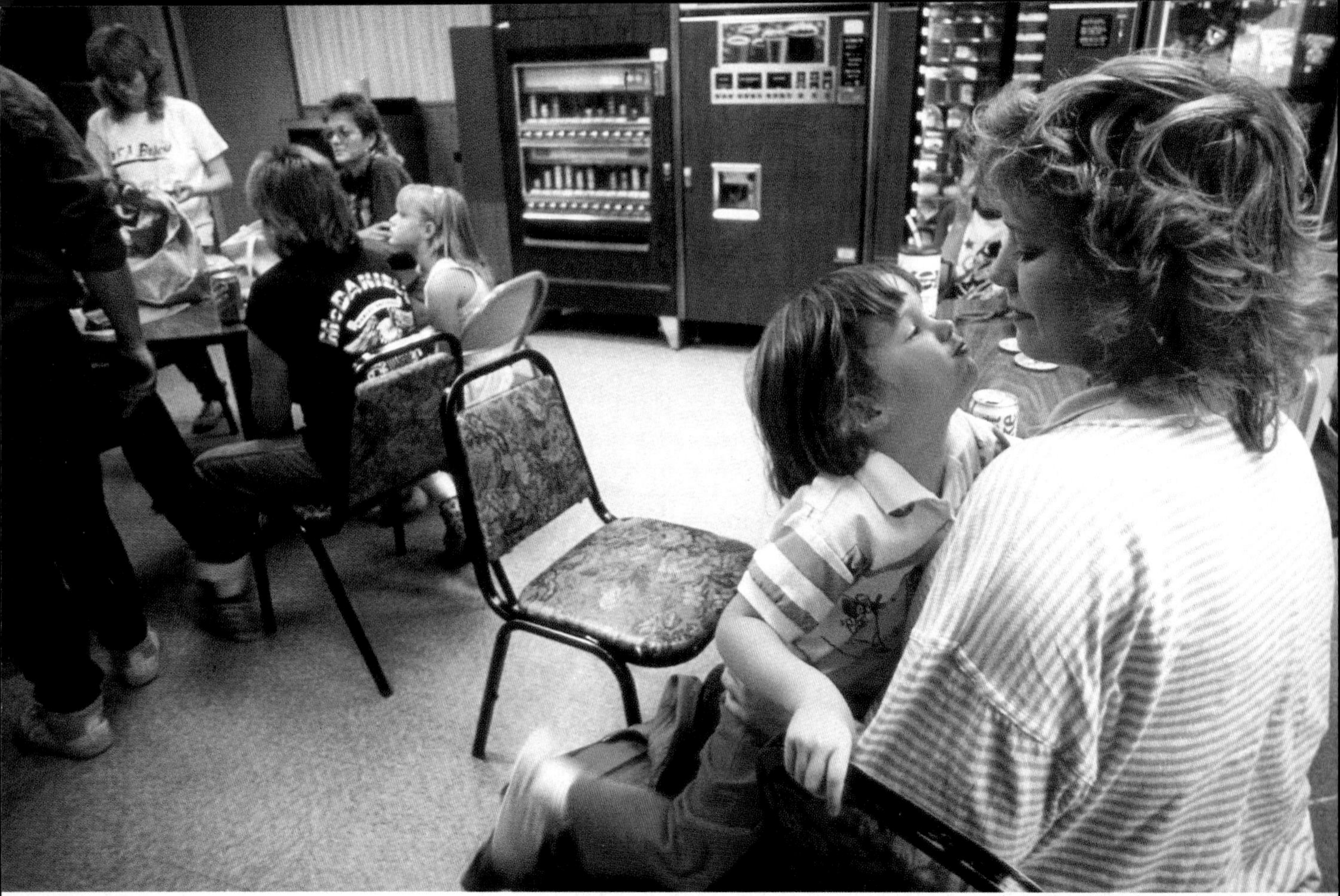

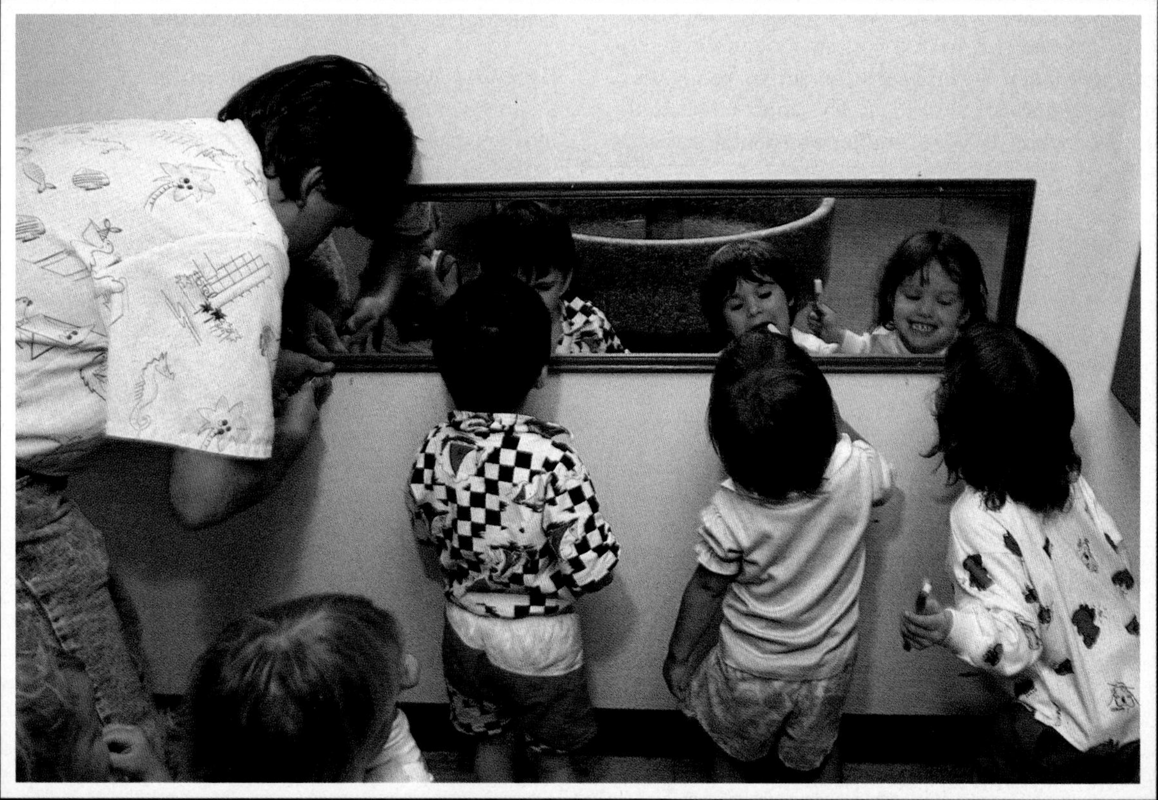

Care Around the Clock

A corporate child care center subsidized by Nyloncraft, an Indiana auto parts factory, operates 24 hours a day, catering to employees on three shifts. Top left, employee Pam Marlow says good-bye to her three-year-old daughter Megan before starting her four-to-midnight job. After playtime and supper, Megan participates in a supervised toothbrushing session, bottom left; a two-hour nap, top right, completes her evening. Around midnight Megan is transported, in her nightgown, back to the factory in time to greet her mother at the end of her shift.

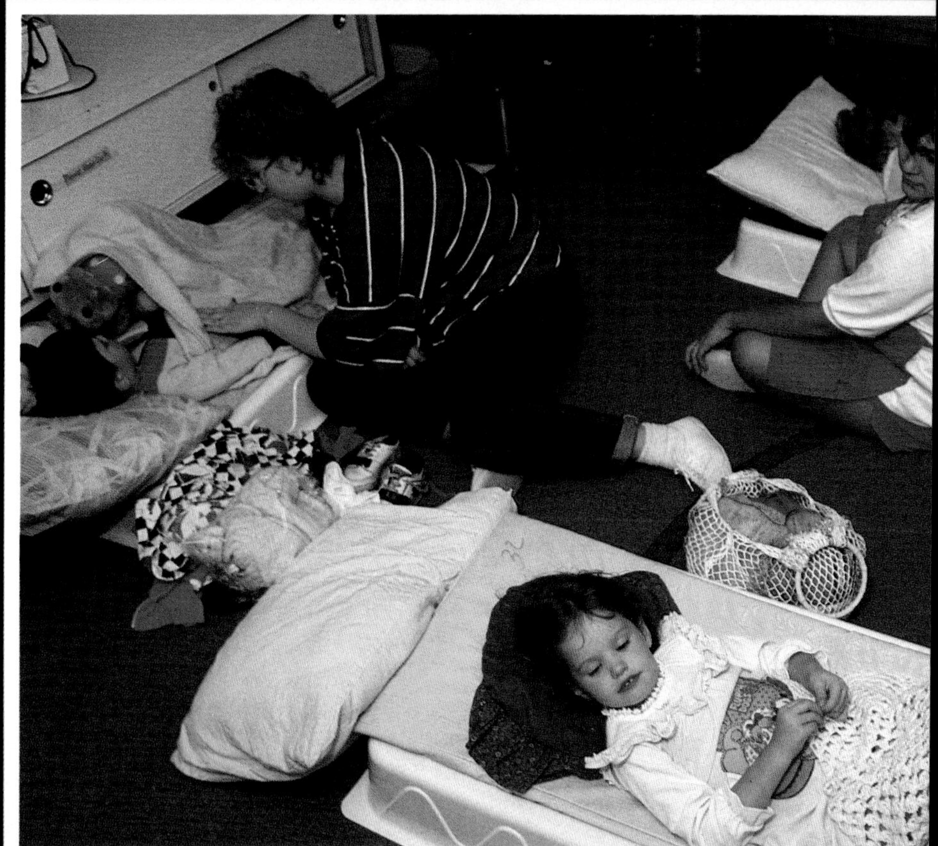

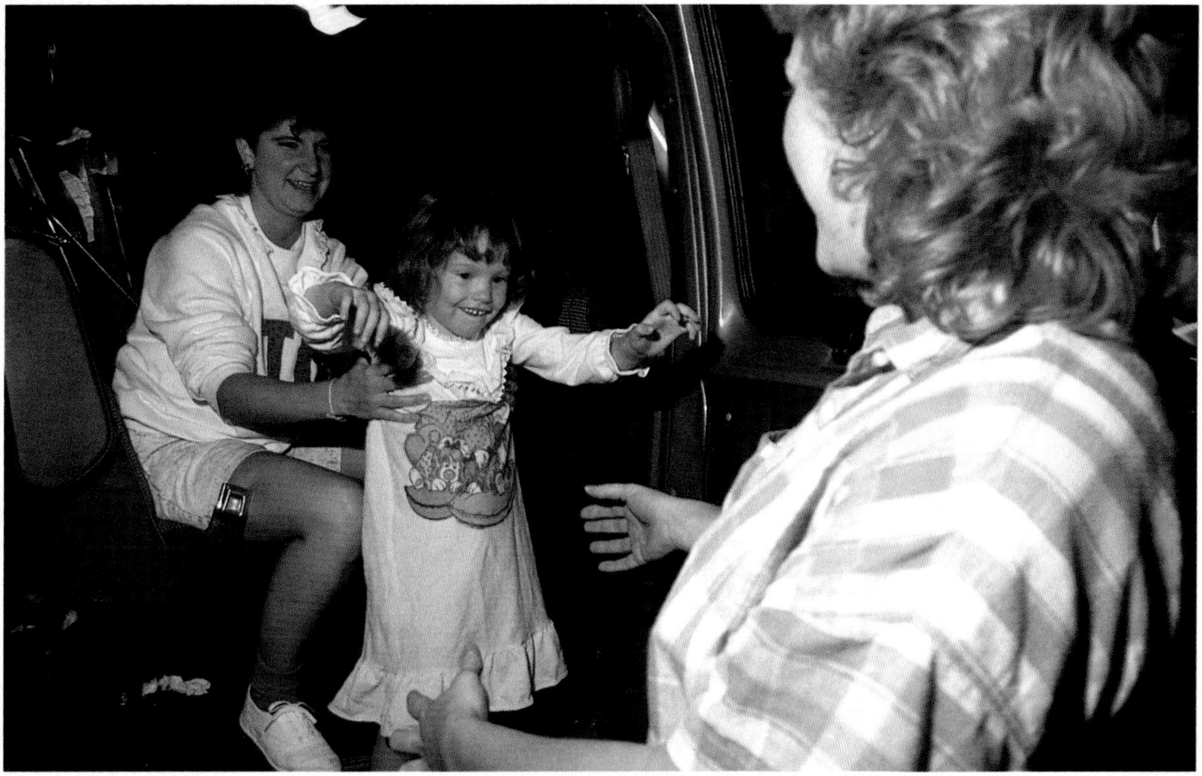

ents with child care can benefit the company by reducing the on-the-job stress that lowers productivity and causes accidents, according to the U.S. Department of Labor's Women's Bureau. Some companies also find that child care benefits help to recruit workers, reduce absenteeism, and lower the rate of turnover.

Although only a small percentage of U.S. employers (mostly large corporations) currently provide child care for their workers, the number is growing. Often this care, available at or near the worksite, is at least partially subsidized by the employer, with workers paying on a sliding scale according to income.

Company-sponsored child care centers are usually of high quality, says Dr. Aronson, because the businesses don't want to be associated with a poorly run program.

Some companies cooperate in public/private partnerships with government or education authorities at the state or local level, providing grants or seeking donations to increase the availability of child care centers and family day care homes. Many run seminars on choosing child care for prospective parents in their work force. In 1990, IBM announced that it would provide a total of $3.5 million toward child care facilities in various U.S. communities where it has offices and plants: $3 million to establish five new day care centers and $500,000 to improve existing facilities and recruit and train family day care providers. (IBM will not, however, subsidize its employees' child care costs directly.) The five day care centers, some jointly financed by IBM and other corporations, will be operated by companies specializing in child care, with at least half the enrollment open to the entire community. The centers will set their own fees.

This center in San Juan Bautista, Calif., offers day care for sick kids—a rare but vital service.

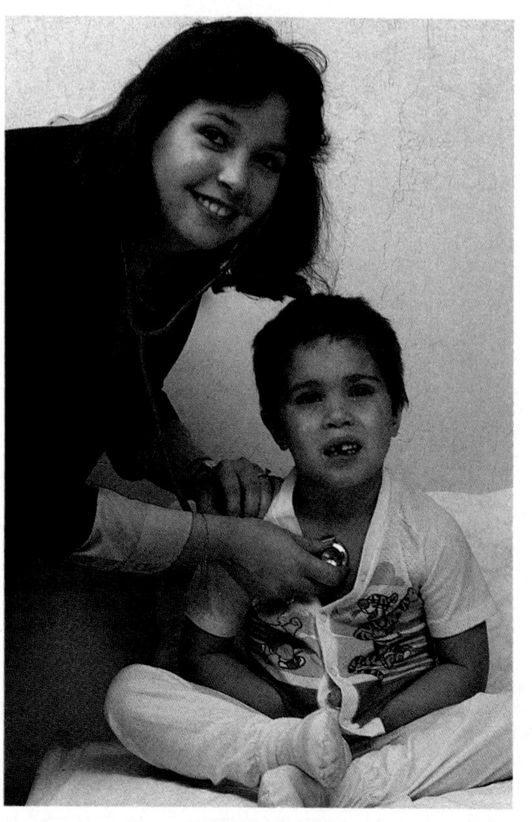

When Children Are Sick

Arranging care for sick children is one of the most difficult challenges for parents and caregivers alike. Some child care centers and family day care providers will care for mildly ill children, but youngsters with communicable diseases, high fevers, or severe coughs should not be admitted to a child care program. Parents should find out ahead of time what kinds of care are available should their child become sick.

The best solution is usually to arrange for a relative or a paid caregiver to come to the child's home. Sometimes experienced sitters who don't want to work steadily will work for a few days during a child's illness. Child care centers can sometimes recommend an appropriate person whom the parent can contact—or may even send a trained aide to the child's home to care for the youngster.

Arranging for the care of sick children has become a concern for many businesses because of the cost of lost productivity when parents miss work to care for them. A group of New York City businesses has contracted with Child Care, Inc., which sends licensed home health aides to an employee's home when a child is ill or emergency child care is needed, such as when a caregiver is ill. Some of these employers pay the aide's full cost for a limited number of days per year; others ask employees to pay part of the fee. The limitation of this service is that aides are not allowed to give medication, nor will they provide care for children with diarrhea, vomiting, or a fever of over 102 degrees.

A program at Providence Hospital in Holyoke, Mass., that provides care for sick children has received praise from area workers, their employers, and hospital officials who are able to make use of pediatric beds that might otherwise be empty. Parents are urged to register their children in advance, so that the hospital will have a record of their immunizations and any chronic conditions or allergies. During an illness, parents pay the hospital $3 per hour for care that is supervised by registered nurses. Many employers are so pleased to have their workers on the job instead of home with sick children that they will reimburse part of the fee.

But when children are seriously ill, or have a communicable disease like measles or chicken pox, many parents find there is no alternative to taking a few days off. Some employers allow workers to miss a few days' work each year for family illness; but many workers must lose pay if they are absent for this reason.

After-School Care

Some parents breathe a sigh of relief when their child enters school, only to realize that arranging for their caregiving may become even more difficult than for younger children.

A growing number of public and private schools have arranged for early morning drop-off and after-school care, usually for an hourly or weekly fee. This eliminates the need for transportation between school and the caregiver and also ensures that youngsters will have after-school playmates their own age.

School officials can sometimes recommend a family child care provider who will meet children at the school when the dismissal bell rings, or who is located either within walking distance of the school or within range of the school's bus service. Reliable high school or college students might also be available as after-school sitters if their own classes end before the younger child's school day is over.

There are no firm rules for deciding when a child is ready to be left unsupervised after school. Considerations include the child's maturity, the safety of the neighborhood, and the proximity of a helpful neighbor. Another factor is the length of time the child will be alone.

Workplace Policies

Sometimes changes in the way people work allow parents to spend more time with their children or give them access to more satisfactory child care arrangements. Parents who have access to a telephone during working hours can call a "self-care" youngster to be sure he or she returned home from school on schedule. Employees who can take personal days or vacation time in hours, instead of days, can leave work early occasionally if the caregiver has to leave. Companies that allow flexible work schedules enable workers to plan their work hours around those of a caregiver. If both parents have flexible work hours, they may be able to limit their need for paid help to just a few hours each day. Some employers even allow workers in appropriate jobs to put in all or some of their work hours at home.

Child Care Contracts

Most child care centers have written contracts. As with any legal document, these contracts should be read carefully. Parents should be sure they understand exactly what services are being purchased and what the price will be. Does the center close down during holiday weeks for staff vacation? Is there a reduction of the charges when a family goes away on vacation or a child is out sick for an extended time? What is the fee if parents pick up a child later than usual?

In the case of family day care, the National Council of Jewish Women suggests that parents write a contract if the child care provider doesn't have one. Like a child care center's contract, it should specify policies about payment, late pickups, holidays and vacation, and illness (the child's and the provider's). The council also suggests specifying a child's schedule, meal and snack arrangements, and any agreements relating to discipline, trips, and substitute caregivers. Arrangements with in-home caregivers should also be specified in a signed contract, which should cover most of the same issues. □

SOURCES OF FURTHER INFORMATION

American Academy of Pediatrics, 141 Northwest Point Boulevard, P.O. Box 927, Elk Grove Village, Ill. 60009-0927. Tel.: (708) 228-5006.

National Association of Child Care Resource and Referral Agencies, 2116 Campus Drive SE, Rochester, Minn. 55904. Tel.: (507) 287-2220.

National Association for the Education of Young Children—Child Care Information Service, 1834 Connecticut Avenue NW, Washington, D.C. 20009. Tel.: (800) 424-2460.

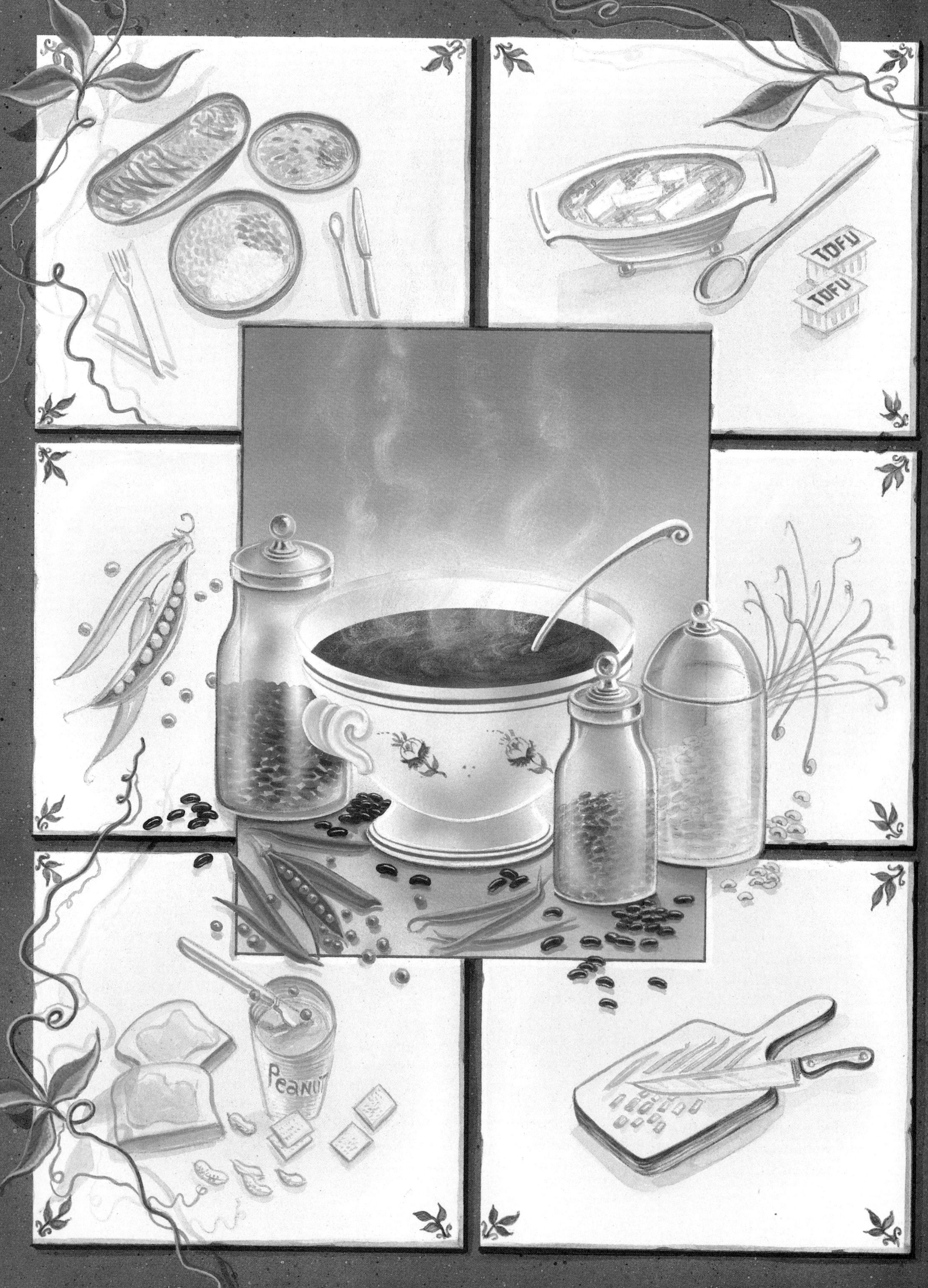
TOFU
TOFU
PeaNUT

Peas, Beans & Other Legumes

Nancy Polk

ILLUSTRATION BY ROBERT PASTERNAK

Edible legumes—peas, beans, lentils, and peanuts—have played an important part in the human diet for millennia. Peas and beans found in a cave on the border between Thailand and Myanmar (Burma) have been carbon dated to 9750 B.C.. Wild runner beans were gathered by cave dwellers in the Tamaulipas Mountains of Mexico between 7000 and 5000 B.C. Bean cultivation began in Ocampo, Mexico, in 4000 B.C. and in Huaca Prieta, Peru, in 3000 B.C. Remains of peas and beans found in Halicar, Turkey, show they were being eaten there even earlier.

In *Food in History*, Reay Tannahill writes about Alexis of Thurii, a fourth century B.C. Greek poet who described the diet of a poor family as pulses (legumes), greens and turnips, iris rhizomes, beechnuts, grasshoppers, wild pears, and, for a treat, dried figs.

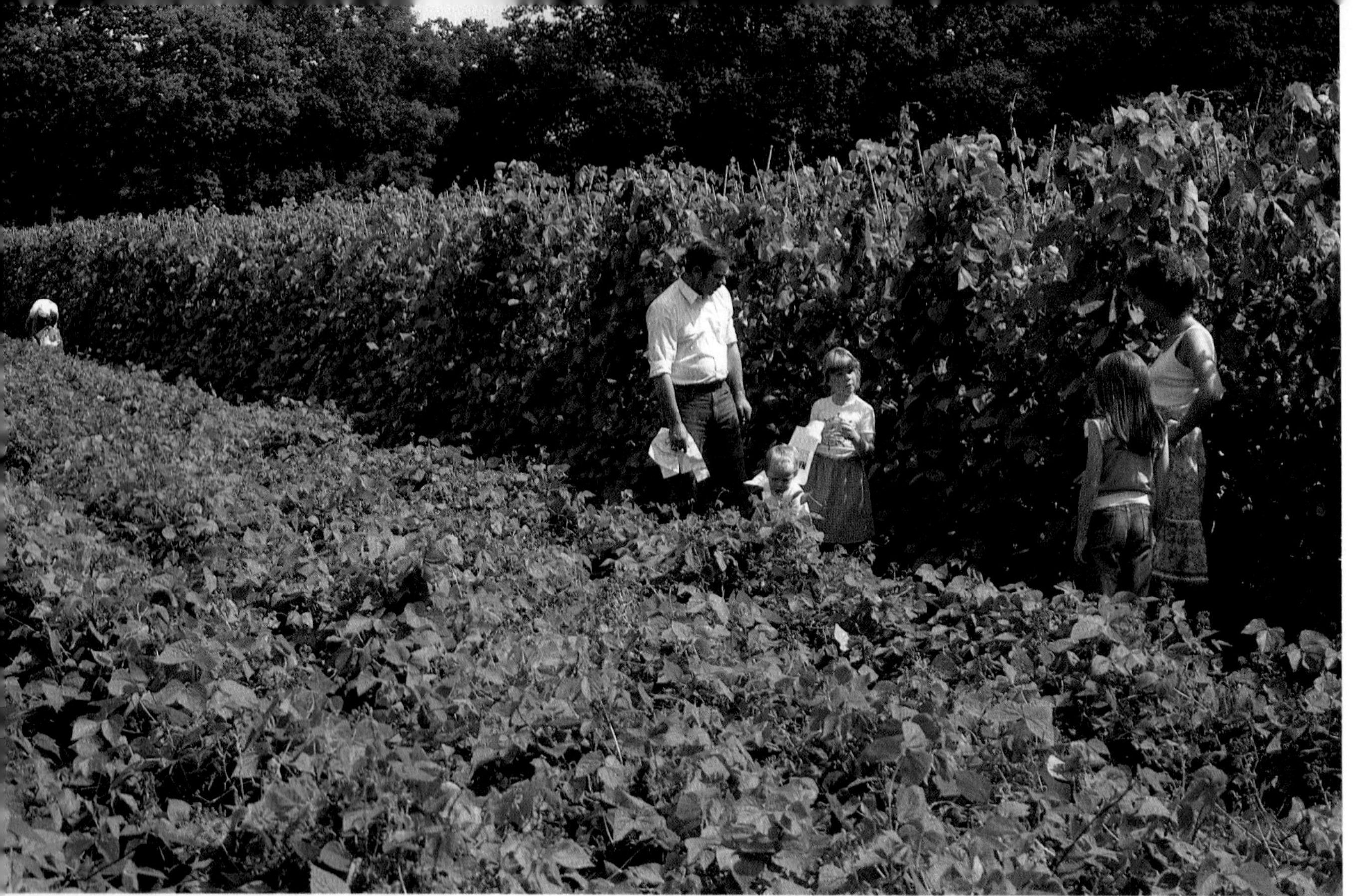

Christopher Columbus told of sampling unfamiliar beans on his historic journey to the New World in 1492. In the early 17th century the Pilgrims ate their first kidney beans in New England. In 1792, Thomas Jefferson, statesman and gardener, recorded the cultivation of another legume, the peanut.

A True Health Food?

It is no accident that edible legumes have such a long history. Our ancestors may not have understood why legumes were so important in a healthful diet, but they did know a good thing when they ate it.

Although some legumes are eaten fresh, it is in their dried form that they have the most nutritional value. First and foremost, dried legumes are an excellent source of protein, which plays an important role in the human body. To build and maintain its tissues, the body needs two kinds of amino acids. It can make one kind, called the nonessential amino acids, but the only source of the other kind, called the essential amino acids, is the protein in food. The highest quality proteins—complete proteins, which contain all the essential amino acids—are found in animal foods such as meat or dairy products. The proteins in plant foods such as legumes—incomplete proteins—contain only some of the essential amino acids. This seeming drawback is readily compensated for, however. The trick is to supplement a plant

---

Nancy Polk is a free-lance writer with a particular interest in issues related to health and home.

Worldwide Favorites

Beans, either fresh or dried, are popular in both the Old World and the New. Left, a family expedition to a pick-it-yourself bean field in England; right, picking string beans in Florida.

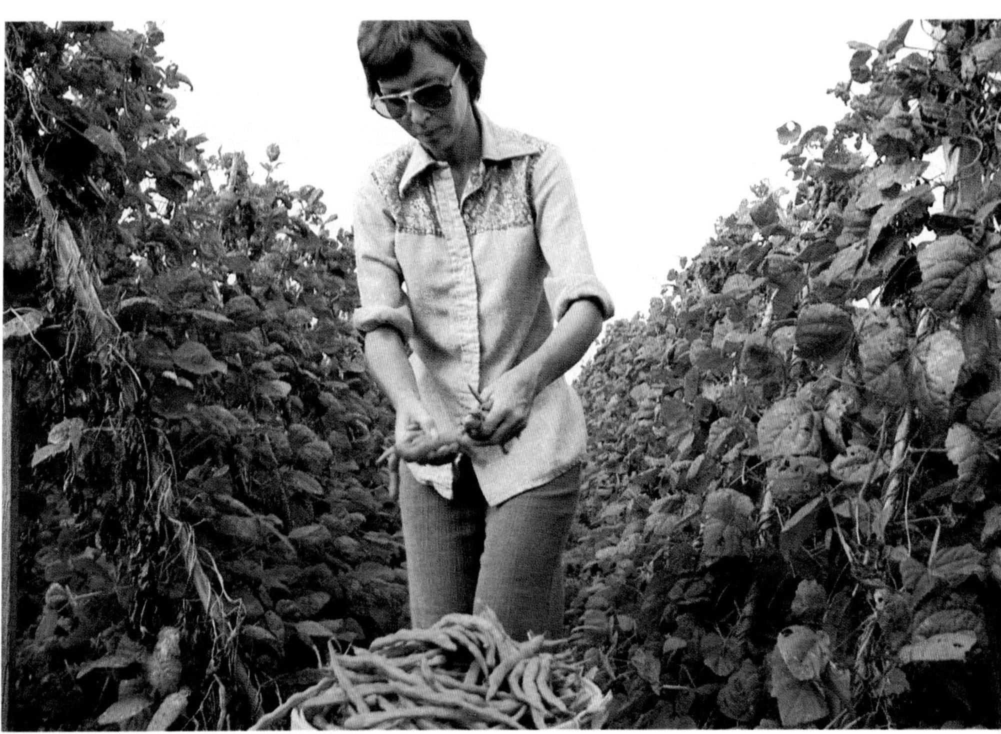

food with a small amount of animal protein or to combine two types of plant foods—legumes with grain, for example—so that the amino acids missing in one are provided by the other. This idea, which today is called complementary protein nutrition, was understood intuitively by ancient peoples. Such traditional combinations as corn tortillas and beans, red beans and rice, black-eyed peas and rice, lentil or pea soup with bread, baked beans with corn bread, and rice and tofu are examples of complementary protein. Dishes like these are often the staples of developing nations today.

Another important characteristic of legumes is that, except for peanuts and soybeans, they are very low in fat. A cup of cooked kidney beans has less than 1 gram of fat, which constitutes less than 4 percent of the total calories one gets from the beans. In contrast, more than 60 percent of total calories in most red meats and 70 percent in hard cheese come from fat. And legumes, unlike animal foods, are cholesterol free.

Dry legumes are also excellent sources of minerals and vitamins including iron, potassium, a number of B vitamins, phosphorus, magnesium, zinc, and calcium. At the same time they are low in sodium.

Legumes are rich in complex carbohydrates—starches, complex sugars, and dietary fiber. Starches and sugars provide energy. The high fiber, or roughage, content of legumes (they provide, on average, 6 to 8 grams per half cup) is of particular interest. Fiber is indigestible organic material found in plant food. Insoluble fiber absorbs water and speeds food through the digestive system. Although the evidence is inconclusive, scientists theorize that this might help prevent colorectal cancer by limiting the time carcinogens stay in the digestive tract.

The Legume Family

The legumes are a family of plants that bear several seeds in a pod. Some legumes are picked while the pods are immature and the seeds small and can be eaten fresh, seeds, pods, and all; examples are string beans, yellow wax beans, and snow peas. Others are picked when the seeds are plump but still unripe and only the fresh seeds are eaten; an example is garden peas. A third group is picked when the seeds are hard and fully ripened, and only the seeds are eaten. Seeds left to mature on the plant in this way are known as dry legumes; examples are kidney beans, pinto beans, and chickpeas. This article deals with dry legumes, unless otherwise noted.

Water soluble fiber, which is abundantly available in legumes (they have more than any other food) appears to lower cholesterol levels in the blood, thereby reducing the risk of heart disease. It is not clear how this works, but it is possible that soluble fiber traps cholesterol in the gastrointestinal tract and then carries it out of the body.

Adult Americans now average about 11 grams of fiber daily; the U.S. National Cancer Institute recommends increasing that to 20 or 30 grams, and other medical authorities, while not suggesting definite amounts, also recommend increased fiber consumption. It is important, however, not to assume that if a little is good more is better. There are problems associated with excessive fiber intake (over 35 grams per day). Gassiness and diarrhea can occur if too much fiber is ingested or if the increase is too abrupt. Gradually increasing the amount of dietary fiber and drinking more fluid to prevent intestinal irritation is the best way to go. (It is also important not to assume that taking fiber supplements will give the same benefits as increasing the amount of fiber-rich food one eats. What is known or suspected about the benefits of fiber is based on studies of diets containing large amounts of high-fiber food and relatively small amounts of meat and fat. No one knows for sure whether the benefits come from the fiber itself or from the presence or absence of some other dietary factor.)

For people concerned about their weight, fiber-rich foods have a further attraction—they are filling. It is easier to stick to a sensible diet regimen if one feels full.

Some other advantages of dried legumes are that they can be stored for long periods without losing their flavor or nutritional value, and they are infinitely cheaper than animal foods.

Hail to the Queen

The soybean is sometimes called the Queen of Beans and with good reason. It is the most versatile legume and possibly the most versatile

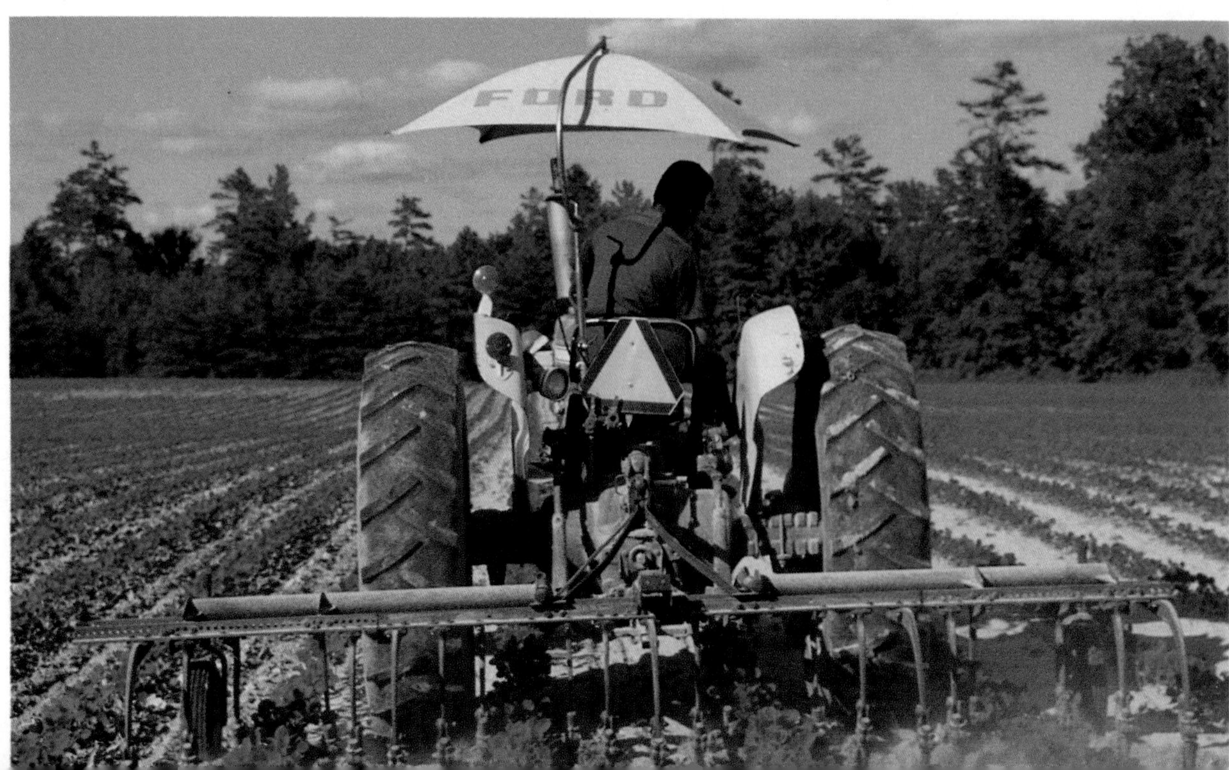

food on earth. Although soybeans as soybeans are not very popular, they have become the most important beans in the world's economy, used in forms as diverse as soy sauce, cattle feed, tofu, oil, flour, and baby formula. Foods made from soy protein concentrate, like textured vegetable protein, are used as meat substitutes that mimic breakfast sausage and burgers.

Soybeans have the highest quality protein of all the legumes, with an amino acid balance almost as good as that of meat. One cup of cooked soybeans provides about 20 grams of protein, about one-third of the Recommended Dietary Allowance (RDA) for an adult male, 25 percent of the RDA for thiamine, over 80 percent of the RDA for iron, and 15 percent of the RDA for calcium. It also contains half the calories of the same amount of beef with much less fat and no cholesterol. (Its high oil content is largely removed by processing.)

Soybeans originated in China, where they have been raised since around the 11th century B.C. Today the United States is the largest producer of soybeans, growing more than 60 percent of the world's crop, mostly on huge Midwestern farms. U.S. soybeans are used primarily in three things: oil (the soybean is the most widely used oilseed in the United States), soybean meal for livestock feed, and protein products for humans.

Granola bars, breakfast cereal, and pasta are just three of the many processed foods that are frequently fortified with soy protein products. Since soy protein offers high quality protein at a low cost, over 50 million pounds of it are used in the U.S. school lunch program.

A soybean product that has been a staple for centuries in Asia has slowly been gaining in popularity in Western countries. This is tofu, which resembles a soft cheese or baked custard. Also called bean curd, it is sold in blocks, unpackaged and floating in water, packaged in water, or vacuum packed. Having a naturally mild flavor, tofu takes on the characteristics of the sauces, spices, and other ingredients with which it is mixed. It is commonly used in Chinese and Japanese cui-

Soybeans are the most important—and most versatile—legumes in the world's economy. The beans being grown in this Florida field (left) may end up being processed (right) into any of a number of products, including oil, baby formula, even imitation ice cream.

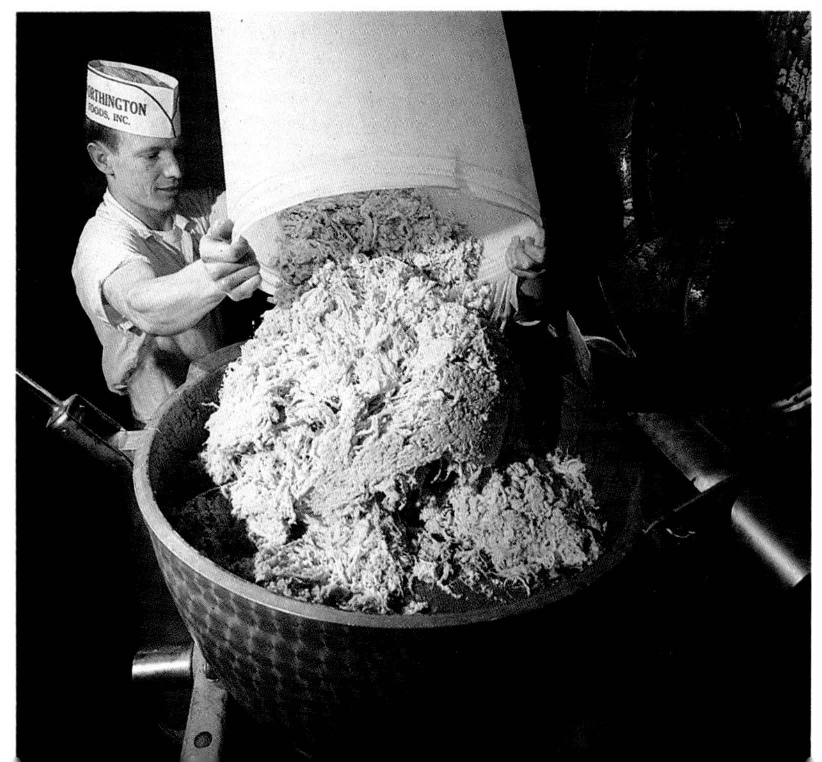

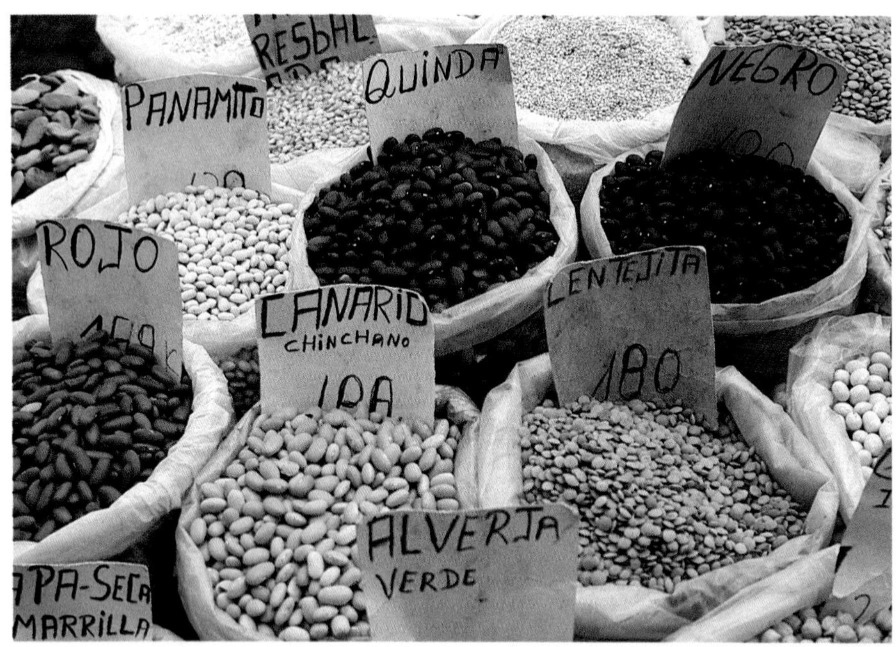

Beans Galore

Colorful displays of dried beans are typical sights in the open air markets of developing countries, where the bean is a staple food (left, Lima, Peru; right, Ixtapan de la Sal, Mexico).

sine. Chinese-style tofu is firm; Japanese-style tofu is soft, with a higher percentage of water.

Tofu is also an ingredient in dairy-free ice cream, imitation cheese, and frozen lasagna. Tofu products are popular with vegetarians, people allergic to dairy products, and those consciously reducing dietary fat and cholesterol. Since it is easy to digest, it is a good food for babies and people with digestive ailments. Tofu contains around 150 calories per 8 ounces (this varies depending on how firmly packed the tofu is), and is low in saturated fat in proportion to unsaturated fat.

Making tofu at home is not difficult. Soybeans, which can be bought at a health food store, are soaked in water and blended to a puree. The puree is then boiled and strained. The liquid part is simmered and a coagulant, also available at health food stores, is added. The coagulant causes curds and whey to form. The curds are filtered and molded to make tofu.

Another soy food with a long history is tempeh, an Indonesian staple available in health food and specialty stores. To make tempeh, soybeans are split and boiled and a starter is added to ferment the beans. The resulting crunchy, solid white bean cake, which is slightly more flavorful than tofu, is a third higher in protein than the original beans. Like tofu, tempeh is very versatile and can be used in foods ranging from sandwiches to casseroles.

Miso, also made by fermenting soybeans, is used in Asian cooking to flavor sauces, salad dressings, stews, soups, and gravies. Sweet miso, a satisfying dairy substitute used to thicken and flavor sauces, and the saltier red miso, used for soup, are the two basic types. Delicate, clear miso soup is typically eaten in Japan as a breakfast food. Another fermented soybean product is the popular soy sauce, made by fermenting and aging soybeans, cracked roasted wheat, salt, and water. Tamari, which, like soy sauce, is used in stir-fried vegetable, meat, and tofu

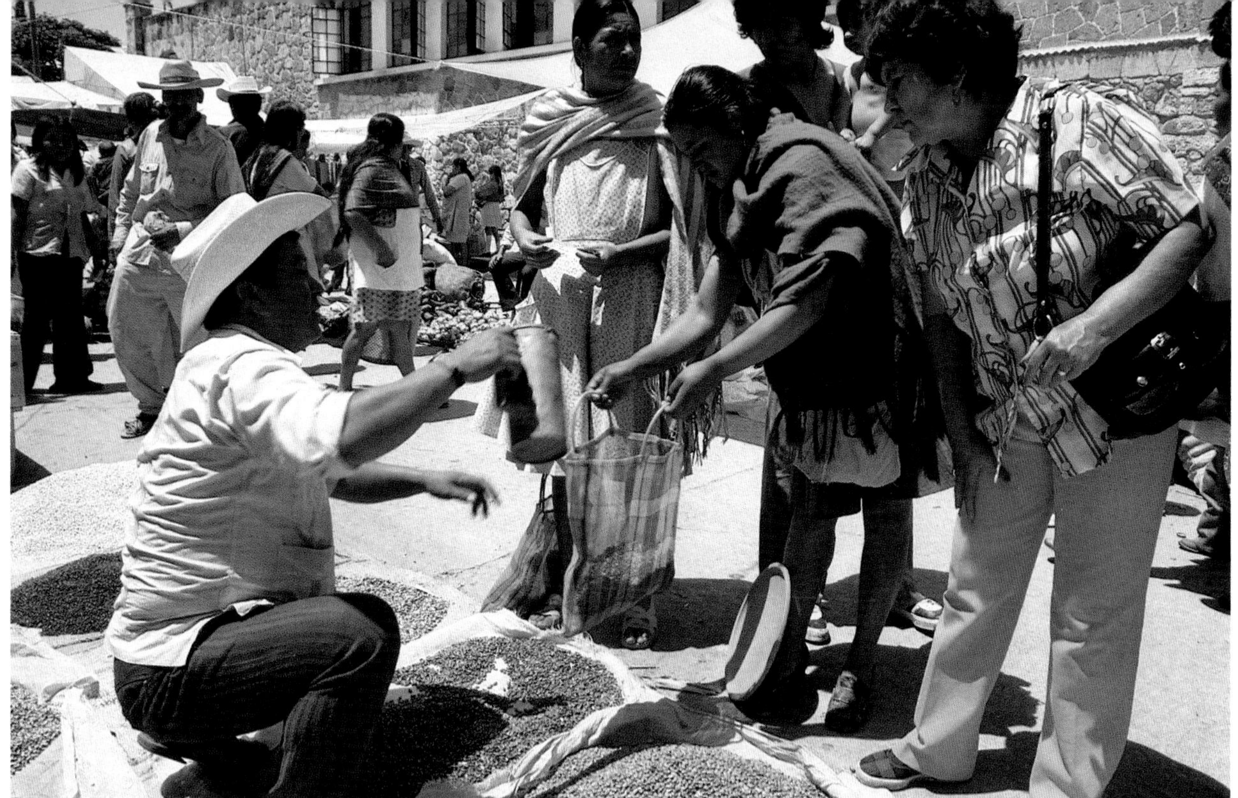

combinations and in soups, stews, and marinades, is similar but is made without wheat. Tamari has a richer flavor, is darker in color, and contains glutamic acid, a natural tenderizer.

Lentils

In Genesis, Esau sold his birthright to Jacob for bread and a pottage (thick soup) of lentils. The ancient Egyptians, Greeks, and Romans also enjoyed lentils. The Romans got their lentils from Egypt, an early import-export transaction. An ancient Chinese tomb, the final resting place of the Lady of Han, wife of the Marquis of Tai, held red lentils dating back to the second century B.C.

Today many of the world's peoples, particularly in Southwestern Asia, depend on lentils for their protein. Lentils flourish in poor soil and harsh climates where nothing else will grow, which probably accounts at least in part for their popularity.

There are two types of lentils, the large Chilean and the small Persian. In India a dish called dhal is made by combining soup stock and pureed lentils. Served with rice, it provides a well balanced vegetable protein.

Peas and Beans Around the World

There are many species of edible peas and beans. Here are some of the most popular types.

Bright red adzuki (aduki, azuki) beans are a favorite in Asia. In Japan mochi, a ball of sweet rice dough filled with a paste of sweetened mashed adzuki beans called ahn, is served at holidays and festivals. It is not as sweet as Western desserts but is a national favorite with the Japanese. The Chinese have a similiar snack called ma yung

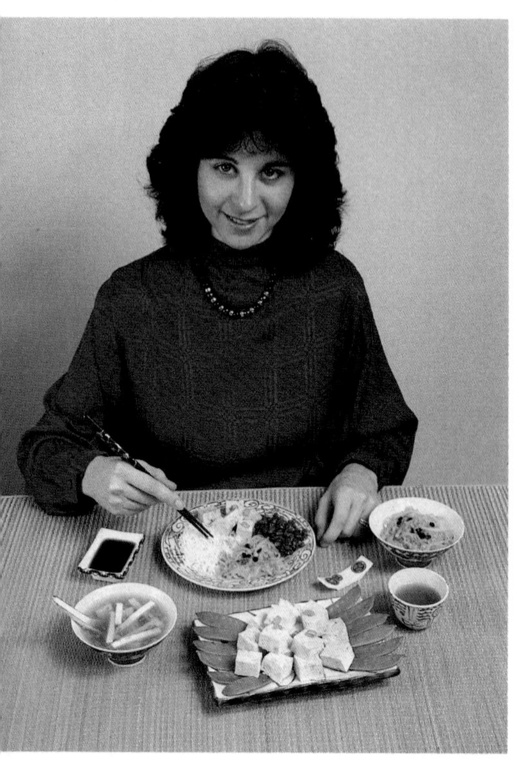

A legume lover's delight—preparing to dine on bean curd soup, tofu, red beans, snow peas, and bean sprouts with black beans, with soy sauce on the side.

bao, steamed sweet bean buns, made from wheat flour and stuffed with bean paste.

Black-eyed peas, tan in color with one black eye, originated in Nigeria. They are a great favorite in the American South. Hoppin' John, a savory mixture of black-eyed peas, onions, rice, and either bacon or chicken stock, is traditionally served throughout the region on New Year's Day. Black-eyed peas with ham hocks and okra is a traditional Southern black dish. Today, about 90 percent of the black-eyed peas grown in the United States are raised in California.

Broad beans (favas) are eaten fresh or dried, particularly in Mediterranean countries. Large dried seeds are available in Middle Eastern stores and enjoyed like popcorn. People whose ethnic origins are Mediterranean or Asian may be genetically susceptible to a rare blood disease called favism caused by eating undercooked fava beans or inhaling the plant's pollen.

Among the best known beans in the Americas are many belonging to the common bean species. The common bean is also called the kidney bean, but most people use that name for two particular common beans, the red kidney bean and the white kidney bean. Other common beans are the string bean and the wax bean (both eaten fresh, pod and all) and many dry varieties, including the navy, Great Northern, and pea bean (all of them white), the black bean, the red bean, and the speckled pinto. Red kidney beans are used in chilis and bean salads. Red beans are favored in the cooking of the Caribbean islands. Either navy or Northern beans are used in caldo gallego, a Spanish/Portuguese stew. Pea or navy beans are used in baked beans, a traditional Saturday night dish in New England. Black beans (turtle beans) are popular in the tropics, particularly in Cuba, where they are made into a richly flavored soup. The classic Brazilian dish feijoada uses black beans, onions, meat, cassava root flour, and orange slices. In Guatemala black beans are boiled and pureed and served for breakfast. In Mexico black beans are served as a separate course. In India and Pakistan they are used in spicy vegetarian dishes, and they frequently appear in curries.

Cranberry beans (Roman beans), which are round and reddish with a sweet strong flavor, probably originated among South American Indians. They are popular in South American and Italian cuisine. A favorite Chilean dish uses these beans with tomatoes, corn, and squash. In Italy they are cooked with cabbage.

Garbanzos (chickpeas, cecis, Bengal grams) are hard, round, and light tan colored. They originated in Mesopotamia and later spread into India and Asia. They are commonly found in Middle Eastern cuisine and often appear on American salad bars. In India flour made from garbanzos is used for an almond flavored sweet.

The garden pea, which may have originated in ancient Egypt, is widely grown throughout the world. The variety known as field peas has smooth hard seeds of various colors; some of the yellow or green kinds are sold as split peas, commonly used in hearty soups. Other varieties are softer and sweeter and are eaten fresh. They include snow peas or sugar snap peas, which are eaten pod and all. (Another name is edible podded peas.) These are often used in Japanese and

Chinese stir fry dishes. They are cooked briefly and never allowed to lose their bright green color and crispness.

The Goa bean (asparagus pea, winged bean) originated in India and is popular in Asia. Although not well known in the United States, it is grown and eaten in the warm weather states of Florida, California, and Hawaii. The pods, which are square with ridges, are eaten along with the seeds. Goa beans are used for sukiyaki. The Indonesians eat the roasted seeds with rice.

Jack beans (swordbeans, Chickasaw limas) were known in ancient Peru and are now cultivated in the tropics, including the West Indies and Mauritius. Jack bean pods are eaten in Japan either preserved in salt or boiled. The dried beans can be ground into a coffee substitute.

Lima beans (butter beans, Madagascar beans) are native to Central America. Remains of these beans have been found in Peruvian excavations dating back thousands of years. They occur in two types, large seeded or small seeded (baby limas). They grow wild throughout the tropics and are raised commercially in California, India, Myanmar, and wet forest areas of Africa. Fresh limas are combined with corn to make succotash, a dish that was familiar to the American colonists and that is still eaten today.

Mung beans, small green balls, are known primarily in the West for sprouting, but in Asia they are used for a variety of dishes. In Thailand they are used to make golden bean cakes, a dessert served in sugar syrup. A Korean recipe for bean pancakes mixes mung dhal—the beans skinned and split in half—with pork, onions, and kimchi, a pungent cabbage.

Pigeon peas (dhal, congo peas) grow in the tropics. They can be eaten fresh or milled into flour. Dried split pigeon peas are used in soup and eaten with rice. They are popular in Thailand and North Bengal.

Scarlet runner beans (multiflora beans) grow easily in the tropics and temperate regions. The blossoms are red. The plants climb on poles or fences to great heights. Runner beans are eaten whole in Europe and Central America.

Yard long beans (asparagus beans, pea beans) are climbers grown in India, Africa, and the Caribbean. The pods, belying their name, can grow to 4 feet long and remain thin and delicately flavored. In Indonesia they are included in rijstafel, a classic meal that is composed of many dishes and sauces.

Peanuts

There's more to peanuts than peanut butter and jelly sandwiches in the lunchboxes of America's youth. Peanuts are not nuts at all but legumes. No one knows for sure where they originated, although the Americas are now believed to have had peanuts before the rest of the world. Ancient Incan tombs contained jars filled with peanuts to provide nourishment after death. Peanuts were cultivated in Mexico at the time of the Spanish conquest in the 1500s. Spanish explorers brought peanuts home, where they are still cultivated. Spanish traders used peanuts in exchange for spices and elephant tusks in Africa,

Storing and Cooking Legumes

After purchasing dry peas, beans, or lentils, try to store them in a cool dry place. They will take longer to cook if stored at high temperature or humidity. There is no need to refrigerate them. When presoaking is necessary, as it is, for example, for garbanzos and split peas, add about 6 cups of cold water per pound of dry legumes and let stand overnight. Or use the quick soak method: boil for two minutes and then let stand for an hour. Whichever method you use, the next step is to drain, rinse, and add fresh water. Draining improves digestibility by getting rid of certain carbohydrates that the body cannot digest well and that may cause intestinal discomfort and flatulence. Cooking dry legumes at high altitudes takes longer because water boils at lower temperatures. Dry legumes cooked in hard water also take longer than times given in recipes. Cook dry beans and peas on medium heat to avoid bursting their skins and getting mush. Once they are cooked, they can be kept refrigerated for four to five days, frozen for several months.

Peanuts are considered as American as apple pie.

where peanuts are now widely grown and are known as groundnuts. Many delicious African soups and stews include groundnuts.

It is not clear how peanuts, today considered as American as apple pie, got to what is now the United States. It was once thought that they arrived in North America in the holds of slave ships, a theory probably based on the peanut's nickname, goober, which is derived from nguba, the Congolese name for peanut. (Other names for peanuts are earth nuts, goober peas, pindars, monkey nuts, and Chinese nuts.) But Native Americans are known to have offered peanuts to the early colonists, who were apparently already familiar with them. Whatever the case, for a long time peanuts were considered "poor people's food." Although by the 1700s they had been firmly established in the colonies, it was as feed for pigs. One hundred years later peanuts were being widely consumed by Americans, who were also using peanut oil and enjoying a drink made from the "milk" presssed out of peanuts. During the Civil War, soldiers on both sides developed an appreciation for peanuts' portability and flavor.

But as long as bits of stem and waste found their way into packaged peanuts, they did not fare well on the general market. This changed with improved harvesting, and demand soared. During the First World War peanuts were used for oil, peanut butter, and candy and as a roasted and salted treat.

Four different types of peanuts are grown in the United States, the world's largest producer of edible peanuts. Runner, the dominant variety since it is so productive, accounts for 68 percent of total U.S. production. Virginia peanuts have the largest kernels, which are commonly roasted and salted in the shell. Spanish peanuts have small kernels covered with reddish-brown skin; they are used predominantly in peanut candy and also for salted nuts and peanut butter. Valencias are very sweet and usually roasted and sold in the shell.

While peanuts are a good source of carbohydrates and protein, they also contain up to 50 percent oil by weight and should be used in moderation.

Peanut Butter. Peanut butter was first recorded in the cuisine of South American Indians. Today, half of all edible peanuts consumed in the United States are used in peanut butter. Legally, peanut butter must contain at least 90 percent peanuts. The other 10 percent may be salt, sweetener, and an emulsifier (or stabilizer), that is, hardened vegetable oil used to prevent separation.

It takes about 546 peanuts to make a 12 ounce jar of peanut butter. The peanuts are roasted and blanched to remove their skin, and a stabilizer is added. ("Old fashioned" or "natural" peanut butter omits the stabilizers—and often the salt and sweetener as well—so it must be kept refrigerated to prevent separation and rancidity.) The nuts are then ground smooth. For crunchy peanut butter the peanuts are also ground smooth, but small chunks of peanuts are added.

Eating More Legumes

To increase consumption of legumes, substitute small amounts of soy or other legume flour in recipes. Soy flour is very strong tasting, so just a few tablespoons are probably enough for a bread or muffin recipe. All dry beans and peas can also be milled into flour, but such flours, primarily used as protein supplements in the developing world, are not easy to find in the United States. They can sometimes be found in health food stores and can also be ground at home.

Don't be afraid to experiment when you cook with legumes. Many types of legumes are interchangeable in recipes; for example, try substituting lentils for kidney beans in chili recipes. Try adding legumes to recipes that include meat and gradually reducing the meat portion to condiment levels. This will both save money and reduce the amount of fat in the diet. Use bean or pea puree to thicken soups or sauces.

For complementary protein nutrition, serve legumes with grains, nuts, and seeds or with dairy products, preferably low-fat ones like yogurt or farmer cheese. Since protein synthesis requires that all amino acids be available together, foods that complement each other should be eaten at the same meal or at least on the same day.

One of the appeals of legumes is their blandness, which means they lend themselves nicely to the addition of herbs, strong spices, and hot sauces. Lentils and curry, kidney beans and salsa, pinto beans and chilis, and the Middle Eastern dish using chickpeas mashed into falafel and sauced with tahini (a combination of sesame seeds, lemon juice, and garlic) are all good examples of this. Investigate ethnic foods. Visit your local library and study cookbooks from unfamiliar cuisines. Foods from India, China, Mexico, Israel, Japan, and Africa all use legumes in imaginative and nutritious ways.

Sprouts

Legume sprouts have more vitamin C and fewer calories than dry beans. They make a tasty addition to sandwiches and are frequently used to decorate the tops of salads and omelets. Mung bean sprouts are often used in Chinese and Japanese stir-fry dishes. Sprouts are now widely sold in supermarkets and produce stores. Seeds especially marked for sprouting at home, including alfalfa, lentil, soybean and chickpea, can be bought at supermakets and health food stores. (Do not use seeds intended for planting; they may have been treated with chemicals to prevent fungal diseases.) Soak the seeds overnight, drain, cover with damp paper towels, and rinse frequently. In only three or four days the seeds have sprouted and the sprouts are ready to eat. Young children particularly enjoy this "planting" and eating experience.

Eating more legumes can help both budget and body.

Other Edible Legumes

Some other edible legumes are licorice, used for sweets and to flavor medicine; carob, a common substitute for chocolate; tamarind, used to flavor a lemony drink in Latin America; fenugreek, a popular spice used in curry powder and chutney and as a flavoring agent in imitation maple syrup; and guar, which yields a gum used as a thickening agent in ice cream and other processed foods. □

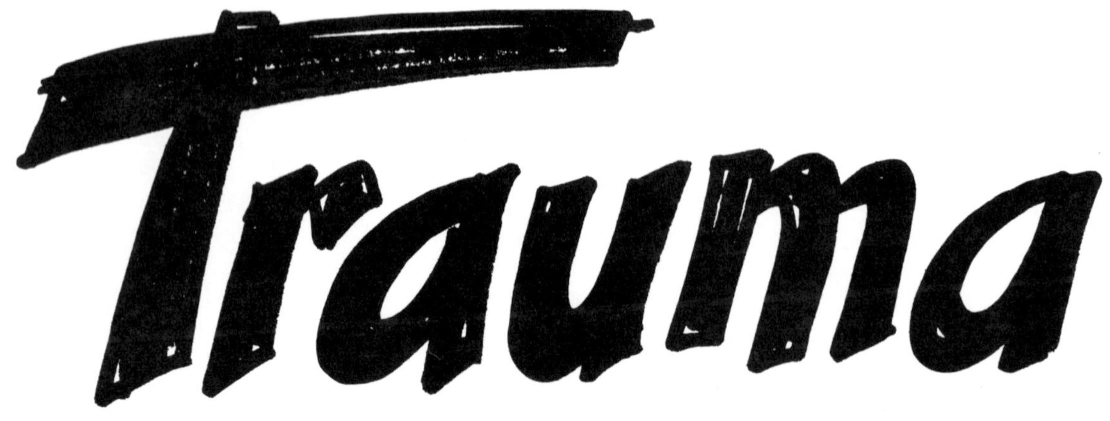

THE EMOTIONAL AFTERMATH

Kim T. Mueser, Ph.D.

The psychological aftermath of severe traumatic events such as war, torture, rape, assault, accidents, fire, and natural disasters can be devastating. The everyday lives of those who have experienced these violent events are often disrupted. Frequently, people are plagued by nightmares, frightening memories, sensitivity to loud noises, and difficulty trusting others. These problems can interfere with the ability to work, care for oneself, and enjoy close relationships. In recent years a specific cluster of symptoms has been identified in some persons who have experienced a traumatic incident. If these symptoms become chronic or develop suddenly a long time after the event, the person has a psychiatric syndrome called posttraumatic stress disorder (PTSD).

Most of the symptoms of PTSD are related to anxiety and hypervigilance (a continuous state of excessive alertness or alarm), although depression and emotional numbing are also common. People with PTSD are usually aware that something is wrong, and family members and close friends may notice changes in their behavior, but often those involved do not realize that the symptoms indicate a specific psychiatric disorder for which treatments are available. If PTSD persists untreated over a long period of time, it becomes more difficult to treat effectively, and the victim suffers more.

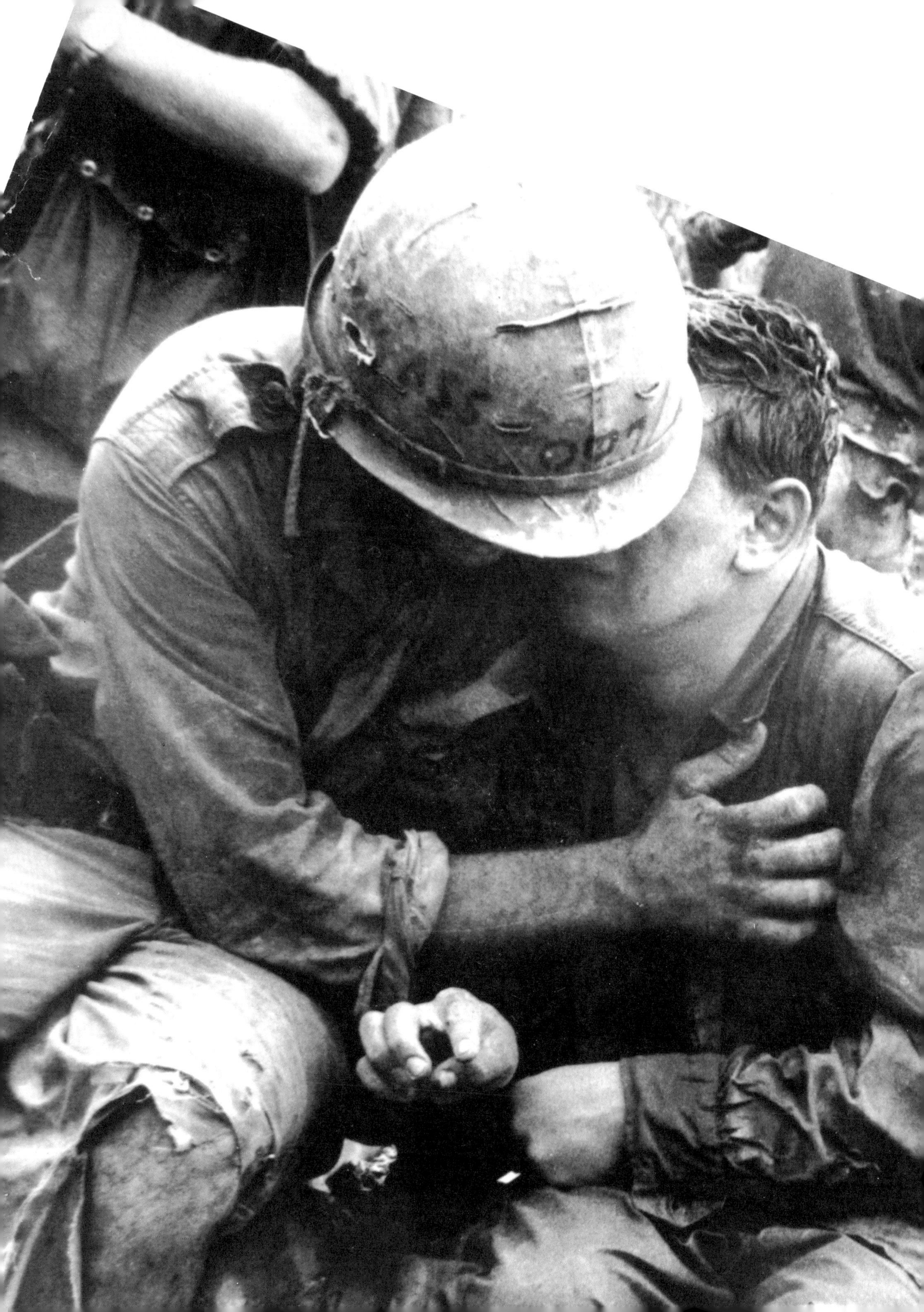

Responding to Trauma

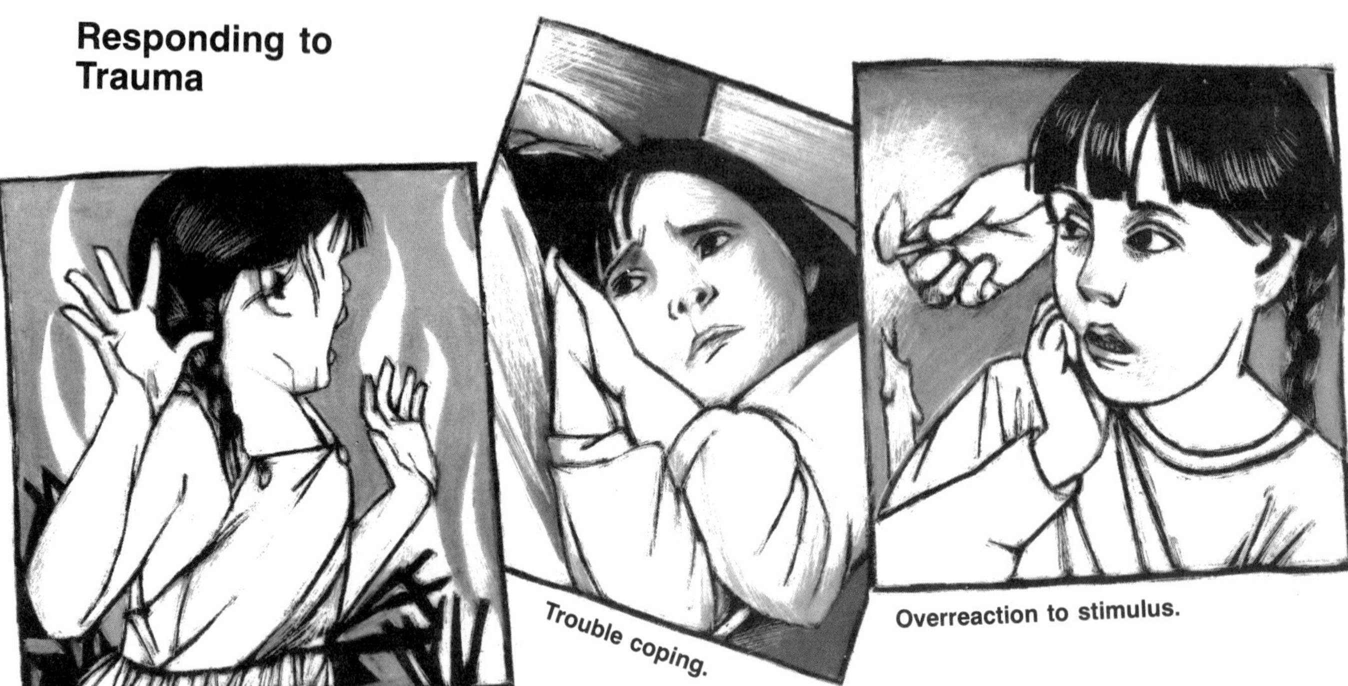

The traumatic event.

Trouble coping.

Overreaction to stimulus.

Detecting the early symptoms of posttraumatic stress disorder is crucial—rapid treatment can prevent the symptoms from worsening, and in many cases the disorder itself can be cured. The risk of developing PTSD in the first place can be lessened if efforts are taken immediately following a trauma to help the person cope with the psychological distress of the experience.

How Common Is PTSD?

It is difficult to estimate the prevalence of PTSD because systematic attempts to define the disorder and assess its presence have occurred, in the main, only over the past 15 years. Recognition of PTSD as a serious consequence of war and other traumas developed slowly following the end of the Vietnam War, as young combat veterans experienced difficulties reintegrating into a society divided about the morality of the war. The term "posttraumatic stress disorder" was accepted into the U.S. psychiatric diagnostic system only in 1980. However, PTSD is not a new disorder, and similar syndromes have been described throughout the years but under different names. The psychological casualties of war were said to be suffering from battle fatigue, shell shock, combat exhaustion, or war neurosis. When the disorder was the result of other types of trauma, it may have been called compensation neurosis, hysteria, traumatophobia, and rape trauma syndrome. What is common to both new and old definitions of the disorder is the recognition that it develops following exposure to a

---

Kim T. Mueser is associate professor of psychiatry at the Medical College of Pennsylvania at Eastern Pennsylvania Psychiatric Institute.

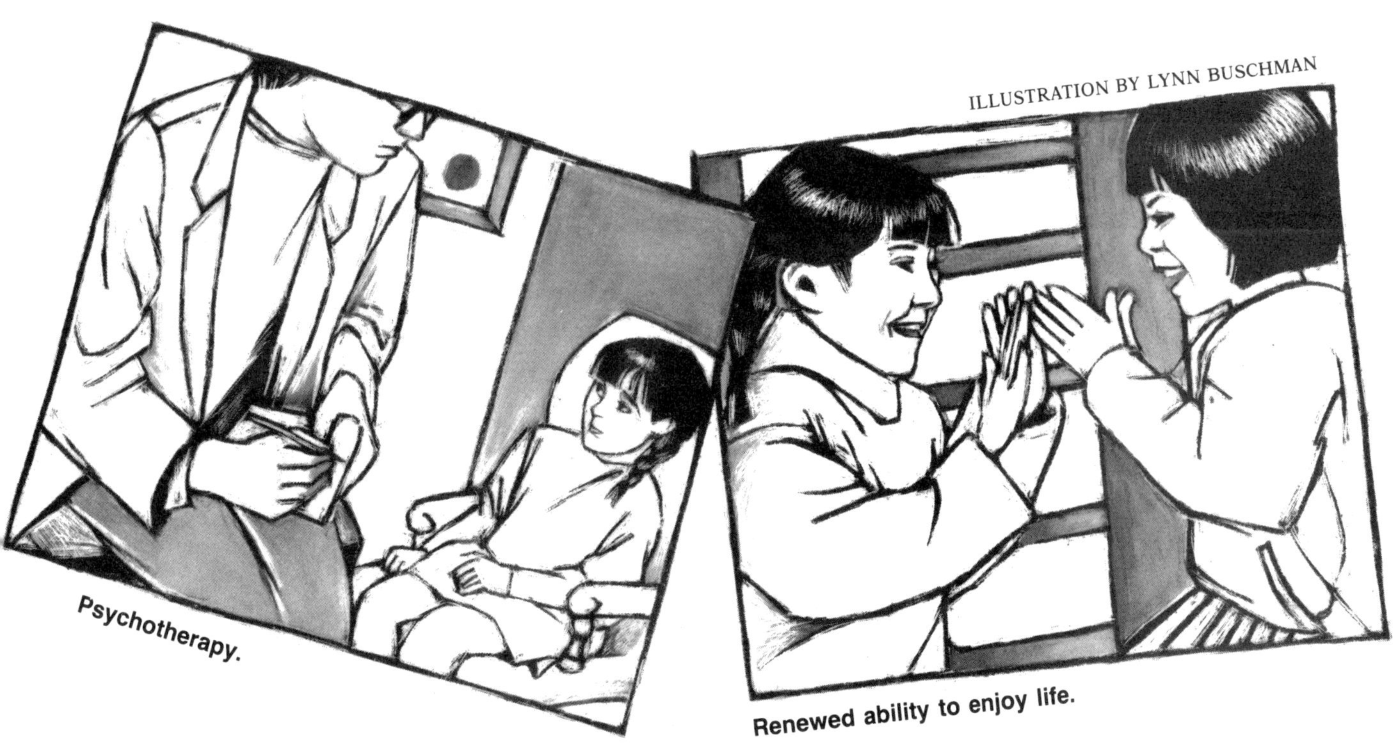

Psychotherapy.

Renewed ability to enjoy life.

specific trauma or series of traumatic events and that its victims experience severe anxiety and problems with daily functioning.

The best estimates suggest that approximately 1 to 2 percent of adults in the United States are afflicted by PTSD. This is equivalent to the rate of schizophrenia in the U.S. adult population, but it may be an underestimate because many people who suffer from the symptoms of PTSD never seek professional treatment. Valid estimates of PTSD among children are not available. However, the problem of physical and sexual abuse of children, compounded by the exposure of many children to domestic violence, suggests that the disorder may be even more common in children than in adults.

Whether or not a person develops PTSD is determined mainly by the extent of exposure to violent incidents, as well as by the nature of these incidents and by the person's perception of imminent danger. Thus, a soldier who has actively participated in combat is more likely to develop PTSD than another soldier with less time on the battlefield. Estimates of PTSD among Vietnam veterans generally range between 15 and 30 percent, but among veterans with high combat exposure the rate is much higher, between 35 and 50 percent. Similarly, a person who is the victim of a crime has a greater chance of suffering from PTSD if the crime is a particularly violent or vicious one, such as rape. Persons who have been the victim of rape have at least a 50 percent chance of developing PTSD if they do not receive psychological treatment. For many people, these symptoms can last for years. Indeed, one study found that about 17 percent of rape victims had the symptoms of PTSD an average of 17 years after the crime. And if people believe that their lives are in danger, they have a larger risk of developing PTSD, even if this belief occurs after the traumatic event. One woman developed PTSD several months after she was raped when she found out that her assailant had killed one of his victims. In this case, the change in the woman's perception of her danger influenced the onset of PTSD.

Diagnosis and Symptoms

Symptoms of PTSD can be delayed for months or years.

There is no blood test, X ray, or any other laboratory measure that can be used to diagnose PTSD. The disorder can be diagnosed only through a careful, structured clinical interview to evaluate whether a person has experienced the specific symptoms used to define PTSD. The person need not have all the symptoms in order to have PTSD, but certain types of symptoms must be present.

In order to be diagnosed with PTSD the person must have been exposed to a traumatic event. The event should be outside the scope of ordinary human experiences, such as simple bereavement or chronic illness. It should also be so intense that it would be psychologically distressful to almost anyone who experienced the event. The immediate response to the event is usually one of terror, helplessness, and fear for one's own personal safety or that of another person. Following the event, three general types of psychological symptoms can emerge: reexperiencing the traumatic event, avoiding stimuli associated with the event or becoming emotionally numb, and experiencing marked increases in one's level of arousal, including suffering from sleep disturbances, irritability, and hypervigilance. These symptoms can develop immediately after the trauma, or the onset can be delayed, sometimes for as long as months or years. Whether the onset is immediate or delayed, symptoms must persist for at least one month before the person can be diagnosed as having PTSD.

Reexperiencing the Traumatic Event. This can occur in several different ways. Unpleasant, intrusive images or memories of the event are common. Sleep may be disturbed by nightmares or dreams about the experience. Sometimes the person may have flashbacks and act or feel as though the traumatic event were occurring again. Events or places that remind the person of some aspect of the trauma—its anniversary, or a location resembling the one where the event occurred—can produce intense psychological distress. Such experiences produce a feeling of never being safe from the disturbing memories of the trauma, so that the event is relived countless times during a person's waking and sleeping life.

Avoiding Stimuli. A consequence of frequently reexperiencing the trauma is that the person attempts to avoid stimuli that recall the event, including activities or situations, thoughts or feelings. For example, a person involved in a serious auto accident might avoid driving or riding in a car. In some cases, the person may be unable to recall important aspects of the trauma that were especially disturbing at the time. Emotional numbing can take the form of an inability to experience the normal range of emotions, such as love, curiosity, or anger. The person may feel detached or estranged from others and lose interest in activities that were previously enjoyable.

Increased Arousal. An increased level of physiological arousal is an important symptom. The person may have difficulty sleeping or con-

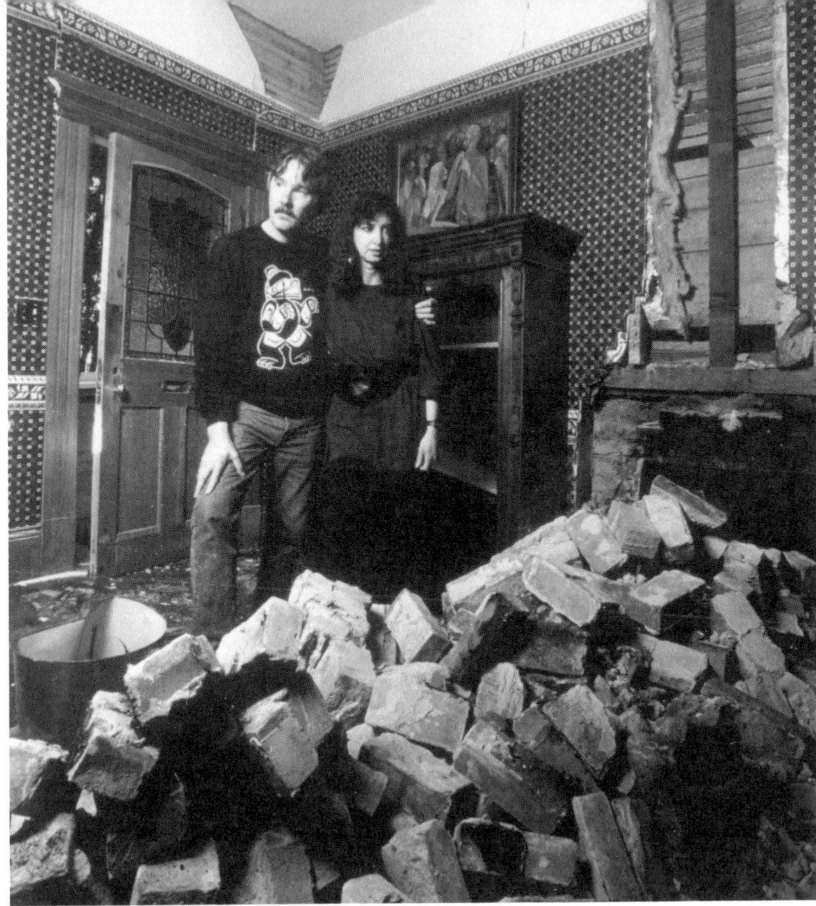

A natural disaster like an earthquake can cause terror and helplessness. Here, a San Francisco couple surveys the rubble that was once the safe haven of their home.

centrating on a task, may be irritable or hypervigilant, or display "startle responses" to sudden noises. A combat veteran may react to the sound of a car backfiring with an exaggerated startle response followed by "hitting the deck," as though a missile had just exploded. Often the person will experience physiological signs of high arousal—increased sweating, tense muscles, shortness of breath, heart palpitations—when exposed to events that are reminders of the trauma. A man who was in a train wreck may tense up and experience a racing heart rate when he approaches a train station.

Common Secondary Symptoms. In addition to these telltale symptoms, many other psychological problems (referred to as secondary symptoms) can arise as a consequence of PTSD. Depression and suicidal thoughts are common. Difficulty trusting others can interfere with relationships and prevent a person from getting close to people, including family members. Feelings of guilt are also common, particularly for combat veterans. Soldiers who killed civilians or children or who participated in war atrocities are often racked with guilt. Sometimes these symptoms emerge a long time after the war, such as when the veteran has his own children. Those who narrowly escape injury or death but lose comrades in battle often experience "survivor guilt." Frequently, people abuse alcohol and drugs to try to escape their unpleasant memories of the trauma. Unfortunately, these attempts at "self-medication" usually backfire, and intrusive memories of the trauma inevitably return when the person's guard is down.

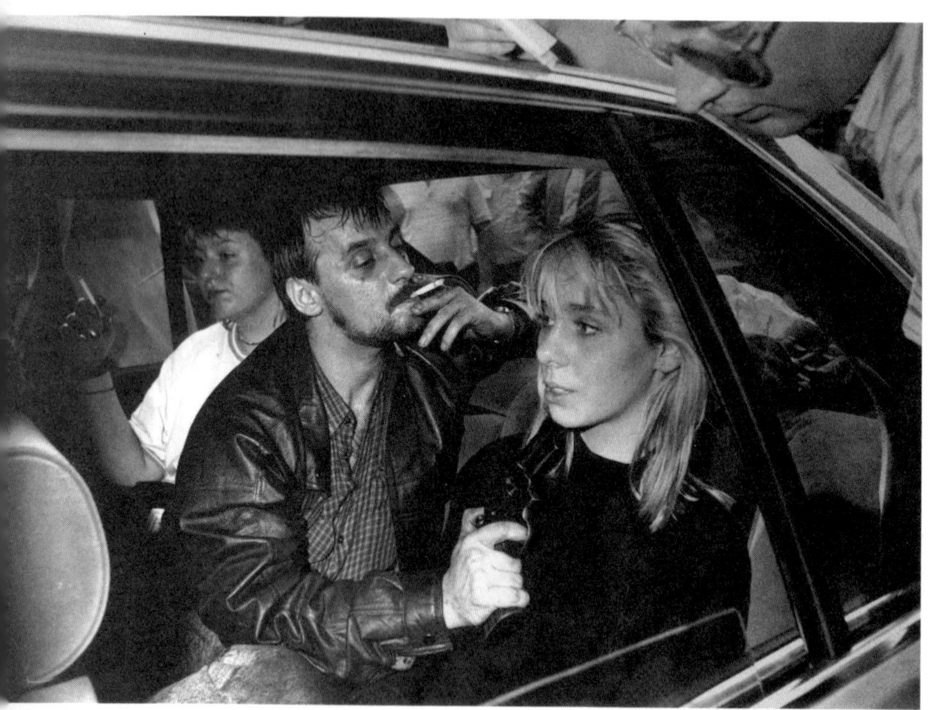

Threats to Life Can Cause PTSD

Innocent passersby can suddenly find they are hostages, with their lives in danger. At left, a German bank robber holds a gun to the chin of one of his hostages. At right, a policeman helps a girl run to safety after her escape from a house in which she had been held hostage by a gun-wielding teenage boy.

The Cause of PTSD

PTSD is different from most other psychiatric disorders in that it is the consequence of an extremely disturbing, often life-threatening, event or series of events. This is in contrast to other illnesses such as major depression, manic-depressive illness, schizophrenia, obsessive-compulsive disorder, or simple phobias—in which no single event can be blamed for causing the disorder. Two theories of learning, classical conditioning and operant conditioning, have provided valuable clues to understanding the development of PTSD. While these theories are unable to explain all of the symptoms, they account for many of them and have paved the road to effective treatments for the disorder.

Classical Conditioning. This refers to learning through the principles of association. Ivan Petrovich Pavlov, the famous Russian physiologist, observed that when an animal was given a shock it would recoil and show other behavior changes suggesting fear. Pavlov found that after the shock had been presented simultaneously with a previously neutral stimulus (such as the ringing of a bell) on repeated occasions, the neutral stimulus alone (the bell) would eventually evoke the same fear response originally caused by the shock. Within the classical conditioning framework, the shock is referred to as the unconditioned stimulus; the neutral stimulus (the bell), as the conditioned stimulus.

When classical conditioning theory is applied to the development of PTSD symptoms, the original trauma serves as the unconditioned stimulus because it immediately evokes the fear response. Other previously neutral stimuli present during the trauma become conditioned stimuli, and it is these that can eventually evoke the same fear response as the original trauma. For example, a helicopter pilot was shot down in

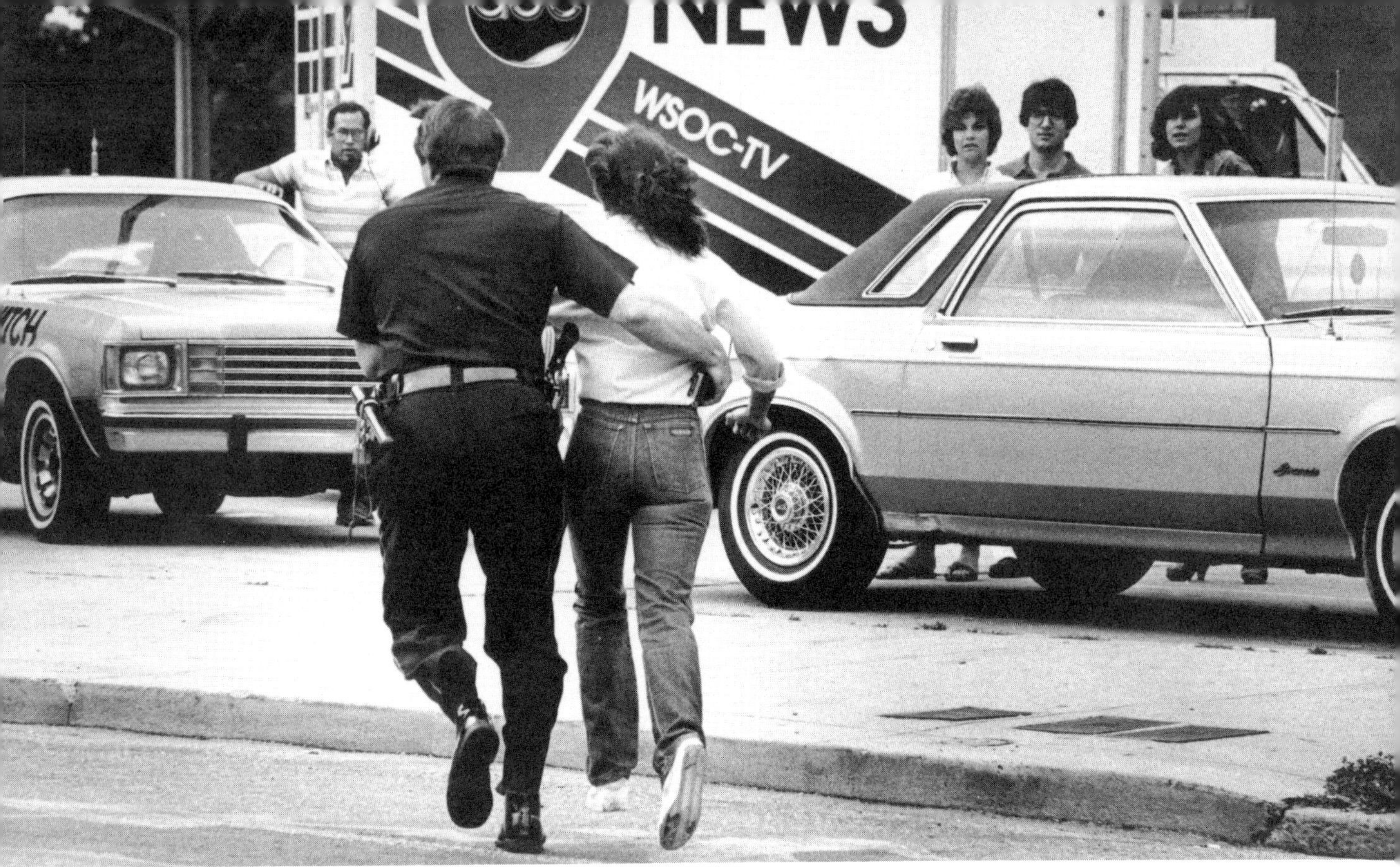

Vietnam by enemy fire during a reconnaissance flight, and most of his crew members were killed. Following treatment of his injuries, the veteran experiences flashbacks, severe anxiety, and intrusive images whenever he hears a helicopter fly overhead or encounters a humid, green area that reminds him of the jungle. In this situation, the original trauma is the helicopter being shot down. The sounds of a helicopter and humid, green areas are the previously neutral stimuli that become conditioned stimuli.

Operant Conditioning. While classical conditioning explains how previously neutral stimuli can evoke the same fear responses as the trauma, operant conditioning accounts for how the fear reaction can persist and occur in an even wider range of situations. Operant conditioning is a type of learning based upon the principles of positive and negative reinforcement. If a behavior is followed by a positive consequence, either some sort of reward or the reduction of something unpleasant, the chances of the person's engaging in that behavior again are increased. Conversely, if a behavior is followed by a negative consequence, like a punishment, the person will be less likely to engage in that behavior again. In PTSD previously neutral stimuli initially elicit fear responses through the process of classical conditioning. Once this fear response has been learned, the person reacts to these "threatening" situations by immediately attempting to escape or by trying to avoid the situations altogether. When a situation is successfully avoided, the person feels temporarily relieved, and the relief becomes the reward, or positive reinforcement, for the escape behavior. Because this behavior is consistently reinforced by a reduction in anxiety, the person learns to avoid more and more stimuli and situations.

The classical and operant conditioning theories of learning account for why people with PTSD avoid stimuli that remind them of their trauma and why they experience strong anxiety in situations only remotely resembling the event. However, not all persons who experience a traumatic event develop PTSD. Furthermore, the symptoms of heightened arousal in PTSD—including sleep problems, hypervigilance, startle reactions, and irritability—are not clearly due to the effects of conditioning. One possible explanation is that people who display more symptoms of overarousal before they are exposed to a trauma may be more vulnerable to developing PTSD than others. This theory is supported by research showing that overarousal is related to vulnerability to other anxiety disorders.

Psychotherapy can improve PTSD symptoms.

Treatment

As recognition has grown that PTSD is more prevalent than was once thought, various treatment programs have been developed. Many programs focus on treating a specific type of trauma victim, such as combat veterans, former prisoners of war, victims of rape and other violent crime, and sexually abused children or adults who were abused as children. Two broad approaches to treatment of PTSD have been explored: treatment with medication and psychotherapy.

Medication. Treatment of PTSD with medication has met with limited success, although it is occasionally useful. Antidepressant medications can alleviate some of the depression that often follows PTSD, but they rarely have a direct effect on the anxiety that is at the root of the disorder. Antianxiety medications, such as a group of drugs called benzodiazepines, which include diazepam (brand name, Valium), or hypnotic drugs (including barbiturates), produce only temporary improvements in anxiety. These medications have the added disadvantage that they may be addictive. Physical tolerance of the medication develops rapidly, so that larger and larger amounts are required to achieve the same relief from anxiety. Other medications used for psychiatric disorders—including antipsychotic drugs, lithium, and anticonvulsants—have not been shown to have beneficial effects on the symptoms of PTSD.

Psychotherapy. Unlike the various medications tried, recently developed psychotherapeutic treatments have been found to improve symptoms substantially. Sometimes the treatments are so effective that they completely eliminate all the symptoms of PTSD, enabling the person to resume a normal life-style.

Group therapy has been found to be of some benefit for the treatment of PTSD. Groups vary in the frequency of their meetings, ranging from once a week to daily, depending on the members' needs. The primary focus is on developing social support among the group members. This is often facilitated by members' sharing their traumatic experiences with each other, discussing current feelings and perspectives on their difficulties, and talking about strategies for coping with ongoing problems.

One treatment based on learning theory that has been found, in carefully controlled clinical studies, to be especially effective at reducing PTSD symptoms is called exposure therapy (also referred to as implosion therapy or flooding). The rationale for exposure therapy is that PTSD is an anxiety disorder in which potentially threatening or fearful stimuli are avoided and that exposure to these threatening stimuli in a "safe" environment is necessary to break the cycle of avoidance. Other anxiety disorders, such as phobias or fear of interacting with people, can be effectively treated by encouraging people to confront the very situations they fear most. This can be accomplished by first helping people imagine themselves in the feared situation and then later exposing them to the actual situation. While their initial reaction is one of fear, anxiety gradually subsides if they continue to be exposed to the object of their fear, and they learn to no longer be afraid of it.

The type of exposure treatment used with persons with PTSD, imaginal exposure therapy, is usually relatively short-term. Treatment sessions generally last one to two hours and are conducted at least once a week and often more frequently for anywhere from several weeks to several months. Therapy is conducted by focusing on the traumatic event and having the person imagine and describe this event repeatedly to the therapist. The therapist helps the person remain focused on the event and monitors anxiety levels to ensure that some reduction in anxiety occurs during each treatment session. When individuals become capable of imagining and describing traumatic events without suffering debilitating anxiety, they cease avoiding the situations that remind them of the event, and other symptoms subside.

People may require exposure treatment for more than one traumatic experience. In such cases, after the anxiety about one traumatic event has been eliminated or substantially reduced, anxiety related to other specific traumatic events is assessed. If the person is still suffering

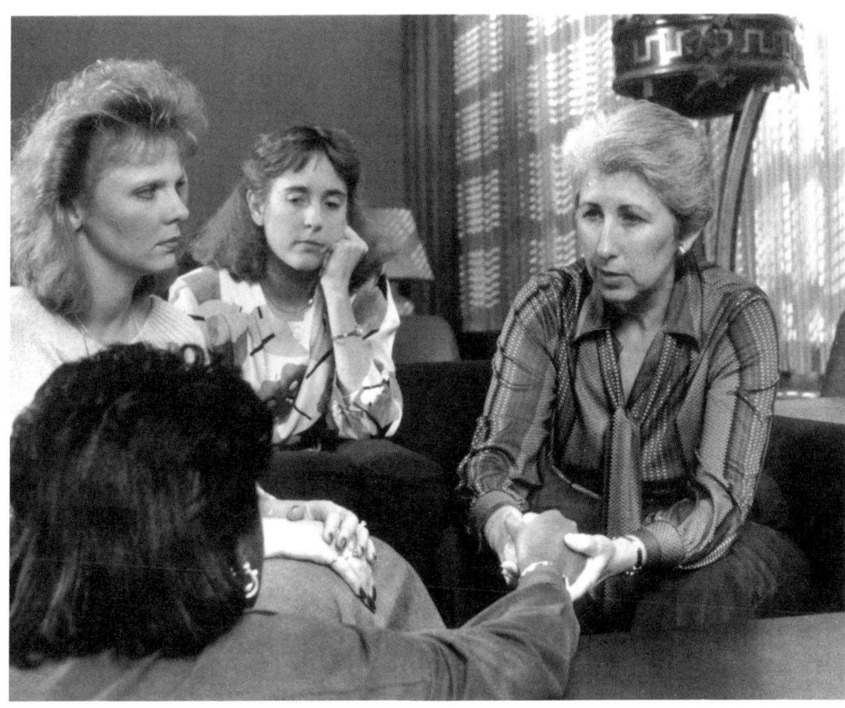

In a group session, a therapist counsels a victim of rape. Through sharing their experiences and feelings, group members can provide social and emotional support for one another.

from anxiety, imaginal exposure treatment is continued on an event by event basis.

Treating Chronic Cases. For some people PTSD is a chronic disorder that cannot be cured. Current treatments, including medications, imaginal exposure therapy, and group therapy, may produce some improvements, but the person may still suffer symptoms. One reason for this is that when the traumatic event occurred long ago, the person may have developed problematic behavior patterns to cope with symptoms. These patterns may help relieve the person's anxiety in the short run, but cause many other problems in the long run. For example, many people with PTSD become dependent upon alcohol or drugs to relieve their symptoms. Effective treatment of PTSD symptoms cannot be conducted until the addiction problem is first treated. A person who was sexually abused as a child may avoid close interpersonal relationships and suffer from depression. Effective treatment would need to address this person's social skills and issues regarding intimacy, in addition to reducing anxiety related to memories of the original traumas. Treatment of PTSD is most effective when it occurs soon after the trauma. People whose lives have been disrupted by a trauma that happened long ago need comprehensive psychological treatment to cope with the memories of the trauma and to overcome other obstacles interfering with normal functioning.

Treatment is most effective when begun soon after the trauma.

Prevention of PTSD

PTSD develops when people are unable to successfully integrate traumatic experiences into their lives—the core symptoms of anxiety, avoidance, and intrusive memories mean they experience the trauma as too painful to accept. The most effective strategy for preventing PTSD from developing is to take steps to help a person come to grips with the experience as soon as possible after the traumatic event. This can be accomplished by encouraging the person to talk about the event and to express feelings, thoughts, and concerns about what happened. If the traumatic event affected a group of people (a natural disaster or a hostage-taking situation), group discussion is frequently helpful, although individual counseling may also be necessary. A single discussion about a traumatic event is probably not sufficient to prevent PTSD. Several discussions are preferable, particularly soon after the event, and people often benefit if some discussions are arranged months or even years later.

A strong social support system—ranging from family and friends to groups set up especially for people exposed to traumatic events—is also crucial for preventing PTSD. Evidence indicates that people with weak social supports are more vulnerable to developing PTSD. This may be partly due to the fact that people are more likely to talk about a traumatic life experience if a close, supportive person is available. Thus, if PTSD is to be prevented in people exposed to traumas, existing support systems must be strengthened and new ones set up—perhaps through family therapy (to improve family members' understanding of the situation) or by encouraging the traumatized individual to seek out a supportive person, such as a member of the clergy. ☐

CHILDREN'S HEART PROBLEMS

Samuel Kaplan, M.D.

Nearly one in every hundred children born in the United States has a heart abnormality. Other heart problems can develop later in childhood as a result of illness. Many heart abnormalities are so minor they need no treatment, and some even heal on their own. But for a number of defects, medical or surgical intervention is essential. In the past physicians generally waited until a child was five or older to operate on the heart. But the field of pediatric cardiology has changed dramatically in recent years, and today surgical repair of heart defects is often done with infants.

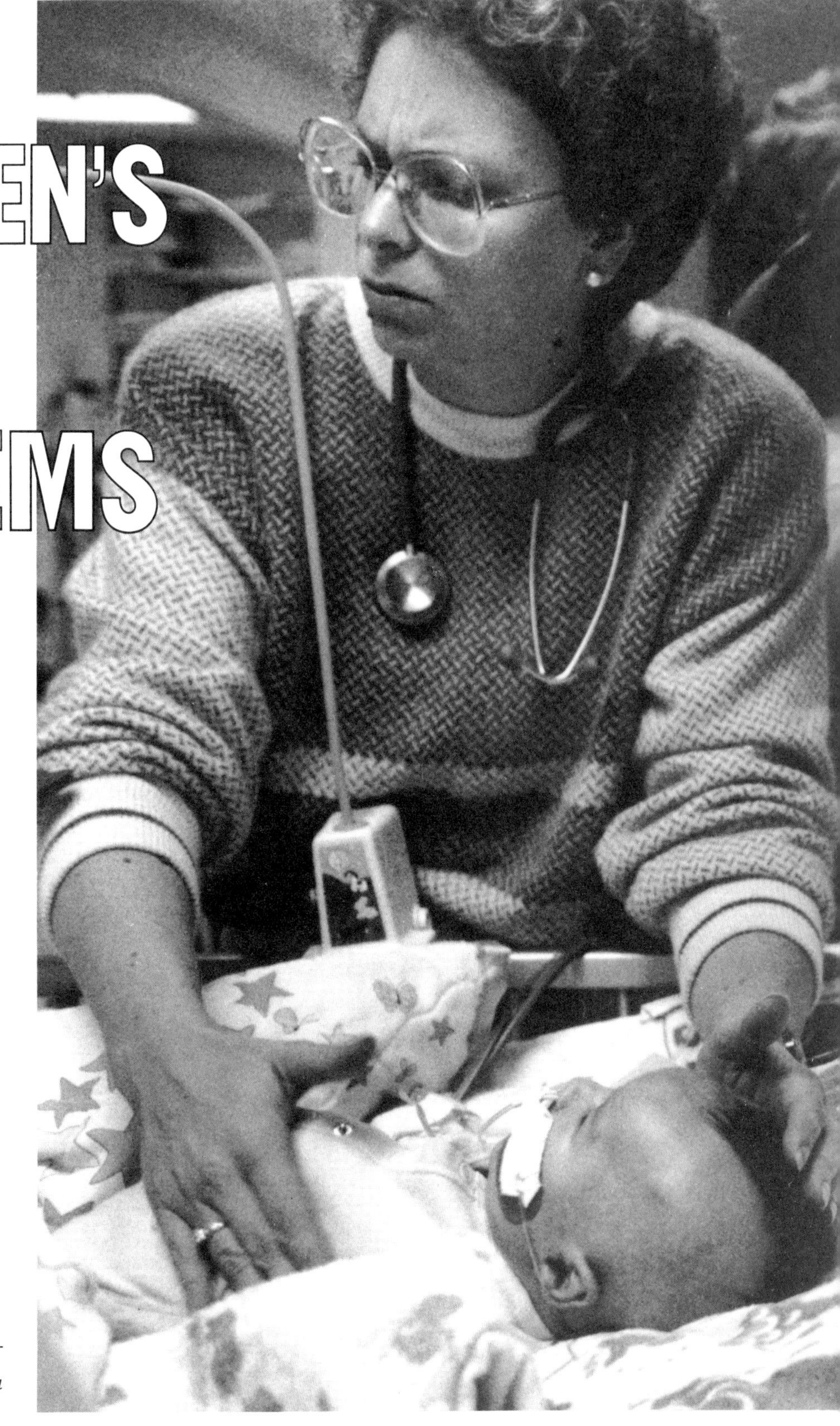

A doctor monitors a baby with a heart defect.

Congenital Heart Problems

The major focus of pediatric cardiology is on the diagnosis and treatment of congenital heart disease, conditions with which the child is born. The heart is basically two pumps, side by side. Each has an upper chamber, or atrium, linked by a valve to a lower chamber, or ventricle. (A valve is a flap of tissue that allows blood to flow only one way.) Normally, "used" blood—blood that has made a full circuit of the body, depositing oxygen in the tissues and picking up waste gases such as carbon dioxide—comes back to the right atrium, passes through the tricuspid valve into the right ventricle, and is then pumped to the lungs through the pulmonary arteries. In the lungs the blood deposits the waste gases and picks up a fresh supply of oxygen. The reoxygenated blood is carried by the pulmonary veins to the left atrium and passes through the mitral valve into the left ventricle; it is then pumped out through the aorta to the rest of the body.

Most congenital heart defects are diagnosed in infancy or early childhood.

When major congenital heart abnormalities are present—in the form of holes in the partitions (septa) between the heart chambers, valve obstruction or leakage, or abnormal connection to the heart of the major arteries or veins—blood does not circulate normally. These abnormalities may occur alone or in combination; for example, a child may have both septal defects and valve obstruction. Most defects are diagnosed in infancy and early childhood, but others may escape recognition until later in life because the child or adolescent has no symptoms and the problem is difficult to detect with a routine physical examination. One defect sometimes not diagnosed until adult life is an atrial septal defect, a hole in the septum between the upper heart chambers through which blood can leak. Because the left ventricle is stiffer than the right and therefore more difficult to fill, the blood is shunted from the left to the right atrium, overloading the right heart chambers and putting a possibly lethal strain on them.

Another common condition sometimes not diagnosed until later in life is an abnormality of the aortic valve, which is located between the left ventricle and the aorta. The aortic valve normally has three leaflets, or divisions, resembling a cloverleaf. In some individuals there are only two leaflets. While the valve may function normally for many decades, it frequently degenerates, slowly thickening and narrowing the valve opening so that not enough blood passes through and also allowing some leakage, or backward flow of blood. Approximately one-half of the aortic valves replaced surgically in adults are found to have this congenital abnormality.

The most common congenital heart abnormality is a ventricular septal defect, a hole between the two ventricles. The prognosis for a child with this problem depends on the size and location of the defect, the volume of blood shunted from left to right ventricle, and how much the circulation in the lungs is affected. The majority of small defects close spontaneously, usually in the first year or two of life. Large defects cause serious problems. Normally the pressure in the right ven-

---

Samuel Kaplan is a professor of pediatrics at the University of California-Los Angeles School of Medicine.

The Normal Heart and Two Congenital Defects

The Normal Heart

In the normal heart newly oxygenated blood travels from the lungs to the left atrium via the pulmonary veins. After passing through the mitral valve into the heart's main pumping chamber, the left ventricle, it is pumped through another valve, the aortic valve, into the aorta and from there to the body. After it has circulated through the body it comes back to the right atrium and passes through the tricuspid valve into the right ventricle. It is then pumped through the pulmonary valve into the pulmonary arteries and back to the lungs.

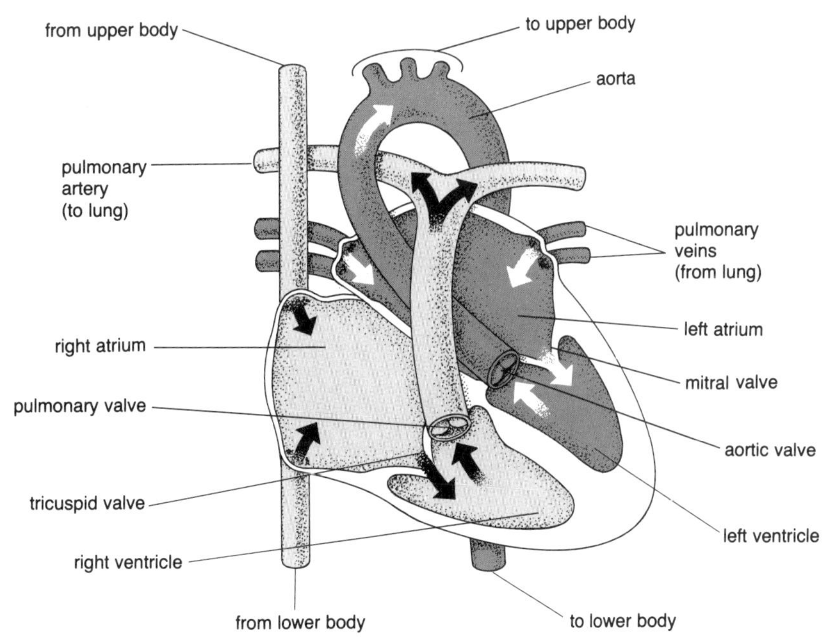

Patent Ductus Arteriosus

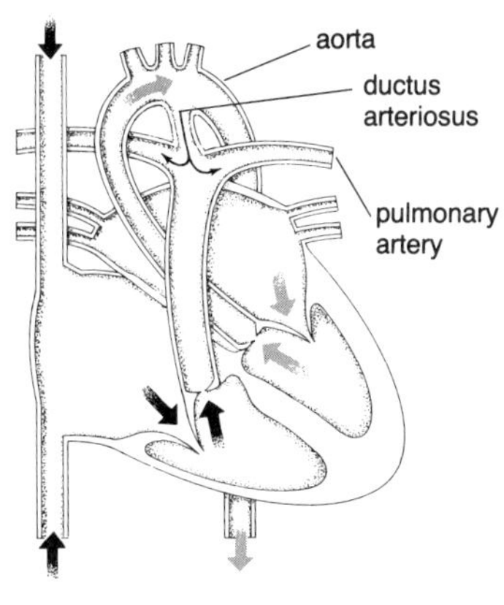

Before a baby is born, the ductus arteriosus channels blood from the baby's pulmonary artery directly to the aorta. The connection is supposed to close after birth. If it does not, oxygenated blood on its way through the aorta to the body leaks back into the pulmonary artery, and the left ventricle has to pump harder to supply enough oxygenated blood to the body.

Ventricular Septal Defect

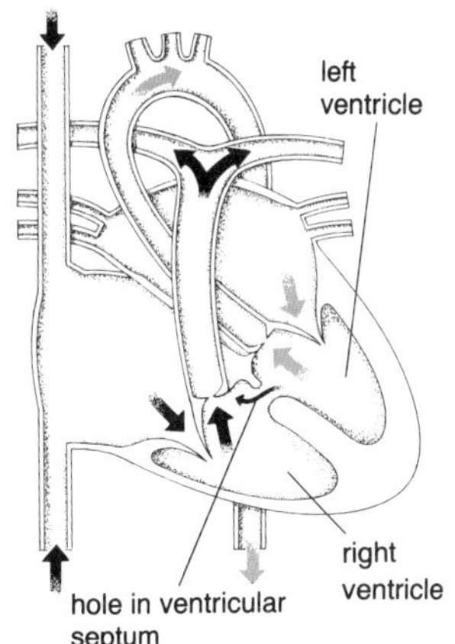

A hole in the septum between the left and right ventricles allows blood to leak from the left to the right. More blood than normal to deal with puts a strain on the right side of the heart.

---

tricle is less than one-quarter of that in the left, but a large defect, besides allowing a large shunt of blood from the left to the right ventricle, equalizes the pressure in the two. The significant pressure increase in the right ventricle puts abnormal pressure on the pulmonary artery. Babies with large defects breathe much faster than is normal, are poor feeders (because it is not possible to breathe and swallow at the same time), and grow slowly.

A major concern is the effect on the circulation in the lungs. If the pressure in the pulmonary arterial system rises significantly, the system may be permanently damaged. Another danger is that the overstressed heart may fail altogether. Thus, surgical closure of the defect is advised when medical treatment fails. Fortunately, the risk of surgery is low (generally less than 3 percent). Infants with large defects who survive without surgery are destined to a restricted life-style with permanently limited physical capacity.

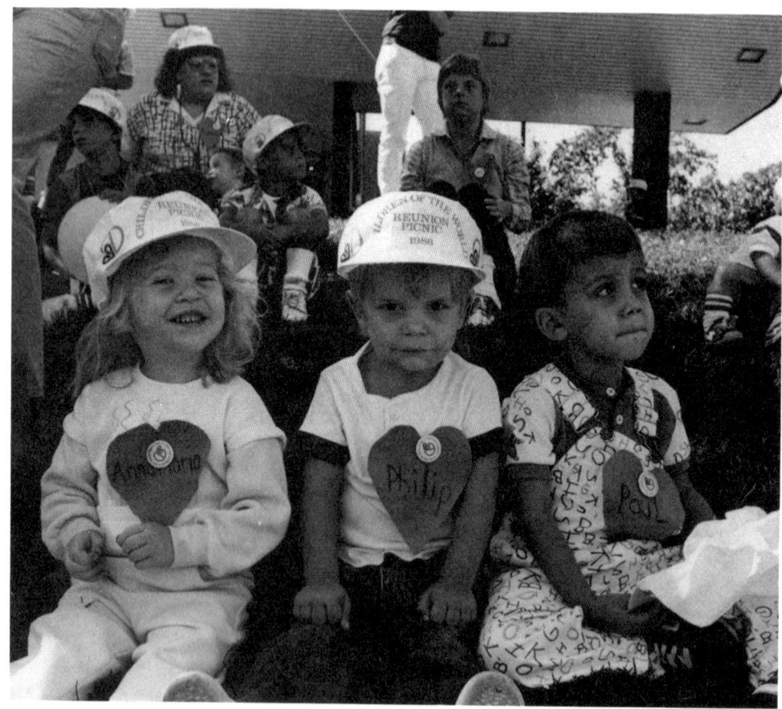

Former pediatric heart surgery patients of the Deborah Heart and Lung Center in New Jersey gather for a reunion picnic.

Diagnostic Procedures

For many years cardiac catheterization has been the most valuable diagnostic procedure for evaluating the functioning of the heart. A thin tube, or catheter, is inserted into a vein or artery (usually in the groin) and threaded to the heart. With X rays monitoring its movements continuously, the catheter is manipulated into the veins entering the heart, the heart chambers, and the arteries leaving the heart. The procedure allows physicians to measure pressure within the heart, take samples of blood to determine its oxygen content, and calculate the pumping power of the ventricles and blood flow through the valves. Fluid that shows up on X rays can also be delivered rapidly through the catheter to heart chambers and blood vessels so that the course of blood flow can be recorded on film. Analysis of data from catheterization procedures helps physicians make correct diagnoses and plan surgical procedures.

Recently, other techniques have been developed that allow imaging of the heart and blood vessels as well as evaluation of heart function. Diagnostic ultrasound (also called echocardiography) uses sound waves to display the anatomy of the heart and measure blood flow through the various chambers and valves. The technique is an attractive alternative to X rays because ultrasound has no known harmful biologic effects. Echocardiography is noninvasive; images are obtained from a device placed on the chest, and no equipment needs to be inserted into the body.

Magnetic resonance imaging (MRI) has been used to provide a "picture" of the heart, veins, and arteries, especially branch pulmonary arteries and the aorta. Radionuclide imaging, in which a radiation-emitting material is injected into the bloodstream and traced with a special camera, allows the physician to determine the size of the heart chambers and the changes produced by contraction of the ventricles. Radionuclide imaging is used primarily to assess heart function at rest and during exercise.

Most evaluations of heart function, including physical examinations and sophisticated tests, are done while the patient is at rest. But the resting state is not "normal" for the growing, active child. Heart function is now evaluated before, during, and after exercise (on a stationary bicycle or treadmill) and note is made of any changes in heart rate, blood pressure, electrocardiogram readings (which measure the heart's electrical activity), the amount of blood pumped by the heart per beat or per minute, the amount of oxygen consumed, and the amount of carbon dioxide produced. These tests of cardiovascular performance may unmask abnormalities that are not detectable at rest or during ordinary activities. They also help to determine the type and form of exercise that may be undertaken by the growing person with heart disease.

Treatment With Prostaglandins

Prostaglandins are hormonelike substances that are produced by nearly all types of cells in the body and play a role in almost all biologic processes. They are also used therapeutically for a number of conditions, one of which is a heart problem in newborns. Prostaglandins can relax the smooth muscle in the walls of arteries, including the ductus arteriosus, the artery connecting the aorta and pulmonary artery in the newborn baby. This connecting artery is essential in fetal life when circu-

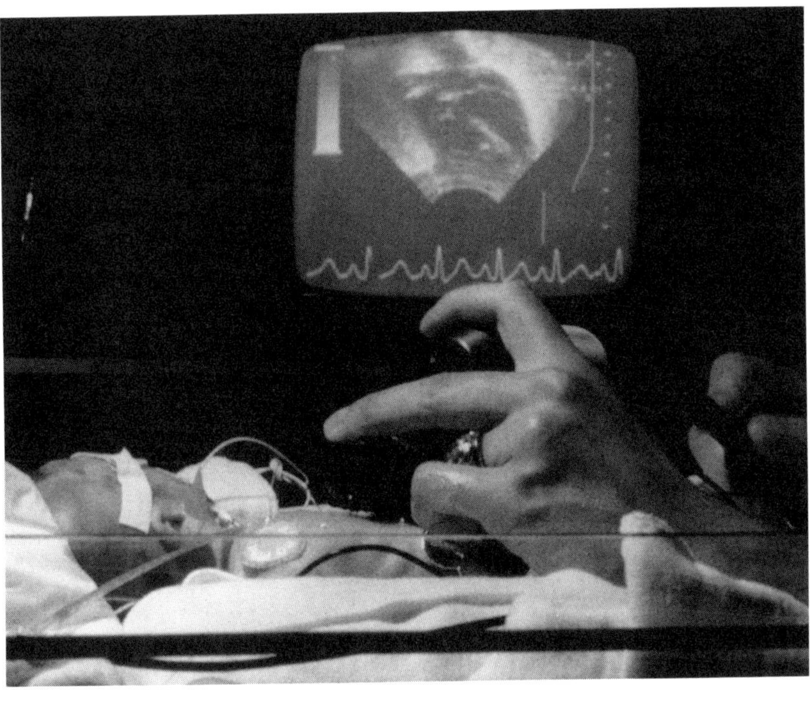

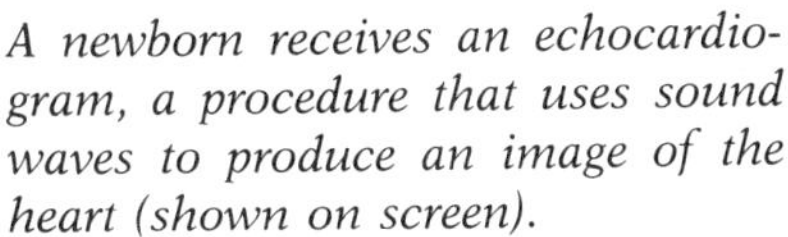

A newborn receives an echocardiogram, a procedure that uses sound waves to produce an image of the heart (shown on screen).

lation to the lungs is unnecessary, but it usually closes soon after birth. Its failure to close can cause respiratory problems. However, some babies are born with complex heart diseases in which blood cannot flow to the lungs unless the ductus arteriosus remains open. If blood flow is not maintained, the condition is generally lethal. Once the newborn's heart abnormality is diagnosed, prostaglandins are given intravenously to keep the ductus open and stabilize the baby's critical state. This allows more leisurely planning of surgery to be done when the baby's condition has improved significantly.

Balloon Catheter Treatment

Balloon-tipped catheters are used to treat obstructed valves and blood vessels.

During the past decade balloon-tipped catheters have been developed to treat congenital obstructions in heart valves and blood vessels. The first type of valve to be successfully relieved of obstruction was the pulmonary valve, which is located between the right ventricle and the pulmonary artery. The balloon-tipped catheter is threaded through a vein or artery and placed in the obstructed valve. The balloon is then repeatedly rapidly inflated for a few seconds and rapidly deflated, until the obstruction is relieved. This method of treating pulmonary valve blockage is attractive because it is usually successful, does not require open heart surgery, does not leave a scar on the chest and is less expensive than open surgery. Follow-up after about eight years has shown that the valve usually remains unobstructed. The procedure is usually not successful if the valve is thick and immobile.

Balloon catheter treatment has also been used on obstructed aortic valves. While the obstruction may be relieved, the procedure may produce or increase leakage of the valve. Balloon catheter treatment does not cure aortic valve obstruction. It is too early to be sure, but pediatric cardiologists expect that in later years aortic valves treated with balloon-tipped catheters will need to be replaced with artificial valves or with valves that are made of human tissue obtained from a donor after death.

Recurring obstruction after surgery for congenital narrowing of the aorta (coarctation of the aorta) has also been alleviated by treatment with balloon catheters. In some medical centers balloon treatment of coarctation of the aorta that has not been surgically corrected has been successful.

Balloon catheter treatment of obstruction of the mitral valve, which is located between the left atrium and left ventricle, has also been successful. Mitral valve obstruction may follow acute rheumatic fever, which is still frequent in less industrialized countries. Balloon treatment is especially attractive in these countries, where open-heart surgical facilities are limited.

Devices have been mounted on the tips of catheters to close the ductus arteriosus if it fails to close on its own after birth (a condition called patent ductus arteriosus) and to close holes between heart chambers, especially atrial septal defects. Although these devices have been used extensively in some medical centers, the procedures were still considered experimental in early 1991 and had not been approved by the U.S. Food and Drug Administration. Abnormal connections between blood vessels have also been treated with specially designed catheters that place plastic material or coils to block blood flow.

Surgical Advances

Successful surgical treatment for some types of congenital heart disease has been available for decades. Patent ductus arteriosus was first operated on successfully in the late 1930s. Coarctation of the aorta was being corrected in the 1940s; the dramatic blue baby operation, which increases blood flow to the lungs in children with decreased flow caused by a variety of abnormalities, was introduced in the same decade. In the mid-1950s the introduction of open-heart surgery allowed heart chambers and blood vessels to be opened while the function of the heart and lungs was temporarily taken over by an artificial heart-lung machine.

Results of surgical procedures such as these are dramatic. They make it possible for children who are frail, have a blue tinge to their skin, and live sedentary lives because of limited tolerance of exercise to begin leading nearly normal lives. It should be pointed out, however, that these operations are not curative. Sometimes the original problem recurs or a new one develops in its place. Annual or more frequent examinations may be necessary to check for such complications.

Surgery for congenital heart defects can have dramatic results.

Recent major advances in surgery include the development of techniques for operating on newborns and young infants. One complex defect correctible through open-heart surgery is called transposition of the great arteries. The aorta and the pulmonary artery connect to the wrong ventricles, so that "used" blood circulates through the body and oxygenated blood goes back and forth between the heart and the lungs. This relatively common condition can now be treated in the first few weeks of life by disconnecting the great arteries from the heart and reconnecting them to their proper ventricles. At the same time the arteries nourishing the heart, the coronary arteries, are reconnected to the new aorta. The results of this operation, immediately and five or more years later, are encouraging.

Another complex heart condition, in which there is virtually only one ventricle, is now amenable to surgical correction. Surgeons can route "used" blood returning from the body to the right side of the heart directly to the pulmonary artery, which will transport it to the lungs for oxygenation. In properly selected patients this operation results in dramatic, immediate improvement. However, complications include temporary retention of fluid and heart rhythm abnormalities. Long-term results are not available, and it is not known whether this type of circulation can be maintained indefinitely.

To treat a condition in which the main stem of the pulmonary artery—before it divides to go to the left and right lungs—is missing, a number of prostheses, or artificial devices, have been developed over the years to connect the right ventricle and what exists of the artery. The early devices were not durable and deteriorated with time. The common practice today is to use human tissue—an aortic valve and aorta or a pulmonary valve and artery obtained from a donor after death. These human tissue prostheses have good immediate results, are

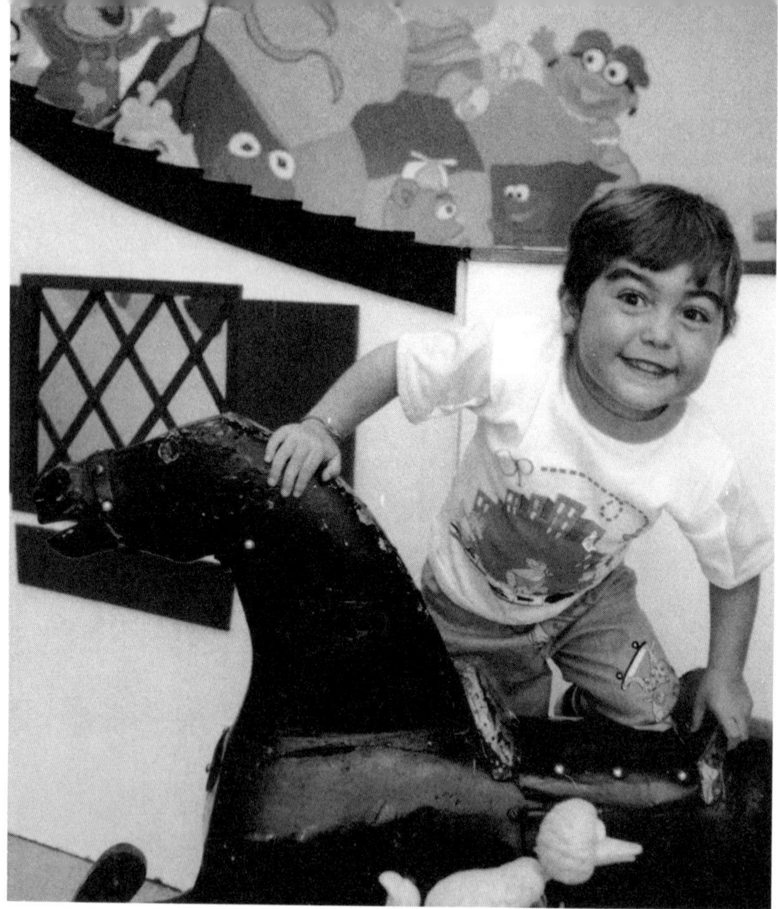

Transplant Recipients

After a heart transplant, children's energy levels bounce back to near normal, as seen in the four-year-old at left. However, like the girl at right, they must take antirejection medication religiously for the rest of their lives.

not subject to rejection, and are more durable than those used previously. However, it is expected that they will need replacement after a number of years.

Heart Transplants

About one-tenth of all heart transplants performed in the United States are done in children who because of heart muscle disease or complex congenital heart abnormalities might not otherwise survive. A problem that requires treatment in early life, usually in the first month, is severe underdevelopment of the major pumping chamber of the heart, a condition called hypoplastic left heart syndrome. Two surgical options are available, heart transplantation or a staged procedure consisting of at least two operations. A number of considerations apply to pediatric heart transplantation. The number of donors is limited so that many infants and children die while waiting for a suitable organ. The child who gets a new heart is committed to a lifetime of treatment and observation to prevent rejection of the heart. Additionally, the treatment to prevent rejection suppresses the immune system, placing the child at risk for infection. The drugs used to prevent rejection have other important side effects, too. For example, the drug cyclosporine significantly reduces episodes of rejection but can affect the kidneys in such a way as to produce sustained high blood pressure, which requires medical treatment. Other potent antirejection medications are being studied at this time, but their availability is limited and their long-term effects unknown. For many years steroids have been used to prevent rejection, but they can stunt a child's growth.

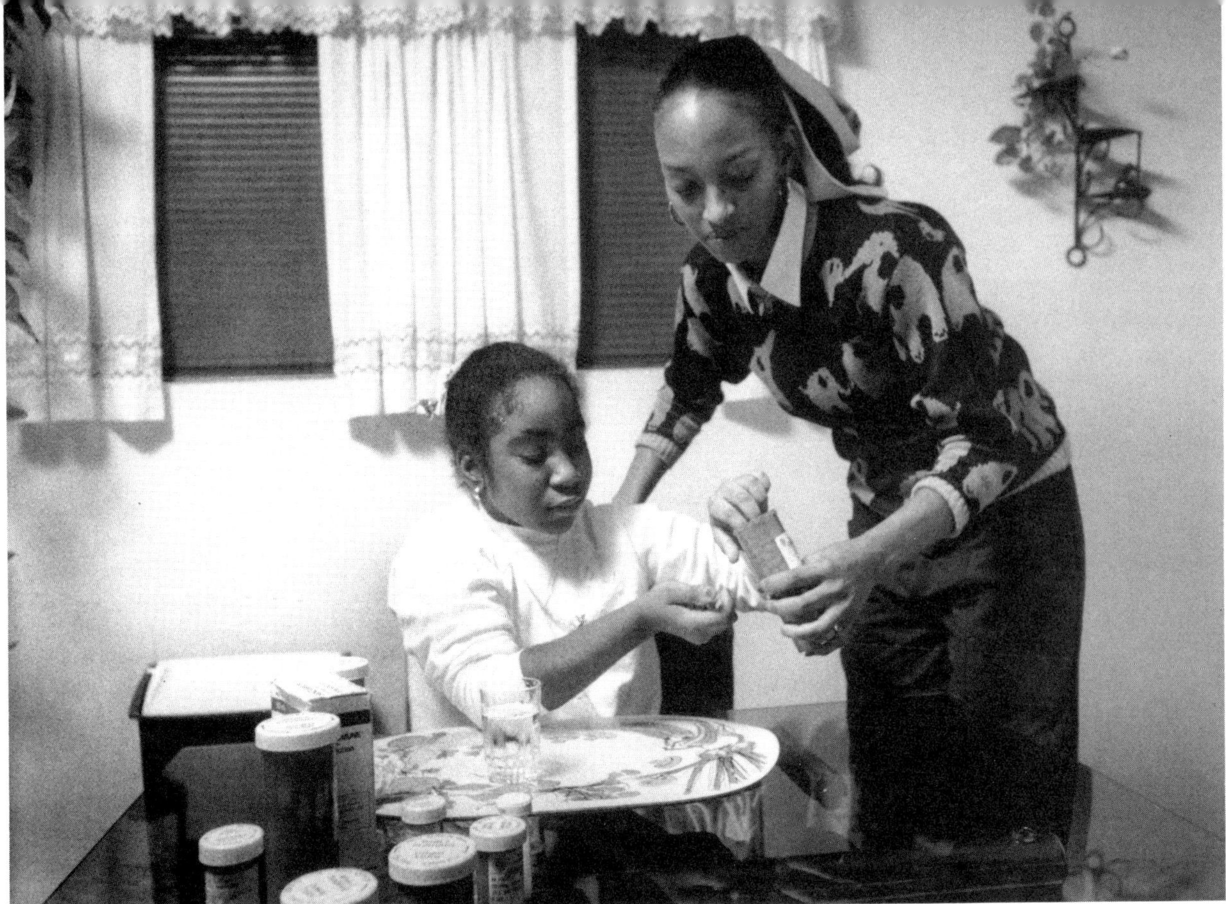

Another important complication of heart transplantation is the development of hardening of the coronary arteries (atherosclerosis) in the transplanted heart, which causes it to pump less efficiently. Why this happens has not been determined, but it may be part of a chronic rejection process.

A problem most frequently encountered in treating teenage transplant recipients is that they cut back on their medicine or stop taking it entirely. Within a few months after a transplant, the improvement in quality of life is so striking that many teenagers believe their body has accepted the new heart and they no longer need antirejection medication. As a result, the number of rejection episodes is higher in teenagers, and they may require frequent hospitalization for treatment of acute rejection.

Lung Transplants

A major complication of many types of congenital heart disease is the development of pulmonary hypertension, or severe high blood pressure in the arteries carrying blood to the lungs. This results in irreversible damage to these arteries and makes surgical treatment of the congenital heart disease inadvisable. Children with pulmonary hypertension can survive into adulthood, but their life span is usually shortened. In the mid-1980s combined heart and lung transplantation was used successfully to treat these patients. However, there were not enough donor hearts and lungs for everyone who needed them, and many patients died while waiting for the operation. Fortunately, methods have been developed for transplanting one or a pair of lungs and correcting

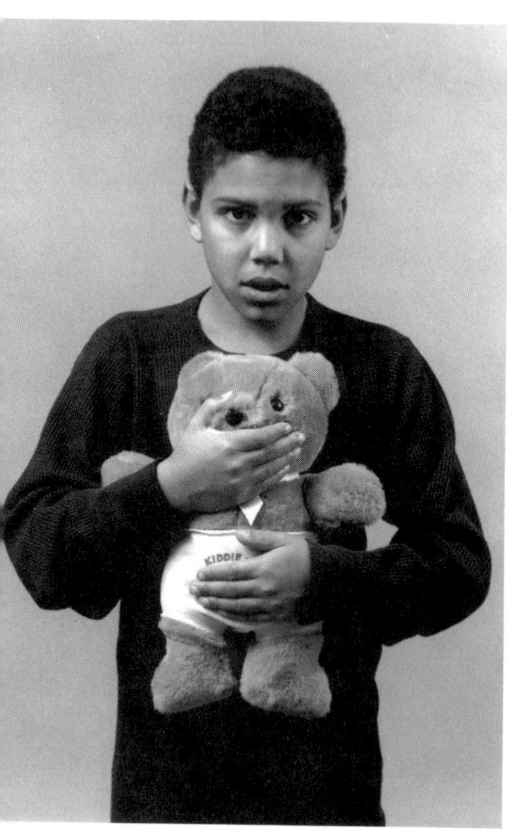

A stuffed bear called the Kiddie Kub helps young open heart surgery patients do the essential deep breathing and coughing exercises that prevent complications. Here, a boy demonstrates how the bear is pressed against the chest.

the heart abnormality during the same operation. Immediate results of these procedures are encouraging, but long-term evaluation is not available.

Fetal Cardiology

Ultrasound examination of the developing fetus is used frequently in obstetric practice and has improved prenatal diagnosis and the monitoring of problem pregnancies. In the past decade diagnostic ultrasound evaluation of the developing fetal heart has become available and has been used to detect congenital heart disease in fetuses considered at risk for such problems. One risk factor is heredity, since the prevalence of congenital heart disease is somewhat increased in families with known heart abnormalities. Other risk factors are that the pregnant woman has a chronic controlled disease such as diabetes or vascular disease, has been exposed to German measles, requires medication for chronic diseases such as epilepsy, or abuses alcohol during pregnancy. When serious congenital heart disease is diagnosed in the fetus, parents and physicians have time to contemplate the need for specialized medical care and to anticipate cardiac problems during the first few days of life. Knowing ahead of time may also prevent the misunderstanding, the confusion, and the anger that may occur in families who are suddenly faced with a newborn who has a potentially fatal heart problem.

Sometimes fetal heart problems can be treated in the womb. An exciting advance is the recognition that heart failure in the fetus can result from a persistently abnormal rapid heart rate and that this condition can be controlled by giving the mother heart-rate stabilizing medication that passes across the placenta to the fetus. The normal fetal heart rate varies from about 120 to 160 beats per minute toward the end of pregnancy. Rates that persist above 240 beats per minute compromise the fetal heart's ability to eject normal volumes of blood. This results in fluid accumulation in the abdomen, the pericardium (the sac that surrounds the heart), and the surface tissues of the body, especially the scalp. The increased demand on the heart results in significantly enlarged heart chambers. Other symptoms include a placenta that is larger than normal and a large volume of amniotic fluid. All of these findings are readily recognized by ultrasound examination. Heart rate can be measured by ultrasound by noting the number of times per minute that the aortic valve opens and closes. A discrepancy between the rate of beating of the ventricles and of the atria that is typical of this condition can also be observed. If the fetal heart rate can be controlled, signs of heart failure disappear, and a normal baby is delivered. If not, the newborn arrives swollen, breathless, and severely ill.

Noncongenital Heart Problems

In addition to congenital abnormalities, there are a number of illnesses that can cause cardiovascular disease and cardiovascular system malfunctioning.

Rheumatic Fever. Rheumatic fever is generally preceded by an acute streptococcal throat infection. About one to two weeks after the strep throat has subsided, an attack on the heart begins which frequently results in long-term, significant valve damage and weakening of the heart muscle. In the first five to six decades of this century, disability and death from rheumatic heart disease were common. Around the time of World War II it was learned that acute rheumatic fever could be prevented in young military recruits by early treatment of streptococcal throat infection with penicillin and that recurrences could be prevented by monthly injections of long-acting penicillin. This practice was soon applied to the treatment of strep throat in children. This first implementation of preventive cardiology significantly reduced the prevalence of rheumatic heart disease in the United States and other industrialized societies so that acute rheumatic fever is now rare. Vigilance must be maintained, however, because in the past decade clusters of patients with the disease have again been recognized in the United States. In less developed countries where facilities for diagnosis and treatment of strep throat are lacking, rheumatic heart disease is still one of the common causes of disability and death among children, adolescents, and young adults.

Kawasaki Disease. In the 1960s a Japanese pediatrician recognized a disease that now carries his name. The cause of Kawasaki disease is unknown, but it is associated with abnormal functioning of the immune system, probably triggered by an infection. It affects mostly children under age five. Pediatric cardiologists became involved when it was recognized that about 20 percent of children with Kawasaki disease also developed weakening of the walls of the coronary arteries that results in aneurysms, ballooning of segments of the arteries. These aneurysms can heal without apparent residual effects or can progress to narrowing or obstruction of the coronary arteries, leading to later heart attacks.

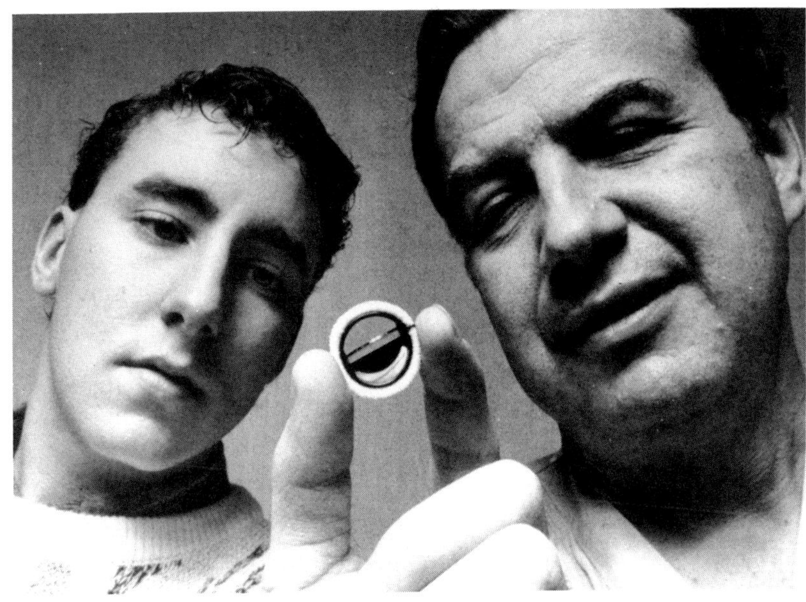

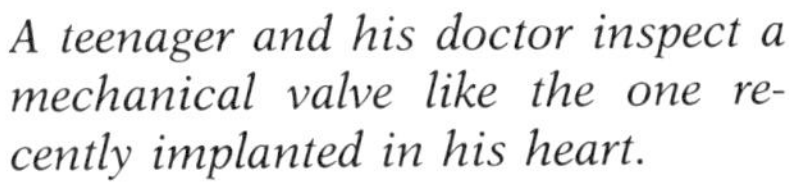

A teenager and his doctor inspect a mechanical valve like the one recently implanted in his heart.

Diseases such as rheumatic fever, Kawasaki disease, and AIDS can damage children's hearts and blood vessels.

The initial symptoms of Kawasaki disease are a persistent fever, red eyes, fissuring and crusting of the lips, a tongue with the appearance and color of a strawberry, a body rash, swelling of the hands and feet later followed by peeling of the skin, and enlarged lymph nodes. After about one to three weeks aneurysms of the coronary arteries show up (they can be detected by ultrasound). The incidence of coronary disease is reduced significantly, but not eliminated, by treatment with intravenous gamma globulin and aspirin. This treatment also improves the general symptoms of the disease.

Heart Muscle Inflammation. Inflammation of the heart muscle, called myocarditis, can be caused by a number of microorganisms (including bacteria and parasites) but is most commonly caused by a viral infection. In most instances a specific viral disease cannot be pinpointed as the cause because the heart muscle problem may become apparent only weeks, months, or even years after the infection. In some cases, shock and heart failure resulting from myocarditis accompany the viral infection. Myocarditis in newborns is generally caused by certain viruses that can inhabit the bowel of children and adults without causing disease. It is assumed that newborns are infected from their mothers during or soon after birth or from outbreaks of infection in hospital nurseries.

Late effects of myocarditis in children and adolescents are the result of poor heart muscle function—the heart cannot pump enough blood and nutrients to meet the body's demands. Symptoms include shortness of breath during moderate or minimal exercise, retention of fluid with swelling of the ankles and legs, enlargement of the heart, and heart rhythm abnormalities. Most children respond well to the medications used to treat heart failure, but the ultimate outcome is unpredictable. A minority do not respond to medications and need a heart transplant.

AIDS. Recent evidence indicates that infection with the human immunodeficiency virus (HIV)—the virus that causes AIDS—is associated with disorders of the cardiovascular system. These disorders affect fetuses and babies who acquire AIDS from their infected mothers during pregnancy or immediately after birth.

Heart muscle function can be affected as a result of inflammation from HIV or from unusual organisms to which these children are susceptible because of their compromised immune systems. Inflammation can lead to inadequate pumping of blood by the heart muscle, resulting in heart failure.

Frequent abnormalities in heart rate (usually significant increases) and in blood pressure (usually decreases) have been attributed to disease of the nerves that stimulate the heart and blood vessels, nerves which are affected early in AIDS. Heart rhythm abnormalities may also occur. Fluid collecting around the heart may further compromise its functioning. Lung disorders that are common in babies with AIDS may also affect heart function. Heart and vascular abnormalities may not be apparent because they are overshadowed by the infections that accompany AIDS. However, involvement of the heart and blood vessels is frequent and can be detected by ultrasound examination of the heart and heart rhythm monitoring. □

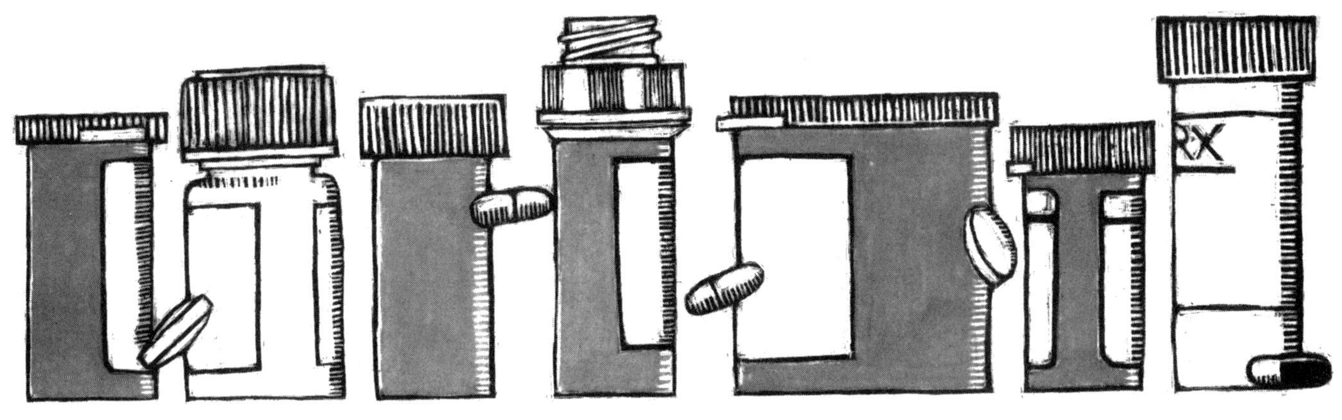

ANTIBIOTICS

Thomas H. Maugh II, Ph.D.

Humans have been battling bacterial infections since the dawn of time. Harmful bacteria can enter the body through the respiratory system, the digestive system, the genitals, or breaks in the skin; they then multiply and produce toxins that may cause serious illness or even death. The development of the class of antibacterial agents called antibiotics was thus one of the greatest achievements in medicine.

Antibiotics are chemical substances produced by or derived from microorganisms that inhibit the growth of or even kill disease-causing bacteria. They are effective against a wide range of illnesses, from ear and throat infections to meningitis, tuberculosis, and most cases of pneumonia. Arguably, they are a primary reason that the average life span of humans has increased from less than 40 years at the end of the 18th century to nearly double that today in the developed nations.

Early Research

Although humans have used molds to treat infections at least since the beginnings of civilization, the first major breakthrough in fighting infection did not come until 1865. In that year, surgeon Joseph Lister of the Glasgow Royal Infirmary, concerned about mortality rates following surgery, began using a synthetic chemical called phenol (carbolic acid) to disinfect instruments, wounds, and incisions; he also sprayed a phenol solution into the air to kill microorganisms, or microbes. (Phenol is too poisonous to be used internally.) By 1869 the mortality rate on Lister's ward had dropped from 45 percent to 15 percent. His achievement is all the more remarkable because, although French scientist Louis Pasteur, a giant in the field of microbiology, had earlier theorized that there was a connection between microorganisms and disease, it was not until 1876 that German doctor Robert Koch first *proved* that bacteria cause disease.

Another pioneer in the field of bacteriology was the German physician Paul Ehrlich. In the early 1900s, Ehrlich, then director of the Royal Institute for Experimental Therapy in Frankfurt, unsuccessfully tried 605 different arsenic compounds against

---

Thomas H. Maugh II is a science writer for the Los Angeles Times.

microbes. But number 606, arsphenamine, was a winner: it killed the microorganism that causes syphilis. Ehrlich theorized that some chemicals, which he called "magic bullets," might bind to and kill bacteria without harming human cells.

German pathologist Gerhard Domagk of the I.G. Farbenindustrie Laboratory for Experimental Pathology and Bacteriology tried thousands of different dyes to test their therapeutic effects against bacteria before announcing in 1932 that he had found one compound, prontosil, that cured streptococcal infections in mice. Research soon demonstrated that enzymes in the mice converted the compound to sulfanilamide, the first of the sulfa drugs. Domagk won the 1939 Nobel Prize for his achievement. Known as the first of the wonder drugs, sulfa drugs were used in the 1930s to treat a variety of infectious diseases, including pneumonia and blood poisoning. The drugs saved countless lives during World War II.

Penicillin Discovered

But nature proved a more effective chemist than man, as shown by a chance discovery in 1928 by British pathologist Sir Alexander Fleming of St. Mary's Hospital in London. Fleming observed that spores from a bread mold called *Penicillium notatum* had contaminated a laboratory dish in which he was growing bacteria, killing the bacteria. Although he realized the significance of the growth-inhibiting substance, which he called penicillin, he did not have the funds to isolate it for testing.

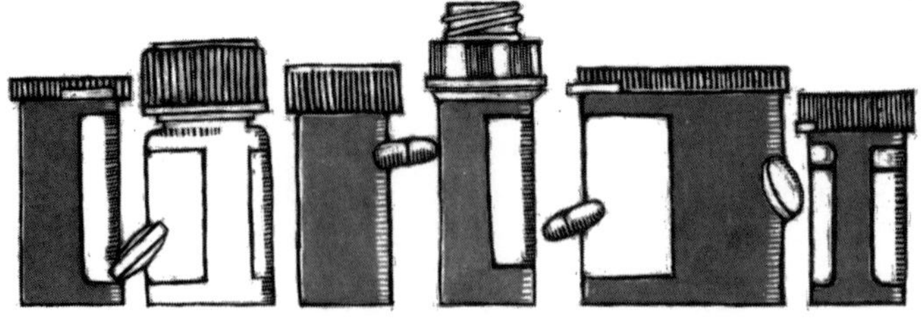

That task fell to two other scientists. Prompted by the need for antibacterial drugs during the early days of World War II, Australian pathologist Sir Howard W. Florey and British biochemist Ernst B. Chain did isolate penicillin from the mold. They tried this antibiotic on humans for the first time in the winter of 1940-1941, with encouraging results. The penicillin family of drugs soon became the single most important group of antibacterial agents. Fleming, Florey, and Chain shared the 1945 Nobel Prize for their work.

Further Advances

New antibiotics were isolated in quick succession in the mid-20th century. Among them, to name just a few, were gramicidin, isolated from a soil bacterium in 1939 and the first antibiotic to be produced commercially; streptomycin, found in 1943; chloramphenicol, isolated in 1947 in a soil microorganism from Venezuela and useful against life-threatening infections such as typhoid and meningitis; aureomycin, the first of the broad-spectrum tetracyclines (effective against a wide range of bacteria), found in 1948 in a mold; and rifampin, produced in 1957 by chemical modification of another mold product and useful against tuberculosis and meningococcal infections.

By the late 1950s, for the first time, physicians had the choice of a wide range of antibiotics in fighting infections. Each of them, as well as many others discovered later, worked against a particular group of microbes, which is why antibiotics are classified according to their effectiveness against specific bacteria rather than against certain illnesses. Some illnesses, for example, pneumonia, can be caused by more than one type of microorganism. Depending on the bacterium causing the disease, different antibiotics may be given.

If an infection is viral, no antibiotic will knock it out. For, as effective as they are against bacteria, these drugs are virtually useless against viruses—the cause of such illnesses as colds, influenza, hepatitis, and AIDS (and certain types of pneumonia).

Penicillin Pros and Cons

Penicillin, the prototype antibiotic and the progenitor of the family of antibiotics that is still most widely used, was found to have an unusual chemical structure. It is characterized by a ring, called a beta-lactam, containing three carbon atoms and one nitrogen. Because the beta-lactam ring, and a second ring fused to it, make penicillin look like a natural constituent of the cell walls of bacteria, the bacterial enzymes that construct the walls mistake penicillin for this constituent and bind to it. This binding action stops the growth and reproduction of the bacteria. Penicillin and the drugs derived from it have remarkably few side effects on humans, although some patients develop severe allergic reactions. Penicillins are so safe for most people, however, and so effective, they have become the most widely used family of antibiotics.

Researchers have produced a variety of penicillin derivatives that are much more effective than the original penicillin. They are, however, primarily effective against certain types of bacteria only: aerobic bacteria, which require oxygen for growth, and gram-positive bacteria, so called because they can be stained purple by certain chemicals. (The purpose of the staining technique is to classify the bacteria for various reasons.) Gram-negative bacteria, which cannot be stained purple and have a more complicated cell wall than gram-positive bacteria, and anaerobic bacteria, which die when they are exposed to oxygen, are generally insensitive to most penicillins.

When the penicillins were first introduced, the most common disease-producing bacteria were gram-positive, aerobic, or both. Now, most species of those bacteria can be controlled by penicillins. However, other antibiotics are usually preferred for treatment of infections caused by gram-negative organisms. The discovery of streptomycin in 1943 was important primarily because it was the first antibiotic to attack gram-negative and anaerobic bacteria, including the gram-negative organism that causes tuberculosis.

A problem with penicillins is the presence in certain bacteria, both gram-positive and gram-negative, of enzymes known as penicillinases or beta-lactamases. These enzymes break apart the beta-lactam ring, making the bacteria resistant to these and other antibiotics.

One approach to the problem of resistance has been to use penicillinase inhibitors—compounds that bind to the enzyme and inactivate it so that it cannot destroy the beta-lactam ring of the antibiotics. One such compound is clavulanic acid, which has a structure similar to penicillin, but very little antibiotic activity. By inhibiting penicillinase, however, it allows a beta-lactam antibiotic to destroy the penicillinase or beta-lactamase producing bacteria.

A product marketed as Augmentin, a combination of amoxicillin (a type of penicillin) and the potassium salt of clavulanic acid, has been shown to kill

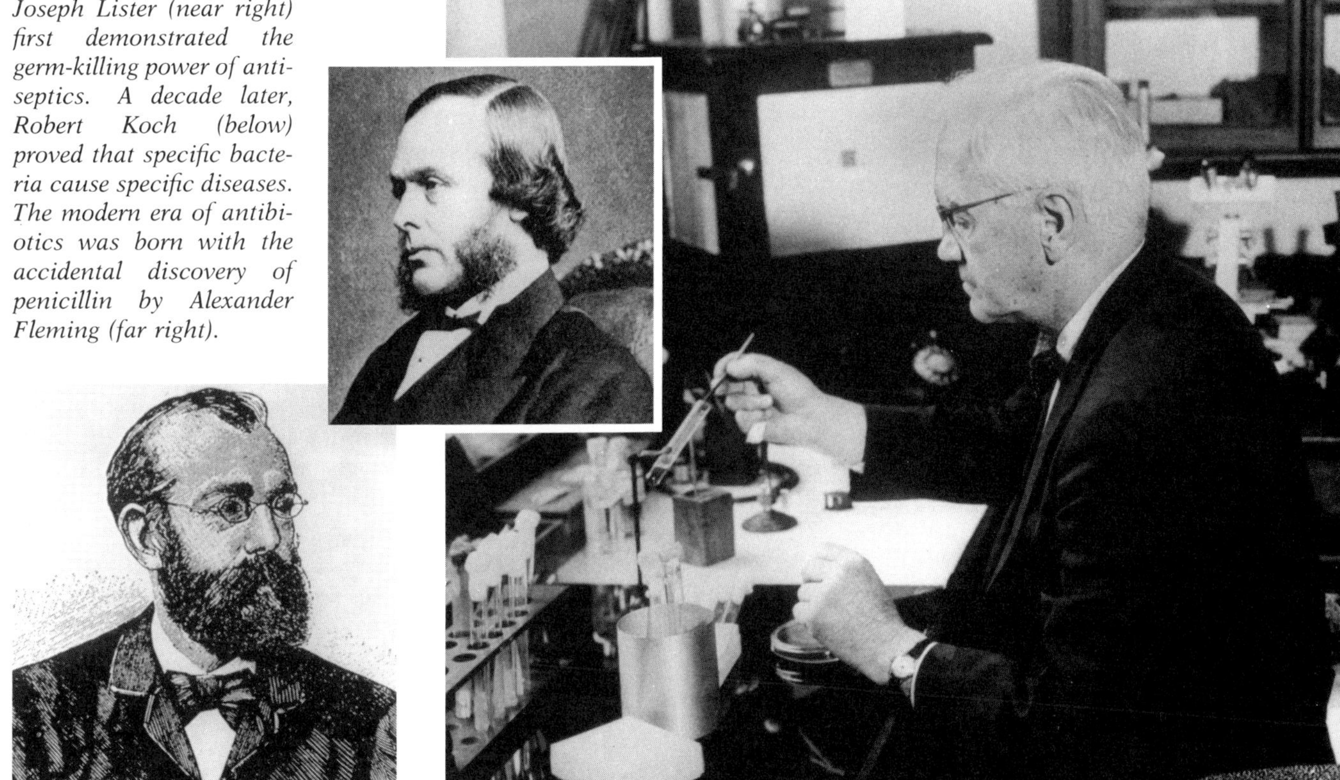

Joseph Lister (near right) first demonstrated the germ-killing power of antiseptics. A decade later, Robert Koch (below) proved that specific bacteria cause specific diseases. The modern era of antibiotics was born with the accidental discovery of penicillin by Alexander Fleming (far right).

amoxicillin-resistant microorganisms. Similarly, a product marketed as Timentin, a combination of a penicillin derivative called ticarcillin disodium and the potassium salt of clavulanic acid, has been shown to kill ticarcillin-resistant microorganisms.

Alternatives to Penicillin

A broader answer to the problems with penicillin was the development of another class of beta-lactam antibiotics called cephalosporins. The prototype cephalosporin was isolated from a fungus found at a sewage outfall off the coast of Sardinia.

The cephalosporins are active against a much broader range of bacteria than penicillins and have a greater intrinsic resistance to beta-lactamase enzymes. Researchers have further improved these useful properties by synthetically enhancing the drugs' chemical structure. On the down side, people who are allergic to the penicillins may also be allergic to the cephalosporins.

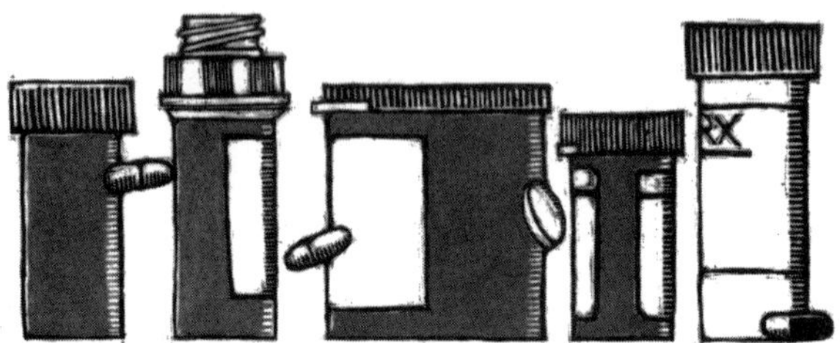

Pharmaceutical companies have been testing soil and water samples from all around the world looking for other potential antibiotics produced by microorganisms. Ironically, one of the best was found by researchers with the Squibb Institute for Medical Research in Princeton, N.J., in a soil sample from the Pine Barrens of New Jersey—only 50 miles from their laboratory. Dubbed monobactams, the newly discovered substances had only limited antibacterial activity when isolated from nature. But the Squibb scientists have made several totally synthetic monobactams that are much more effective. The first, called aztreonam, was approved by the U.S. Food and Drug Administration in 1986.

Aztreonam is active against gram-negative and aerobic bacteria but has almost no activity against gram-positive and anaerobic bacteria. This means that aztreonam will not kill naturally occurring gram-positive bacteria in the intestines, which is an advantage. Many researchers believe that the destruction of these and other beneficial bacteria during conventional antibiotic treatment allows resistant bacteria that might be present to increase in number, thereby helping to spread them through the population. Aztreonam requires intravenous or intramuscular administration.

How Antibiotics Work

Antibiotics work by a variety of different mechanisms. As explained earlier, the penicillins prevent the formation of new cell walls, so the bacteria can no longer grow and multiply. A number of other antibiotics work in the same way, including the cephalosporins and bacitracin. Some antibiotics work on the bacterial cell membrane, which lies immediately beneath the cell wall and controls the passage into and out of the cell of vital substances. Polymixin-type antibiotics are among those that kill bacteria by increasing the leakiness of cell membranes. Members of other groups of antibiotics block the synthesis of proteins vital to the growth of the bacteria. Included here are the tetracyclines, erythromicin, and aminoglycoside-class antibiotics such as streptomycin, gentamicin, and tobramycin.

Resistance

Certain bacteria are resistant to penicillins, as was discussed earlier. But penicillins are not the only antibiotics to which resistance exists. Researchers are not yet completely sure how resistance develops in all cases. Some bacteria may simply undergo mutations that allow them to adapt to the effect of certain antibiotics. In other cases, there may be a small naturally resistant population whose growth is favored when all the sensitive bacteria are killed by the antibiotic; many researchers believe that the widespread use of antibiotics as growth promoters in cattle contributes significantly to the development of resistance in this way. The unnecessary use of antibiotics (for example, against viral illnesses) also exacerbates the problem. Of even more concern to researchers is the finding that genes from one species of resistant bacteria can be transferred to nonresistant species during a specialized form of bacterial reproduction, thus conferring resistance on them.

Resistance can present severe problems for physicians and patients. Such is the case with tetracycline, which is widely used against acne, periodontal disease, and urinary tract infections because it is inexpensive and has relatively few side effects. A 1990 study of 200 women patients showed that anywhere from 20 to 90 percent of the bacteria in the women's urinary tracts were resistant to tetracycline. The solution to such resistance is to use other antibiotics and antibacterials, alone or in combination.

Resistance has also been a problem in the case of the organism that causes gonorrhea. Until recently, gonorrhea was usually treated with penicillins or, in patients allergic to them, with tetracycline. Against penicillin-resistant strains, however, physicians preferred to use spectinomycin. A study carried out in the late 1980s showed that the number of gonorrhea strains resistant to one or more of these drugs had increased tremendously. The antibiotic ceftriaxone is now recommended for treatment of gonorrhea.

Side Effects

A wide variety of side effects are associated with antibiotics, ranging from relatively mild to serious and life threatening. Some oral anitbiotics, for example, cause diarrhea. Some antibiotics administered by injection or applied directly to the skin cause skin reactions such as rashes or swellings. Some sensitize patients so they cannot be treated with them—or related ones—again. As noted earlier, penicillins and cephalosporins can cause serious allergic reactions in some people. Tetracycline stains children's teeth. Streptomycin and other aminoglycoside-class antibiotics can damage the kidneys and both the hearing and balance mechanisms of the inner ear and must be closely monitored. With all of this in mind, physicians who are deciding what antibiotic to prescribe in a particular case take care to weigh the desired benefits against the possible side effects.

Beyond Today's Antibiotics

To combat the infections caused by resistant bacteria, physicians are turning to certain synthetic anti-infective drugs. Among the most promising of these are the antibacterial quinolones. The first quinolone, a drug called nalidixic acid, has been available since 1962, but it was relatively ineffective unless large doses were given, which caused a wide variety of side effects. In the early 1980s, however, Japanese researchers found that by adding a fluorine atom to this and other quinolones, they could prepare more effective drugs that can be given in lower doses with fewer side effects. The new fluoroquinolones, ciprofloxacin and norfloxacin, have been shown to be particularly effective against gram-negative bacteria that cause persistent urinary tract infections. As of early 1991 they were being used by some physicians against the organism that causes Legionnaires' disease, although they were not formally approved for this use by the U.S. Food and Drug Administration.

For the future, researchers are looking at a number of new possibilities for fighting infections. Swedish researchers have developed what they call a "Trojan horse" antibiotic, a powerful drug that bacteria take inside their cells because it is camouflaged by being attached to a bacterial nutrient. And immunologists at the University of California at Los Angeles have isolated powerful antibacterial compounds called defensins from the white blood cells of animals, including humans. These drugs should eventually add new weapons to the physician's armamentarium against disease-causing bacteria. □

How to Take Antibiotics

As with any drug, it is important to read the label and follow directions. Some antibiotics are not absorbed well by the body in the presence of food or dairy products. Such drugs should be taken on an empty stomach. Although many drugs should not be taken in conjunction with alcohol, drinking alcohol is not generally a problem with antibiotics. If you're not sure about when to take an antibiotic or whether any foods should be avoided, ask your doctor or pharmacist.

The most important consideration in antibiotic therapy is to take all the medicine your physician prescribes (for many infections, a ten-day course of medicine). This is crucial to eradicate the bacteria completely. However, some patients stop taking their antibiotic when they begin feeling better, leaving themselves open for a relapse.

If you suffer side effects, such as nausea, diarrhea, or secondary infections like yeast infections, or if you experience allergic reactions such as a rash or a fever (which may occur with penicillin, for example), alert your physician at once so that your treatment can be changed if necessary.

Don't use an antibiotic you happen to have around the house when you get a cold or the flu. The antibiotic will not do you any good because it does not affect the viruses that cause these illnesses, and indiscriminate use of antibiotics contributes to the development of antibiotic-resistant organisms.

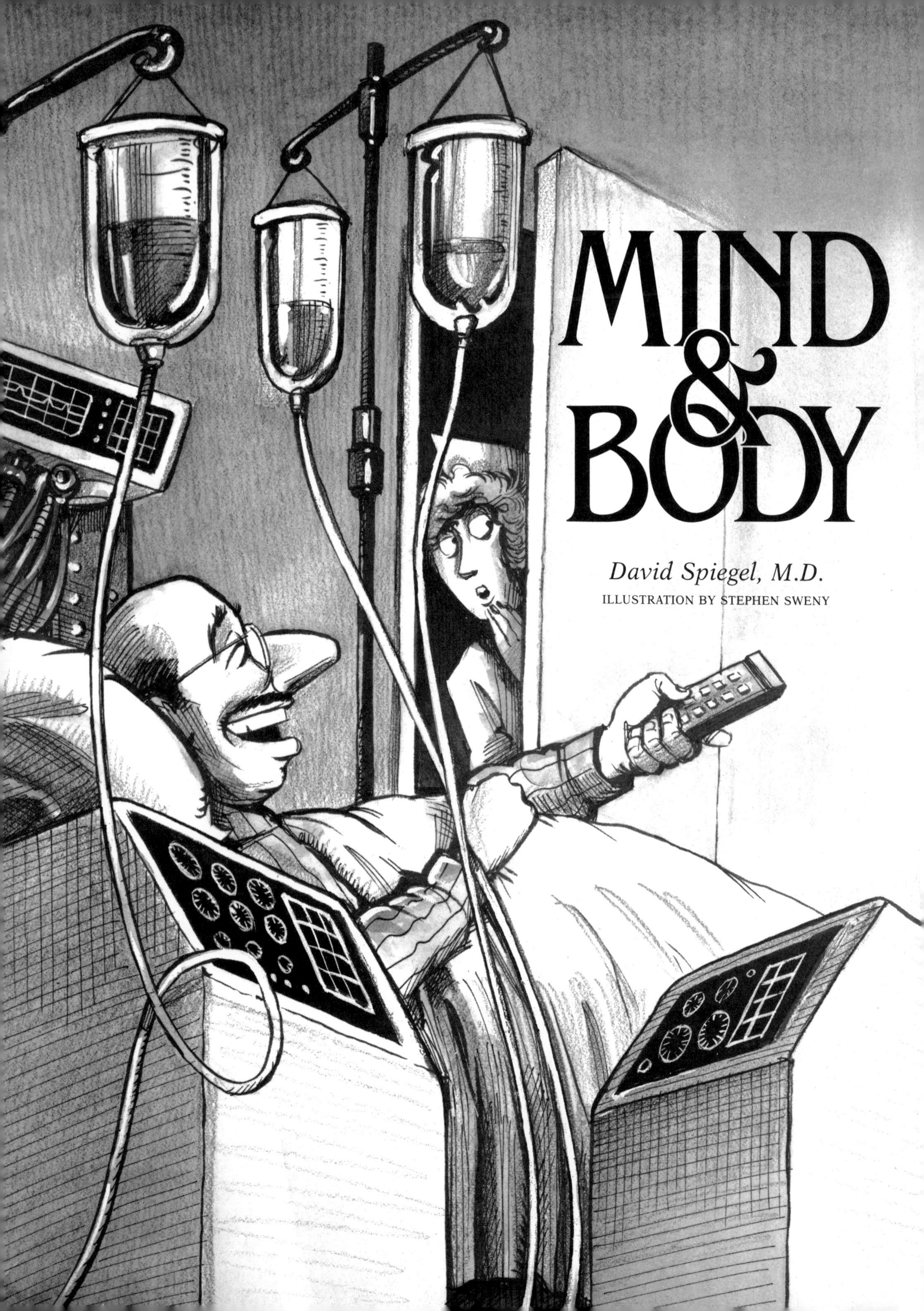
MIND & BODY
David Spiegel, M.D.
ILLUSTRATION BY STEPHEN SWENY

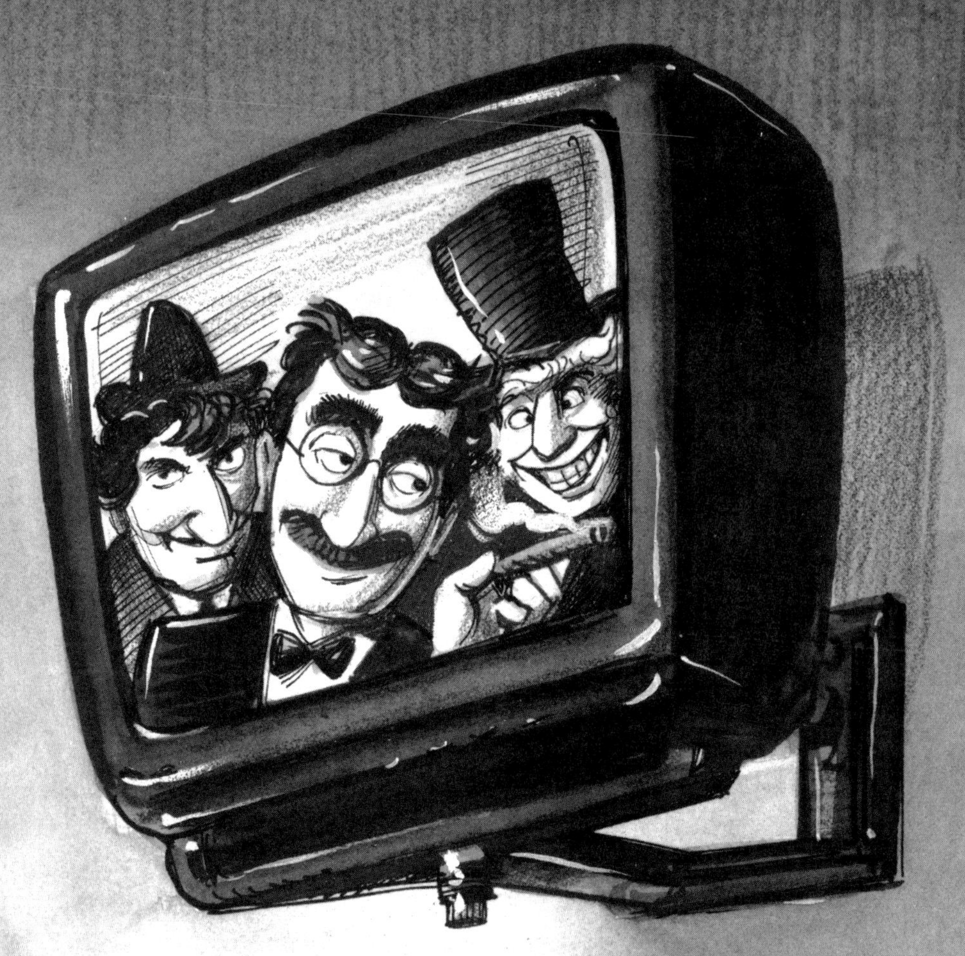

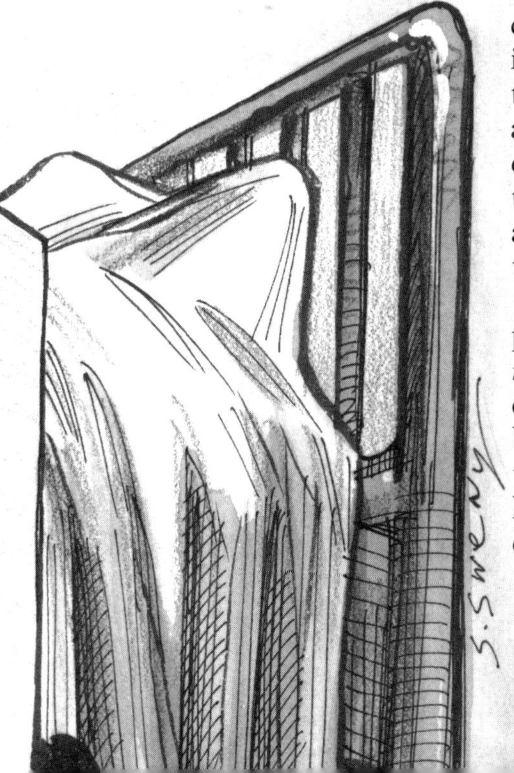

In the past few years there has been an upsurge of interest in what might be called the "inner game of illness," or the effect the mind has on the body and the way it copes with disease. Is the mind instrumental in, detrimental to, or irrelevant to the way we get diseases or the way we fight them? There have been tantalizing hints that factors such as attitude and social support can affect susceptibility to disease or the course of an illness. At the same time, there has been an enormous amount of misinformation and overselling of the "mind over matter" approach to treating illness.

There are two extreme positions regarding the interdependence, or lack of it, between mind and body. *Mindless materialism* is the theory that diseases are purely physical events which may affect the mind but are not influenced by it. At the other extreme is *disembodied spiritualism,* the belief that simply imagining a cure will cause it to happen. Imagine your white blood cells killing cancer cells, the theory goes, and that will somehow make

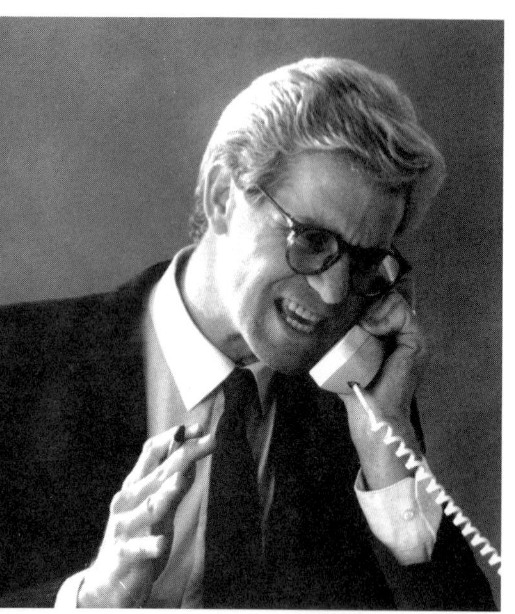

The personality type most often associated with heart attacks is Type A—hard-driving, impatient, and quick to anger.

the process occur in the body. Both extremes are incorrect, but in between lies evidence of complex, two-way interactions between mental and physical events.

Interest in this area has been sparked by both scientific research and popular books suggesting that the old Cartesian adage "I think, therefore I am" has new meaning in modern medicine. In 1979 author Norman Cousins published an account of how his intensive exposure to old movies that made him laugh while he was suffering from an autoimmune disease helped him recover. And investigators have studied personality traits that seem to predispose a person to some illnesses.

Personality Type and Illness

In the 1970s cardiologists Dr. Ray Rosenman and Dr. Meyer Friedman asserted there was a link between risk of heart disease and the now-famous Type A personality. Type A individuals are hard-driving, impatient, especially about matters of time, and hostile, or quick to anger.

More than 2,000 studies have now been published on the Type A personality. Early work showed that Type A individuals did indeed seem to be prone to heart attacks. But more recent research has led to modifications of the original observation. Some studies found that, ironically, Type A people seem to be somewhat more likely to recover from heart attacks than their less-competitive, Type B peers. Other studies, conducted by Dr. Carl Thoresen at Stanford University, showed that training heart attack patients to modify their Type A characteristics by restraining their impatience and hostility leads to improved outcome. Indeed, some recent research by Dr. Dean Ornish has shown that a combination of such training and relaxation exercises like meditation, along with strict control of fat in the diet, moderate and well-supervised exercise, and group support, not only lowers the risk of having a second heart attack but also actually reduces (albeit by a small amount) narrowing of the coronary arteries.

Those investigating the Type A personality and heart disease have concluded that the characteristic of most relevance is hostility. Heart-attack prone individuals seem to get angry easily and are unduly expressive of their anger. This is exactly the opposite of the personality trait most often associated with cancer. Since the early days of formal medicine in ancient Greece, doctors have observed that many cancer patients seem to be polite to a fault, in other words underexpressive of hostility. In a 1975 study by English researchers Steven Greer and Tina Morris, women having a biopsy for a breast lump were given psychological tests before the biopsy results were known. Those who turned out to have cancer were far less likely than those with benign lumps to admit to ever having expressed anger. This study has been corroborated by several other researchers.

David Spiegel is associate professor of psychiatry and behavioral sciences at Stanford University School of Medicine. He coauthored the study of the effects of support groups on women with breast cancer that is described in this article.

More recent research in England and the United States has shown that once patients get cancer, those who have what has been described as a "fighting spirit" tend to live longer. In one study at Johns Hopkins, cancer patients rated as uncooperative were more likely to live longer than those who were considered "good patients." Some of this increased longevity may be attributable to the feistier patients' being perhaps less ill to begin with. However, the consistency with which studies point to the absence of expressed hostility as a factor that increases the likelihood of getting cancer and decreases the odds of surviving with it suggests that the phenomenon should be regarded as worth looking into.

A recent study in Belgium found that women with a more serious type of breast cancer were significantly more anxious, suspicious, and generally symptomatic on psychological tests than patients who had the less serious form of breast cancer. Another recent study from England demonstrated an association between severe life stress, for instance the loss of a spouse, and recurrence of breast cancer.

Investigators have also found that lack of assertiveness is associated with faster disease progression in malignant melanoma, a serious skin cancer. However, not all the studies are consistent. One found that while being socially outgoing predicted longer survival of breast cancer patients, low rather than high levels of anger predicted better outcome.

Cancer patients with a fighting spirit tend to live longer.

Several early studies reported that depressed patients seemed more prone to develop cancer, but a major recent study published in the *Journal of the American Medical Association* found no relationship at all between scores on two scales of depression and the likelihood of getting cancer at a later time. It is also worth noting that not all studies show a relationship between psychological variables and cancer progression. Two major studies reported no link between the psychological factors they measured and length of survival time after a diagnosis of cancer.

What can one conclude from this cancer research? While contradictions remain and not all studies agree, there seems to be some evidence that suppression of anger may be associated with getting cancer and that assertiveness (a fighting spirit) and social integration (wide social contacts and strong personal relationships) are associated with longer survival once someone has cancer.

Social Integration

A related line of investigation has provided clear evidence that social integration is an important factor in health generally. Studies of large numbers of people across the United States have shown that there is a strong correlation between having a large social network and a reduced risk of death from illnesses of all types. In these studies the number of friends and family members available and the frequency of contact with them were found to be strongly associated with lower mortality.

The strength of the correlation between the size of the social network and mortality has been compared to that between smoking and death from lung and heart disease and to that between cholesterol levels and death from heart disease. In other words, it is very strong.

Interestingly, the kind of social support that best predicts survival in men is marital status—married men live longer. Longevity in women, however, is best predicted not by marital status but rather by relationships with female family members and friends. In other words, it is good for your health to have a relationship with a woman, regardless of your own gender, and alas, it does not seem to do your health much good to have a relationship with a man, regardless of your gender. Other research has shown that married cancer patients tend to live longer than unmarried cancer patients. In all of these studies there have been controls for differences in health habits and other factors that might account for differences in survival.

In addition to the size of the social network, the quality of social support has been shown to affect the outcome of illness. In a recent study at Yale of patients with heart disease, those who felt more sup-

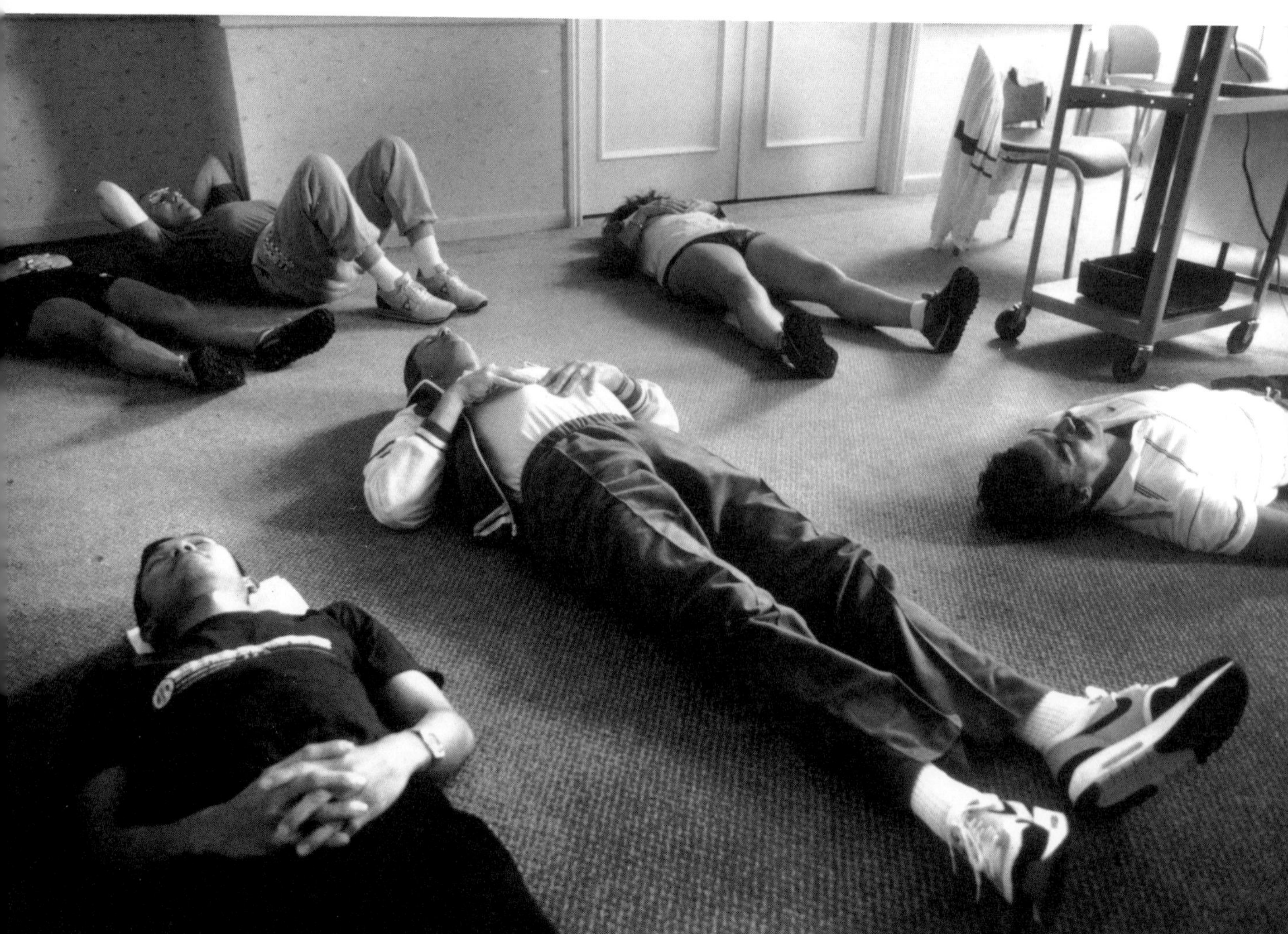

ported by their spouses, family, and friends tended to live longer. Social support is critical in getting through a crisis like the threat to life that is an inevitable part of having a heart attack.

Putting Theory Into Practice

If the absence of social support increases the risk of dying from disease, it makes sense that providing additional social support might reduce that risk. Several attempts have been made to study the effect of providing social support to patients with cancer. In one recent study, 86 women who had breast cancer that had spread to some other part of the body were randomly assigned to one of two groups. Fifty of the women attended weekly support groups for a year while the remaining 36 had just their usual cancer care. The women in the support groups were encouraged to form strong supportive bonds with one another. When one was hospitalized, the others visited her. They grieved when a member of the group died and were encouraged to openly discuss their fears of dying and death. They were asked to examine having a terminal illness as a series of problems, each of which could be addressed. For example, concerns about increasing pain, loss of control, helping family members cope with the illness, and the thought of being separated from loved ones were discussed openly. One member likened the experience of having cancer to looking down into the Grand Canyon with a fear of heights. She said, "You know

THE MIND-BODY LINK

Learning to meditate and control emotions, together with exercise, group support, and changes in the diet, lowers the risk of heart problems for Type A personalities.

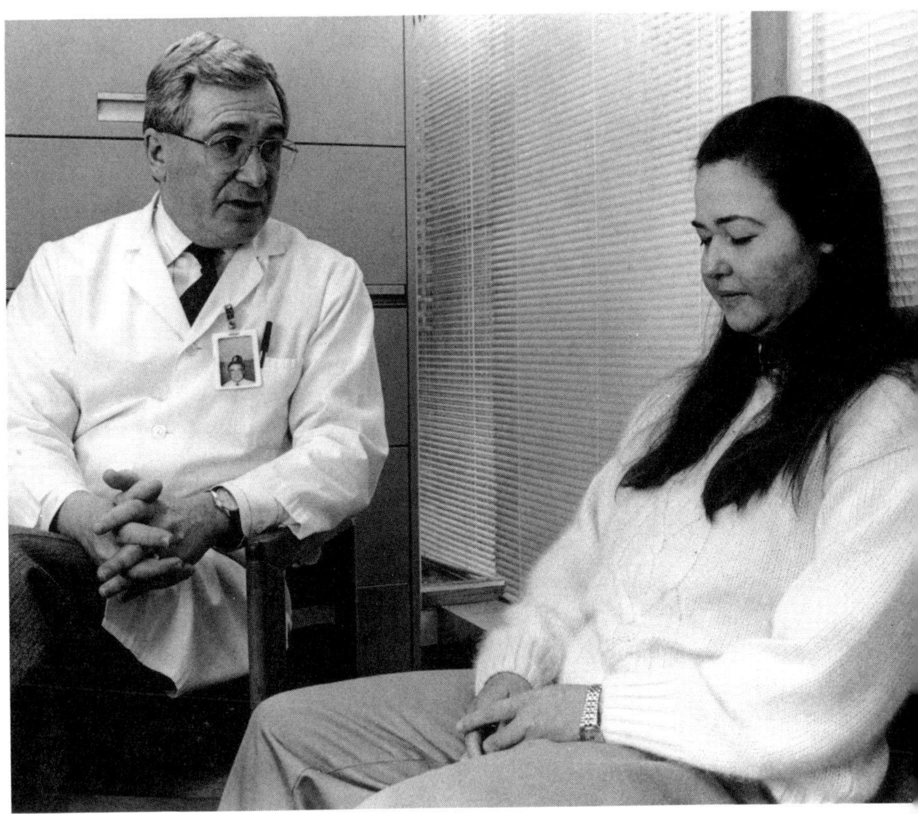

that if you fell down it would be the end, but you feel better about yourself because you can look." The patients were also encouraged to be more assertive with their physicians, actively negotiating how they would take their chemotherapy and making sure that their questions were clearly answered. In addition, monthly family group meetings were held to allow husbands and children to express their concerns and problems. The patients were also taught a self-hypnosis exercise for the purpose of helping them control pain.

Breast cancer patients in support groups cope better with the disease.

The effect of the support groups on the participants' emotional state was quite good. The women in these groups proved to be less anxious and depressed, were coping better with the disease, and had half the pain of those receiving standard cancer treatment only. But much more surprising was the effect on the disease itself. The patients in the support groups lived an average of 18 months longer. Four years after the study had begun, all of the 36 patients not assigned to a support group had died, but one-third of the 50 women who had participated in a group were still alive.

The focus of the support groups was on living better rather than living longer. Through their discussions, the women came to feel like experts in living, sorting out the trivial from the important in their lives, then offering meaningful support to their friends in the group and to family and friends outside the group. Something happened that seemed to make a difference in the amount of time they survived, although it is important to note that all but five of the patients did eventually die of breast cancer.

The finding of prolonged survival in cancer patients offered group support is all the more surprising in that at no time did the group leaders convey to the patients that participation in the group would lead to any change in the progression of the illness, nor did the group members seem to think that their involvement in the group would help them live longer. In fact, a great deal of time was spent talking about dying and death and about changing life priorities, given the fact that the time available to the members was limited at best. The emphasis was on making life as rich and full as possible. This meant intensifying relationships with family and friends, determining to impart important values to children while it was still possible to do so, and finishing projects that had been put aside.

There have been only a few other studies of the effects of psychosocial treatments on cancer survival time. One showed a similar enhancement of survival time in breast cancer patients but the value of the results was limited by the fact that the patients were free to choose whether or not to get chemotherapy and radiation. Half of the women chose neither, which is highly unusual. Another study, which initially purported to show extended survival for cancer patients offered psychotherapeutic treatment, concluded that the differences were attributable to the fact that the treatment patients had had cancer for a shorter period of time.

"Positive" Thinking

Although there are psychological as well as physical things people can do to help themselves cope with illness, there is no evidence that serious illnesses can simply be wished or laughed away. And there is no justification for blaming patients if diseases get worse. Human beings simply do not have such mental control over physical disease. Some patients seem to get the message—from friends, family, popular literature, and some types of therapists—that they have the power to heal their bodies through psychological means. This idea not only may build false hopes but often causes the patient to feel responsible and guilty when a disease worsens. A woman in a breast cancer support group previously mentioned, who went to a visualization program for the treatment of cancer, returned to hear bad news from her oncologist: her cancer had spread substantially. When she broke the news to her counselor at the visualization program, she was asked, "Why did you want your cancer to spread?" This doctrinaire application of the disembodied spiritualism theory adds a burden of guilt that is an unwarranted and unnecessary complication for a person who is already coping with a progressive and very often fatal illness.

Serious illnesses cannot simply be laughed or wished away.

A related danger in the emphasis on psychological treatment of physical illness is that well-meaning family members may censor the slightest show of sadness or depression in a patient, accusing the person of worsening the disease. Patients themselves may feel they are betraying their bodies and their families if they experience the natural despair that comes at times with serious illness. One woman with cancer likened it to "something sitting on my chest late at night." That fear is real and must be confronted from time to time.

Helping Loved Ones Cope

The patient is not the only one who suffers when serious illness strikes; family and friends suffer too. Openly discussing topics like the illness itself, the feelings it arouses, feelings for one another, the future, and death can benefit all involved. However, some patients, in a vain quest for the technique which will make them exceptionally resistant

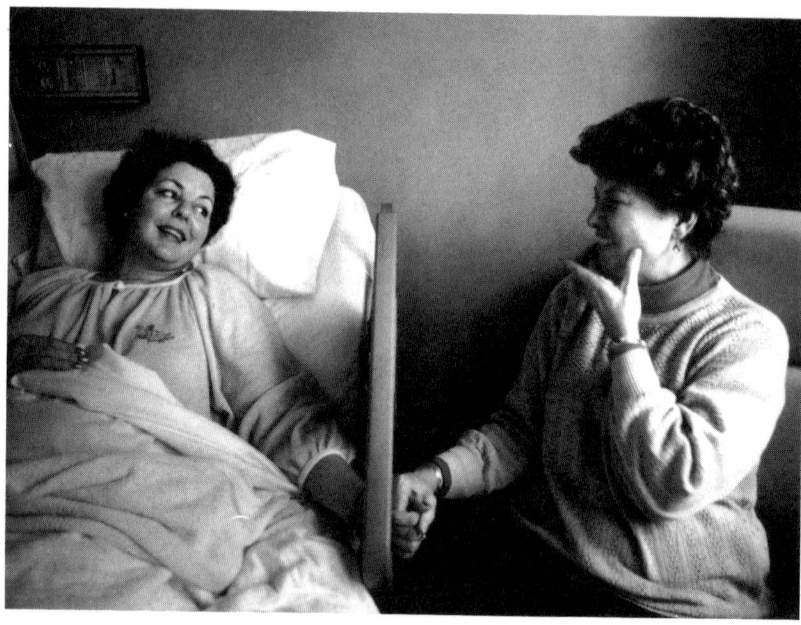

Loving support from family and friends is important for cancer patients.

to disease, ignore loved ones and the emotional pain they are experiencing. One man with cancer of the colon was so determined to overcome cancer that he was reluctant to pay any attention to his relationship with his girlfriend, who had lost her father to the same disease the previous year. She begged the patient to help her deal with her feelings and fears, but he felt this would mean "giving in" to the disease. A man whose wife has cancer may not be able to discuss with her his fears of loss and loneliness because she would interpret this as proof of lack of faith in her efforts to conquer the disease.

When close family and friends are thus cut off from expressing their emotional reactions, relationships can be limited just at the time that they should be deepened. This can create isolation and self-absorption in patients, preventing them from helping their families deal with the illness and from reducing their own sense of isolation by talking directly about their fears of dying.

In the breast cancer support groups, the direct expression of fears and concerns coupled with strong emotion led to a powerful sense of closeness among the groups' members. With family, as with friends, silent absorption in personal problems with a veneer of normalcy leads to distancing. During a crisis such as the development of a serious illness in a family member, relationships either get better or get worse. It is a time of great opportunity to deepen and share feelings about one another, instead of wasting precious time through preoccupation with wishful thinking.

How Social Support Helps

Doctors can only speculate about why patients with good social support live longer. It could be that because they are less depressed, such patients have a better diet, nourish their bodies better, and thus enable their bodies to contend with the illness more effectively. They may be more active, get adequate exercise and rest, and have fewer sleep problems.

Another possibility is that patients who are less depressed, with better communication skills, can work more effectively with their doctors, eliciting more vigorous treatment that is more closely attuned to their needs.

Research indicates that having friends and family helps alleviate stress. In studies conducted at Stanford University by Dr. Seymour Levine, animals show less increase in the hormone cortisol in response to a stressful stimulus when other familiar animals are near them. Humans react in much the same way. Walking through a dangerous neighborhood alone is much more stressful than taking the same walk with several friends. Even if the danger is not much reduced, the subjective and accompanying physical experience of stress is reduced by the presence of friends. The hormones that are produced in response to stress have many effects on the body, including suppression of the immune response. Thus, it is possible (although by no means proven) that social support, by buffering stress, allows the body to fight illness better.

Open discussion of an illness can benefit both patient and family members.

A related, still controversial theory is that psychological events can directly influence the activity of the immune system. Studies have shown, for example, that medical students experience reductions in immune system activity during examination periods unless they have good social support. People caring for a spouse with Alzheimer's disease show reductions in the activity of their white blood cells. Bereaved individuals show similar changes, as do older, severely depressed patients. While it is not certain that efficiency of immune system functioning plays much of a role in fighting off advanced cancer, infection can be quite dangerous in cancer patients, and any enhanced ability of the immune system to ward off infection might inhibit the progression of the disease and thereby increase a patient's survival time.

Whatever the mechanism, studies of cancer and other illnesses, ranging from arthritis to heart disease, are providing some initial evidence that improved social support and psychological well-being are not only ends in themselves but means of enhancing patients' ability to combat the disease. Good social support and emotional state are no replacement for traditional medical treatment. But the evidence of their importance may help redefine medical treatment to include a psychosocial component. □

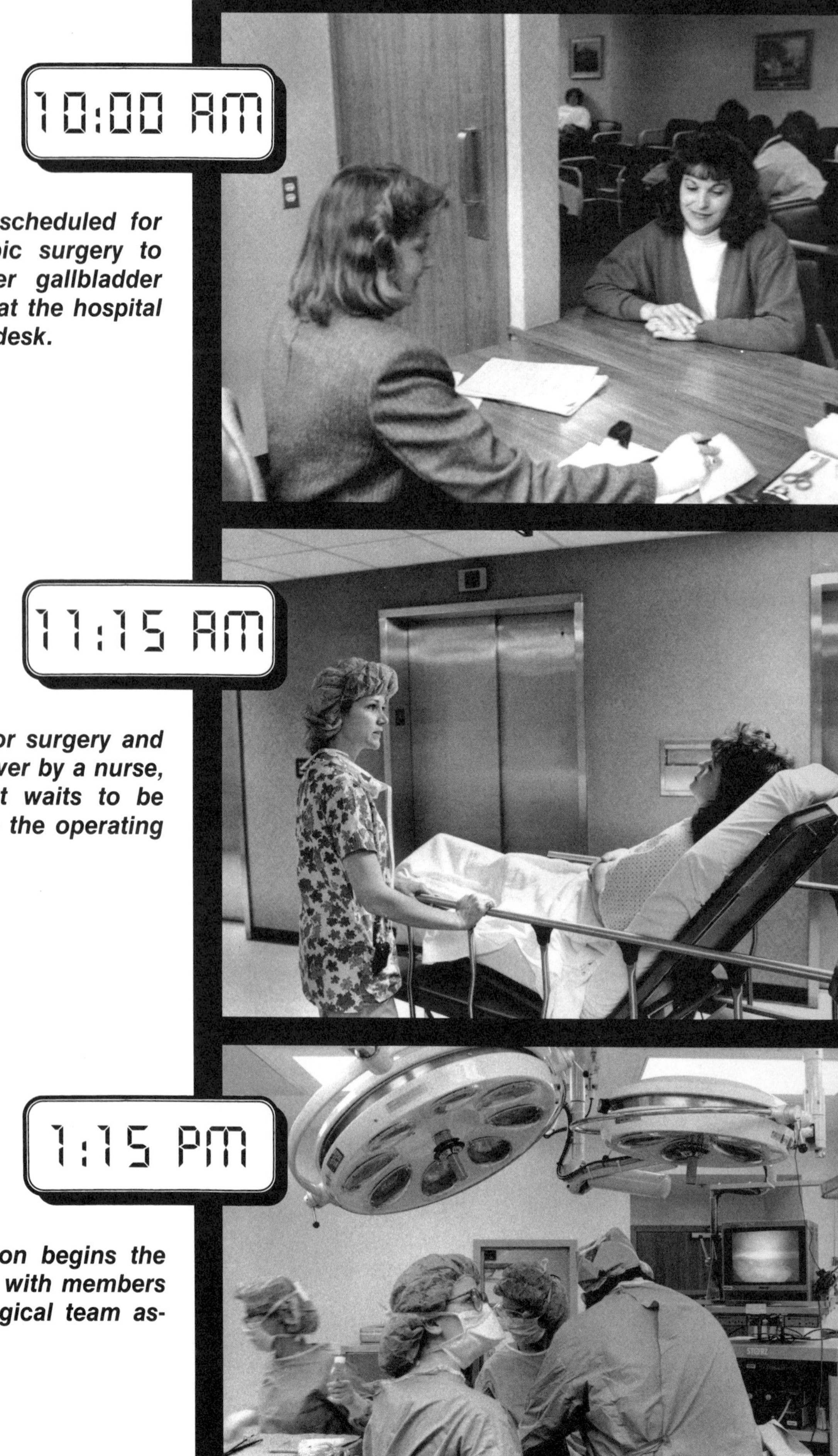

A patient scheduled for laparoscopic surgery to remove her gallbladder checks in at the hospital admitting desk.

Prepped for surgery and watched over by a nurse, the patient waits to be called into the operating room.

The surgeon begins the operation, with members of the surgical team assisting.

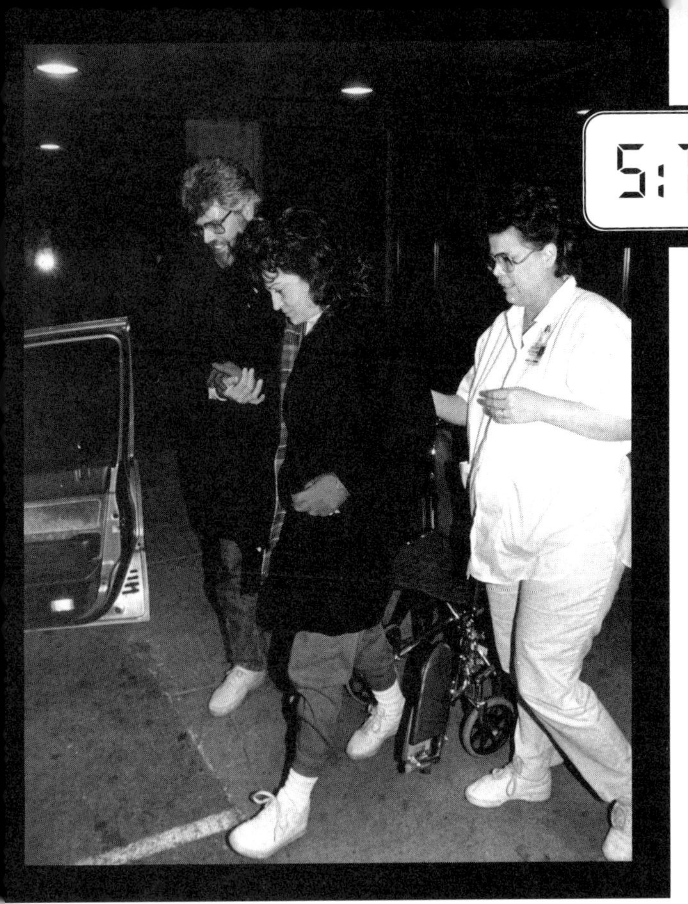

5:15 PM

Helped by her husband and a nurse, the patient leaves the hospital, ready to be driven home.

7 HOURS, 15 MINUTES IN THE HOSPITAL

MODERN SURGERY TECHNIQUES

Michael R. Treat, M.D.

Modern surgery got its start in the latter part of the 19th century, when there was a great spurt in the development of surgical techniques. This was made possible by such factors as the availability of reasonably safe general anesthesia, new ways to control infection, and a growing understanding of anatomy and physiology. It was during these years that abdominal surgery was transformed from an often lethal procedure chosen only in extremis to the preferred way of dealing with a wide range of problems and that many of the basic surgical tools and procedures used today were developed.

The Legacy of Large Incisions

A fundamental surgical principle that emerged from this surgical heritage was to make a large enough incision to do the job safely. Too small an incision may inadequately expose vital organs and lead to mistakes and complications. An adequately sized incision is one that permits the surgeon's hands, the assistants' hands, and the various instruments such as scissors, scalpel, tissue clamps, and retractors to be placed where they are needed. However, large incisions impose a physical cost on the patient. To offset this cost, tremendous improvements have taken place over the past hundred years in what is called surgical support: improvements in antibiotics, cardiovascular drugs, and anesthetics; better monitoring of the patient's body functions during the operation; availability of blood products; and new equipment and techniques for postoperative care, such as intensive care units. These advances permit modern surgeons to accomplish safely larger and more complex operations than would have ever been possible before. They have also permitted the performance of surgery on patients who would have been considered too old or sick for surgery in the past.

Technical advances have made it possible for surgeons to do more complex operations.

A New Way of Operating—and Thinking

Recently, certain technological developments have contributed to a shift in surgeons' attitudes toward the necessity of large-incision surgery. It is now possible to perform procedures through very small incisions or punctures or through natural body orifices with the aid of an endoscope, a slender fiber-optic instrument used for looking into and working within body cavities or hollow organs. There is a new awareness that using this technology greatly reduces the stress on the patient's body.

Although it is still easier to do an operation through a large incision than through a very small one, the benefits to the patient of what is called "minimal access" surgery are so great that surgeons are compelled to find less invasive ways to accomplish surgical goals. In a very real sense, surgeons are making it harder on themselves in order to make it easier on the patient.

If the surgical giants of the late 19th century could come back to a contemporary operating room and see the advances in the safety and efficacy of surgery that have been made on the basis of their legacy, they would probably be most impressed by endoscopic procedures. Imagine their amazement when looking at a large video monitor and seeing the inside of a patient's colon, while the patient is lying comfortably on the examining table, perhaps watching the same monitor. Or picture their surprise at seeing a laser fiber appear from the end of the endoscope and, almost magically, produce an intense burst of light

---

Michael R. Treat is associate professor of clinical surgery at Columbia University and attending surgeon at Columbia-Presbyterian Medical Center.

to remove the diseased tissue. Or at watching a gallbladder being removed by a surgeon whose hands are actually outside the patient's body the whole time.

Colonoscopy and Gastroscopy

Two now-common procedures that employ the techniques of minimal access surgery to treat problems in the digestive system are colonoscopy and gastroscopy. Colonoscopy is the use of a long flexible endoscope (a colonoscope) to examine and operate on the inside of the colon, or large intestine. Since colonoscopy is done from within a lumen, or hollow space within an organ, it is an example of what is called intraluminal minimal access surgery.

The technological development that made colonoscopy possible was the ability to transmit images along specially arranged bundles of glass fibers that can transmit light even when bent around a curve. Each single fiber in the image bundle is very tiny (approximately 10 microns, or millionths of a meter, in diameter), and each transmits just one point of light from the scene under view. There are many thousands of fibers in the bundle, to make up a complete picture. In order to obtain a true image from one end of the fiber bundle to the other, the fibers have to be arranged in an orderly array, or coherent bundle. Colonoscopes also contain incoherent bundles, sheaves of fibers not arranged in any particular way. An incoherent bundle is used to transmit light from an outside source to illuminate the area being examined or worked on. The ability of an incoherent bundle to transmit an intensely bright light inward from an external light source is just as important as the ability of a coherent bundle to transmit an image from inside to the operator of the instrument.

Minimal access surgery reduces stress on the patient's body.

Scientists have long known, in principle, how light can be transmitted around a curve by means of glass fibers. But it takes a tricky bit of manufacturing to construct a coherent array of the many thousands of fibers required to obtain a high-resolution image. The first flexible fiber-optic endoscope (actually it was a gastroscope, an endoscope for examining the stomach) was developed by Dr. Basil Hirschowitz at the University of Michigan and was manufactured by American Cystoscope Makers in the late 1950s.

A colonoscope is about a half inch in diameter and about 70 inches long, with what could be thought of as two eyes and a little mouth at the distal end (the end that goes into the patient). One eye is the opening for the light brought along an incoherent fiber-optic bundle to illuminate the scene, and the other eye is an opening covered by a lens that focuses the scene onto the distal end of the coherent fiber-optic bundle. The mouth is a small hole at the end of an internal channel that runs the length of the scope. In the proximal (operator's) end of the scope are an eyepiece plus an opening through which accessory instruments can be passed along the scope's internal channel. A video camera may be attached to the eyepiece to permit viewing on a monitor. The distal tip of the scope is bendable in all directions in response to control dials or knobs located at the proximal end of the scope. The proximal end also contains buttons to activate suction or water/air inflow. (Suction is used to remove excess fluid that interferes with the view; water is used to wash away debris; air is used to distend the colon so it can be examined more readily.) It takes a lot of smart engineering to package all of these things into an instrument with a reasonably small diameter.

Before the colonscope is used, the patient's colon must be emptied. This is generally accomplished with a combination of liquid diet, laxatives, and enemas. The operator introduces the colonoscope into the rectum and pushes it carefully along the colon while watching its progress through the eyepiece or on a video monitor. The view resembles what one sees while moving along a tunnel. Frequent adjustments must be made to steer the tip of the scope around the turns. It takes a skilled operator to make this procedure reasonably comfortable for the patient, who is generally awake but sedated. The mechanics of advancing the scope are rather subtle, since one is endeavoring to push a floppy tube (the scope) into another floppy tube (the colon), which is tethered to the body at some places, free to move and stretch at others.

The object of passing this long scope along the inside of the colon is to see if any abnormalities are present and, if appropriate, to correct them. For example, colonoscopes are frequently used to remove polyps (benign but premalignant growths) from the large intestine. The first colonoscopic polypectomy (removal of a polyp) was done in the early 1970s. Today polyp removal is done rather routinely on an outpatient basis, and patients are able to go back to work the next day. Before the availability of colonoscopic polypectomy, a full-scale abdominal operation had to be done to remove a polyp. The operation involved opening up the abdomen and then opening up the colon to snip off the polyp. The mortality rate, chance of complications, postoperative pain, and time lost from work with this large-incision approach were all far higher than when a colonoscope is used.

Some colonoscopic surgery can be done on an outpatient basis.

Similar long flexible instruments called gastroscopes (inserted through the patient's mouth) can be used to view and perform therapeutic procedures in the esophagus, stomach, and duodenum (the upper part of the small intestine). In addition to removing polyps, it is possible to use colonoscopes and gastroscopes to stop bleeding occurring from conditions such as ulcers or abnormal blood vessels, to open up blockages caused by malignant tumors, to dilate passageways narrowed by a variety of conditions, and to remove foreign bodies. Specially modified gastroscopes are used to remove stones from the bile ducts and to relieve benign and malignant obstructions of the biliary tract (the gallbladder and bile ducts).

Laparoscopy

As fascinating and useful as colonoscopy and gastroscopy are, they are not able to solve all the problems the general surgeon encounters. Many problems, such as gallstones, are often best approached by opening up the abdomen. However, even these cases need not involve a large incision. A rigid type of endoscope called a laparoscope makes it possible to operate in the abdomen through very small incisions.

For general surgeons, laparoscopy has always been a kind of step-

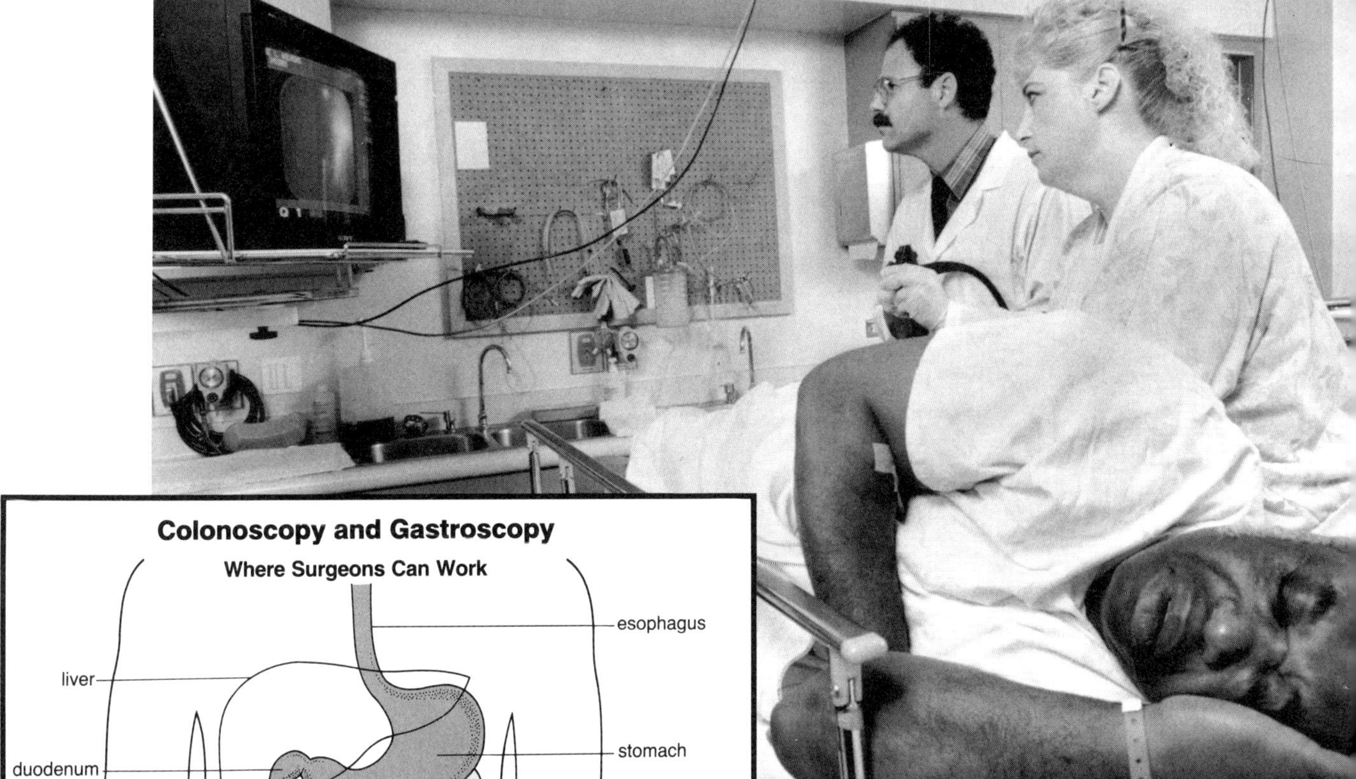

Using colonoscopes and gastroscopes, physicians can view and perform certain procedures in the colon, esophagus, stomach, and duodenum. Above, as a patient lies quietly on the operating table, medical personnel examine a video image of his colon.

child of endoscopic procedures, although gynecologists have long been aware of its great diagnostic and therapeutic utility. Especially in Europe, gynecologic surgeons have for more than a decade been refining and extending the possibilities of intra-abdominal endoscopic surgery to levels of accomplishment that were (until recently) quite surprising to general surgeons schooled in the belief that one needs to make a large incision in order to accomplish complex technical tasks. Although there have been a few advocates of laparoscopy among general surgeons, it is only very recently that laparoscopy has really caught the eye of the rank and file general surgeon. In 1990 a procedure called laparoscopic cholecystectomy, or gallbladder removal using a laparoscope, generated more excitement and interest among general surgeons and potential patients than any other surgical advance in the preceding decade. This increased awareness of the technical possibilities of laparoscopic surgery was due in large measure to the brilliant efforts of Dr. Eddie Joe Reddick from Nashville, Tenn., in successfully performing a large series of laparoscopic cholecystectomies and also to the pioneering work of Jacques Perissat, from Bordeaux, France.

Although general surgeons have only recently rediscovered it, the laparoscope itself is not a new device. The first laparoscopies were done around the turn of the century. Since laparoscopic optics are based on conventional lenses, laparoscopes existed long before the development of the fiber-optic technology required for flexible endoscopes. For intra-abdominal endoscopy, most surgeons feel that a flexible instrument is of no advantage. A laparoscope measures about 16 inches in length and less than half an inch in diameter and contains a series of lenses that convey the image from the distal end to a camera or operator's eye at the proximal end. It is really a sort of telescope with optics designed to provide a wide-angle, close-up view. Using sophisticated modern laparoscopes, the intra-abdominal organs can be seen with breathtaking clarity.

Although the basic laparoscope has been available for a long time, it is the coupling of the laparoscope to high-resolution color video systems that has opened up the possibilities of laparoscopic surgery. A video camera on the laparoscope allows visual coordination among the several team members required to carry out complex surgical procedures such as gallbladder removal. In open surgery it is taken for granted that surgical assistants are able to see the field, or the area being operated on, well enough to help effectively. In complex laparoscopic surgery the entire team depends on intelligent positioning of the laparoscopic video camera, and often two video monitors are employed so that all can see what is going on. Thus the "cameraman" in the

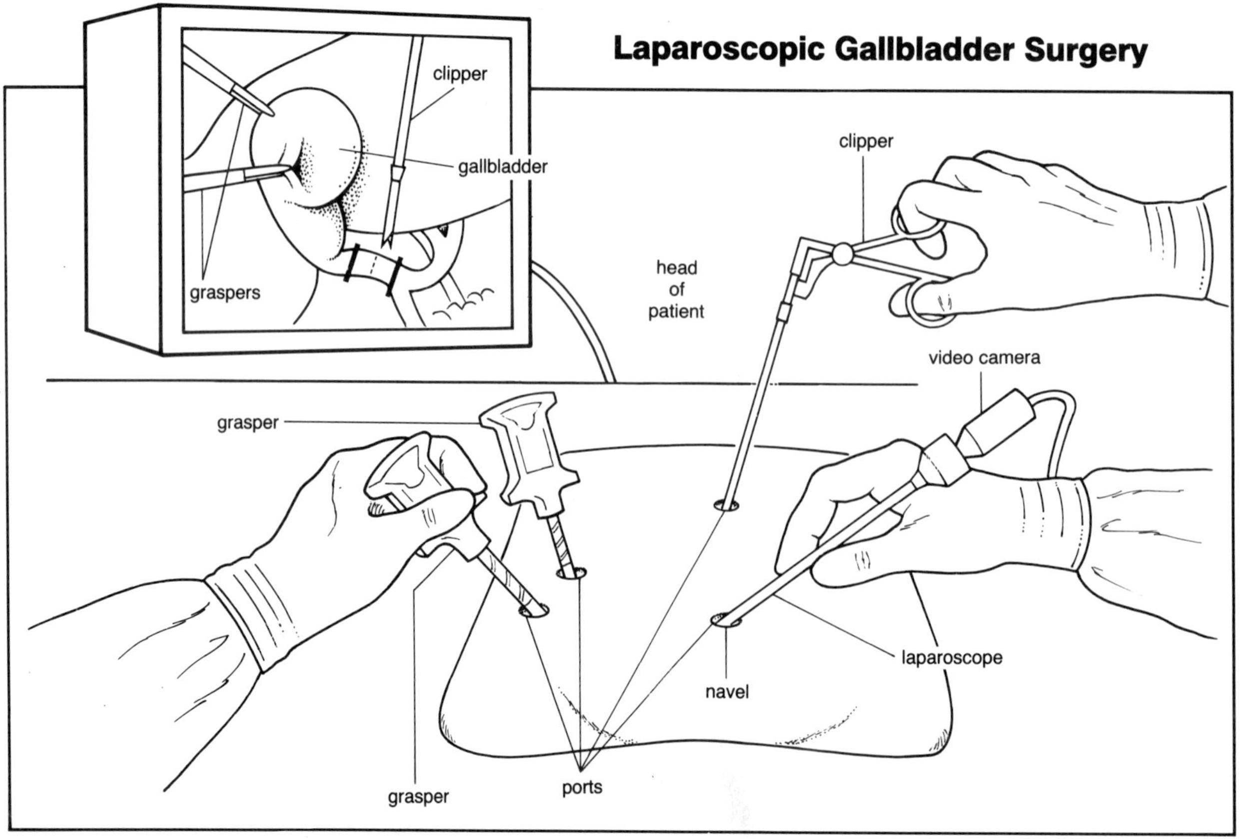

laparoscopic surgical team plays an essential role in the smooth performance of the operation.

For laparoscopic cholecystectomy the patient is placed under general anesthesia, and the abdominal cavity is filled via a needle puncture with a harmless gas (usually carbon dioxide) in order to lift the abdominal wall away from the organs in the abdomen and thus provide room to maneuver the instruments. Several, usually four, punctures or ports are made in the abdomen. Through one of the ports the laparoscope with attached video camera is placed. Through two other ports, graspers are placed to lift the gallbladder in order to expose the place where its duct, the cystic duct, joins the main (common) bile duct and where the cystic artery enters the gallbladder. (The common bile duct is the channel through which bile flows from the liver to the gallbladder and the small intestine, where it is needed to digest fats.) One assistant is in control of the laparoscope with video camera and one assistant holds the graspers to position the gallbladder.

The primary surgeon then begins a careful examination in order to identify and isolate the cystic duct, cystic artery, and common bile duct. Accurate identification of these structures is the crux of the operation, and an error here can cause major problems for the patient. Once they have been positively identified, the surgeon, operating through one of the ports, uses special clips to close off the cystic duct from the common bile duct and to close off the cystic artery. Then, the cystic duct and artery are severed. Next, the gallbladder's attachment to the underside of the liver is severed. Finally, the tip of the gallbladder is pulled through one of the ports and cut so the bile can be removed, allowing the now-deflated gallbladder to be pulled completely out. The punctures are each closed with one or two stitches. Patients are usually able to eat the same day and often can go home the next morning (in fact, some go home the same day). Return to normal work routines can take place within a few days. The difference in postoperative recovery between laparoscopic gallbladder removal and open surgery is impressive and is the chief reason why this procedure has become so popular.

Although amazingly well accepted by surgeons and patients alike, laparoscopic cholecystectomy still has some areas where further improvement and evaluation are needed. As with an open cholecystectomy, there are inherent risks. A major concern in performing cholecystectomy is that the vitally important common bile duct not be harmed in the course of separating the cystic duct from the common duct. Because there are variations in anatomy from one person to the next, extraordinary care must be taken to locate these structures, so that complications do not arise. The rate of major ductal injury with open cholecystectomy is quite low, and in time it should be possible to match or better that complication rate when the procedure is done through the laparoscope. Although some surgeons have expressed skepticism, the fact that the procedure is being done through the laparoscope does not mean that the visualization of important structures is less adequate than that obtained through an open cholecystectomy. In fact, many surgeons are coming to believe that the visualization may be superior through the laparoscope/video combination.

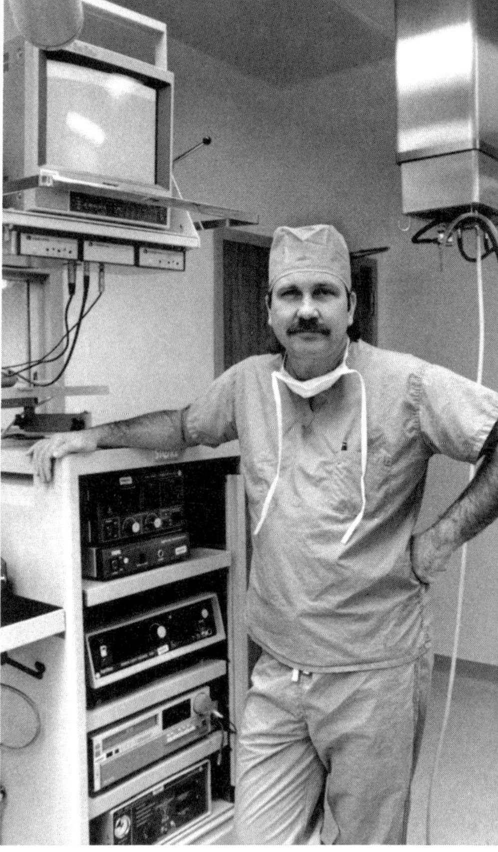

Dr. Eddie Joe Reddick, whose success in removing gallbladders has increased awareness of laparoscopic surgery's technical possibilities. One of Dr. Reddick's patients is featured in the pictures on pages 152 and 153.

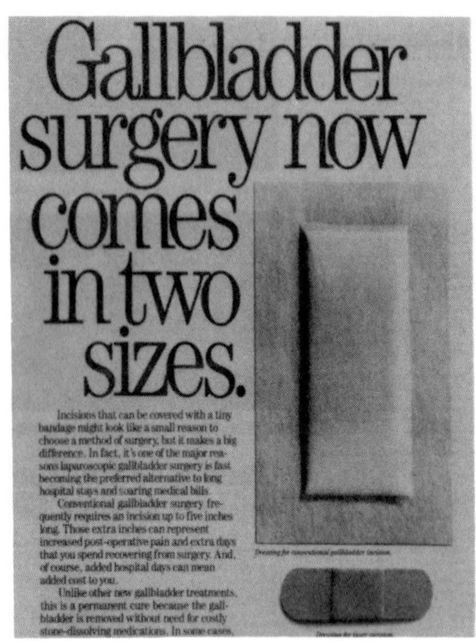

A major reason for the popularity of laparoscopic gallbladder surgery is that it shortens recovery time.

However, laparoscopic cholecystectomy does call for somewhat different skills on the part of the operating surgeon, even if the surgeon is already very experienced in removing gallbladders. Approximately 500,000 open cholecystectomies are done in the United States every year and many more around the world. Thus, there is a tremendous volume of experience with this procedure. Open cholecystectomy is probably the most thoroughly understood major operation performed by general surgeons today, and it has a long and excellent track record. In terms of complication rate, it is a hard act to follow. For open cholecystectomy, the bitter lessons have essentially all been learned and are passed along to surgeons-in-training. Laparoscopic cholecystectomy is unique in modern surgical experience in that it represents a very rapid change to a technically more complex and demanding procedure in the face of a very well established and simpler traditional alternative. Unfortunately and inevitably, there is a learning curve for this new procedure as with all new procedures. Fortunately, excellent courses have been developed for teaching surgeons the necessary skills.

The Future

Minimal access surgical procedures, once viewed as isolated technical tricks or special purpose procedures, are becoming widely accepted as routine extensions of general surgery. Surgeons are increasingly willing and able to use high technology methods to spare their patients the pain and possible complications associated with large incisions. One of the by-products of this evolution may be the erosion of traditional boundaries between medical specialties, as surgeons with particular technical skills apply them to operations they would not normally perform. This trend will probably be strongly resisted by those physicians who feel that they have special training and knowledge to work in a particular area. I personally believe that it is not in the patient's best interests to have a surgeon perform a procedure unless that surgeon knows a great deal not only about the tool or process being used but also about the medical problem needing correction. There is more to being a surgeon than knowing how to handle the instruments. One should know why and when to use them, as well as when not to.

Several new surgical societies have arisen as a result of the development of new types of endoscopic surgery. In the United States, there is the Society of American Gastrointestinal Endoscopic Surgeons, and in England, the Minimally Invasive Therapy Society.

For minimal access surgery to reach its full potential, many technical problems must be solved. At present, anyone who performs endoscopic surgery cannot help but feel at times that he or she is operating with one hand tied behind the back. It is difficult for the endoscopic surgeon to obtain the same degree of control over the surgical field as the open surgeon. Although skill and practice can overcome the limitations imposed on the endoscopic surgeon by the equipment, the open surgeon has a number of advantages. The open surgeon employs natural vision, can easily look at the operating field from a variety of angles, and has the best surgical instrument on the planet, the human hand. The endoscopic surgeon is looking at a two-dimensional representation of the field and is working with instruments that have only a few degrees of freedom of motion and are capable of only simple opening and closing actions. These instruments, as wonderful as they are, do not come remotely near to the flexibility, dexterity, and tactile sense of the hand. There is a long way to go before endoscopic surgical tools are truly extensions of human senses and hands.

In the near future, the kinds of technology that will improve endoscopic surgery will be borrowed from industry and aerospace. Two important areas of technology are lasers and "tele-operating."

Lasers and Endoscopes. Laser technology has already found its way into the operating room. However, for open surgery, many of the existing applications of lasers—to cut or burn away tissue—do not offer the patient much advantage over cheaper conventional surgical tools such as scalpels or electrocautery. In addition, any small advantage gained by the precision with which lasers can be used on tissue is outweighed by the overall negative impact of a conventional large incision.

For endoscopic surgery the situation is different, and lasers make more sense. From the technical standpoint, it is more difficult (though certainly not impossible) for the endoscopic surgeon to do certain basic things, such as place stitches and tie knots, that are very easy in open surgery. Lasers, long used to cut tissues, more recently have begun to be used to join them. This phenomenon, called laser tissue "welding," is being used in limited clinical testing and may prove to be of great value to the endoscopic surgeon. The laser energy can be brought to the target area through a thin fiber-optic conduit that can easily be passed through an endoscope, even a flexible one. Although development work is still being done, it may well turn out that laser tissue welding will replace mechanical methods (clips, stitches) of joining tissues together, at least for endoscopic applications.

Endoscopic procedures are becoming widely accepted as routine extensions of general surgery.

Tele-operating. The concepts of "tele-operating," currently being applied to the proposed exploration of other planets by robots or robot-like systems, also have potential for endoscopic surgical application. Tele-operating systems are not true robots, since they are not designed to function independently of human control. They link operator and machine so as to obtain the benefit of human intelligence in directing mechanical systems that can go into environments where it would be difficult to send a human being. Clearly, the same concepts that apply to directing a robotic arm collecting samples on the Martian surface could also apply to a tiny device that might explore the human intestine or remove a gallbladder. The way in which endoscopes are used now, while reasonably effective, is pretty crude compared to some of the tele-operating prototypes being developed by the aerospace industry. Instead of relying on endoscopic devices that have to be pushed manually into the patient through a natural orifice or small incision, surgeons may someday use miniature, self-propelled "endosurgical robots" that will convey to the operator by a thin fiber-optic link a full-color, full-sound, tactile "virtual world" image of the operating field. If society is willing to pay for these improvements, there are many imaginative and beneficial medical uses for tele-operating technology. □

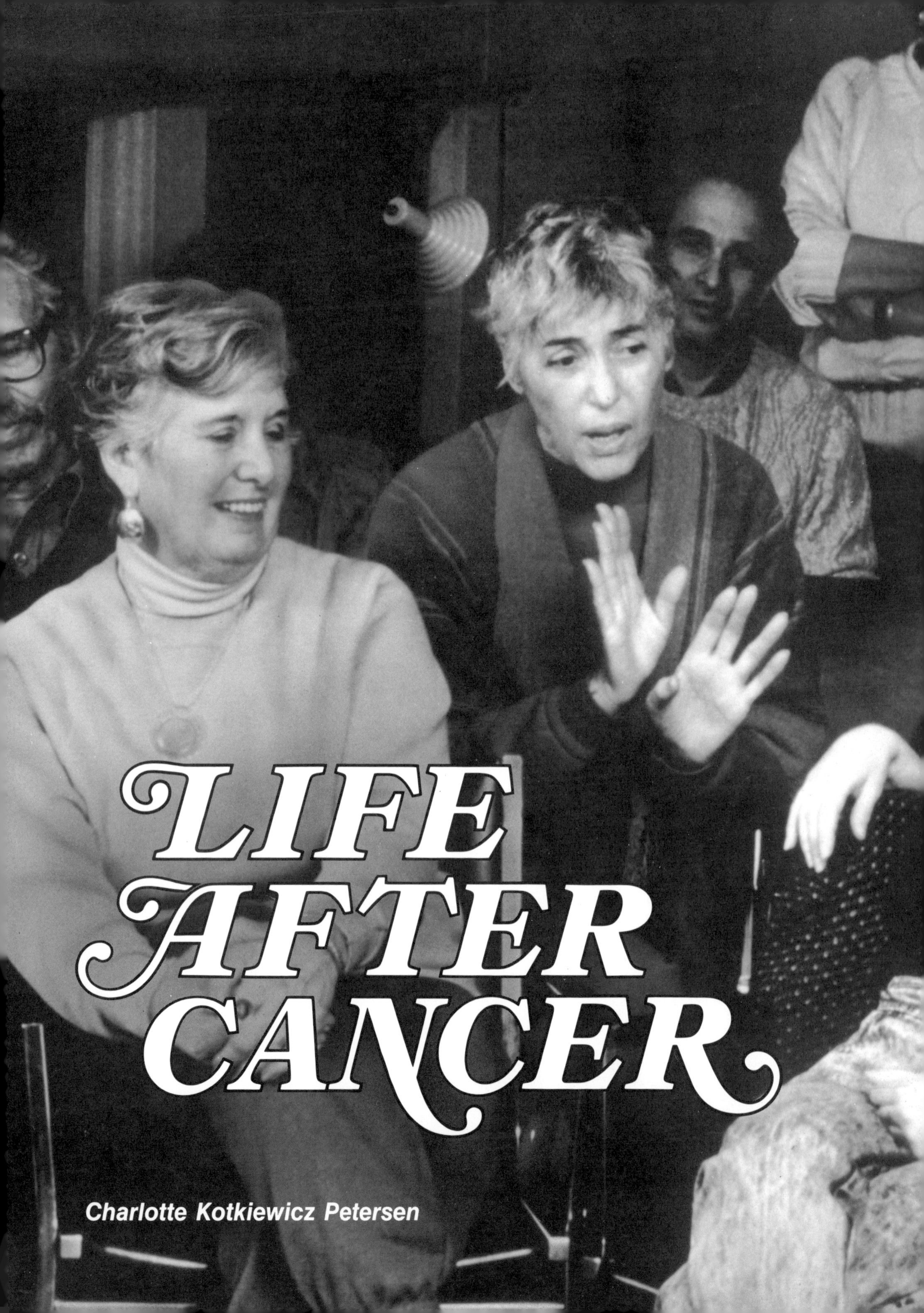

LIFE AFTER CANCER

Charlotte Kotkiewicz Petersen

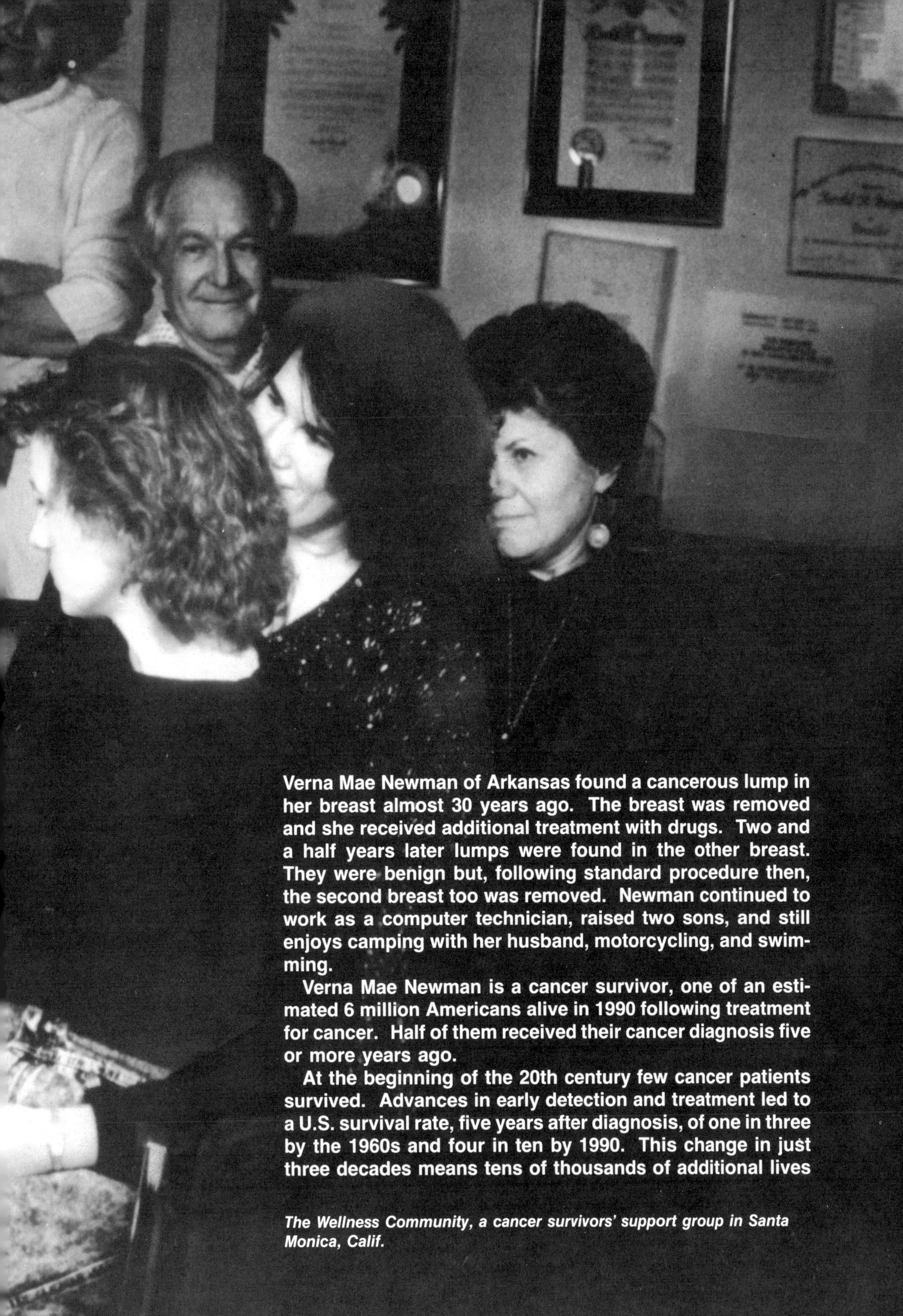

Verna Mae Newman of Arkansas found a cancerous lump in her breast almost 30 years ago. The breast was removed and she received additional treatment with drugs. Two and a half years later lumps were found in the other breast. They were benign but, following standard procedure then, the second breast too was removed. Newman continued to work as a computer technician, raised two sons, and still enjoys camping with her husband, motorcycling, and swimming.

Verna Mae Newman is a cancer survivor, one of an estimated 6 million Americans alive in 1990 following treatment for cancer. Half of them received their cancer diagnosis five or more years ago.

At the beginning of the 20th century few cancer patients survived. Advances in early detection and treatment led to a U.S. survival rate, five years after diagnosis, of one in three by the 1960s and four in ten by 1990. This change in just three decades means tens of thousands of additional lives

The Wellness Community, a cancer survivors' support group in Santa Monica, Calif.

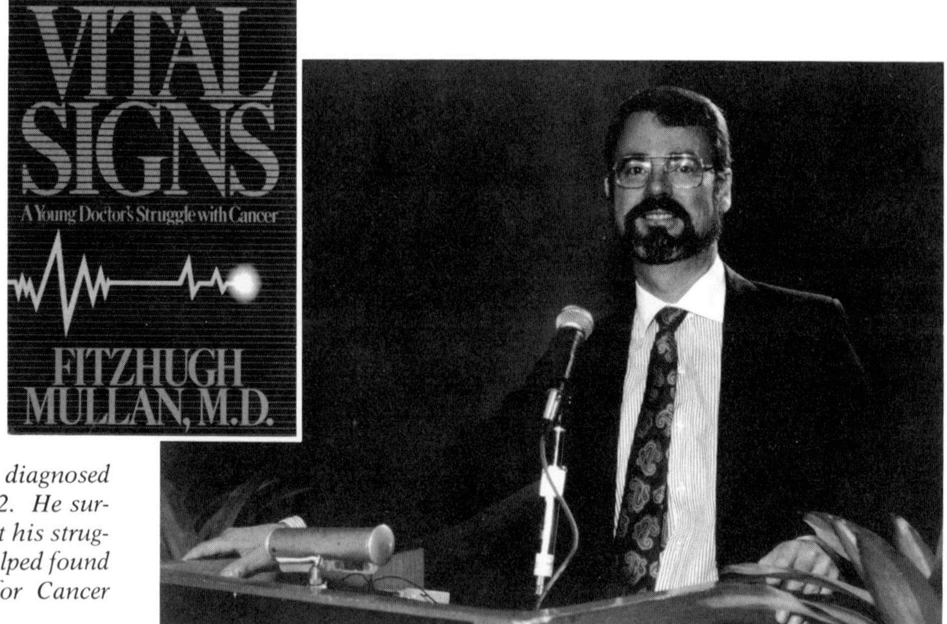

Dr. Fitzhugh Mullan was diagnosed with lung cancer at age 32. He survived to write a book about his struggle with the disease and helped found the National Coalition for Cancer Survivorship.

are saved each year. When the 40 percent rate is adjusted to take into account deaths from other diseases and accidents, a "relative" five-year survival rate of 50 percent is arrived at for all cancers in the United States. This figure is commonly used to measure progress against cancer and as an estimate of the proportion of potentially curable cancer patients.

Many cancer survivors can be considered cured—they have no evidence of any remaining cancer and have the same life expectancy as someone who never had cancer. Others are living with cancer still present in their bodies. Whichever category they are in, many, if not all, survivors have had to adjust their life-styles because of the medical, pyschological, practical, and financial problems cancer can cause.

These problems can be severe. Permanent effects of treatment could include loss of a body part, such as a leg, breast, or larynx (voice box), with accompanying mobility, self-image, or communication problems. Even the less drastic side effects of treatment with radiation or chemotherapy, such as nausea, vomiting, fatigue, and hair loss, can compromise the quality of life while treatment is in progress. Cancer patients who require extensive treatment or who have recurrences may face the loss of a job, and with it, their health insurance. Added strains on family life can lead to emotional and financial crises.

Being a survivor, then, is not easy, and, as every survivor knows, there is no guarantee that it will last. Yet many survivors have stated that their experiences with cancer gave them a deeper appreciation of life, while forcing them to focus their energies on what was truly important to them.

Survivorship Defined

Who are the cancer survivors? The National Coalition for Cancer Survivorship, a network of organizations and individuals throughout the United States concerned about life after cancer, believes that survivorship starts the moment the diagnosis is made, because it is then that one's life starts to change. "From the time of its discovery and for the balance of life, an individual diagnosed with cancer is a survivor," reads the NCCS charter.

Dr. Fitzhugh Mullan, a founding member of the NCSS, is a cancer survivor. He was a 32-year-old physician practicing in Santa Fe, N.M., when a routine chest X ray revealed a tumor in his right lung. He had two operations, separated by a round of chemotherapy (treatment with anticancer drugs). It was during the most debilitating part of the treatment that his wife discovered she was pregnant

---

Charlotte Kotkiewicz Petersen is a medical writer and editor who has worked for the American Cancer Society, Memorial Sloan-Kettering Cancer Center, and Oncology *magazine.*

with their third child. Mullan wrote a book about his ordeal, helped found the NCCS (in 1986), and was named its president.

While the experiences of each cancer survivor are unique, there are some common elements in the course of events each individual confronts following the diagnosis. Mullan has called this course of events "the seasons of survival." The first, or acute, stage starts at diagnosis and is a time of concentrated medical treatment, of concern about the effects of treatment on body and mind, and of fear of death. The second, or extended, survival stage begins when concentrated treatment stops. It is a time when an individual is relinquishing the role of patient and beginning to resume everyday activities, even if these must be modified to adjust for the effects of cancer and its treatment. The third, or permanent, survival stage begins when cancer no longer plays a dominant role in a person's day-to-day routine. (Some cancer patients, of course, never reach the second or third stage.)

Five-year Cancer Survival Rates for Selected Cancers*
(all stages of disease)

Cancer	Rate
Bladder	75%
Breast	75%
Cervix	67%
Colon-Rectum	52%
Leukemia	34%
Lung	13%
Melanoma (skin)	80%
Oral	52%
Ovary	38%
Prostate	70%
Testis	87%
Uterus	85%

*In the United States; figures are for cases diagnosed from 1974 to 1985.

Source: National Cancer Institute

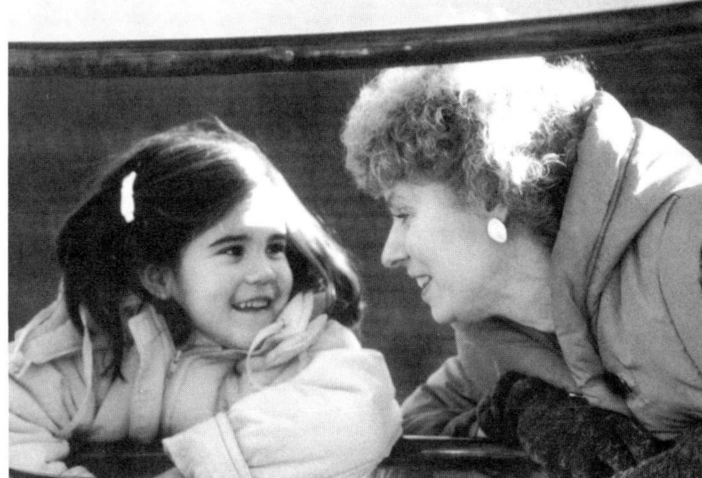

Overcoming her post-treatment depression after breast cancer, Nancy Hoeltzel resumed her teaching career.

Some Common Fears

The diagnosis of cancer can be psychologically devastating. It typically provokes a set of fears known as the five "Ds": death, disfigurement, disability, dependence, and disruption of key personal and professional relationships. The strength of any of these fears depends not only on the type of cancer and the treatment planned, but also on the individual. While an adult might fear disability leading to loss of a job and to dependency, an adolescent might be more concerned with disfigurement and disruption of social relationships. Although these fears may seem overwhelming, they are normal for someone confronting a major disease. Excessive fear could, however, lead to inability to act, and further problems.

Once a person has been successfully treated there is always the fear of recurrence. For example, breast cancer caught before it has spread has a 30 percent rate of recurrence following surgery and radiation. The fear is usually greatest during the first two years after treatment but may continue for years and cause panic attacks, sleep problems, and even thoughts about suicide. Some patients become hypochondriacs, and others avoid necessary follow-up healthcare.

Nancy Hoeltzel is a cancer survivor whose son helped her overcome her post-treatment fears. In 1975 this Michigan woman discovered a lump in her breast that proved to be cancerous. After having her breast removed, she suffered from depres-

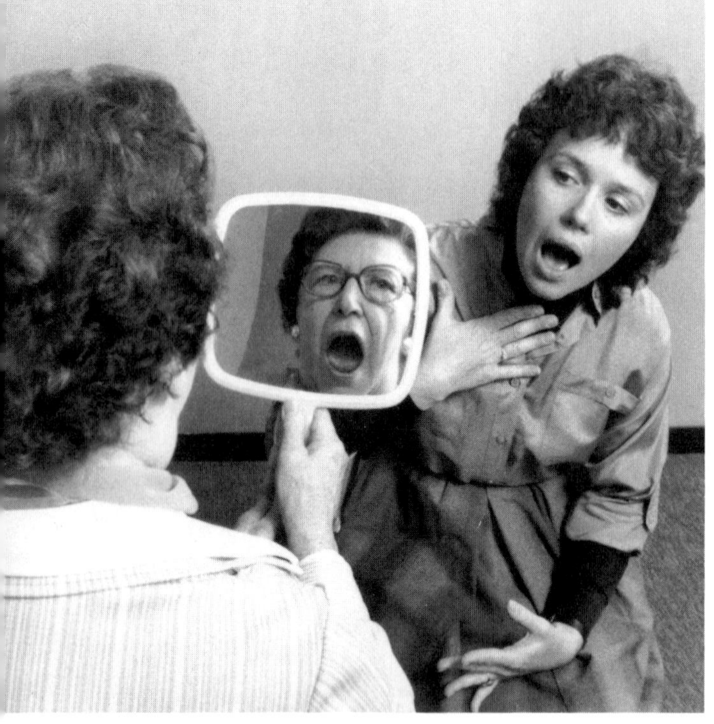

A cancer survivor whose larynx has been removed learns to speak by using swallowed air and forming words in the throat.

sion. Finally, a statement by her youngest son, "Mommy, I don't want you to die," made her realize that she would have to learn to deal with her negative feelings and go on. She set goals for herself, including returning to school for a master's degree in elementary education, and began teaching kindergarten. She founded a local chapter of Make Today Count, a self-help group for cancer survivors, families, and friends, and she lectures for the American Cancer Society.

If cancer does recur, the patient once again faces fear and depression and may not be able to function normally for a week or two. On the hopeful side for these patients is that new treatment methods may be better able to control the cancer than the methods used when the cancer was first diagnosed.

Physical Changes

Cancer and its treatment can leave a legacy of physical problems. The nausea and vomiting, dryness or soreness of the mouth, hair loss, redness or itching of the skin, fatigue, and increased susceptibility to infection that radiation and chemotherapy can cause generally disappear once active treatment ends or shortly afterward.

Some other side effects of cancer treatment, however, are irreversible. Certain drugs may cause lasting damage to the heart or bladder. Surgery for some cancers of the colon or rectum may necessitate an ostomy, a surgical opening in the abdomen for elimination of body waste (although this is not necessary in many cases). Treatment for some types of cancer can result in loss of a body part. If this is the larynx, the patient can learn to speak again using a form of speech known as esophageal, in which air is swallowed and then expelled through the mouth. At least two-thirds of all those whose larynxes have been removed are successful in learning this speaking technique. Others may rely on products such as an electric larynx or a mechanical device that fits into the opening left in the throat and uses exhaled air to create speech.

Limbs lost, primarily to bone cancer, call for major adjustments in getting around and performing daily activities, perhaps with the help of artificial limbs. Surgery for advanced cancers of the head and neck region can not only cause problems with chewing, swallowing, and speaking, but also result in facial disfigurement. Using implants and some of the survivor's own tissue, a plastic surgeon may be able to at least partially restore both appearance and function.

This was the case for Wilcie Skaggs of West Virginia, who, the week after he was diagnosed as having cancer of the nose, was told that he would die if his nose wasn't surgically removed. He had the operation in October 1984 and the next year endured three months of complicated reconstruction and plastic surgery. He survived to become an active volunteer for the American Cancer Society and a city councilman.

Changed Relationships

Having cancer is an experience that can point out the true friends, the ones who will rally around the survivor and stay as long as needed. Others may not be able to deal with changes in the survivor's appearance, or they resist being reminded of their own mortality. Some survivors themselves withdraw, embarrassed by their condition or appearance and afraid of rejection. If the cancer survivor is a parent, there may be increased financial stresses and changed family roles as others try to take over some of the cancer victim's responsibilities. If the cancer patient is a child, the parents may become overprotective and indulgent, causing jealousy among siblings. Yet with all these added strains and stresses, studies have shown that cancer can be a catalyst for a closer family relationship.

Changes in body image and impairment of bodily functions can alter relationships between sexual partners. Women who have been treated with radiation to the uterus, cervix, or vagina may have pain or discomfort during intercourse. Women who have had a hysterectomy may feel "incomplete" and miss the sensation of the uterus contracting during orgasm; if both ovaries were also removed, women who had not yet reached menopause will experience the sudden onset of menopausal symptoms. Women who have had a breast or portion of a breast removed may feel unattractive to their partners, unworthy, and less feminine. Men treated with radiation or surgery for prostate cancer may experience problems with erections. These physical problems can be compounded by misconceptions, among them a belief that cancer may be transmitted through sexual intercourse and that radiation can make a patient radioactive and hence unsafe to touch. Health professionals counseling cancer patients can clear up such misconceptions and provide practical advice on overcoming limitations.

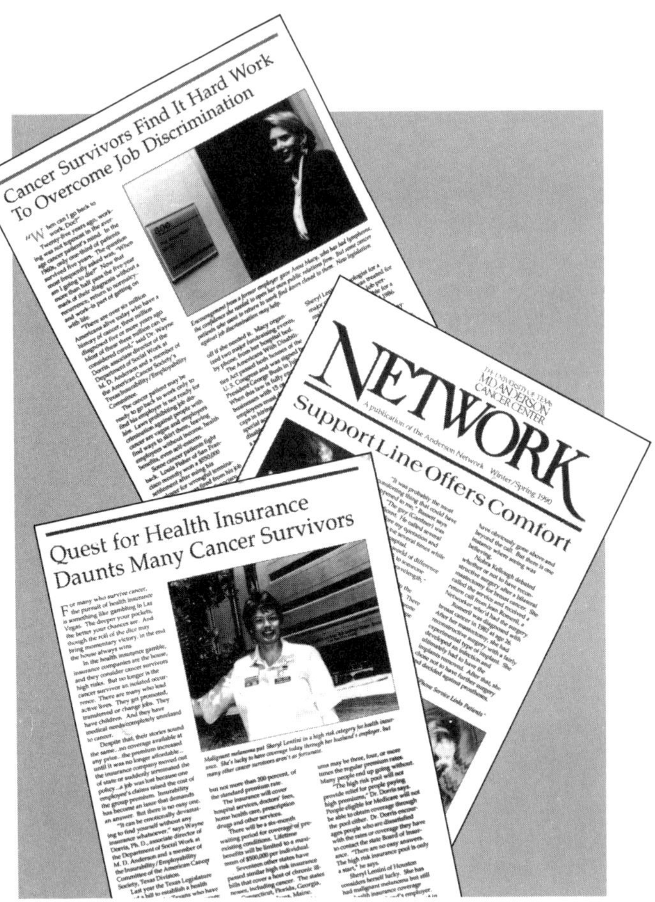

Cancer Survivors Find It Hard Work To Overcome Job Discrimination

NETWORK

A publication of the Anderson Network

Support Line Offers Comfort

Quest for Health Insurance Daunts Many Cancer Survivors

The Anderson Network, a volunteer program run by former patients, offers nonmedical support to cancer survivors at the University of Texas M. D. Anderson Cancer Center. Its hospitality room in the hospital, below, provides a cheerful setting for informal discussion; its publications highlight such concerns as health insurance and job discrimination.

Can Survivors Have Children?

Chemotherapy can impair the reproductive system; among its possible effects are failure of the ovaries and premature menopause. Cancer of the reproductive organs may cause sterility, but this is not always the case. Women treated for early cervical cancer can later conceive, and some men treated for early-stage testicular cancer can retain fertility. Cancer survivors whose reproductive organs may have been affected directly or indirectly are advised to have genetic counseling and to wait two years after completing treatment before attempting to become parents. This allows the patient to recover from the physical and psychological effects of treatment and ensures that any potential recurrence of the cancer has been adequately delayed. Pregnancies that begin more than two years after treatment have the same chance of being successful as those among people not treated for cancer.

Many of those who survive childhood cancer can look forward to having children. A U.S. National Cancer Institute study found that treatment for childhood and adolescent cancer given before 1975 reduced female fertility by 7 percent and male by 24 percent. By type of cancer, a significant reduction in fertility was found for males and females

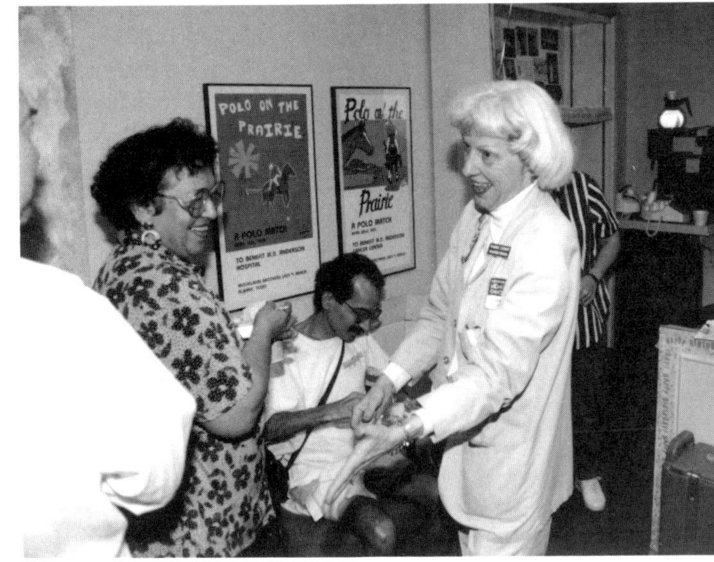

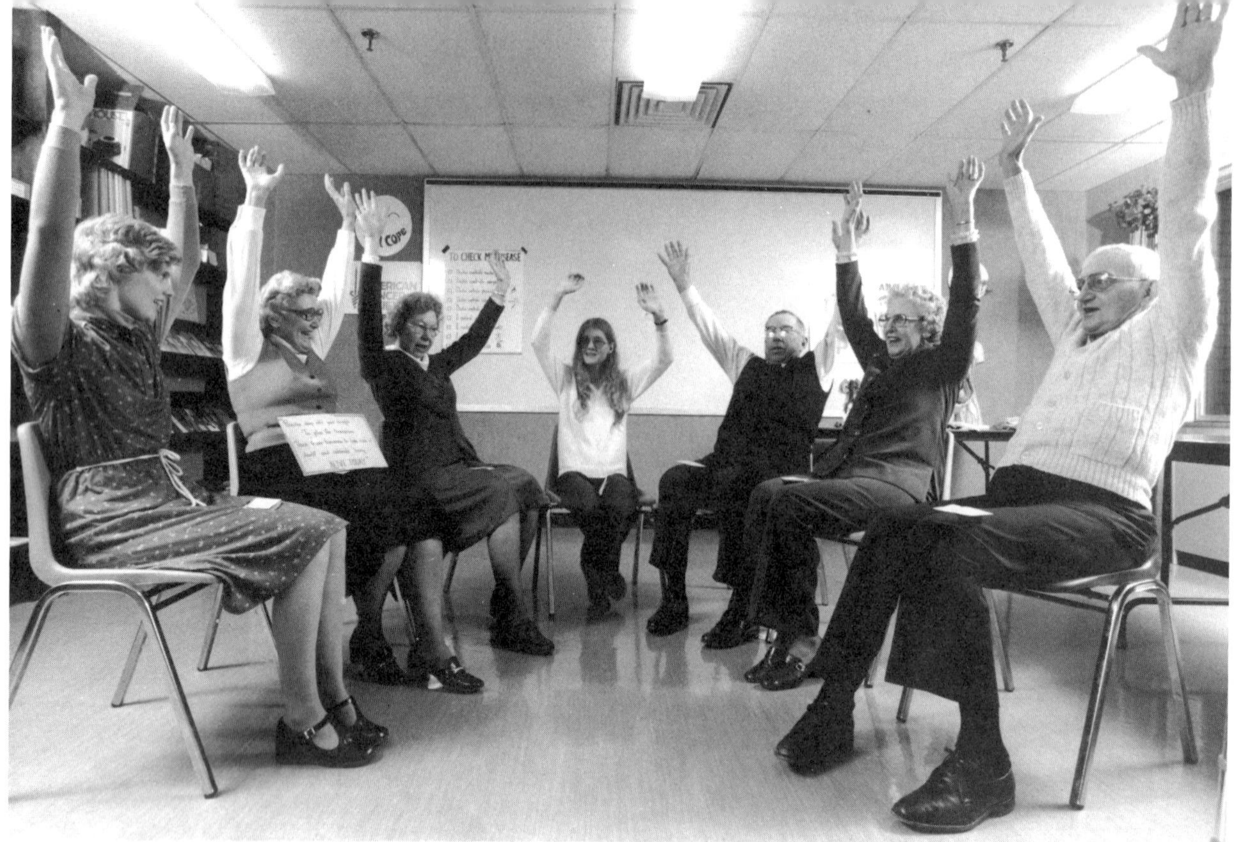

A Minnesota class of I Can Cope, a national patient education program of the American Cancer Society, focuses on remaining active in both mind and body.

treated for the form of lymph system cancer called Hodgkin's disease (23 percent) and for males treated for genital cancer (55 percent). The study, published in 1987, looked at cancer patients treated before 1975 to assess the long-term impact. Newer treatments, however, are often more toxic and given in higher doses.

Another National Cancer Institute study, also published in 1987, showed that children of cancer survivors are generally not at increased risk for developing cancer because of their parents' cancer treatment. The cancers that did occur among the children of cancer survivors were primarily directly inherited types, such as retinoblastoma (an eye cancer), or those for which family history is a known risk factor, such as breast cancer.

Employment Concerns

New York City police officer Vivian Potter was diagnosed with cancer of the lymph glands in 1983 and continued to fulfill her duties in the Narcotics Unit while receiving chemotherapy. A year and a half after her diagnosis, the Police Department tried to fire her because of the cancer. She fought the department for a year, until it abandoned its effort to force her resignation.

Michael W. Lamb, Sr., received his diagnosis of Hodgkin's disease at his Air Force precommissioning physical examination. During his treatment the Air Force declared him unfit for duty, but he fought to remain on active duty. Finally, the Air Force ruled to reinstate him as a test case. He was later promoted to captain, and the Air Force changed its policy concerning cancer patients.

A study conducted some years ago by the Metropolitan Life Insurance Company among its own employees showed that cancer patients had the same turnover and absenteeism rates as other workers and could continue to do the job they were hired to perform. Yet, although attitudes and policies about cancer survivors have improved, some job discrimination persists. This is mainly attributable to three myths about cancer—that it is a death sentence, that it is contagious, and that cancer survivors are unproductive.

Most cancer survivors are capable of doing the jobs they held before diagnosis. In three studies conducted in California, 71 percent of white-collar workers, 69 percent of blue-collar workers, and 40 percent of young people returned to where they worked before their cancers were diagnosed. A survey of employers found that it was their usual practice to bring back those who had been on leave for cancer treatment, although there were cases where the person was told not to return. Some employers also indicated that they adjusted working hours and conditions if needed.

Velma Jean Mabey of Idaho was able to return to her job after a small, painless lump in her left arm and shoulder turned out to be fibrosarcoma, a form of soft-tissue cancer. Both her arm and her shoulder had to be removed. Within six days she was back at work as office manager for a local doctor. That was in the mid-1970s. She uses a one-handed typewriter at work.

Some problems encountered in the workplace are related to the disease or its treatment, others to the reactions of coworkers. Treatment with drugs or radiation may cause the person to tire more easily or become nauseated. Pain may cause difficulties in moving or reaching for something. Coworkers may feel uncomfortable being around someone who has had cancer, particularly if there is physical evidence. Some persons return to their old job only to find they have suddenly been shifted onto another career track.

Trying to get a new job can be more discouraging. In the California studies, 13 percent of the blue-collar workers, 22 percent of the white-collar workers, and 45 percent of the young people reported being rejected for a job. It is not possible to say how many of these rejections were due to cancer, but about 6 percent of those interviewed for the employer survey said that cancer is usually a reason to disqualify a person. An analysis of all these and several other studies concluded that employers tend to think of all cancer survivors as having similar capabilities and expected survival times, and that employers often do not realize that the prognosis for many cancer patients has greatly improved.

The Rehabilitation Act of 1973, designed to prevent discrimination against persons with disabilities in the United States, covers those who have been treated for cancer. The law applies to most firms with contracts or subcontracts from the federal government. These employers must have affirmative action plans to hire and retain persons with disabilities, including cancer survivors. Under this law, cancer survivors cannot be discriminated against in hiring, promotions, transfers, layoffs, or termination, among other areas. Employment tests must be related to the job. Another section of the law applies to all institutions, such as schools, colleges, and hospitals. Schools must accept as students qualified children and adults with disabilities and cannot discriminate against adults with disabilities in hiring. Under the law, physical and medical examinations cannot be required before a job is offered and can be required after a job offer only if required of all employees. Many U.S. states have their own antidiscrimination laws as well.

The Americans With Disabilities Act of 1990, which likewise applies to cancer survivors, extends the 1973 law. The act requires employers to make "reasonable accommodations" to persons with disabilities, unless the employer can demonstrate that this would create "undue hardship." These changes might include making existing facilities accessible and usable to those with physical limitations, restructuring work schedules, and modifying equipment, training, and policies.

Health Insurance

Insurance issues are closely related to employment concerns, because a lost job often means that insurance is lost just when it is needed most. Some survivors feel trapped in jobs because they fear they might not qualify for new insurance if they change jobs. This can be particularly distressing for young people who may be looking for career advancement or new experiences. Many insurance companies do allow employees changing jobs to convert from the current employer's group plan to an individual policy, but the coverage is usually more limited and the price higher.

Obtaining or renewing individual insurance coverage on one's own can be difficult. Cancer survivors may face outright rejection by insurance companies, or be issued policies with very high premiums or restricted coverage. In many cases the policies specifically exclude coverage for "preexisting conditions" such as cancer for months or even years. A 1985 federal law known as COBRA provides many employees with the option of continuing to be covered under the employer's insurance plan for up to 18 months after leaving a job—at the employee's expense. This can buy time to find the best available insurance policy without loss of coverage.

Continuing Support

Most cancer survivors need some form of rehabilitation to resume a normal or near-normal life-style.

This can include physical rehabilitation to improve mobility and endurance so that everyday activities can be carried out; psychological rehabilitation to address concerns such as the fear of death or recurrence, depression, and low self-image; social rehabilitation to lessen the strain cancer imposes on personal and business relationships; and financial and vocational rehabilitation.

Psychological support groups for cancer patients are now generally recognized as important means of comfort and aid. The groups, which may be led by a psychiatrist, psychologist, social worker, nurse, or cancer survivor, provide patients with an opportunity to share their anxieties and concerns with those who have had similar experiences. In a 1989 study of 86 women with breast cancer that had spread to other organs, those randomly assigned to a special support group reported less depression and anxiety and survived an average of 18 months longer than a control group.

The Post-Treatment Resource Program at Memorial Sloan-Kettering Cancer Center in New York City, one of the most comprehensive programs for cancer survivors, offers educational seminars and workshops on topics of concern to cancer survivors; provides individual, family, and group counseling; and runs informal support groups and social hours. According to Program Director Karrie Zampini, the immediate post-treatment time is often very difficult for cancer survivors because, although they have completed the difficult treatment phase, they are no longer under direct medical care and must adjust to more active management of their own lives again. When the close medical supervision that goes with cancer treatment ends, patients can feel abandoned.

Because the first survivors to draw on Memorial Sloan-Kettering's program tended to be breast cancer patients, separate discussion groups were instituted for them. A group for adults aged 20 to "30-something" addresses the issues that confront younger cancer patients, such as dating, socializing, and dealing with overprotective parents. There are also separate groups for those over 40 and for senior citizens.

At group meetings of cancer survivors, participants often offer personal accounts of their struggles and usually introduce themselves not only by name, but also by type of cancer and date of diagnosis, the cancer having become so much a part of

The Walker Cancer Support Group at Stanford University Hospital in California stresses self-help and encourages survivors to be aware of their feelings in coping with the disease.

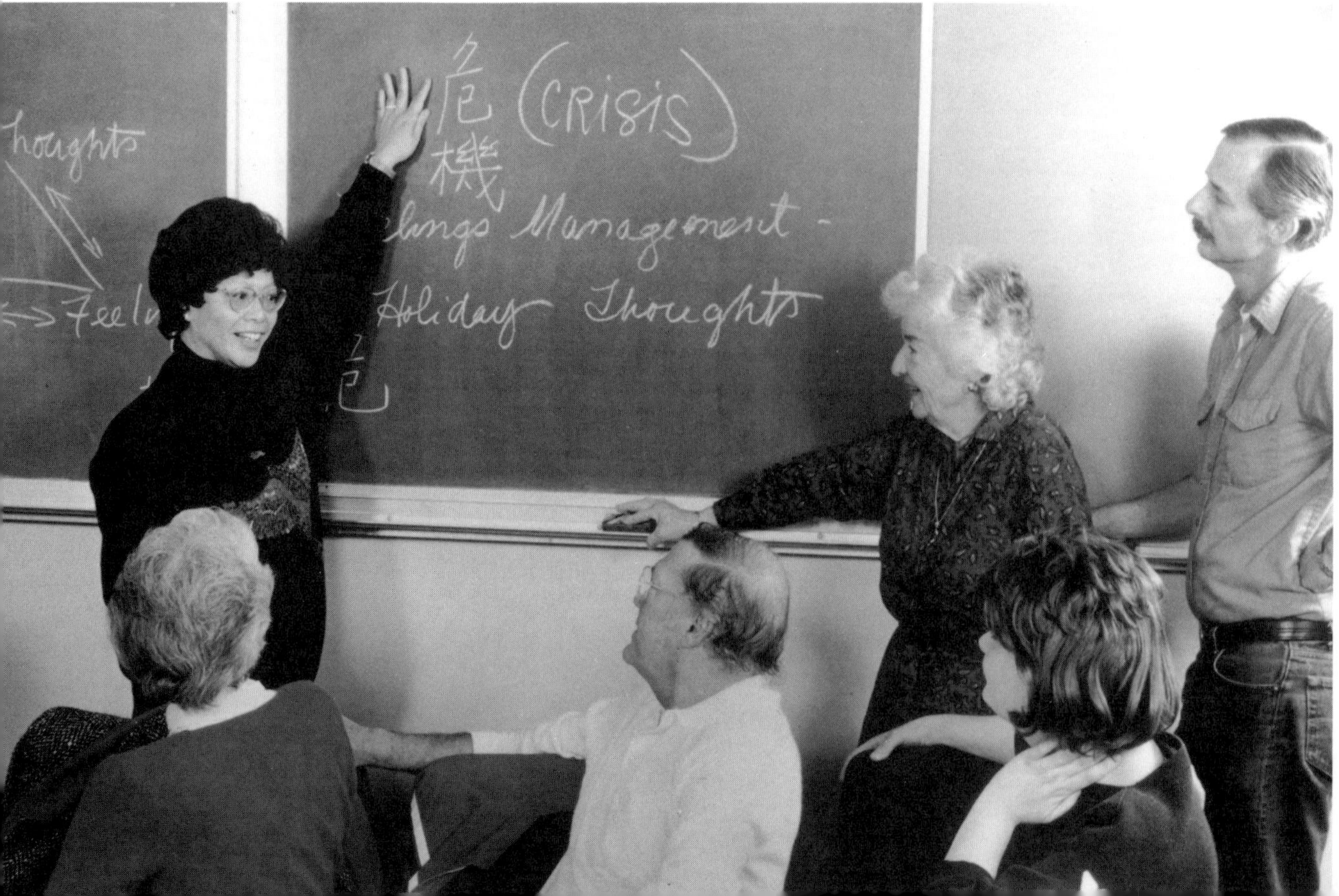

their identity. No matter how much support a patient has received from family, Zampini notes, a real camaraderie develops among survivors. They need to be reassured that concerns with such issues as recurrence and self-image are normal. Especially in the United States, she said, with its "go for it" and "be tough" attitude, cancer survivors sometimes feel pressured to be "model" survivors and deal with all their problems immediately. Yet many patients need time to grieve, whether for loss of health, a changed appearance, or loss of a body part. At the post-treatment program, survivors are reassured that there is a psychological healing process and that it takes time to integrate the cancer experience into their lives and go on.

Many U.S. and Canadian hospitals, including Memorial Sloan-Kettering and the University of Texas M. D. Anderson Cancer Center in Houston, have patient-to-patient volunteer programs in which former patients visit those recently diagnosed. The Texas program, known as the Anderson Network, has hundreds of members in Texas and other states who provide support via telephone and operate a hospitality room at the cancer center. CanSurmount is a short-term visitor program run by the American Cancer Society, with volunteers making visits in hospitals or at home. The volunteers do not answer medical questions but can offer emotional support and practical advice on living with cancer. Programs run by the National Coalition for Cancer Survivorship also rely on this technique of what NCCS President Mullan calls "the veterans helping the rookies." In Canada, the Canadian Cancer Society's Patient Services program sponsors practical and emotional support networks for survivors, including one-to-one visiting programs.

Self-help groups are directed by the survivors themselves. These groups stress self-reliance and fellowship. It was once feared that such groups would foster negative attitudes toward physicians and cancer treatment, but these concerns have not been substantiated. Many members seek professional help as well. In an evaluation of an Alabama self-help group, TOUCH (Today Our Understanding of Cancer is Hope), participants reported significant gains in knowledge about cancer, in the ability to talk to doctors, family, and friends about the disease, in relationships, and in coping with the disease. What they most valued about the group were altruism, sharing, and the feeling of hope.

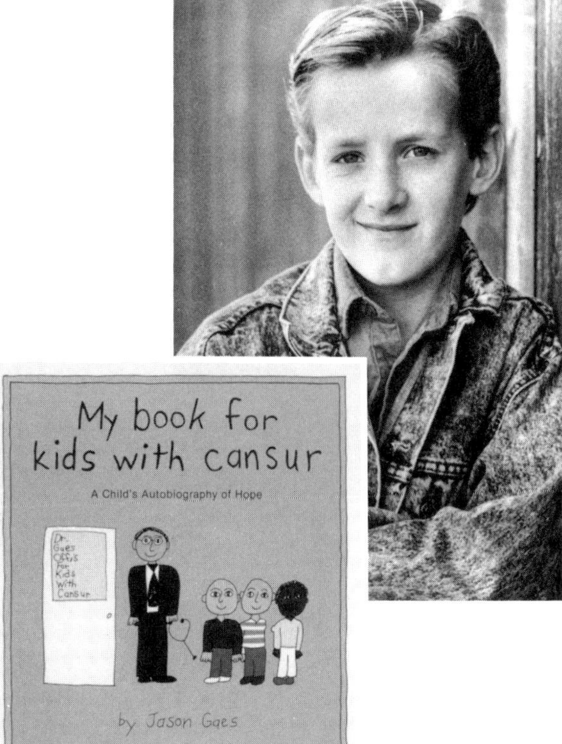

My book for kids with cansur *by Jason Gaes, having inspired countless young cancer patients since it was first published in 1987, appeared in paperback in 1991. Its author, who was eight when he wrote the book, hopes to become a pediatric oncologist.*

In the United States, Make Today Count is a nationwide network of more than 200 chapters that meet informally to provide mutual emotional support for members. Its goal is to assist patients and families to "live each day as fully and completely as possible."

Special Concerns of Children

While six-year-old Jason Gaes of Worthington, Minn., was visiting relatives in June 1984, his uncle discovered a lump in Jason's mouth that, along with four additional tumors found by a physician, was diagnosed as Burkitt's lymphoma. Jason was not expected to live past his seventh birthday, but he refused to give up. He went through two painful years of surgery, radiation, and chemotherapy. When he was eight, he wrote *My book for kids with cansur*, which describes how these treatments affected him, how he dealt with his fears, and his stays in the hospital. Years later Jason is still answering letters generated by the book and by his other public activities aimed at telling those diagnosed with cancer to keep fighting.

In the United States there were an estimated 7,600 new cases of cancer among children in 1990; in Canada, an estimated 3,500 people under 21 years old underwent treatments for cancer in that year. U.S. children's five-year survival rates range from 51 percent to 89 percent, depending on the specific type of cancer. By the year 2000, one in every thousand young adults seeking a job will be a survivor of childhood cancer.

Children with cancer face special challenges. Some aggressive cancer treatments may later cause sterility, thyroid problems, curvature of the spine, dental problems, learning difficulties, and emotional problems. Children who survive cancer have a 10 percent chance of developing another type of cancer after 20 years, although as treatment improves the chances are reduced. A follow-up study of childhood cancer survivors who were treated with radiation and the anticancer drugs known as alkylating agents suggests that these individuals are at increased risk of developing bone cancer and that the risk rises with increasing amounts of radiation or drugs.

Another study showed that children and adolescents who survive cancers of the central nervous system are more likely than their brothers and sisters to have physical, social, and intellectual problems as adults. Compared to their siblings, these survivors were 11 times more likely never to have been employed and 6 times more likely to have had a health condition affect their work. They were 29 times more likely to be unable to drive and 4 times more likely to have remained single.

A study involving more than 2,000 survivors of childhood and adolescent cancer and more than 3,000 siblings who did not have cancer found that both female and male survivors were less likely to marry than their siblings, but most of the difference was accounted for by male survivors of cancers of the central nervous system. For other cancer survivors, the difference was slight.

Long-term survival for cancer patients is still a fairly new reality. While in the past the major effort was understandably directed toward treatment, newer efforts also try to ease the transition from being a patient to being a child again. One such program is the Pediatric Star Community at the M. D. Anderson Cancer Center. Emphasis is placed on maintaining as much normalcy as possible for these young cancer survivors, both while in the hospital and after returning home. This includes schooling, and expectations for good grades are not put on hold while the child is receiving treatment.

Childhood cancer can be considered a family disease, because the whole family is involved. Schedules must be changed to arrange for treatment, and family relationships are altered. Self-help groups

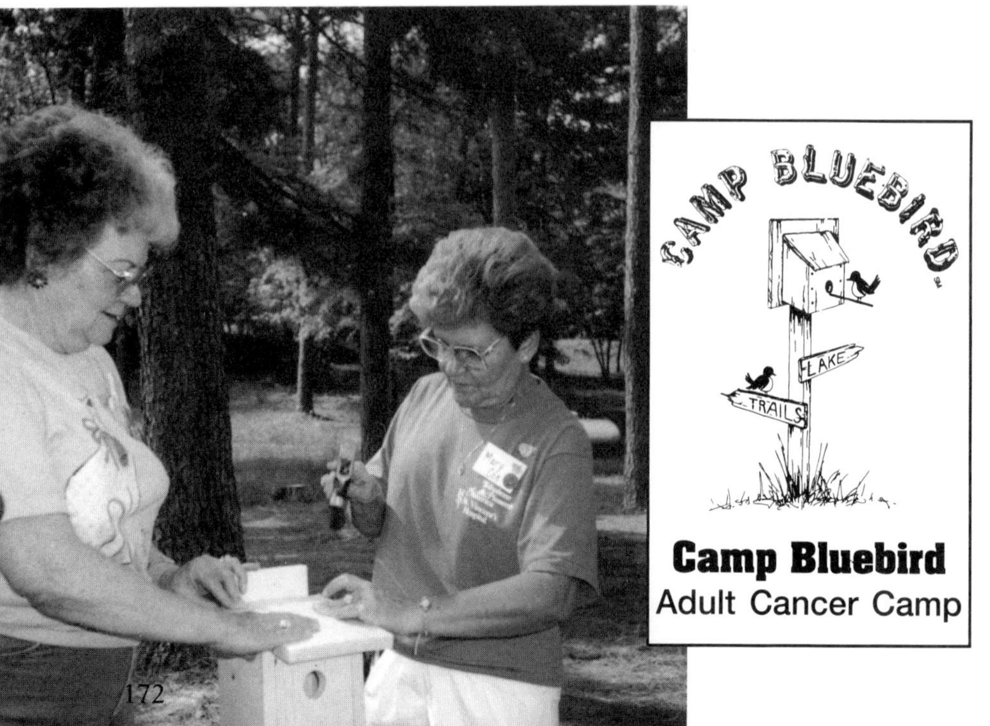

Camp Bluebird, sponsored by a Birmingham, Ala., hospital and Telephone Pioneers of America, offers three-day retreats for adults in all stages of cancer. Its wide variety of recreational activities and the group support sessions all focus on enjoying life. As a special interest, the group has joined a local campaign to preserve the bluebird population (photo at left: campers building birdhouses).

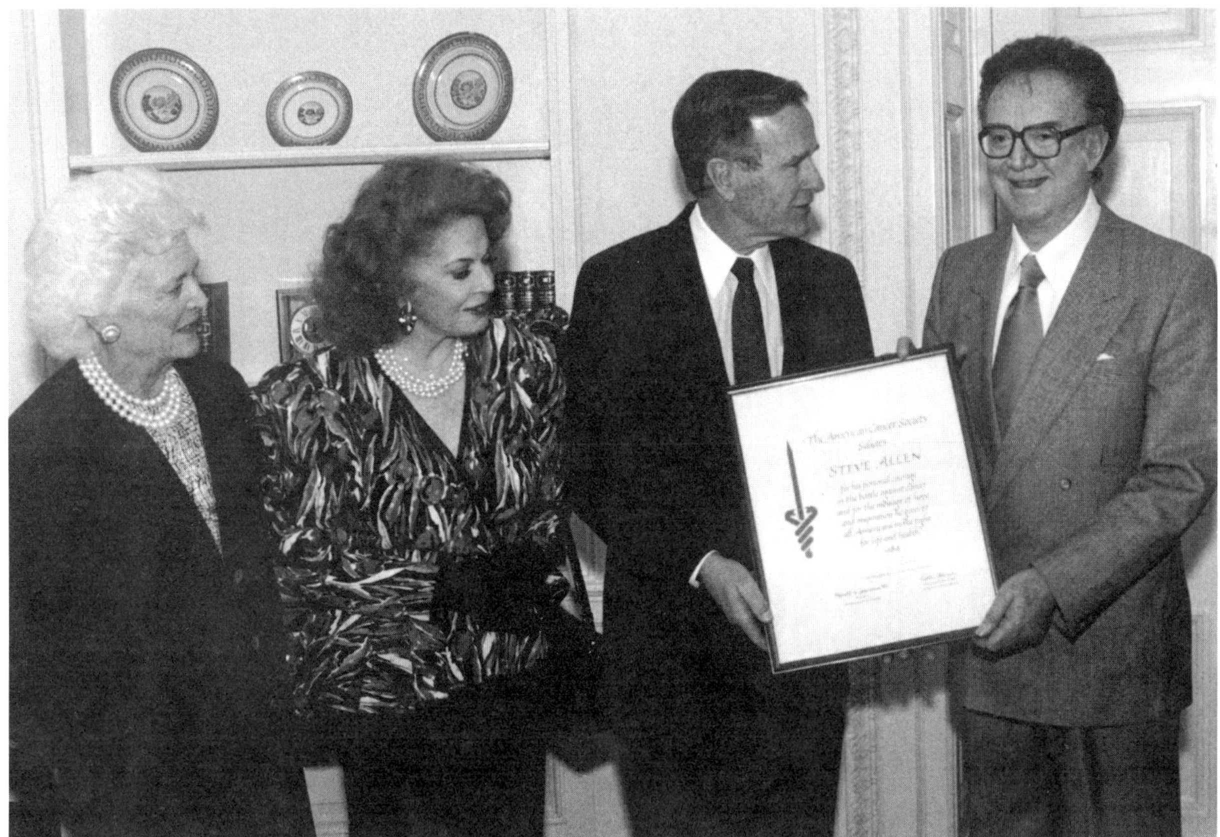

For his brave struggle against cancer, Steve Allen, right, received the American Cancer Society's Courage Award for 1989 from President George Bush. Watching with Barbara Bush (left) was Allen's wife, Jayne Meadows.

can be an important part of the support system for older children and their families. Peer counseling offers an opportunity to discuss shared experiences and gain practical advice. The Candlelighters Childhood Cancer Foundation is an international network of more than 250 parent support groups. It includes parents of the newly diagnosed and those of long-term survivors.

The Long-term Follow-up and Health Maintenance Clinic at M. D. Anderson was established in the mid-1970s to meet the special needs of former childhood cancer patients. The clinic provides thorough physical examinations to monitor long-term side effects of cancer treatment and to check for the development of second malignancies. It also provides instruction on healthful life-style practices to reduce the risk of recurrence. Patients who develop medical problems are referred to appropriate departments at the hospital or to specialists in their hometowns.

Fighting Back

Cancer survivors are becoming increasingly willing to identify themselves as such and to fight back against the disease and its effects on their lives. Several factors have converged to promote this new sense of empowerment. More effective and less devastating treatments mean greater hope of continued survival with a good quality of life. For example, young patients with primary bone cancer who in the past might have been subjected to an amputation of the arm or leg can now be successfully treated by removal and replacement of only a section of the bone.

The success of other special interest groups in fighting for their rights and a greater willingness to challenge authority, including medical experts, have helped make cancer patients more willing to take an active part in their treatment. Organizations such as Y-ME, a national breast cancer advocacy group, have begun to lobby for more funds for research and mandatory insurance coverage for mammograms (breast X rays), as well as offering information and support to patients. The stigma of cancer has been lessened by celebrities being candid about having cancer—people such as former First Lady Betty Ford, TV personality Steve Allen, actor Jack Klugman, and actress Jill Ireland (who died of breast cancer in May 1990).

Another prominent cancer survivor is Richard A. Bloch, who along with his brother, Henry, founded the tax preparation business H. & R. Block. Since being cured of lung cancer more than ten years ago, Richard Bloch has been celebrating life as a cancer survivor and encouraging others to do the same. Since 1986, he has staged an annual "Fighting Cancer Rally" in Kansas City, Mo., and in June 1990 he dedicated a Cancer Survivors Park there for which he provided the funds. He has also donated the money for two free cancer centers, one offering group therapy, the other sponsoring a panel of experts who people diagnosed with cancer can consult for a second opinion.

This theme of entitlement and empowerment is embodied in the charter of the NCCS: "The mission of the National Coalition for Cancer Survivorship is to communicate that there can be vibrant, productive life following the diagnosis of cancer; that millions of cancer survivors share a common, transforming experience that has impacted their lives with new challenges and enhanced potentials; and that these survivors, their families and supporters represent a burgeoning constituency and a powerful, positive force in society." □

SOURCES OF FURTHER INFORMATION

American Cancer Society. Tel.: (800) ACS-2345 or contact your local chapter.

The Anderson Network, the University of Texas M. D. Anderson Cancer Center, 1515 Holcombe Boulevard, Houston, TX 77030. Tel.: (713) 792-2553 or (800) 345-6324.

The Canadian Cancer Society. Contact your provincial office.

Canadian Candlelighters Childhood Cancer Foundation, 148 Quinn Street, Felixburg, Que. J0J 1N0. Tel.: (514) 248-3341.

The Cancer Information Service (a U.S. nationwide telephone information system). Tel.: (800) 4-CANCER.

Candlelighters Childhood Cancer Foundation, 1312 Eighteenth Street NW, Suite 200, Washington, DC 20036. Tel.: (800) 366-2233 or (202) 659-5136.

Make Today Count, 101½ S. Union Street, Alexandria, VA 22314. Tel.: (703) 548-9674.

National Cancer Institute, Office of Cancer Communications, 9000 Rockville Pike, Building 31, Room 10A24, Bethesda, MD 20892. Tel.: (301) 496-6641.

The National Coalition for Cancer Survivorship, 323 Eighth Street SW, Albuquerque, NM 87102. Tel.: (505) 764-9956.

SUGGESTIONS FOR FURTHER READING

BEATTY, ROBERT O. *Still a Lot of Living: Coping With Cancer.* New York, Macmillan, 1978.

BLOCH, RICHARD. *Fighting Cancer: A Step-by-Step Guide to Helping Yourself Fight Cancer.* Kansas City, Mo., Cancer Connection, 1985.

BLOCH, RICHARD, AND ANNETTE BLOCH. *Cancer... There's Hope.* Kansas City, Mo., Cancer Connection, 1981.

GLASSMAN, JUDITH. *The Cancer Survivors and How They Did It.* New York, Dial, 1983.

HOLLEB, ARTHUR I., M.D. ET AL., EDS. *The American Cancer Society's Complete Book of Cancer.* Garden City, N.Y., Doubleday, 1986.

LESHAN, LAWRENCE. *Cancer as a Turning Point: A Handbook for People with Cancer, Their Families, and Health Professionals.* New York, Dutton, 1989.

MORRA, MARION, AND EVE POTTS. *Choices: Realistic Alternatives in Cancer Treatment* (revised edition). New York, Avon, 1987.

MULLAN, FITZHUGH. *Vital Signs: A Young Doctor's Struggle With Cancer.* New York, Farrar, Straus & Giroux, 1982.

NATIONAL COALITION FOR CANCER SURVIVORS. *Charting the Journey: An Almanac of Practical Resources for Cancer Survivors.* Mount Vernon, NY, Consumers' Union, 1990.

PEPPER, CURTIS BILL. *We the Victors: The New Lives of 100 People Who Conquered Cancer and How They Did It.* Garden City, NY, Doubleday, 1984.

SIEGEL, MARY-ELLEN. *The Cancer Patient's Handbook.* New York, Walker and Company, 1986.

SPINGARN, NATALIE DAVIS. *Hanging in There.* New York, Stein & Day, 1982.

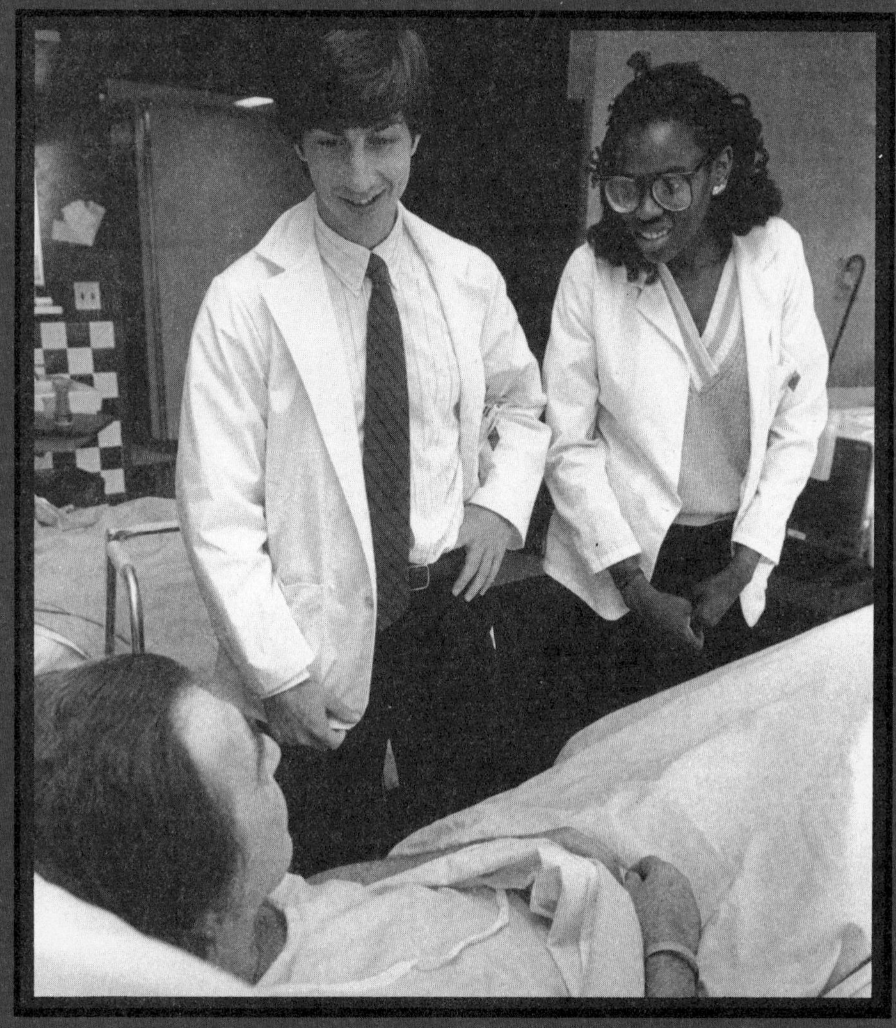

SPOTLIGHT ON HEALTH

Contributors

Authors of articles in the Spotlight on Health section

Barrett, Janet. Writer specializing in health, social services, and education issues. STEROIDS AND TEENAGERS.

Bloomfield, Louise A. Staff Editor. THE VIRTUES OF OLIVE OIL.

Bondi, Edward E., M.D. Associate Professor, Department of Dermatology, University of Pennsylvania. ATHLETE'S FOOT.

Cohn, Jeffrey P. Writer specializing in health issues. LEG CRAMPS.

Dickson, Jesse H., M.D. Professor, Chief of Spine Service, Division of Orthopedic Surgery, Baylor College of Medicine; Deputy Chief of Service, Orthopedic Surgery, The Methodist Hospital; President, Scoliosis Research Society; Head of Hip Service, Shriners Hospital for Crippled Children, Houston unit. SCOLIOSIS.

DiDonato, Roberta M., M.S.P.A. Supervisor, Speech Pathology Service, The Methodist Hospital; Clinical Instructor, Department of Otorhinolaryngology, Baylor College of Medicine. VOICE PROBLEMS (coauthor).

Donovan, Donald T., M.D. Assistant Professor, Baylor College of Medicine; Deputy Chief of Service, The Methodist Hospital. VOICE PROBLEMS (coauthor).

Finkelman, Martin L., M.D. Attending Physician, Long Island College Hospital; Fellow, American Academy of Pediatrics. CIRCUMCISION: PROS AND CONS.

Fisher, Jeffrey, M.D. Associate Professor of Clinical Medicine, Division of Cardiology, New York Hospital-Cornell Medical Center, New York City. CONGESTIVE HEART FAILURE (coauthor).

Gustaitis, John W., M.D. Chairman, Department of Radiology, The Community Hospital, Munster, Ind. THE SAFETY OF X RAYS.

Gustaitis, Joseph. Staff Editor. EATING OUT WISELY.

Iseman, Michael D., M.D. Chief, Clinical Mycobacteriology Service, Division of Infectious Diseases, National Jewish Center for Immunology & Respiratory Medicine; Professor of Medicine, University of Colorado School of Medicine. TUBERCULOSIS.

Jones, James F., M.D. Staff Member, Department of Pediatrics, National Jewish Center for Immunology & Respiratory Medicine; Associate Professor of Pediatrics, University of Colorado School of Medicine. CHRONIC FATIGUE SYNDROME.

Klippel, John H., M.D. Clinical Director, National Institute of Arthritis and Musculoskeletal and Skin Disease. LUPUS.

Koren, Michael J., M.D. Assistant Attending Physician, New York Hospital; Fellow in Cardiology, Cornell University Medical College. CONGESTIVE HEART FAILURE (coauthor).

Mandel, Irwin D., D.D.S. Professor of Dentistry, Director, Center for Clinical Research in Dentistry, Columbia University School of Dental and Oral Surgery. PREVENTING GUM DISEASE.

Noble, Robert C., M.D. Professor of Medicine, Division of Infectious Diseases, University of Kentucky College of Medicine. THE RESURGENCE OF SYPHILIS.

Ober, William B., M.D. Former Clinical Professor of Pathology, Mount Sinai School of Medicine, New Jersey College of Medicine. WHAT AUTOPSIES REVEAL.

Russo, Paul, M.D. Attending Surgeon, Memorial Sloan-Kettering Cancer Center; Assistant Professor of Surgery, Cornell University Medical College. INCONTINENCE: A TREATABLE PROBLEM.

Sternfeld, Leon, M.D. Medical Director, United Cerebral Palsy Associations and United Cerebral Palsy Research & Education Foundation. CEREBRAL PALSY.

Strauch, Ingrid J. Staff Editor. ATHLETIC SHOES: NOT JUST SNEAKERS ANYMORE; COPING WITH MORNING SICKNESS; FAINTING; SAFE COOKWARE.

Work, Janis A., Ph.D. Medical writer and editor. THE NEW MEDICAL EDUCATION.

Coping With MORNING SICKNESS

Ingrid J. Strauch

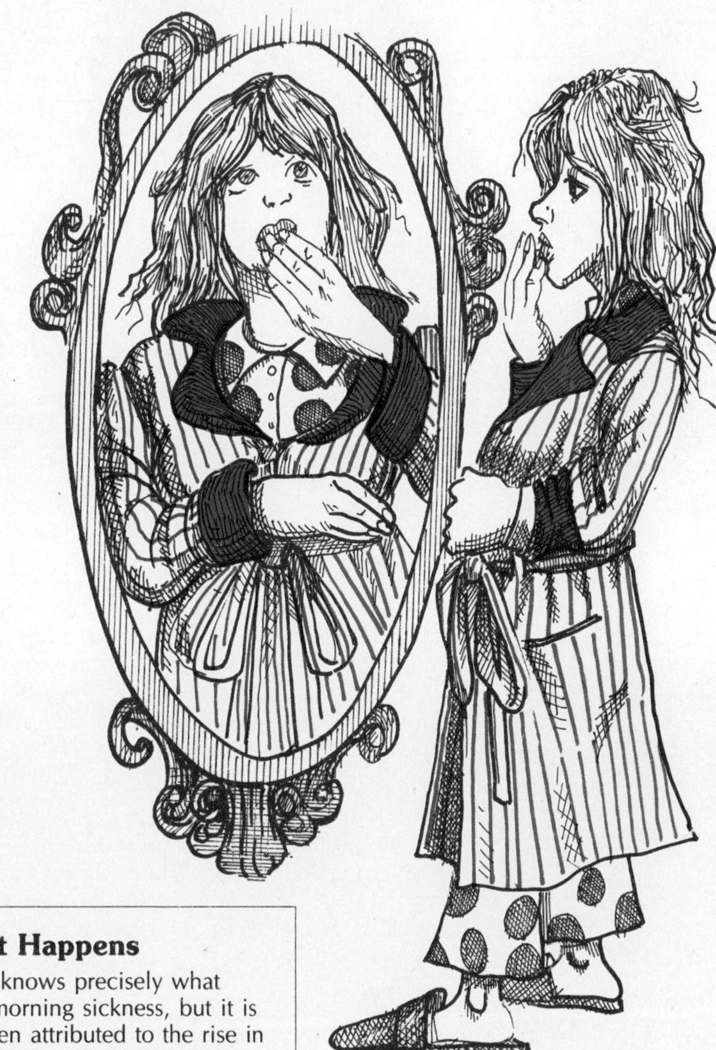

Sometimes it may be the first sign that a woman is pregnant: a wave of nausea sweeps over her as she climbs out of bed, or her stomach turns when someone lights a cigarette, or she feels the urge to vomit at the whiff of a greasy hamburger.

Morning sickness is the name given to the nausea and vomiting that affect over 50 percent of pregnant women in their first trimester (the first three months of pregnancy). As the name implies, the problem is most often experienced in the morning, but the symptoms may occur at any time of day or may persist throughout the day.

For most women morning sickness begins in the early weeks of pregnancy and generally subsides between the 12th and 16th weeks. In rare cases it remains throughout the entire pregnancy. The degree of discomfort varies from one individual to the next. Only about a third of those who suffer from morning sickness experience vomiting, which sometimes occurs without nausea. Excessive salivation occasionally accompanies the nausea or vomiting.

Because morning sickness afflicts so many women, it is considered a normal, if unpleasant, part of pregnancy. In most cases it goes away by itself and needs no treatment, and it usually has no lasting effects on either mother or fetus.

Why It Happens

No one knows precisely what causes morning sickness, but it is most often attributed to the rise in blood levels of two hormones—human chorionic gonadotropin (hCG) and estrogen—that occurs with pregnancy. (The body steps up production of both hormones about ten days after conception.) The level of hCG falls off in the 14th or 15th week of pregnancy, which is when morning sickness abates in most women.

Women carrying twins or triplets may suffer from especially severe morning sickness, since multiple gestation can lead to very high hormone levels.

In women prone to morning sickness, various factors can bring on or prolong a bout of nausea. Tobacco smoke, cooking odors, and fried or spicy foods are the most common culprits. Eating too much sugary food is another potential cause, and emotional stress appears to make morning sickness worse.

Feeling Better

No cure has been found for morning sickness despite centuries of trial and error by both physicians and patients. Perhaps it is fortunate for women that some of the attempted remedies—such as rubbing lard on the skin, bleeding with leeches, or applying cocaine to the cervix—didn't work. However, a few things do seem to help.

Since nausea tends to be worse when the stomach is either completely empty or overly full, it can sometimes be relieved by eating several small meals during the day rather than three large ones. Eating a cracker or a piece of dry toast before getting out of bed in the morning can alleviate the surge of nausea that often accompanies getting up, and a small snack right before bedtime can have a similar effect. If nausea is worse in the morning, it may help to allow more time for morning routines, since hurrying and feeling pressured can aggravate the problem.

It is best to stick to foods that are appealing even if they don't add up to a balanced diet, since it's important to eat *something*. Pregnant women generally find that bland foods high in complex carbohydrates, such as rice, bread, or pasta, go down most easily. If possible, they should avoid preparing for others foods with odors that provoke nausea.

Pregnant women are also advised to drink plenty of fluids to help neutralize stomach acid and prevent dehydration from vomiting. Drinking between rather than with meals may be more beneficial, because this helps prevent a too-full stomach.

Eating a dry cracker before getting out of bed can alleviate the surge of nausea that often accompanies getting up in the morning.

Moderate exercise can help control nausea, but movements that involve considerable bending and stretching tend to upset the stomach. Walking is a good choice because it also confers the benefits of aerobic exercise.

Although vomiting may relieve nausea to some degree, it is generally recommended that women suppress the urge to vomit whenever possible. Frequent vomiting can cause various medical problems. If vomiting does occur, it's important to rinse the mouth with water afterward since the acid in the stomach's contents can cause tooth decay.

Severe Cases

Occasionally a woman will develop such severe nausea and vomiting that she becomes dehydrated. When this extreme form of morning sickness (hyperemesis gravidarum) occurs, the woman may need to be hospitalized for intravenous feeding. Because emotional factors appear to play a significant role in this disorder, IV feeding is usually accompanied by psychological counseling, and in some cases drugs are administered to reduce nausea. With treatment, most patients cease vomiting within a few days and can begin eating small amounts of bland food, then eventually return to a broader diet. In rare cases serious medical complications arise, and the pregnancy must be terminated to protect the health of the mother.

A woman should consult her doctor if any of the following occur: she cannot eat or drink for 24 hours, she is vomiting three or four times a day, or she has lost weight because of nausea and vomiting. A woman whose diet has changed radically because of morning sickness should discuss this with her doctor even if she is not losing weight, to ensure that she and her unborn baby are receiving proper nutrition.

Drugs

There are no drugs on the U.S. market specifically formulated for morning sickness. In 1956 the U.S. Food and Drug Administration approved the drug Bendectin for morning sickness, but in 1983 the manufacturer, Merrell Dow Pharmaceuticals, ceased production because of hundreds of lawsuits claiming that Bendectin caused birth defects. Although an FDA panel found no association between Bendectin and birth defects, the drug has not been reintroduced in the United States. (It remains available in Europe.) In Canada a product identical to Bendectin, called Diclectin, has been on the market since 1979 and continues to be available. Studies of the drug are ongoing, but to date none have shown it to cause birth defects.

Other drugs that have been prescribed in the past include antinausea medications, sedatives, tranquilizers, and antihistamines. But the safety of such drugs for pregnant women has not been proven; in fact, some have been associated with fetal abnormalities in animal studies. Because the human fetus is particularly susceptible during the first trimester to any tendency of a drug to cause developmental malformations, a pregnant woman should ask her doctor about the risks involved before taking drugs—including over-the-counter products—for any medical condition.

A pregnant woman who is vomiting three or four times a day, has lost weight, or cannot eat or drink for 24 hours should consult her doctor.

The Good News

The good news about morning sickness (other than that it has to go away sometime) is that it may be a sign of a healthy baby to come. In a recent study of some 9,000 pregnancies, it was found that women with morning sickness had a slightly lower rate of premature deliveries, miscarriages, and stillbirths. Researchers theorize that women with nausea have higher levels of the hormones needed for a successful pregnancy. □

VOICE PROBLEMS

Roberta M. DiDonato, M.S.P.A.
Donald T. Donovan, M.D.

The voice is a wonderful tool that allows us to communicate our thoughts, emotions, and personalities. It is produced by many of the same structures that serve as pathways for air or food. Only humans have developed the ability to produce speech with these structures. The voice is considered to be adequate if it sounds pleasant, is appropriate in pitch for an individual's age and sex, and has the correct amount of loudness without strain. Some individuals have gone far beyond adequacy and developed special skills in using their voices: singers produce exquisite tones, and actors can manipulate their voices to carry great distances and to convey the personality of a role. However, most people take the voice for granted. It is not until a voice problem arises that the delicacy and sensitivity of the vocal mechanism is recognized.

Dysphonia

Voice specialists call voice problems dysphonia, *dys* for disorder and *phonia* for voice. Dysphonia can affect anyone, although women and the elderly are most often afflicted. Frequently dysphonia is simply a result of misusing the voice, by shouting too much, for example. Hoarseness caused by an isolated instance of loud talking or yelling usually disappears without treatment within a few days, provided the voice is not strained again during that time. Laryngitis—inflammation of the larynx (voice box)—also causes temporary hoarseness or loss of the voice. Laryngitis is most frequently caused by upper respiratory infections, such as a cold, and by allergies. Its symptoms, too, generally clear up spontaneously as the infection passes or the allergy season ends, or they can be alleviated with proper treatment of the allergy.

However, some cases of dysphonia pose serious problems. Chronic dysphonia can have a devastating effect on normal communication and social interactions. Sometimes dysphonia is the first symptom of life-threatening illness, such as cancer or neuromotor diseases (diseases of the nerves and muscles). Depending on its cause and severity, dysphonia may be treated medically or with voice therapy.

The Vocal System

In order to understand how the voice functions and what causes voice disorders, some knowledge of the three mechanisms that create the voice—the phonatory, respiratory, and resonatory systems—is important.

The Phonatory System. This is what actually produces the sound that is shaped into voice. It is composed of the larynx, a structure whose shape is visible from the outside of the neck and is often referred to as the Adam's apple. The larynx consists of the two vocal cords, or vocal folds—folds of tough, elastic tissue covered by mucous membranes—along with strands of cartilage, approximately 17 muscles (9 outside and 8 inside the larynx), and 4 nerves.

Voice is produced when muscles attached to the strands of cartilage cause the vocal cords to move closer together (an action called adduction) and air from the lungs passing through the narrowed space makes them vibrate. Other muscles can lengthen, shorten, tense, or relax the vocal cords, and these movements, along with variations in the force of the air pressure passing through the vocal cords, help to change the pitch, loudness, and quality of the voice.

The Respiratory System. Professional speakers and singers know the importance of the respiratory system in producing the most pleasant-sounding voice. This system consists of the lungs, trachea (windpipe), throat, mouth, and nose. As air is inhaled, or breathed into the lungs, through the mouth and nose, the lungs expand to fill the enlarged chest cavity created by the contraction of the chest muscles and the diaphragm (a broad flat muscle that separates the chest cavity from the abdominal cavity). Air is squeezed out of the lungs as the diaphragm and chest muscles relax again, making the chest cavity smaller. It is during this second part of the breathing cycle that voice is produced, as the air expelled from the lungs travels up the trachea and past the vocal cords. The air from the lungs provides a "pad" of air between the vocal cords to help them vibrate. This pad of air acts like a cushion and prevents the vocal cords from banging into each other with too much force.

The Resonatory System. This controls the sound of the voice; without it the voice would be thin, weak, and unimpressive. The system is composed of muscles and nerves that can alter the size and shape of the resonating chambers—the throat, mouth, and nose. By tensing or relaxing muscles in the throat, repositioning the tongue, lips, and jaw, or moving the soft palate to close or open the nasal passage, one can alter the sound of the voice. Even minor muscle tension can alter the shape of these chambers and dramatically modify the sound.

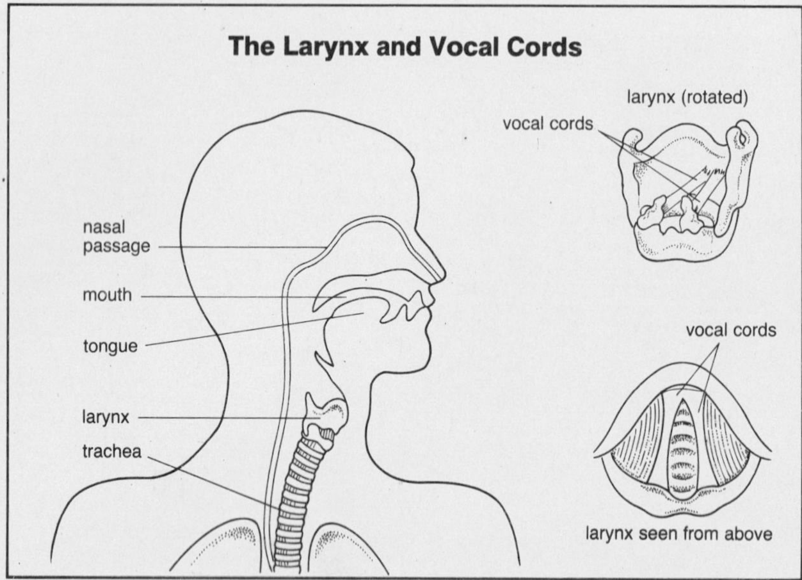

Singers have referred to this technique of altering sound by controlling the resonating chambers as placing the voice in either the head or the chest register. The ideal voice has the correct proportions of throat, mouth, and nose sounds; too much or too little of any of them detracts from the vocal quality.

Symptoms of Voice Disorders

The most common symptoms of dysphonia are hoarseness, a weak voice that is fatigued by the end of the day, an inability to project the voice, and chronic throat clearing. Less common symptoms include sudden, involuntary pitch changes, tightness in the throat, and catches in the voice. Various medical conditions can affect the muscles and nerves involved in the many parts of the voice system. A person experiencing any of the above symptoms—except for brief hoarseness with an obvious cause, such as having strained the voice—should consult an otolaryngologist (a physician who specializes in the ears, nose, and throat) to determine what is causing the problem.

The otolaryngologist examines the mucous membranes of the mouth, nose, and larynx to assess whether any abnormalities such as growths, masses, or lesions are contributing to the voice disorder. In addition, the doctor checks the mobility and symmetry of motion of the tongue, palate, and structures in the larynx, to see if the patient is suffering from paralysis of the vocal cords or from misuse of the muscles involved in speaking. This part of the examination is done with special mirrors or with an endoscope—a flexible, tubular instrument attached to a bright light that magnifies whatever the doctor is looking at.

Benign Growths

If a growth or lesion is present, it's important to find out whether it is benign or malignant. Some benign disorders are listed here.

Vocal Nodules. People who abuse their voices with constant loud talking or screaming may get vocal nodules, small, hard, callus-like nodules that make the voice sound raspy. This also occurs when muscles of the vocal system are strained—for example, if an individual tenses the muscles in the mouth and throat and holds back the sound or if the muscles in and around the larynx are overly tensed.

Vocal nodules generally occur in pairs on opposing surfaces of the vocal cords. They can be surgically removed but may recur if vocal abuse continues. The doctor may recommend that the patient visit a speech pathologist for voice therapy to learn how to use the voice without harming it. The nodules may disappear spontaneously if proper techniques are learned. (In the United States speech pathologists are certified by the American Speech-Language-Hearing Association and usually licensed by the state they practice in.)

Vocal Cord Polyps. These blister-like swellings occur on the mucous membranes of a single vocal cord. They interfere with the vibrations of the vocal cords, causing chronic hoarseness and a breathy voice quality. Polyps often develop in people who abuse their voices or who chronically inhale smoke or other fumes. Usually, the polyps must be surgically removed. If the cause is vocal abuse, voice therapy is then needed.

Vocal Cord Papillomas. Infection by a certain strain of the human papilloma virus can cause small, wart-like growths in the larynx. The growths cause hoarseness and require removal with a laser to restore the voice. Unfortunately, removing the warts does not eradicate the virus, and in many cases they recur chronically, requiring repeated surgery. In some patients the growths become so large that they obstruct the airway.

Vocal Cord Granulomas. Areas of granulation tissue may develop as a result of trauma to the vocal cords. This is tissue rich in blood vessels that forms during the early stages of wound healing and is red and granular in appearance. These granulomas are most common in patients who must have tubes inserted in the airway for prolonged periods while on a respirator. They may also be seen in patients with severe heartburn, which occurs when acid from the stomach backs up into the throat, causing chronic inflammation and breakdown of tissue. Surgical removal of granulomas is often required, with medical treatment of the underlying cause where this is appropriate.

Malignancies

In a small percentage of patients with chronic hoarseness, the cause will be found to be cancerous ulcerations or masses on the vocal cords. Cancer of the larynx occurs most commonly in patients with a long history of cigarette smoking. Untreated, the malignant growths will result in progressive loss of the voice, difficulty swallowing, eventual airway obstruction, and death. Appropriate treatment includes a surgical biopsy (removal of part of the growth) to make a definitive diagnosis and then treatment with either radiation or further surgery to eradicate the cancerous cells. The type of treatment depends on the location and stage of the disease at the time that it is diagnosed.

If the cancer is caught early, radiation therapy can often cure it without affecting the voice. If it has advanced, however, and surgery is required, it may be necessary to remove structures vital to normal voice production. Voice therapy is then an essential part of treatment. In cases where the entire larynx must be removed, an operation called a total laryngectomy, voice therapy is necessary so that patients may create a new voice. This can be done by using an artificial larynx called an electrolarynx or by learning one of two ways in which the esophagus can be used as a substitute for the larynx.

Vocal Cord Paralysis

Paralysis of one or both vocal cords can result from trauma to the neck, thyroid surgery, tumors in the chest or neck, or inflammation (following a viral infection) of the nerves that control motion in the vocal cords. It can usually be detected upon careful examination of the nose, throat, and larynx.

Paralysis of one vocal cord results in a weak, breathy voice because the unparalyzed, mobile cord cannot reach the paralyzed one. It also causes difficulty in swallowing, characterized by coughing or choking on liquids, but in general does not significantly interfere with breathing. Paralysis of both vocal cords causes only slight changes in the voice if the cords are immobilized close to one another, but it does obstruct the airway, resulting in noisy breathing and shortness of breath upon physical exertion.

If a single cord is paralyzed, the mobile cord may strengthen spontaneously over time and eventually be able to reach the paralyzed cord, restoring the voice to near normal. Alternatively, the paralyzed cord may be enlarged by injecting it with Teflon, allowing the two cords to meet. In the case of two paralyzed cords, surgical separation of the cords is often necessary to maintain an adequate airway. Such a separation will make the voice sound hoarse, and sometimes voice therapy is needed to help a patient make the most of the vocal functions that remain.

Muscle Tension Disorders

There are two types of voice disorders associated with the muscles of the vocal system. Hyperfunctional disorders result from too much muscle tension. They lead to a hoarse, strained voice or to vocal nodules (see above). Hypofunctional disorders result from inadequate muscle tension. For example, if the tongue muscles are lax and the tongue is positioned in the front of the mouth, the voice will sound thin and weak. If the palate muscles do not move to close off the nasal passage during speeech, the voice will sound nasal. If the vocal cords do not have adequate tension, the voice may sound breathy, since more air than is usual escapes through the opening between them. If there is too little air supply from the lungs, the voice will sound soft and may have a fry-like sound at the end of phrases. Muscle tension disorders can be treated with voice therapy to develop more appropriate techniques for vocal use. □

TAKING CARE OF YOUR VOICE

1. Speak and sing in normal tones. Pitching the voice unnaturally high or low will create a strain on it.
2. Don't try to yell above background noise. In a noisy jet or train this may mean keeping quiet for several hours.
3. Don't smoke, and avoid smoky environments as much as possible.
4. Avoid throat-clearing and coughing habits and noisy gargling. All put pressure on the vocal cords. If you must gargle, do it noiselessly.
5. Try to keep the muscles of the face, throat, and neck relaxed.
6. In a dry environment, such as that in an airplane, drink plenty of water or other fluids to moisten the throat.
7. Before delivering a speech or singing in a performance, avoid dehydrants such as antihistamines or tranquilizers, lozenges flavored with mint or menthol, and alcohol.
8. If you are hoarse, rest your vocal cords by speaking only when necessary and in a soft voice. Whispering puts even more pressure on the vocal cords and should be avoided.
9. See an otolaryngologist if hoarseness that is not associated with a cold, a change in the voice, pain upon speaking, or voice fatigue persists for more than two weeks.

Eating Out Wisely

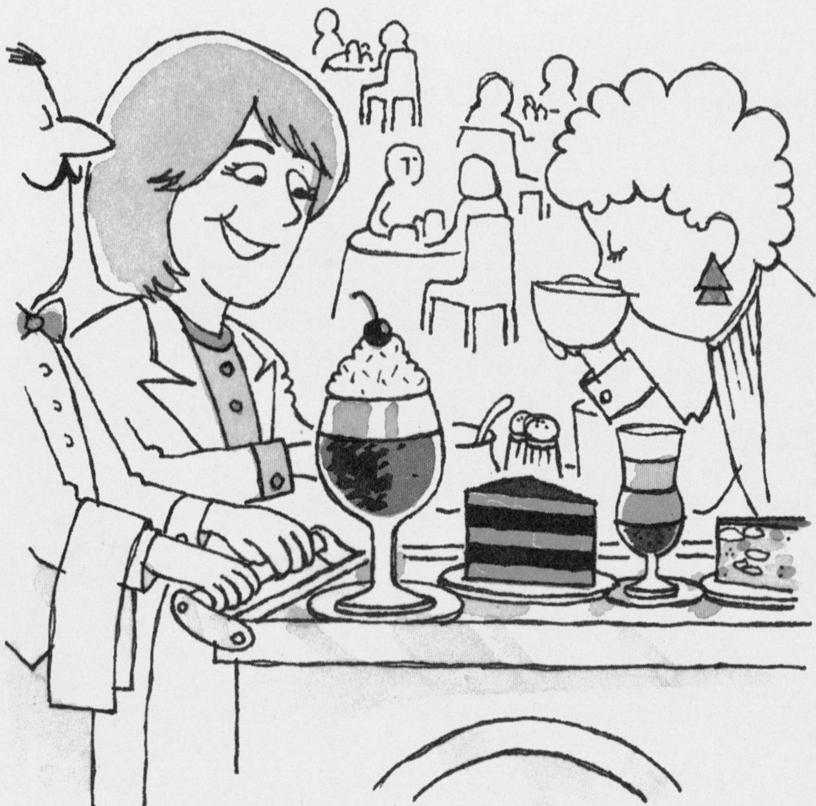

Joseph Gustaitis

Take the skin off the chicken before you eat it. Put yogurt on that baked potato instead of sour cream. Sprinkle your salad with a bit of olive oil and wine vinegar.

When preparing their dinners at home, more and more health-conscious cooks are following these, and other, sensible pieces of nutritional advice. The problem is, when some of these same people go out to a restaurant, they think nothing of tucking into a meal of greasy fried chicken, a baked potato buried under gobs of high-fat sour cream, and a salad drenched in a dressing that deserves to be called creamy cholesterol.

Americans eat out, on average, four times a week, which means that about one out of five meals is eaten outside the home—a rate approximately double what it was in the 1950s. Every day, about 46 million Americans eat in fast food restaurants, which now dispense about 200 hamburgers every *second.* What this boils down to is that many an earnest diet is wrecked upon reefs bearing the sign "Eat Here."

Fat and Sodium

Obviously, it's more than just waistline-expanding calories that are at stake (or steak). The American Heart Association recommends that fat make up less than 30 percent of total calories consumed and that no more than 10 percent of calories be in the form of saturated fat. Found mainly in meat, dairy products, and certain tropical oils, saturated fat is the kind most closely associated with atherosclerosis (hardening of the arteries) and increased risk of a heart attack. Experts would also like to see average daily cholesterol consumption get below 300 milligrams (according to the U.S. Department of Agriculture, it's now 304 for women but 435 for men).

Then there's sodium, a major component of salt—for some people, consuming too much puts them at risk for high blood pressure. The estimated minimum requirement of sodium for healthy persons is 500 milligrams a day, which may sound like a lot until you digest the fact that a fast-food lunch consisting of a double burger with cheese, fries, and a chocolate shake nets you nearly 1,600 milligrams. That same lunch also delivers about 1,500 calories and nearly 200 milligrams of cholesterol—and it's 50 percent fat. That's just about the kind of meal a nutritionist would recommend . . . as a way of celebrating every time you see a solar eclipse.

Sulfites

Calories, fat, salt—these are ingestibles nearly everyone should be monitoring with some care. But for some people restaurants can conceal another danger. About one out of every hundred people (most of them are asthma sufferers) are allergic to sulfites, a group of sulfur-based chemicals used as preservatives in foods and drugs. Allergic reactions can range from mildly irritating to fatal; so far, more than a dozen deaths have been linked to foods or drugs containing sulfites. However, the risk in the United States has been considerably lowered. In 1986, in an action aimed mainly at the threat posed by restaurant salad bars, the Food and Drug Administration prohibited the use of sulfites on raw fruits and vegetables, and in 1990 the ban was extended to fresh potatoes. (Sulfites are also banned on raw fruits and vegetables in Canada, but not on potatoes.) This does not mean that susceptible diners are out of the woods, because sulfites may still be used in fruit juices, shellfish, and wine. To play it safe, people who are sulfite-sensitive would be wise to steer clear of these items when eating out.

Good Sense—and Willpower

For the rest of us, responsible restauranting involves a mix of common sense, nutrition know-how, and willpower. Not that it can't be tricky. For example, a so-called "light" taco can have more calories than a regular one. It can be called "light" because its shell is flakier and easier to chew.

Nevertheless, there are reliable strategies that can help a savvy diner eat out, enjoy it, and stay reasonably close to sound nutritional guidelines.

• Watch out for creamy, rich sauces. If it sounds like gravy, avoid it or ask to have it served on the side. As runners and nutritionists will tell you, pasta is great, but if you drown it in cream sauce, you're loading on fat and calories. Tomato sauce is a safer bet.

• Fish is generally a better choice than red meat, though not if it's fried—a fish filet that's been breaded and fried can be high in both calories and fat. Try the fish that's poached, steamed, broiled, or baked. If you do have meat, trim off the fat.

• Beware the "fat salad." Salad bars *can* be a boon to dieters, what with all those fresh veggies, now without sulfites. But it's all too easy to swamp a salad with bacon bits, fatty dressing, and cheese.

• Words to avoid: *creamed, au gratin, battered, fried, breaded, scalloped, hollandaise*. They can all mean "high fat." Words to welcome: *grilled, broiled, steamed, stir-fried, poached*. If sodium is a concern, beware of *smoked, pickled, barbecued, marinated, Parmesan, teriyaki*.

• This may seem obvious, but an "All You Can Eat" special is just too much of a temptation for practically anyone.

• Chinese and Japanese cuisines, which traditionally emphasize low-fat, high-vegetable dishes, can be wise choices *if* fried foods and salty soups are avoided and soy sauce (high in sodium) is served on the side.

• A restaurant dinner does not have to be a traditional four-course meal of appetizer, soup, main course, and dessert. You may get along fine with just the main dish. Or try sharing some of the meal—an appetizer or a dessert—with a friend.

• A large menu usually means you can find *something* that's a shrewd nutritional option. It also suggests that dishes are prepared to order and, therefore, the chef will be able to honor special requests.

• For fast-food places, the guidelines vary. As a rule, keep it simple. Loading a sandwich with bacon and mayonnaise is an obvious error (hold the mayo on a burger and you can save around 150 calories—most of them from fat). If fruit juice or low-fat milk is available, why not give it a try instead of a shake? A baked potato is a wiser choice than French fries. Pizza can be a sensible fast food if you lay off the high-fat, high-salt pepperoni and other such toppings. Places with salad bars are intelligent choices, as long as the "fat salad" is shunned. And in fact, more and more chains, responding to the public's widening interest in nutrition, now *are* offering salad bars, as well as foods that are baked, broiled, or steamed.

Changing the Menu

That last bit of information may be the best news of all. Restaurants are getting the message and making an effort to serve meals that make nutritional sense. A recent Gallup survey of over 500 restaurants found that three-fourths of them will honor requests for changes in food preparation, such as cooking without salt, serving sauce and salad dressing on the side, broiling or baking instead of frying, using margarine or oil in place of butter, and removing chicken skin. Clearly, you don't have to assume that a harried chef will consider your desires an imposition.

In addition, about 40 percent of American restaurants have changed their menus to reflect the public's growing demand for better nutrition; the National Restaurant Association has even published a guide for members who want to offer more healthful food. This switch is not entirely altruistic. The restaurant business is very competitive, and owners are quick to respond to what they perceive as changing tastes—some even hire consultants to help them create lighter menus. Similarly, cooking schools are now emphasizing nutrition courses for budding chefs, a major change from the days when the cuisine philosophy seemed to be "more is more."

Does this mean that the era of the T-bone steak is no more? That we can bid adieu to hollandaise sauce? That we have seen our last cheesecake? Of course not. Special occasions will remain special. Yet when a person eats out four times a week, not *all* those occasions can be special. But they can be sensible. □

LUPUS

John H. Klippel, M.D.

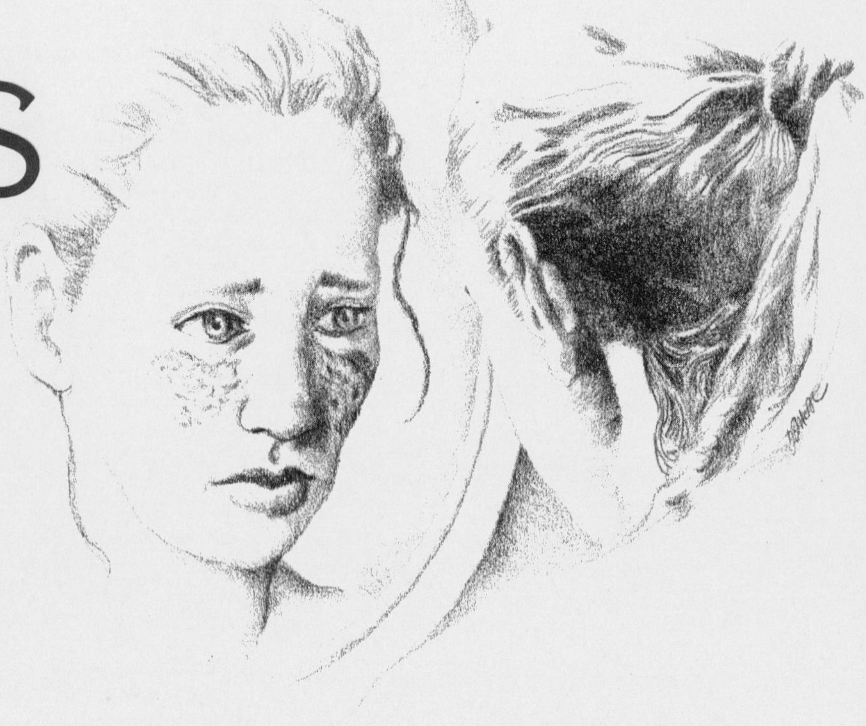

Systemic lupus erythematosus (SLE), more commonly known as lupus, is a chronic disease that affects an estimated 500,000 people in the United States. It is caused by abnormalities in the body's immune system that make it attack healthy tissue. Common signs and symptoms include fever, fatigue, skin rashes, arthritis, and mouth ulcers. In some cases internal organs like the kidneys, brain, or lungs are affected, leading to very serious illness. The disease primarily affects women between the ages of 20 and 40 and is more common in some racial groups than in others. In the United States it is found more often in blacks and Asians than in other groups.

Signs and Symptoms

Lupus is a lifelong condition with periods of remission and relapse. Months, or even years, of good health may be interrupted by episodes of acute, unexpected, and potentially severe illness.

Most patients with lupus have signs and symptoms that are not specific to the disease and make its diagnosis difficult. They include extreme fatigue, unexplained fevers, poor appetite, weight loss, headaches, and weakness and may be so severe that patients are unable to attend school, hold a job, or perform routine household chores.

Skin rashes on the face, arms, and chest are common in patients with lupus. (The rashes lead some people to believe that lupus is contagious. It is not.) Rashes on the cheeks, called butterfly rashes because of their shape, are the best known sign of the disease and affect 50 percent of lupus patients. The rashes are typically intensely red and may appear as a rouge-like blush over the entire surface of the cheeks or may develop as multiple, small blotches. The rash often extends across the bridge of the nose and may spread to involve the forehead or chin. The rash may last for days or weeks, often varies in intensity, and does not cause pain, itching, or scarring of the skin. Another common type of skin rash, called discoid lupus, begins as small red disk-shaped spots covered with whitish scales that usually appear on the nose and cheeks. As the rash enlarges, the area in the center of each lesion becomes depressed and often loses normal skin color. Discoid rashes often itch and may produce extensive scarring of the skin. (There is another, much milder former of discoid lupus in which the skin rash is the only symptom.)

Lupus is difficult to diagnose because many of its symptoms, such as headache and loss of appetite, are found in other illnesses, too.

Most lupus rashes are photosensitive, that is, they are made worse by sunlight. In patients who are extremely sensitive to light, even overhead fluorescent lights may be capable of causing or worsening lupus rashes.

Ulcers may form on the roof of

the mouth or on the mucuous membranes inside the mouth, nose, or vagina. Typically, the ulcerations are not painful, but they may cause bleeding or become infected. In addition, lupus patients may notice increased loss of hair after brushing or washing or increased amounts of hair on the pillow in the morning.

Arthritis—with swelling, pain, and stiffness in the joints, particularly the knees, wrists, and small joints of the hands—is common. Symptoms are typically worse in the morning and gradually improve during the day. The arthritis often tends to migrate from one joint to another and rarely lasts longer than several days in any joint.

Sometimes lupus affects the lungs, the heart, the kidneys, or the central nervous system, causing serious problems.

The membranes lining the lung, heart, or abdomen may become inflamed in patients with lupus. This can cause excruciating chest or abdominal pain that may be confused with a heart attack, a blood clot in the lungs, a fractured rib, or appendicitis. Pleurisy, or inflammation of the lining of the lungs, causes sharp, stabbing pains in the side or back that worsen during a deep breath. The pain from pericarditis, or inflammation of the lining of the heart, is typically located under or to the left of the breastbone. It is often most evident while one is lying down and may be relieved by sitting up.

Swelling of the ankles and legs (edema) may be a sign of kidney involvement or lupus nephritis, in which the kidney's ability to rid the body of wastes is reduced. The progressive loss of kidney function may lead to kidney failure and the need for dialysis or kidney transplantation. Kidney disease is detected by urine or blood tests.

Neurologic involvement, or central nervous system (CNS) lupus, can produce an assortment of symptoms. Mood or thought disorders are common, including depression, anxiety, forgetfulness, shortened attention span, and impaired ability to think clearly. In addition, serious physical problems may develop, from seizures or paralysis of a limb to impairments of sensation or loss of bowel or bladder control.

Role of the Immune System

Although the exact cause of lupus is unknown, a disordered immune system is considered to be central to the disease. In a normal immune system, antibodies attack foreign substances and organisms, such as bacteria and viruses, that enter the body. However, abnormal antibodies formed by the immune systems of patients with lupus attack the body's own healthy tissues. These antibodies are called autoantibodies, or "self" antibodies. Autoantibodies that react with the nuclei of cells, or antinuclear antibodies, are of particular importance and are present in almost all patients with the disease. They can be detected with a blood test and changing levels are frequently used to follow the course of the disease. Other common types of autoantibodies found in patients with lupus include antibodies to blood cells, leading to anemia (a low red blood cell count), a reduced white blood cell count, or increased bleeding from a low blood platelet count. Blood tests can detect these deficiencies in the blood.

The two factors thought to be most important in the production of autoantibodies are hereditary influences and exposure to environmental triggers of the disease. The evidence for the role of heredity includes a greater frequency of lupus in identical twins and within families and the finding that certain genetic traits are weakly associated with the disease. A known environmental trigger in some people is drug therapy for such conditions as seizures or heart disorders. Once the drugs are stopped, both the autoantibodies and the symptoms of lupus disappear. Many researchers believe there are as yet unidentified environmental triggers, such as infectious agents or allergy-causing materials in the food or air, that may set off the abnormal immune system action that leads to lupus.

Treating Lupus

Although lupus may be a very serious disease, with proper treatment most lupus patients can expect to have a normal life span. However, when major organs are involved, there is an increased risk of death from kidney failure, strokes, and infections.

The exact cause of lupus is unknown, but the immune system is believed to play a part, as may heredity and environmental triggers also.

The two most important aspects of the treatment of a patient with lupus are the determination of the extent and severity of the disease and the choice of drugs to be used. Since the symptoms and course of the disease can vary greatly from one patient to another, regular visits to physicians familiar with lupus are essential. The frequency of visits may be as often as daily or weekly in the patient with evolving signs or symptoms of lupus or as infrequently as yearly in the patient who is in remission.

Drugs that suppress inflammation have a major role in the treatment of lupus. Two general classes of anti-inflammatory drugs are used: nonsteroidal agents and corticosteroids. Nonsteroidal medications include aspirin and over-the-counter drugs containing ibuprofen, such as Advil or Nuprin, as well as drugs available only with a prescription. These drugs are most commonly used to treat minor symptoms of lupus such as fever, joint pains, arthritis, weakness, and fatigue. The most common side effects of this group of drugs are gastrointestinal: nausea, vomiting and stomach pain. Taking the medications with food or with an antacid often helps to relieve these symptoms.

Of all the drugs used in the treatment of lupus, corticosteroids are unquestionably the most important, because they tend to inhibit the immune system and help reduce inflammation of the internal organs. Corticosteroids may be taken in pill form or even given intravenously in patients with more serious manifestations of the disease. In addition, creams that contain corticosteroids are useful in alleviating lupus rashes. Most lupus patients experience rather prompt and often dramatic improvement after corticosteroids are started. However, corticosteroids have a number of potential side effects, especially when high doses are used or when the drugs are taken for a prolonged period. Some of the more common are weight gain, fullness in the cheeks, unwanted hair growth, development of stretch marks or bruises on the skin, lowered resistance to infection, osteoporosis, and a serious form of arthritis that affects large joints such as the hips, knees, and shoulders. Another possible complication of corticosteroids is high blood pressure.

Drugs that suppress inflammation, from over-the-counter products like aspirin to prescription-only corticosteroids, are important in the treatment of lupus.

Drugs originally used for the treatment of malaria are valuable in the treatment of certain symptoms of lupus, including fever, fatigue, arthritis, and skin rashes. Of the antimalarial drugs, hydroxycholoroquine (brand name, Plaquenil) given in very low doses is by far the most widely used. Low-dose Plaquenil is generally regarded as quite safe and produces few side effects; gastrointestinal complaints and occasional skin rashes are among the most common. Much attention has been focused on the possibility that the drug will damage the retina of the eye. Fortunately, this is extremely rare. As a precaution, patients treated with antimalarial drugs should have an eye examination every six months to detect any early evidence of damage to the retina.

Therapies that suppress the functioning of the immune system are currently being used in the experimental treatment of patients with serious manifestations of lupus, such as advanced kidney disease or central nervous system disease. The various approaches used include chemotherapy similar to that used in the treatment of cancer patients, radiation therapy, and the removal of abnormal antibodies from the blood by a procedure called plasmapheresis.

Living With Lupus

Lupus can be treated with varying levels of success; nevertheless, it is a chronic disease that requires some adjustments.

Lupus patients are more susceptible to infections than others. Unexplained fever, chills, or sweating may be a sign of infection and requires prompt evaluation by a physician. Several measures can be taken to reduce the risk of infection, such as receiving yearly flu shots (or pneumococcal vaccine in patients who have had their spleens removed) and taking antibiotics when undergoing dental or surgical procedures in which there is a risk of infection.

Lupus patients who are sensitive to the sun must remember to avoid intense sun exposure, as it can trigger a flare-up. This includes adjustment of activities to avoid daylight hours of peak sun intensity (10 A.M. to 4 P.M.), the liberal use of sunscreen lotions, and the wearing of appropriate clothing to reduce sun exposure.

Lupus is a chronic condition and requires some adjustments in life-style, such as avoiding stress.

As stress and insufficient rest may cause flare-ups, lupus patients may have to take it easier than most people and should try to avoid stress as much as possible. The American Lupus Society and the Lupus Foundation of America offer information, counseling, and support groups for lupus patients and their families. They can be contacted at their national headquarters, or local chapters can be found through the telephone directory. □

Sources of Further Information

American Lupus Society, 3914 Del Amo Boulevard, Suite 922, Torrance, CA 90503. Tel.: (213) 542-8891 or (800) 331-1802.

Lupus Foundation of America, Inc., 1717 Massachusetts Avenue NW, Suite 203, Washington, DC 20036. Tel: (202) 328-4550 or (800) 558-0121.

WHAT AUTOPSIES REVEAL

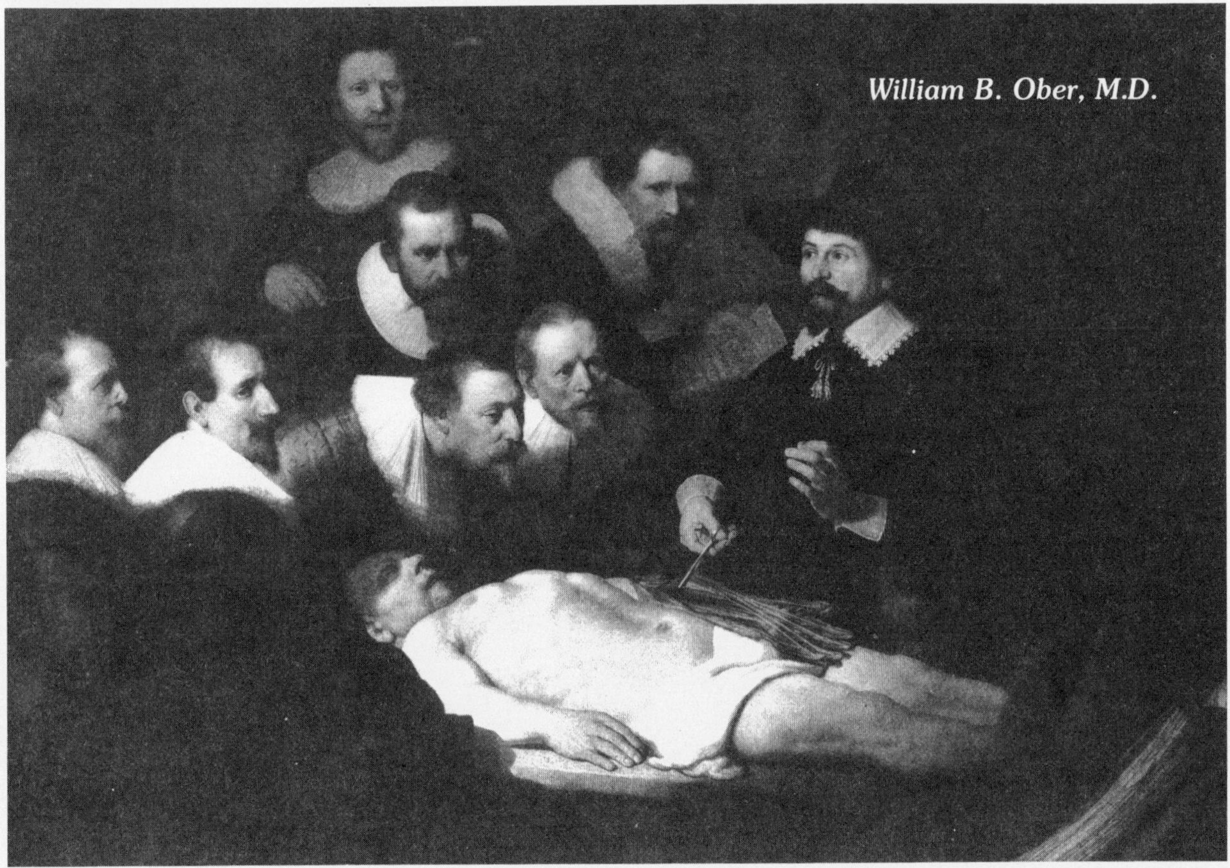

William B. Ober, M.D.

Rembrandt's The Anatomy Lesson *shows the famous 17th-century pathologist Dr. Nicolae Tulp.*

An autopsy, also known as a postmortem (after-death) examination, is the scientific dissection of a body performed to establish either the cause of death or the nature and extent of disease. The word autopsy derives from the Greek and means "to see for oneself." (It is interesting to note that the first sightseeing omnibus from London to Brighton was called the autopsy bus.)

Autopsies have been performed for nearly 700 years. They have added tremendously to medical knowledge as well as revealing valuable information about individual cases—whether it is what (or who) killed the person, why a puzzling set of symptoms occurred, or how likely it is that the same disorder may strike other family members.

Autopsies are generally performed by pathologists, physician specialists who are trained in certified residency programs, most commonly at hospitals affiliated with medical schools or universities. The field of pathology focuses on the nature and causes of disease and the anatomic changes that occur because of it.

A Long History

Autopsies as we know them today probably began in 14th-century Italy, usually when poisoning was suspected, although it is unclear what criteria those who made the dissections (prosectors) could have used to establish or refute the charge. A 14th-century Italian manuscript contains an illustration of a woman's body with the abdomen opened, the major organs displayed around it, and next to it a prosector with a knife. The 15th-century Florentine physician Antonio Bienivieni was probably the first to ask the families of his patients for permission to perform autopsies. In the 16th century more and more autopsies were performed, and the beginnings of a medical literature on their findings can be identified.

French physician Jean Fernel's landmark monograph *Medicina*

(1554) included a section subtitled "Pathologia," which was the first explicit treatise on special pathology based on autopsy results. (Special pathology is the branch of pathology dealing with abnormalities in specific organs.)

Fernel's work was expanded half a century later by Felix Pater of Basel, Switzerland, who in 1602-1603 published an elaborate classification of diseases based on 300 dissections. Another farsighted physician was Volcher Coiter (1534-1590) of Nürnberg, who repeatedly urged the authorities to support a policy of postmortem examinations for people who died of puzzling diseases.

In the 17th century the first competent illustrations of lesions found at autopsy appeared. Typical are the illustrations in *Observationes Medicae* (1641) by Nicolae Tulp, who is familiar to us from Rembrandt's painting *The Anatomy Lesson*. New collections of autopsy reports also appeared, of which the best known is by Théophile Bonet in 1679. His weighty compendium contained the results of 3,000 autopsy reports, classified and cross-indexed. By 1700 a body of verifiable knowledge based on autopsy experience existed; what was lacking was a codification of the accumulated information.

Autopsies were first performed in Italy in the 1300s when poisoning was suspected—though how it could be detected is not clear.

That need was filled with the publication of *De sedibus et causis morborum* (1761) by Giovanni Morgagni (1682-1771), who is rightly credited with being the founder of modern autopsy pathology. His remarkable book was based on over half a century of anatomic pathology studies at Padua. Its claim to fame is Morgagni's meticulous correlation of clinical detail and pathological observations, supplemented by full citations from the existing literature. The book was translated into English in 1769, and it became the basis for anatomic pathology studies for the next century. It is largely due to Morgagni that medical thinking ceased being based on an abstract general concept of "disease" and instead adopted the idea of specific diseases with differing causes and varying anatomical locations.

During the latter half of the 18th century, the Scottish brothers William Hunter and John Hunter established anatomical museums in England where preserved specimens could be studied. Their nephew Matthew Baillie published *The Morbid Anatomy of Some of the Most Important Parts of the Human Body* in 1794, the first textbook in English devoted to anatomic pathology. The development of color printing in the first quarter of the 19th century made it possible to reproduce important illustrated anatomical works. Later in the 19th century three English physicians (all working at Guy's Hospital in London) made major contributions to the understanding of diseases based on autopsy material—Richard Bright to kidney disease, Thomas Addison to adrenal disease, and Thomas Hodgkin to lymphatic disease. Each of these men has given his name to a disease he investigated.

In the latter half of the 19th century advances in bacteriology made it possible to assign specific causes to specific diseases. Pathologists began to be trained to make such diagnoses not only at autopsy but also from surgical specimens and biopsies. The development of aniline dyes in the 1860s made it possible to stain tissue, so that structures such as a cell's nucleus or membrane could be more easily observed; the development of the rotary microtome (an instrument that cuts tissues) in the 1870s enabled scientists to prepare specimens for examination under a microscope—for both diagnosis and teaching. As a result of these advances, the autopsy became an indispensable teaching exercise.

Significant errors in diagnosis are discovered in as many as one out of five autopsies performed in a hospital in the United States.

Types of Autopsies

There are two main types of autopsies: hospital autopsies and forensic autopsies.

Hospital Autopsies. This type of autopsy is performed on patients who die in a hospital, and permission of the next of kin must be obtained. (Most major religions place no prohibition on postmortem examinations, although there are exceptions, including Orthodox Judaism and Hinduism.) In addition to establishing the cause of death when that is not known in advance, the hospital autopsy is designed to detect the effects of treatment and to discover unsuspected diseases or conditions not diagnosed. Significant errors in diagnosis are discovered in as many as 20 percent of hospital autopsies performed in the United States, Canada, and Western Europe.

In the United States the current hospital autopsy rate is 10 to 15 percent of all hospital deaths, a sharp decline from the levels of two decades ago, when hospital accrediting bodies discontinued the requirement that autopsies be performed in over 25 percent of deaths. Another reason for the decline is that doctors and hospital administrators are less eager to call for autopsies, fearing malpractice suits by the families of patients.

Forensic Autopsies. Forensic medicine is the application of medical facts to legal questions—for instance, the use of autopsy results to help determine whether a crime has been committed. In the United States forensic autopsies are performed by medical examiners, many of whom are trained pathologists and a few of whom have additional specialized training in forensic pathology. These autopsies are done when required by the statutes of individual states. Usually included under such statutes are deaths from homicide, suicide, accidents, and drug overdoses, cases that may pose a threat to public health, and cases of patients who die in suspicious circumstances or for whom no physician signed a death certificate. In addition to determining the cause of death, the forensic autopsy is designed to determine the mode of death, be it natural causes, homicide, suicide, or accident.

The Procedure

The pathologist usually performs the autopsy in a room set aside and equipped for that purpose. The physician and trained assistants remove the brain through an ear-to-ear incision at the back of the head and open the torso with a Y-shaped incision from the armpits to the middle of the chest and down to the lower abdomen. They examine the internal organs visually, remove them to weigh and measure them, and supplement their observations by selecting various body fluids and tissues for laboratory analysis, to clarify ambiguous findings as well as to support obvious ones. Depending on the nature of the case, some tissue samples may be examined under a microscope.

The autopsy generally takes place within a day of death, but bodies can be exhumed for autopsy months or years later if a question arises as to the cause of death. (Pathologists can distinguish between tissue changes caused by embalming and those caused by disease.)

The autopsy procedure lasts two or three hours, although the results of laboratory analyses may take days or weeks. A preliminary report is usually available within 72 hours, a full report within a month. Autopsy does not preclude an open-casket funeral should this be desired by the family. Families can request copies of autopsy reports from hospitals and can arrange to discuss the findings with hospital staff. Families can also request that an autopsy be performed. In a hospital autopsy, no matter who initiates the procedure, the cost of the autopsy is absorbed by the hospital.

An autopsy on a gunshot victim can reveal the kind of gun used, the direction of firing, and the distance between victim and attacker.

What Is Learned

The type of information gained from an autopsy depends on the nature of the case. If a patient dies of some form of cancer, an autopsy will establish the extent of the disease's spread. Autopsy material is also valuable in classifying tumors. Autopsies sometimes reveal genetic diseases, serving to warn relatives about predispositions to the same condition. Forensic autopsies can, in the case of gunshot wounds, tell what weapon was used, the direction it was fired from, and at what range.

Some scientific autopsy studies have led to unforeseen medical advances. For example, research done by Monroe Schlesinger, a Boston pathologist, led to the development of techniques to diagnose and treat heart disease. In the 1930s and 1940s, Schlesinger injected the coronary arteries of corpses with a radio-opaque substance that enabled him to locate both by X ray and dissection the areas of narrowing or obstruction caused by arteriosclerosis. By the 1970s and 1980s clinicians were performing in living patients what Schlesinger had done with corpses. Based on Schlesinger's work, physicians began using safely injectable dyes to visualize the coronary arteries of living subjects by conventional radiology. As techniques for open heart surgery were developed, blockages could be localized and coronary bypass surgery performed to relieve arterial obstructions. Later, the same technique of injecting dyes into the arteries for diagnostic purposes was used in conjunction with balloon angioplasty, a method of relieving coronary obstructions by inserting into the blocked artery, and then inflating, a balloon attached to the tip of a catheter.

An autopsy study of soldiers killed in the Korean War provides another example of how autopsies can reveal new medical information. Army pathologists Robert Holmes and William Enos examined the coronary arteries of the young men—most were under 30 years old—and found a surprising degree of arteriosclerosis. This was the first intimation that coronary artery disease often begins early in life and not, as was previously thought, after people have reached their 50s.

The information obtained from forensic autopsies is clearly of direct value. Such autopsies yield evidence that may be used in prosecuting homicide cases and can sometimes help investigators exclude specific suspects. They may also be useful in determining whether a death was an accident or a suicide, a finding of importance to both claimants and insurance companies. □

The Safety of X Rays

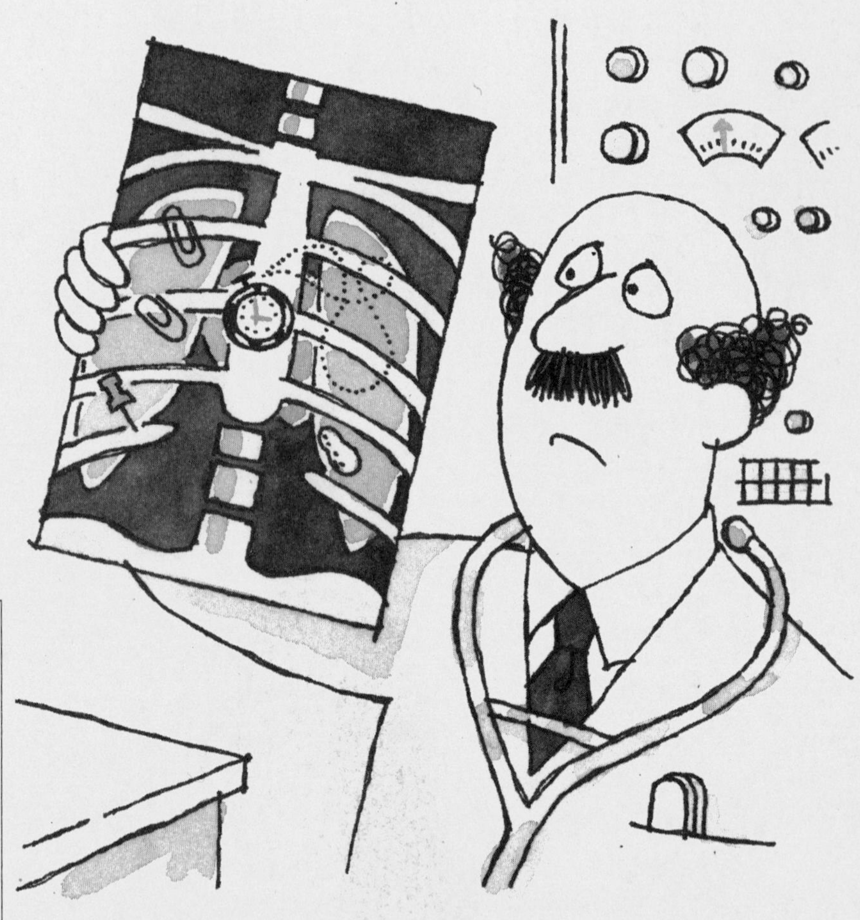

John W. Gustaitis, M.D.

Just about everyone has had some experience with diagnostic X rays—we've either had one ourselves or are close to someone who has. And we know the benefits they offer, such as the detection of fractures, pneumonia, or cancer.

On the other hand, we've also heard about some of the harmful effects that can be associated with radiation, and some people may ask, when their doctor recommends a diagnostic X ray, "Is it really safe for me to have this done? What is the risk to me?"

Fortunately, there have been quite a number of studies which allow some assessment of the potential risk. And though the answers are not definite, the evidence strongly suggests that the risk of diagnostic X rays is small, perhaps inconsequential. It may be of interest to take a look at how some of this information has been obtained, to compare the risks of the radiation doses from diagnostic X rays and other sources, and to compare diagnostic X rays to other procedures, which may or may not use radiation, that produce images of internal organs and tissues.

What X Rays Are

Most people have seen X ray machines and are aware that the rays cannot be seen or felt. Where do they come from? X rays are produced when very high-speed electrically charged particles are absorbed in matter. For diagnostic X rays, they are produced in an X ray tube. The particles are electrons—negatively charged atomic particles. The electrons are accelerated to very high speeds in the tube and made to bombard a metal target. When they do, the electrons are deflected and emit some of their energy in the form of X rays.

The resulting X rays are similar to other types of waves with which we are more familiar—such as light waves and radio waves. These are all members of the same family of electromagnetic radiation, which travel through space in straight lines at the speed of light. The difference is that X rays have more energy than the others, and it is this energy, when transmitted to the atoms or molecules in living tissues, that can produce the effects associated with potentially harmful radiation. This energy can actually change the electron structure of atoms and break the bonds in molecules.

Radiation Hazards

A number of studies and observations have been made to define the injurious effects that X rays may produce, and there is no doubt that very large doses of radiation, much greater than those associated with diagnostic X rays, are harmful. In fact, the very first report of a radiation injury occurred within just a few months of the discovery of X rays by Wilhelm Roentgen in December 1895. But the seriousness of radiation hazards was underestimated for many years, and it was not until the 1920s that the first governmental action was taken, in Great Britain, to limit X ray exposure. More recently, because of the considerable interest in radiation safety, there has been legislation in the United States to control the use of and exposure to radiation.

Although there have been some studies which have tried to define the risk of radiation in low doses—such as those encountered in diagnostic X rays—most of the studies of radiation's effects have come from data obtained from high-dose exposure. Some examples are the follow-up studies of the survivors of the atomic bomb attacks on Hiroshima and Nagasaki, of people exposed to radiation from nuclear bomb tests and the accompanying fallout, of victims of radiation accidents, and of uranium miners and pioneers in radiology.

The radiation from a chest X ray is about 10 to 15 percent of the natural radiation Americans are exposed to in one year.

Since most of the useful studies involve such high-dose exposure—vastly higher than that of diagnostic X rays—attempts have been made to extrapolate the data from the high-dose range to the low-dose range. The precise method for doing this is still being debated. As a result, no one can be certain what the exact risk of diagnostic X rays is, and we may *never* have a definite answer. Nevertheless, it is prudent to assume that there may be at least a statistical risk from small doses of radiation. We have to accept the possibility of adverse effects from small X ray doses.

Weighing the Risks

Fortunately, there are two other methods that can be used to get a better idea of the potential risk of diagnostic X rays. One is to compare the dose of radiation received from X rays to other common sources of radiation. The second is to compare the effects of radiation to *non*-radiation risks which may adversely affect health.

There is naturally occurring radiation to which we are all exposed. Two of the main sources of this "background radiation" are cosmic rays and terrestrial radiation, and the amount of radiation absorbed from this exposure is not usually considered harmful.

Cosmic radiation arises from high-energy particles from outer space which penetrate the atmosphere and create various types of radioactive particles that reach the earth's surface. The higher the altitude, the greater the exposure. Terrestrial radiation originates in soil and rocks containing naturally occurring radioactive materials such as uranium. The dose levels can vary widely depending on geographic location and types of building materials—certain types of stone used in construction, such as granite and limestone, can emit small amounts of radiation.

Several studies have been conducted to estimate the effects on health of natural background radiation, and though it seems that there is a statistical risk to health from this exposure, it is quite small. For purposes of comparison, it is estimated that the radiation dose from a chest X ray is approximately equivalent to 10-15 percent of the average background radiation that Americans are exposed to in a year.

Another way to assess the risk of diagnostic X rays is to relate it to nonradiological risks. Most of our daily activities involve some degree of risk which we take for granted, whether it be driving to work, eating certain types of food, or performing certain occupations. How can we compare the risk from X rays to some of these other common hazards? This has been done by estimating what activities or aspects of life-style might increase the chance of death by one in a million—a risk that most of us would find acceptable.

X rays are similar to light waves and radio waves, but because they have a lot more energy, they have more potential for harm.

Statisticians estimate that a chest X ray involves such a one-in-a-million risk—but so do, among other things, drinking just half a liter of wine, traveling 300 miles by car, or spending as little as two days in a city with a serious air pollution problem. As can be seen from these comparisons, the risk of a chest X ray compares favorably with many everyday activities.

Other Procedures

Simple X rays are not the only types of diagnostic imaging procedures a patient may encounter. There is also nuclear medicine, computed tomography (better known as a CT or CAT scan), diagnostic ultrasound (also called a sonogram), and magnetic resonance imaging (MRI).

Both nuclear medicine and CAT scanning involve the use of radiation (in the former, a radiation-emitting material is taken into the body.) As with chest X rays, there is some degree of risk involved, though it, too, is considered acceptable in light of the obvious benefits.

Ultrasound and MRI do *not* involve radiation. Ultrasound images are produced by sending high-frequency sound waves through the body, and MRI images are created by placing the patient in the field of a high-strength magnet. There is not yet any conclusive evidence that there are any harmful effects from either ultrasound or MRI, though prudence dictates that they be used only when there is a specific medical indication.

Just because you had an X ray when you broke your arm doesn't mean you should avoid another if you develop pneumonia symptoms.

Improving X Rays

Even though the risk from diagnostic X rays appears to have always been small, several technological advances have made it possible to reduce the radiation dose—and there are more such advances to come. New combinations of X ray films and intensifying screens, already available, can reduce the dose needed for a clear image by a factor of four. New types of X ray tube filters may permit the necessary dose to be cut in half, and improvement in X ray film processing can allow a further reduction.

Still greater reductions may be possible with the use of digital imaging. Fluoroscopic images would be stored on computer disks and would be viewed on a TV monitor. This would actually replace X ray film. Since these systems are more sensitive to smaller amounts of radiation, they would employ smaller doses.

But there is a limit. The amount of radiation exposure can be reduced only so much and still allow a satisfactory X ray image to be produced.

An Acceptable Risk

So when your physician says you need a diagnostic X ray, should you be concerned? Current data suggest that the risk to an average patient from a common diagnostic procedure is small. If you compare the risk with other common hazards—including the inescapable presence of natural background radiation—the risk-benefit ratio would appear acceptable, especially when you consider that a diagnostic X ray can be of immense value in detecting, determining the severity of, or ruling out medical problems.

Is there any special cause for concern if you have had a previous X ray a short time before? As a rule, if your physician has a good medical reason to advise a radiological procedure—whether it is a lung examination, an X ray of a painful bone, or an X ray to detect a possible tumor—it's prudent to have the procedure done. Since people's medical histories can vary tremendously, it is impossible to establish a maximum radiation dose from diagnostic X rays which a person should not exceed in, say, one year. Just because you had an X ray when you broke your arm doesn't mean you should avoid another if you develop possible pneumonia symptoms a month later.

Some types of diagnostic X rays, in fact, definitely should be taken repeatedly (at specified intervals) because their value in early diagnosis of possibly life-threatening disease far outweighs the minimal risk from radiation exposure. The classic example is the mammogram. Used to detect breast cancer in its early stages, it is one of a woman's best health safeguards, for when detected early enough, breast cancer can have a cure rate of 85 percent or more. The American College of Obstetrics and Gynecology recommends that women between 40 and 49 have a mammogram every year or two and women 50 and over have one every year. Women aged 35 to 39 are urged to have one baseline mammogram, to be used for comparison with those taken after 40.

One of the most frequently performed radiological procedures is the dental X ray. The American Dental Association does not have an official policy on a recommended interval between these X rays, pointing out that because everyone's teeth and potential dental problems are different, it's best to leave that decision to one's dentist. The association does suggest, however, that since modern dental X ray equipment involves low radiation exposure, a yearly dental X ray is a good rule of thumb.

Some types of diagnostic X rays, like mammograms, should definitely be taken repeatedly.

Although everyone agrees that the potential of adverse effects from small doses of radiation must be recognized and that unnecessary radiation exposure should be avoided, no responsible organization has recommended avoidance of any properly justified radiological procedure on the basis of radiation risk. The final decision on whether the X ray is indicated should be made by patient and doctor. □

THE VIRTUES OF OLIVE OIL

Louise A. Bloomfield

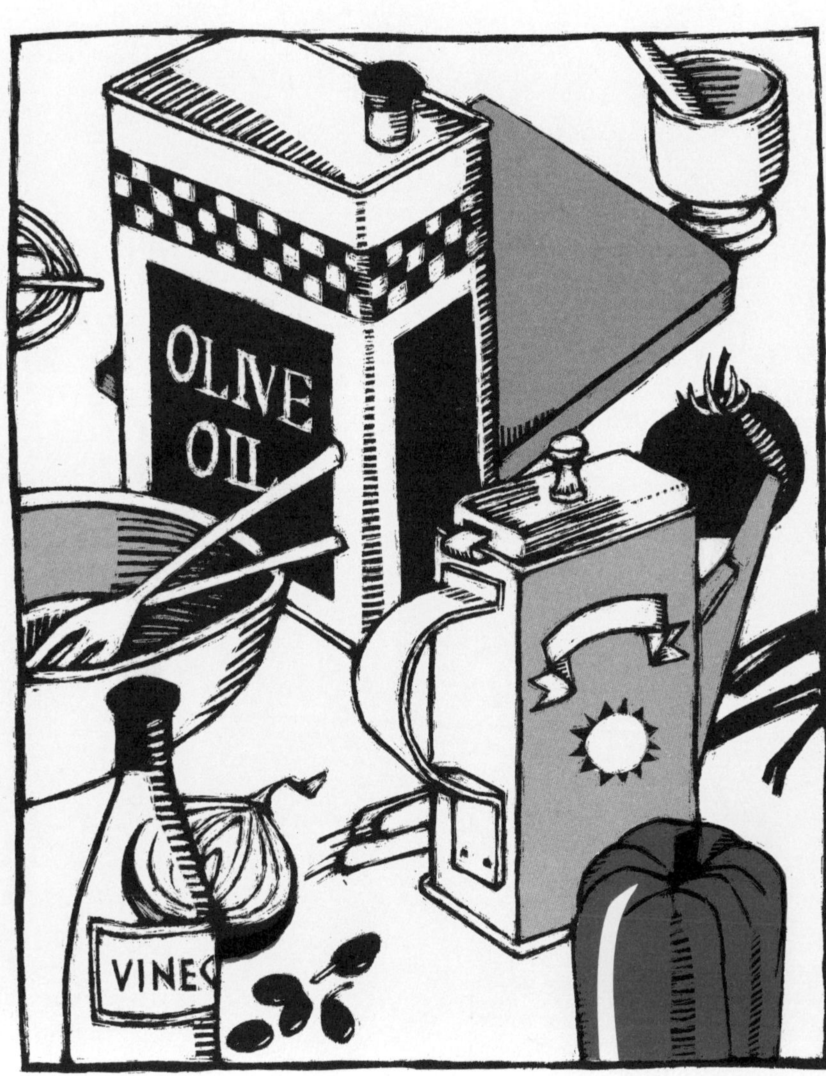

Whether for its widely publicized health benefits, its gourmet reputation, or an increased interest in ethnic cuisine, olive oil has found its way into more and more American kitchens in recent years. Bottles, tins, and jars of olive oil were on the shelves of an estimated 16 percent of American homes in 1989, reflecting a 72 percent increase in sales over the previous five years. With the rising demand, a flood of brands and varieties has come onto the market, giving customers a bewildering array to choose from. Which is better, extra virgin or extra light? Does more expensive mean better for your health, better tasting, or neither of the above?

Though many Americans have come to olive oil only recently, it has been used in cooking since roughly 3000 B.C. when olives were first cultivated in the eastern Mediterranean region. (Other early uses were as fuel for lamps and as a beauty aid.) Raw olives in their natural state are inedible; most of the olives in those jars stacked on supermarket shelves have been pickled and packed in brine. Currently, some 90 percent of all the olives grown are used for oil, not eating. The olives are pressed—sometimes more than once—and the oil they yield may be refined to lower its acidity. Most olive oil is also filtered.

The Golden Remedy?

Medical interest in olive oil began in 1958 with the launching of a study to investigate the connection between diet and heart disease in 12,000 healthy men in seven countries. The study found that Mediterranean diets, which are high in olive oil, could be correlated with lower rates of coronary heart disease, the leading cause of death in the United States. (Other differences in dietary habits, such as less meat and more carbohydrates in the Mediterranean diet than in the American, could also have played a role.)

The key benefit of olive oil is that it consists mostly of the type of fat called monounsaturated. Later studies have found that diets high in monounsaturated fat as compared to saturated fat (found in significant quantities in meat and dairy products, for example) result in lower blood levels of cholesterol.

A waxlike fatty substance, cholesterol is needed by the body for various purposes. But when excess cholesterol circulates in the blood (often because of a diet too high in saturated fat) some of that cholesterol is deposited on artery walls, leading to hardening of the arteries and ultimately, perhaps, to a heart attack or stroke.

Cholesterol is borne through the blood by molecules called lipoproteins. Low-density lipoproteins (LDLs) are associated with the depositing of cholesterol on artery walls, high-density lipoproteins (HDLs) with removal of cholesterol from the bloodstream. Hence, LDL-cholesterol is regarded as dangerous or "bad" cholesterol, while HDL-cholesterol is seen as "good" and a low LDL to HDL ratio as favorable in protecting against heart disease.

Both the monounsaturated fat in olive oil and the type of fat called polyunsaturated, the main fat found in many vegetable oils (like corn and safflower oil), have been shown to reduce LDL-cholesterol levels when substituted for saturated fat. But while polyunsaturated fat has been found in some studies to reduce *both* LDL and HDL levels, monounsaturated fat apparently has no effect on HDL-cholesterol levels, thus improving the LDL to HDL ratio.

Olive oil is high in monounsaturated fat, which may help keep blood cholesterol and blood pressure at low levels.

New Findings

Olive oil is composed of roughly 75 percent monounsaturated, 15 percent saturated, and 10 percent polyunsaturated fat. Two studies published in 1990 added luster to its image.

A team led by Dr. Maurizio Trevisan of the State University of New York School of Medicine in Buffalo surveyed dietary habits in nine different Italian communities whose patterns of fat consumption varied widely. They found that those people for whom olive oil provided the largest proportion of dietary fat not only had the lowest blood cholesterol levels, but also had the lowest blood pressure. Unlike monounsaturated fat, heavy use of polyunsaturated fat did not appear to be linked to lowered blood pressure.

The other study, carried out in the Netherlands, may be of concern for users of margarine, which is eaten by millions as an alternative to butter since butter is high in saturated fat. Margarine is made from polyunsaturated fat that has been hydrogenated, a process that makes it a solid at room temperature. In the process of hydrogenation, trans fatty acids are formed. The 1990 study found that unusually large amounts of these trans fatty acids raised blood LDL-cholesterol levels while lowering HDL levels. Though experts still tend to recommend margarine over butter, some people may see this study as another reason to switch to oils high in monounsaturated fat—with olive oil at the top of the list.

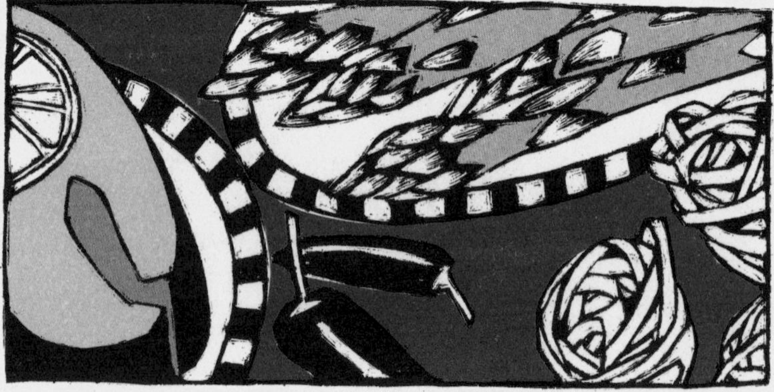

BUT WHAT DO YOU DO WITH IT?

Olive oil's uses in the kitchen are limited only by imagination. As a substitute for butter, it can be used in sautéing, frying, and basting; it is wonderful drizzled over fish before broiling. It can be mixed with herbs and vinegar and/or lemon and lime juice to make a marinade for vegetables, fish, chicken, or red meat. Many Mediterranean dishes, such as ratatouille (a French vegetable casserole using eggplant) and various classic pasta sauces, depend on olive oil for their full effect.

As a condiment it is a fragrant and delicious salad dressing oil, and it can even be used on bread in place of butter (dunking is the preferred method for this purpose). It has even cropped up in baking, where you would hardly expect an oil made from olives to find a place. One zealous manufacturer not only replaced butter with olive oil in a pound cake recipe to promote its light olive oil through supermarket tastings, but also handed out the recipe so customers could go home with their own supplies.

Making the Grades

Once you've decided to make olive oil a part of your diet, the challenge is to choose from the dozens of available products. They can vary tremendously in price and flavor, but there is no difference in their potential health benefits.

The International Olive Oil Council has established labeling regulations for quality oils that are the basis for international standards. Though there are no specific legal requirements governing the labeling of olive oil sold in the United States, most of the oil on the U.S. market (imported from Italy, Spain, or Greece) meets both international standards and similar United States Food and Drug Administration guidelines.

The lowest-grade oil made from olives, frequently sold as "pomace oil," is extracted chemically from the residue of previous olive pressings and then refined. The FDA guidelines prohibit labeling this product as olive oil. It is sometimes called "sansa" and is sold very cheaply; it is not a quality oil.

According to international standards, "pure" olive oil can be made from first or later pressings and can then be refined (by either heat or chemical processes) and flavored with better olive oils. "Virgin" olive oil, of better quality, comes only from first pressings and is unrefined.

Of still higher quality is "extra virgin" olive oil, also from first pressings and unrefined, but with a lower acidity level. The maximum acid content for extra virgin olive oil is only 1 percent.

When they are pressed, olives yield more oil if heated, but the oil is of lesser quality. Oil labeled "cold pressed" has been obtained without heating the olives.

High quality comes at a price; the best extra virgin olive oils can cost as much as $35 a quart in the United States. Some of the better olive oils available have a rich, fruity flavor that can wonderfully enhance salads and pasta dishes.

Within the quality categories there can be wide variations in flavor and color. More than 60 varieties of olives are used for oil production, and both the variety and the climate affect the end product.

In addition, manufacturers have devised oils to suit American palates, blending exoticism with caution. "Light" and "mild" are terms frequently found on these oils, generally meaning that they have been modified to make them taste less like olives—and possibly to lighten their color. Despite their designation, "light" olive oils have no fewer calories than any other fat—all have 40 calories per teaspoon.

"Virgin," "extra virgin," and "cold pressed" are indications of an olive oil's quality; "light" and "mild" refer to color and flavor only.

CONVERTING TO CANOLA

Experts praising the benefits of olive oil often mention canola oil in the same breath. The canola plant, also called rape, is related to cabbages and the mustard plant. Oil from its seeds has been used in cooking for many years in Europe and Canada but was unknown in the United States except as an industrial lubricant until 1985, when the Food and Drug Administration approved it for human consumption.

Canola (or rapeseed) oil contains even less saturated fat than olive oil (6-7 percent as opposed to olive oil's approximately 15 percent) and is almost as high in monounsaturated fat. Unlike olive oil, it does not affect the taste of food and is used only as a cooking oil, not as a condiment. It is sold in supermarkets, for about the same price as corn oil, and is found in commercially packaged products like potato chips, corn chips, and French fries.

A Spoonful a Day?

Experts stress that olive oil should be used as a *substitute* for saturated and hydrogenated polyunsaturated fats, not as a supplement to an otherwise unchanged diet. For example, vegetables can be sautéed in small amounts of olive oil instead of butter.

For all its promised benefits olive oil is still a fat and, like other fats, is best enjoyed in moderation. In addition to being high in calories, diets very high in total fat increase the risk of heart disease and are linked with cancer of the colon, prostate, and breast, according to the U.S. National Research Council's Committee on Diet and Health.

Olive oil can be a healthful gourmet treat but, like other fats, is best enjoyed in moderation as part of a well-balanced diet.

The National Cholesterol Education Program recommends that total fat intake should not exceed 30 percent of the calories in an adult's diet. It further recommends that saturated and polyunsaturated fat should each constitute no more than 10 percent of calories consumed, with the balance coming from monounsaturated fat.

Although olive oil may not be the perfect, all-encompassing health food, it can play a useful role in sound diet practices. And of course, it offers a golden opportunity for experimentation in the kitchens of serious or even casual cooks. □

CEREBRAL PALSY

Leon Sternfeld, M.D.

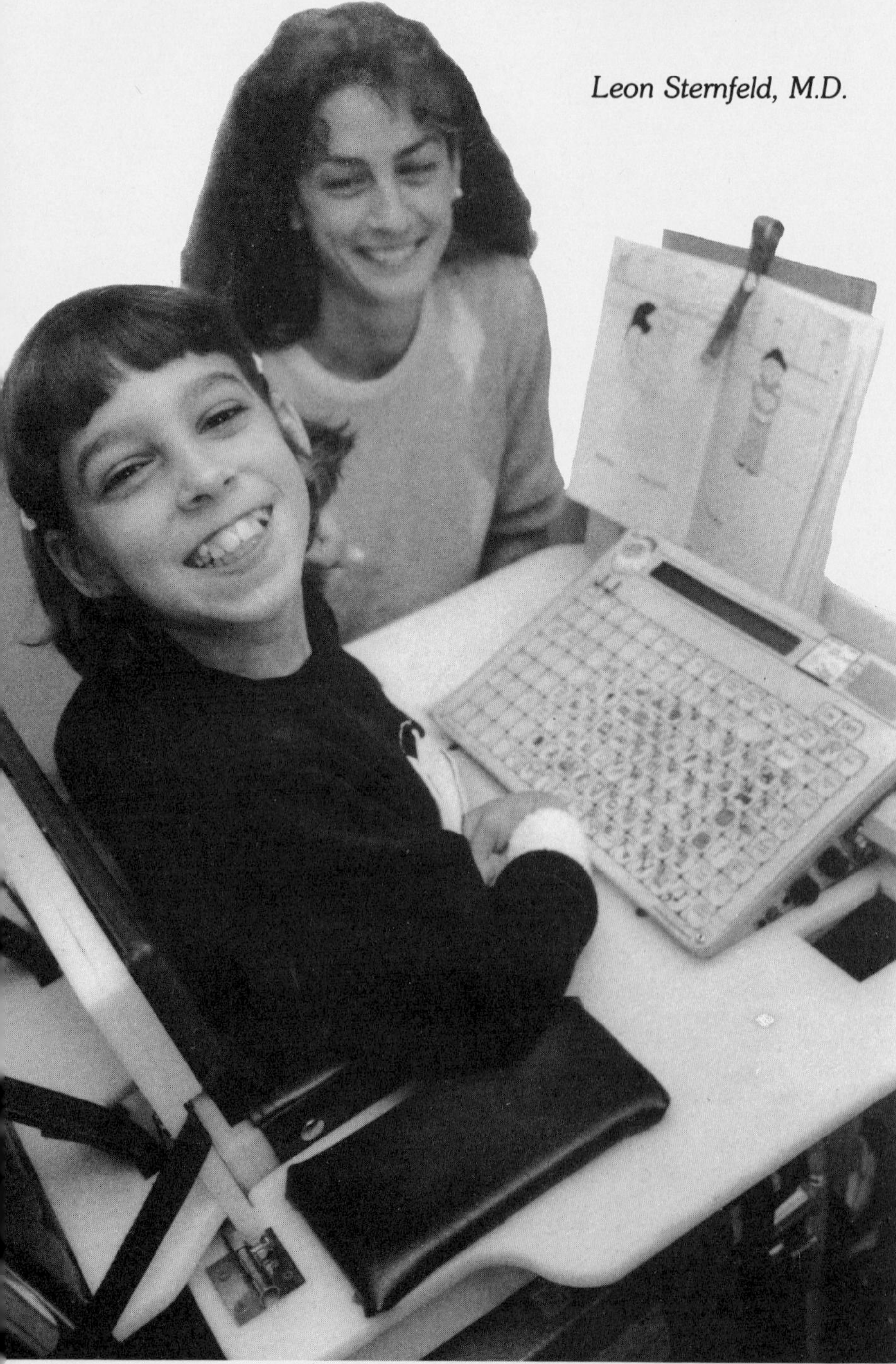

Cerebral palsy is a diagnostic label given to a group of conditions characterized by abnormalities in movement and balance and by delayed physical development. The person with cerebral palsy usually has an awkward and difficult gait, poor balance, and impaired control and coordination of movements, leading to difficulties in handling eating utensils or drinking containers, dressing and grooming, writing, talking, and swallowing. Drooling and facial grimacing are common. In addition, one or more of the following problems often occur: abnormal muscle tone (floppy or very tight muscles), involuntary irregular, startle-like movements, convulsive seizures, absent or poor speech, visual and hearing impairments, poor control of body temperature, and delayed intellectual development.

Why It Happens

More than 90 percent of cerebral palsy cases are congenital, that is, caused by factors related to childbearing. In about 35 percent of these cases, the infant was born prematurely, and usually weighing less than 3.3 pounds (1,500 grams). A premature infant is five times as likely as a full-term baby to have cerebral palsy, although many persons with cerebral palsy have no history of prematurity.

There is general agreement that cerebral palsy is due to a nonprogressive lesion, or injury, in the brain, the location and extent of which determines the exact characteristics of the condition in each individual. There is considerable confusion and disagreement over what causes the brain lesion in congenital cases. Expert opinion currently holds that it occurs early in the pregnancy—rather than in late pregnancy, at the time of labor and delivery, or in the first 28 days of life.

The remaining 10 percent or less of cerebral palsy cases are considered to be acquired, that is, they occur after the 28th day of life and up to the age of five, when the brain is 90 percent matured. Most cases of acquired cerebral palsy are due to head trauma from automobile accidents, falls in and around the home, and child abuse. Other causes are infections of the brain and its linings (meningitis and encephalitis), exposure to toxic substances (lead, household cleaning materials, medications, alcohol, and addictive drugs), and severe malnutrition and child neglect. The clinical characteristics, diagnosis, and management of acquired and congenital cerebral palsy are identical. The essential difference is that most cases of the acquired form are preventable.

Cerebral palsy is not inherited. Some uncommon genetic disorders may be difficult to distinguish from cerebral palsy, and it is important that these be diagnosed correctly since specific treatment may be available for them. Rarely, there may be a second sibling with cerebral palsy in a family, but there have been no reports of a parent or parents with cerebral palsy having children with cerebral palsy.

Types

The most frequently occurring type of cerebral palsy is the spastic type, which is characterized by tightness of the body musculature. In spastic diplegia, the most common form, the lower extremities are the most affected, with a characteristic cross-over of the legs, the so-called scissors gait. Other forms are spastic quadriplegia, a rather severe and generalized involvement of the entire body, and hemiplegia, an involvement of one side of the body. Most persons are either mildly or moderately affected; only a small fraction are severely affected. However, the increasing survival rate for very small premature babies—those between 1 and 2 pounds at birth, and particularly those born to mothers who are drug-addicted or infected with the virus that causes AIDS—is leading to an increase in babies with more severely damaged brains.

Another type of cerebral palsy, the athetoid type, is characterized by involuntary and irregular movements of the head, neck, and face and of the extremities, particularly the upper ones. Balance and gait are unsteady, although most persons with this type are ambulatory, albeit with varying degrees of difficulty. Hearing deficiencies are common, and speech may be garbled or entirely absent. Generally, in athetoid cerebral palsy intelligence is unimpaired.

In recent years there have been almost no new cases of athetoid cerebral palsy (which was once the second most common kind) because its cause, hyperbilirubinemia, has been controlled. In hyperbilirubinemia, too much bilirubin (a pigment produced by the breakdown of red blood cells) accumulates in the blood. Too much bilirubin can damage the brain.

Cerebral palsy is incurable, but physical therapy and other techniques can help people function to the maximum extent possible.

A major cause of hyperbilirubinemia is a blood incompatibility between mother and fetus. In the most common blood incompatibility, the mother's blood is Rh negative and the fetus's Rh positive. This Rh incompatibility does not lead to problems in a first pregnancy. So if a mother with Rh negative blood is given an antibody within three days after each pregnancy ends (whether in a live birth or a stillbirth, a miscarriage, or an abortion), none of her babies should be affected by incompatibility problems.

Jaundice of the newborn, which has a number of different causes, is a sign that bilirubin is not being processed properly. In most cases the condition clears without treatment. If bilirubin levels become high, however, babies are treated by phototherapy, exposure to light, which is highly effective in breaking down the excess bilirubin in the blood and neutralizing its toxic effect. Phototherapy has been investigated extensively and found to be not only effective, but completely safe.

A third type of cerebral palsy, the ataxic type, is characterized by unsteadiness and difficulty with rapid or fine movements. A combination of different types, most often spastic and athetoid, is common.

Incidence

It is generally accepted that 2 out of every 1,000 people have cerebral palsy, which translates in the United States to about 500,000 persons of all ages. About 40 percent of them are under 20 years of age; however, a substantial number are in their 50s and 60s—some are even in their 70s and 80s. The life expectancy of persons with cerebral palsy is comparable to that of the general population, except for a relatively small group that is multiply and severely handicapped and may be institutionalized.

The number of new cases occurring annually appears to have reached a plateau after having decreased in the past quarter-century. The generally accepted rate of new cases at present, for purposes of planning services, is 1 per 1,000 live-born babies, which means somewhere between 3,500 and 4,000 new cases annually in the United States.

Diagnosis

There is no way now to detect cerebral palsy during pregnancy. Nor can it be diagnosed at birth. Infants at high risk, such as those who were premature or had jaundice, should be followed more closely than normal well-baby care allows for.

Usually the mother is the first to suspect that there may be a delay in the infant's development, and astute physicians have learned to heed the mother's suspicions. Signs of developmental delay are floppy or limp body posture or stiffness of arms and legs in the first few months; failure to smile by 3 months; poor head control after 3 or 4 months; inability to sit alone after 8 months; difficulty in standing by 12 months; inability to walk or walking on toes by 18 to 20 months; and poor or no speech by 27 months. Other warning signs are difficulty in maintaining body temperature, extreme irritability, frequent gagging or choking when fed, and tongue thrust (for example, the tongue pushes soft food out of the mouth).

Although there is no definitive diagnostic test for cerebral palsy, an evaluation and assessment by a developmental pediatrician with consultation by a pediatric neurologist and a pediatric orthopedic surgeon will usually rule out other possible conditions and lead to a correct diagnosis when the child is between 15 and 24 months of age. Many children are now being diagnosed at an earlier age, some at under 12 months.

Management

Cerebral palsy is a life-long condition. There is as yet no way to repair the original lesion in the brain, and cerebral palsy is not a disease amenable to treatment and cure. The major goal is to maximize the functional abilities of the person with cerebral palsy and minimize the handicapping effects.

This involves as early intervention as is feasible by physical, occupational, and speech therapists. (Occupational therapy involves learning coordination and how to manage daily routines, such as dressing oneself and eating.) An expert in special education, a nurse, and a social worker frequently join this team. With the active participation of a family member, generally the mother but including both parents if possible, and with input from the medical specialists, the team develops an individual management plan to attain specified goals and objectives. This plan is reviewed periodically and is modified as appropriate.

Many communities now have "early development" programs in centers where, in addition to the professional services for the affected child, parent counseling and support groups are available to help other members of the child's family.

Medications have so far not been effective over long periods of time, except for standard anticonvulsant drugs given to children with seizures. The levels of these medications in the blood must be carefully monitored. So must medications sometimes given to control drooling. Muscle relaxants have not been too effective and do have side effects, serious and dangerous in some instances.

Orthopedic surgery and the use of orthotic appliances such as braces play a significant role in both the prevention and correction of deformities, particularly of the lower extremities and the back. In recent years gait analysis laboratories have accumulated considerable data about normal and abnormal walking. This work has been of great value in enabling orthopedic surgeons, orthotists, and physical therapists to provide better services to persons with cerebral palsy. (Orthotists specialize in the support and bracing of weak or deformed muscles.)

Various neurosurgical procedures have been tried in the past, only to be abandoned because they proved to be ineffective. Currently, a number of pediatric neurosurgeons in the United States are performing a procedure called selective dorsal (or posterior) rhizotomy. In this procedure, the dorsal nerve rootlets emerging from the lumbar (lower) part of the spinal cord are tested to find which of them are causing spastic contraction of the muscles in the legs. Those responsible are then cut, which relieves the spasticity and enables physical therapy to be more effective. The strict eligibility requirements that the surgeons have stipulated are met only by a limited number of children with spastic diplegia. No thorough evaluation of the procedure has been made to date.

Physical, occupational, and speech therapists now teach those with cerebral palsy how to use a number of mechanical and electronic devices that enable both children and adults to be involved in the daily activities of routine living, schooling, and working. These devices help them to dress, groom, and feed themselves and to get around more efficiently both indoors and out-of-doors. One of the most significant technological developments has been that of augmentative communication systems, using computers and voice synthesizers, that enable those with little or no speech to communicate. This has been of major importance in enabling children to obtain a regular education, and as they mature into adulthood, to live independently and be engaged in gainful employment.

During childhood the objective of therapy is to help the child achieve the maximum potential for growth and development—physical, intellectual, emotional, and social. As the child matures into adulthood, additional services are required, such as vocational training, appropriate living accommodations, transportation, and recreation/leisure activities—all essential for any adult. People with cerebral palsy are entitled to the opportunity to live as normal and integrated members in our society.

Prevention

Acquired cerebral palsy can be prevented in part by widespread education about and efforts toward accident prevention, particularly accidents involving automobiles and hazards in the home. Prevention of child abuse and neglect is also important, as is regular pediatric well-child supervision, including complete recommended basic and booster immunizations, monitoring of growth and development, and proper nutrition guidance throughout infancy and the preschool years.

As mentioned previously, prevention of hyperbilirubinemia has almost eliminated the athetoid type of cerebral palsy. There are no specific preventive measures at present for congenital spastic cerebral palsy. There is evidence, however, that good health practices preceding and during pregnancy can to some extent prevent prematurity, which is so closely associated with a substantial fraction of cerebral palsy cases.

Such practices include good nutrition, particularly during adolescence and early adulthood, and up-to-date immunization status, with particular emphasis on German measles (rubella) immunization. (There are a number of American women in the childbearing years who may be susceptible to the rubella virus, as they did not have the disease in childhood and were not in the first groups of children to be immunized when the vaccine was approved for use in 1969.)

Recommended measures for women who are or want to become pregnant also include correction of any physical conditions, such as diabetes or anemia, elimination of infections, particularly those of the genital tract, and avoidance of smoking, alcohol, and addictive drugs. Women who become pregnant before 18 years of age or after 35 face a higher risk of premature delivery. Regardless of age, it is of the utmost importance that prenatal care be started as early as possible and continued under the regular supervision of a qualified obstetrician.

While no guarantee can ever be given, the observance of good health practices both before and during pregnancy will increase considerably the chances of having a sound and healthy baby.

See also the feature article SPORTS FOR THE DISABLED. □

NATIONAL ORGANIZATIONS

United Cerebral Palsy Associations is a nationwide network of some 180 state and local affiliated agencies in the United States. These affiliates provide direct services to persons with cerebral palsy and their families, act as advocates for the disabled, are involved in public and professional information and education, and support research on cerebral palsy and the neurosciences (through the UCP Research and Educational Foundation). Information and referrals can be obtained from UCPA's New York office (7 Penn Plaza, Suite 804, New York, NY 10001; 1-800-USA-1UCP) or its Washington office (1522 K Street, NW, Suite 1112, Washington, DC 20005; 1-800-USA-5UCP).

A similar nationwide network exists in Canada, under the aegis of the Canadian Cerebral Palsy Association. Direct services to those with cerebral palsy and their families, including advocacy services, are provided by the national association's member organizations at the provincial and regional levels. The national association provides the member agencies with educational materials and acts as an advocate at the federal level. Information can be obtained from the association's headquarters at 880 Wellington Street, Suite 612, Ottawa, Ontario K1R 6K7; 1-800-267-6572 (calls from outside Canada can be made to 614-235-2144).

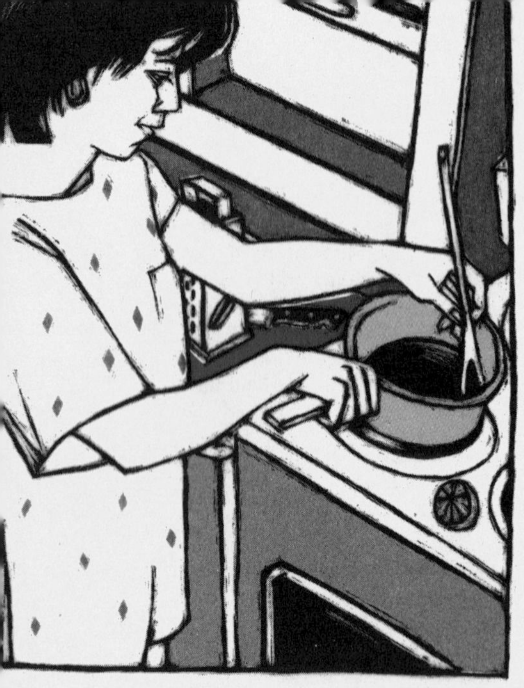

Safe Cookware

Ingrid J. Strauch

Ideally, a cooking vessel should heat food evenly and efficiently, without reacting to it in any way that changes the food's taste or introduces a potentially harmful substance. Among the most common materials for cookware are aluminum, cast iron, stainless steel, ceramics, copper, and enameled iron or steel. As new products, such as nonstick surfaces, appear on the market, consumers often wonder which type of cookware is best and whether some materials used in cookware might be harmful.

No one material is perfect—most are well-suited for certain cooking needs and less appropriate for others—but all are generally safe when manufactured according to proper techniques. However, unlined copper pots and improperly produced ceramics may release toxic substances into food that can be deadly at high enough concentrations.

Aluminum

One of the most popular types on the market, aluminum cookware is relatively inexpensive and is an excellent heat conductor, meaning that it heats evenly without developing hot spots that burn food. However, public concern arose over the safety of aluminum pots when it was discovered that Alzheimer's disease victims have unusually high levels of aluminum in their brains. Although some metal does leach into food during cooking, researchers say there is no evidence that the use of aluminum pots or utensils is linked to the disease. More likely the aluminum in the brain is a result, not a cause, of Alzheimer's.

Manufacturers of aluminum cookware do warn consumers not to store acidic or salty foods—such as tomato sauce or sauerkraut—in aluminum pots because they may cause more of the metal to dissolve. The acid and salt may also cause pitting of an aluminum pot's surface, making food stick more and the pot harder to clean. Severe pitting can cause a pot to heat unevenly.

Anodized Aluminum

Cookware made of anodized aluminum is growing in availability and popularity. Anodized aluminum is put through an electrochemical treatment that renders it harder and more scratch resistant than ordinary aluminum. The process does not diminish the metal's efficiency as a heat conductor, and it creates a surface that causes food to stick less and is easier to clean.

The anodization process also seals the aluminum so that none leaches into food, even acidic foods like tomatoe sauce, rhubarb, and sauces containing vinegar or lemon juice.

Nonstick Coatings

Nonstick coatings, such as Teflon, are made of a tough, nonporous material called fluorocarbon resin that was first used in war machinery in the 1930s. It began showing up in kitchenware in the 1960s. The coating makes it possible to cook with little or no fat, is easy to clean, and is noncorrosive. However, nonstick surfaces are easily scratched, and food then sticks to the damaged areas. To minimize breaks in the coating, manufacturers recommend using wooden or plastic cooking utensils and avoiding abrasive scouring pads and cleansers.

Even with the best of care, nonstick pans sometimes get scratched, and small pieces of the coating can get into food. Fortunately that does not mean the pan has to be thrown out. Flakes of fluorocarbon resin pass through the body undigested, causing no harm.

Fluorocarbon resin will emit fumes if heated for long periods at high temperatures, but studies have shown that the fumes are not harmful. Researchers investigating the possibility that nonstick coatings might break down somehow after long-term use and release toxins into food found that the resin remains safe after years of use.

Iron

Cast-iron cookware has been used for thousands of years and has proved itself safe, strong, and inexpensive. It conducts heat evenly and is especially suited for frying, browning, and baking. However, iron can rust, so the insides of iron pans should occasionally be coated with a thin layer of unsalted cooking oil to protect the surface.

An added—but essentially insignificant—benefit of cooking in cast iron is that it can boost a dish's iron content by a small amount. Acidic foods can dissolve a considerable amount of iron from a pan, but it may not be in a form the body can easily absorb. Persons wanting to increase their iron intake should not rely on iron pots and pans but should include more iron-rich foods in their diet.

Stainless Steel

Cookware made of stainless steel is safe and durable. Stainless steel is an alloy and contains, among other things, iron and chromium. It is the chromium that makes it resistant to rust and corrosion. The drawbacks to stainless steel cookware are that it usually costs more than cast iron and is a poorer heat conductor.

To improve heat conductivity, stainless steel cookware is often made with an aluminum or copper bottom, since both of these metals are much better conductors. Alternatively, stainless steel pots are made very thin, but food is then much more likely to burn. Although anything can be cooked in stainless steel, it is not advisable to store acidic or salty foods in it for long periods because they may pit the surface.

Copper

Copper is an excellent heat conductor and, for that reason, is the choice of cooks for foods, such as delicate sauces, that must be heated at precisely controlled temperatures.

However, many foods dissolve copper easily, and ingesting too much copper can have toxic effects. To avoid medical problems, only copper pans lined with tin or stainless steel should be used in cooking.

Usually copper accumulates gradually in the body, reaching unsafe levels only after repeated uses of unlined copper cookware. Symptoms of copper poisoning include nausea, vomiting, and diarrhea. In extreme cases, consuming large amounts of copper can cause acute anemia and liver damage.

Ceramics

While most ceramic cookware and tableware commercially produced in the United States today is safe for cooking and eating, pottery made in developing countries is a potential source of the highly dangerous metal lead. Lead is commonly used in pottery glazes. If the glaze is fired properly—at a high enough temperature for a long enough time—the lead is sealed and does not leach into food. But when the glaze is improperly fired, toxic and even deadly amounts of lead can end up in food.

In 1971 the U.S. Food and Drug Administration set limitations on the amount of lead permitted to leach from ceramic housewares. Most of the ceramics produced commercially in the United States after 1971 meet these standards, as do ceramics from Japan and the United Kingdom, which have quality control procedures similar to the United States. In 1988 the FDA entered into an agreement with China to ensure that ceramic products shipped to the United States would be inspected for safety, although these products are not tested when sold in China.

The FDA warns consumers to test any ceramics purchased in China, Hong Kong, or India—and especially products purchased in or imported from Mexico—before using them for cooking or eating. FDA inspectors have found tableware and cookware from Mexico leaching quantities of lead up to a thousand times the recommended limit. Test kits similar to those used by the FDA are available for home use.

Certain acidic foods, such as coffee, orange juice, and tomato juice, dissolve lead in large quantities and will speed up the poisoning process when consumed from improperly fired mugs or other tableware. Even in originally safe ceramics, repeated washing in a dishwasher can wear down the glaze and make pottery unsafe.

The price of ingesting lead is high. In adults symptoms of lead poisoning include personality changes, headaches, vomiting, constipation, and abdominal pain. In children symptoms include vomiting, seizures, and lapses of consciousness. Chronic lead poisoning can cause irreversible effects, such as kidney failure in adults and mental retardation and seizure disorders in children.

Enamel

Porcelain (or vitreous) enamel is used to create a smooth, glassy surface on iron and stainless steel cookware. Enamel is resistant to scratches and stains and is also more attractive than bare metal. Unlike the glazes used to color ceramics, enamel glazes do not contain lead.

Before 1971, some enamels contained another potentially toxic substance, cadmium, which was sometimes used in red, yellow, and orange pigments, mainly by manufacturers outside the United States. At the same time that it established standards for lead in housewares, the FDA set limits on the amount of cadmium permitted to leach from enamel glazes. Manufacturers have since ceased using cadmium, so consumers are not at risk from enameled cookware marketed today.

Plastic

Although plastic containers are rarely used for stove-top cooking or in a conventional oven, they are frequently used for microwave cooking. Only plastic containers specifically manufactured to be microwave safe should be used in this fashion. Other types of plastic may melt, and chemicals in the plastic may migrate into food. Substances in plastic wrap, often used to cover food in a microwave oven, can also leach into it. To avoid this problem, the wrap should be stretched tightly over the container so it is not in contact with the contents. □

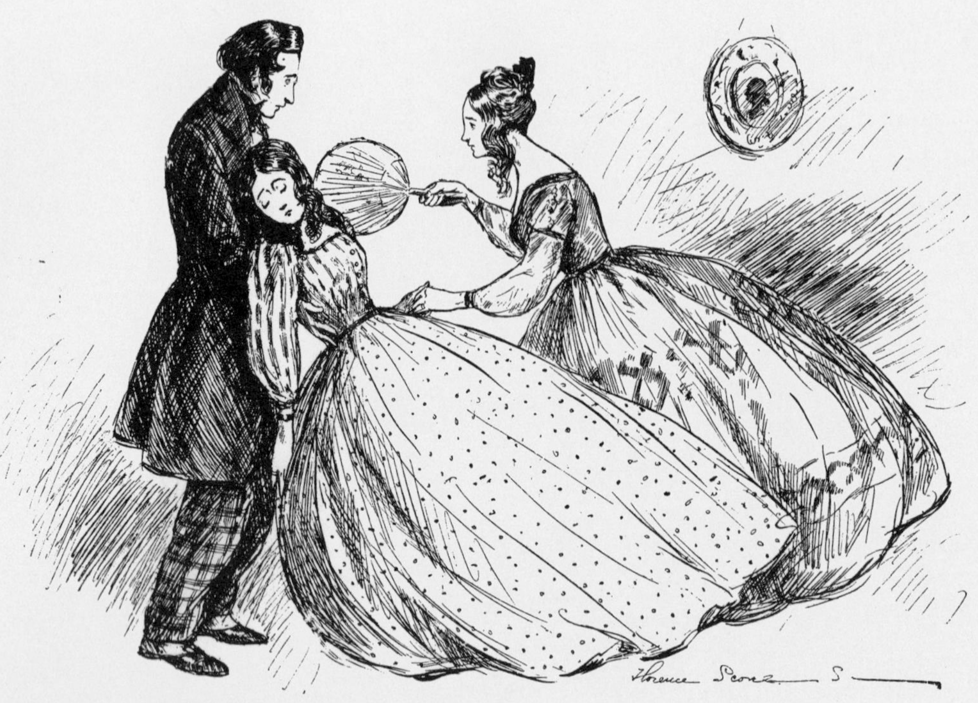

FAINTING

Ingrid J. Strauch

In Victorian times women fainted with astounding regularity. Novels from that era depict women swooning in response to just about any upset: news of war, infidelity, even a social snub. Sometimes just the sound of a crude word sent a genteel lady fluttering for her smelling salts.

Today such a reaction seems absurd. Although emotional shocks can indeed cause fainting, very few people faint with such frequency. But in the 1800s and early 1900s it was fashionable for a woman to be fragile, and a good swoon was evidence that her delicate sensibilities needed protection from the rougher edges of life. It is possible that the clothing styles of the times helped cause the epidemic of fainting—tightly cinched corsets created desirable 21-inch waists, but they also squeezed internal organs out of their natural locations. It is generally thought, however, that such habitual fainting was a learned behavior that served a social purpose at the time.

What Is a Faint?

A simple faint—known by doctors as vasovagal syncope—is a temporary loss of consciousness that occurs when not enough blood reaches the brain because of a drop in blood pressure. While frightening to experience or observe, it is usually harmless.

The cardiovascular and the nervous systems work together to regulate blood flow. When the cardiovascular system is working properly, the heart pumps adequate amounts of blood through the arteries to the brain and throughout the body. The rate at which the heart beats, blood pressure, and indeed circulation as a whole are affected by a part of the nervous system called the autonomic nervous system. Impulses from certain autonomic nerve fibers accelerate the heart rate; impulses from others, in particular, fibers in the vagus nerve, slow down and, to a lesser degree, weaken the force of contraction of the heart.

Together the two types of nerve fibers maintain a balance. When

Fainting is commonly triggered by an emotional shock, pain, the sight of blood, or simply standing in a hot room for too long.

external factors such as exercise or strongly felt emotions (for example, fear or excitement) cause a rise in blood pressure, a reflex occurs that causes the autonomic nervous system to slow the heart rate somewhat and slightly lower the blood pressure. If an external factor such as standing up from a reclining or sitting position causes blood pressure to fall, the system triggers the opposite response: the heart pumps faster and the arteries constrict to raise the blood pressure.

Sometimes, however, the system cannot raise the blood pressure quickly enough. When the vagus nerve is overstimulated by an outside event, the heartbeat slows, the contraction of the heart weakens slightly, and a reduced amount of blood is pumped through the heart, leading to a drop in blood pressure. The system kicks in to raise the blood pressure but is unable to do so right away. This is because the event that caused the blood pressure to drop also had some direct effect on the brain, and the brain partly regulates activity in the autonomic nervous system. In these circumstances, it is not until the "roadblock" in the brain is removed, generally after the person has actually fainted, that the autonomic nervous system is able to finish its work and bring the blood pressure back to normal.

Common Causes

Often, a faint is triggered by an emotional shock or pain; such events overstimulate the vagus nerve. For many people the sight of blood, especially their own, is an emotionally traumatic event.

Other situations that commonly bring on fainting include standing in a hot, stuffy room or in the hot sun for an extended period of time. The body tries to dissipate heat by dilating blood vessels in the skin, which lowers blood pressure. If the individual's heart rate does not rise to compensate, the person faints.

Travelers who must sit still for hours and people, such as guards, whose jobs involve standing in one place for a long time are prone to fainting. This is because, in the absence of physical activity, blood pools in the lower parts of the body.

Some people can faint when urinating or during violent coughing. When urination causes fainting, it is most likely the result of an abnormal nerve reflex sent from the bladder to the brain that affects autonomic nervous system activity. When coughing is the problem, it appears that normal circulation is temporarily cut off when the abdominal muscles contract, preventing the blood in abdominal veins from leaving the abdomen.

In a medical condition called orthostatic hypotension, in which faintness and fainting are the primary symptoms, the autonomic nervous system is unable to compensate for the normal drop in blood pressure that takes place when a person stands up from a reclining or sitting position. Blood pools in the legs and does not circulate adequately to the brain. The condition is often caused by medications, such as drugs for high blood pressure, antidepressants, and antipsychotics. It can also occur when people who have been confined to bed stand up. To alleviate fainting episodes, a physician may adjust a drug dosage, prescribe a drug to raise blood pressure (assuming high blood pressure is not the condition being treated), or simply advise the patient to stand up more slowly.

Fainting and Serious Illness

Sometimes loss of consciousness is a symptom of an underlying, possibly serious, condition. It may indicate that a person is having a transient ischemic attack (TIA), a temporary interruption in the blood flow to the brain. A variety of conditions, including the buildup of fatty deposits in certain blood vessels, can lead to a TIA. A TIA may be a warning sign that the person is at high risk for a major stroke.

Some other conditions that can cause a temporary loss of consciousness include heart arrhythmias (abnormal heartbeats), a pulmonary embolism (a blood clot in the lungs), and a severe allergic reaction. A mild epileptic seizure

First aid for a faint includes making sure the victim is lying down in a safe place with the feet higher than the head and loosening any tight clothing.

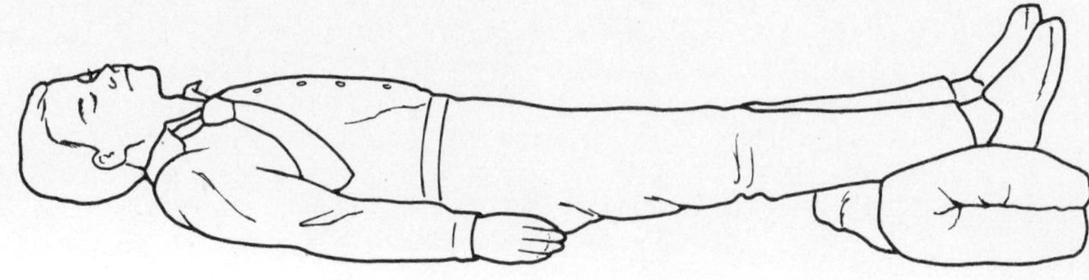

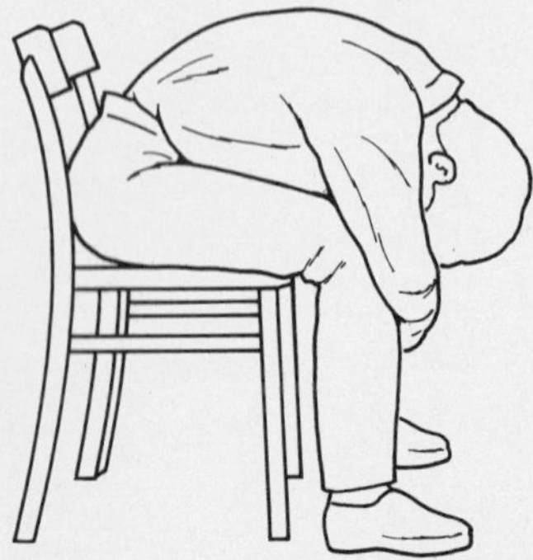

If warning signals are recognized in time, sitting down and bending the head to the knees can sometimes prevent a faint.

might be mistaken for a simple faint.

Because of such possibilities, it's a good idea to consult a physician after fainting. Diagnosing the cause can be difficult because faints typically don't leave many clues behind. The patient may be able to help the doctor by recalling details such as when he or she had last eaten and air temperature at the time of the faint. Witnesses may be able to recall expressions of pain before a faint or convulsions during the time of unconsciousness.

If the cause remains elusive in a patient with repeated fainting spells, the doctor may equip the patient with a portable electrocardiogram (ECG) monitor, which records the electrical impulses produced by the contraction of the heart muscles. The doctor may then be able to discover whether heart arrhythmias are causing the fainting. Arrhythmias occur in a variety of illnesses and are one of the most serious as well as the most common causes of fainting other than the causes associated with the simple faint discussed earlier.

First Aid

Sometimes a faint can be prevented if the warning signs are recognized. Symptoms typically preceding or accompanying a faint include extreme paleness, sweating, cold skin, dizziness, numbness or tingling in the hands and feet, nausea, and tunnel vision, or a narrowing of the full range of vision. A person experiencing these symptoms should try to lie down or sit down with the head at knee level. Doing so will often restore normal blood circulation, allowing enough blood to reach the brain, and the feeling of faintness or dizziness will go away.

First aid for an actual faint includes making sure the victim is lying down in a safe place with the feet higher than the head. If possible, it's best to leave victims lying where they fall. Loosen any tight clothing that might interfere with circulation, such as a necktie or collar.

First aid givers should immediately check for unobstructed breathing and circulation. Breathing can be determined by looking for the rise and fall of the chest, listening for sounds of breathing, and feeling air exhaled on a hand held close to the victim's mouth and nose. Circulation is best checked by feeling for the carotid artery pulse. This is done by placing three fingers in one of the grooves found on either side of the Adam's apple.

Victims who vomit must be rolled onto their sides to prevent inhalation of the vomit. The first aid giver may need to wipe out a victim's mouth, preferably with a cloth.

In a benign faint, recovery should be prompt: the victim should revive within a few seconds or minutes. Otherwise, medical assistance should be sought. Medical help may also be needed if the victim sustained an injury while falling.

Under no circumstances should liquids be given to an unconscious person, nor should water be poured over the person's face in an attempt at revival because the water could be inhaled. Instead, the victim's face may be washed gently with cool water. Once consciousness is regained, the victim should remain in a reclining position for several minutes. A faint may recur if the victim stands or sits up too soon after recovery. □

Because the loss of consciousness is sometimes a symptom of a serious underlying illness, it's a good idea to see a doctor after fainting.

ASTRONAUTS AND FAINTING

Astronauts returning to earth may be prone to fainting because of a phenomenon known as fluid shift. On earth bodily fluids and blood naturally pool slightly in the legs, but in the weightlessness of space, blood and fluids shift to the upper half of the body. The nerves that monitor blood pressure in the chest perceive the increased amount of blood as a rise in blood pressure, and the body reacts by lowering its overall blood volume through increased urination. While the astronaut remains in space, lowered blood volume and fluid shift are not a problem. But when the astronaut reenters the earth's gravitational field, the blood shifts back to the lower body, and with less blood available to circulate, the heart is not always able to keep the brain adequately supplied. Both Soviet and U.S. space travelers have combated this problem with varying degrees of success by periodically wearing, while in space, specially made "vacuum trousers" that suck fluids back into the legs.

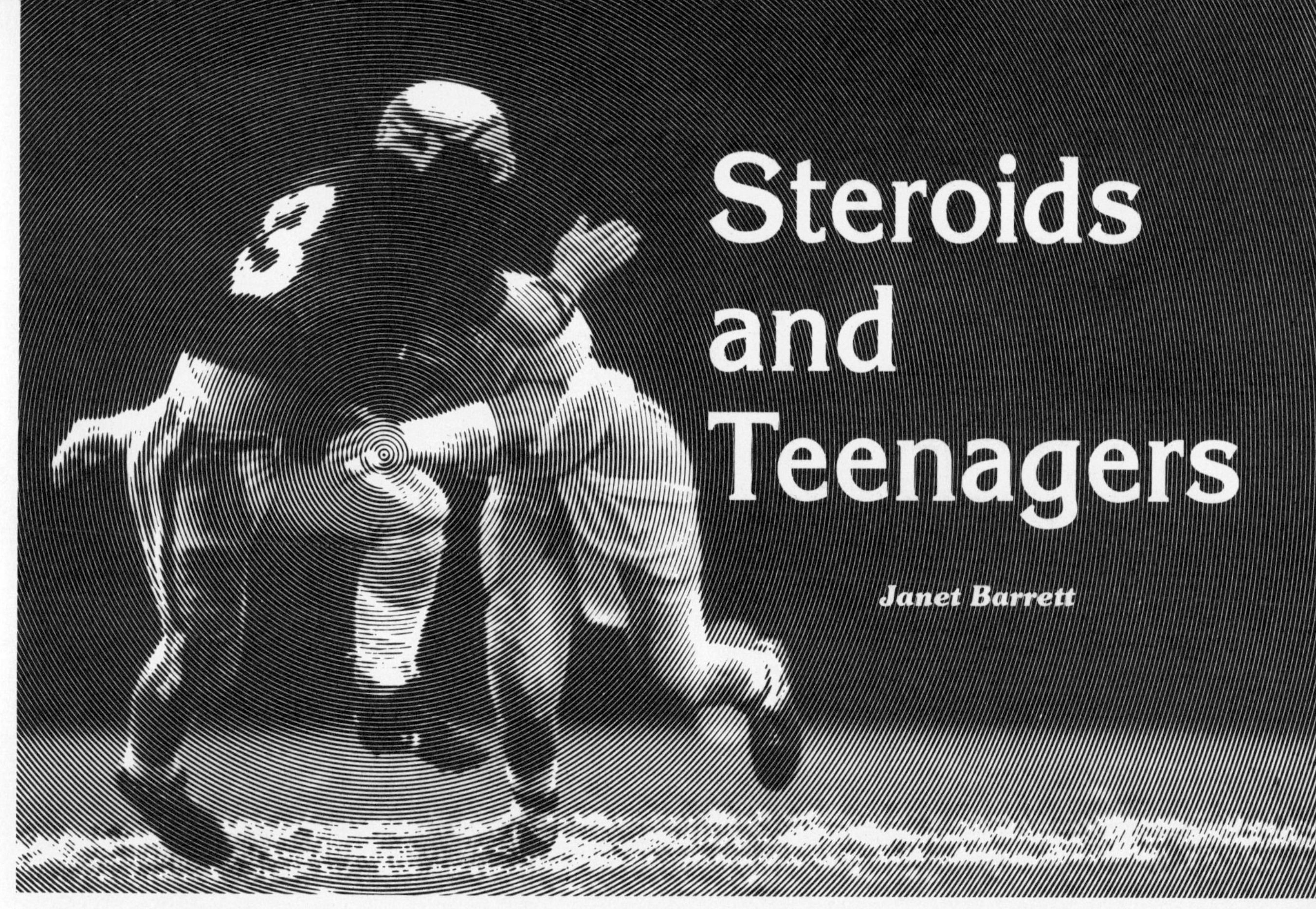

Steroids and Teenagers

Janet Barrett

They are called "roids" and "juice"; using them is known as "bulking up." They are anabolic steroids—a group of powerful, potentially harmful, synthetic hormones that have been used by professional and top-ranked amateur athletes since the mid-1950s to increase muscle mass, strength, and endurance.

Now these steroids are increasingly being abused by high school and college athletes, bodybuilders, sports enthusiasts, and even preadolescents. They all think a pill or an injection will make them perform better—or simply look better.

Steroids, prescribed and monitored by a physician, have legitimate medical uses, but building muscle strength is not one of them. Whether anabolic steroids truly produce such an effect is debatable; that they have unpleasant and often serious side effects is certain.

Young Users

Though there are no firm figures, it is estimated conservatively that, not counting those taking the drugs under a doctor's supervision for medical purposes, there are at least 1 million anabolic steroid users in the United States today. Of that number, 70 percent are male, and more than half are under age 18. One 1989 survey found that besides school athletes, an additional 10 percent of high school students have tried steroids. The practice has even filtered down to grade school, where users may be as young as nine or ten years old.

Whether anabolic steroids really deliver the promised benefits is debatable. The unpleasant and often serious side effects are not.

To some degree, the growing use of steroids is probably linked to an enormously increased interest in the United States in bodybuilding, no doubt fueled by such pop heroes as Arnold Schwarzenegger. Such celebrity hype has sent young men and women to health clubs and gyms in search of more muscle. There, some have found not only exercise equipment waiting for them, but sellers of anabolic steroids, claiming their product is a faster route to a more perfect body.

How They Work

Anabolic steroids are artificial compounds closely related chemically to the male sex hormone testosterone. They were developed in the 1930s to help men whose bodies did not produce enough testosterone, which is responsible for the development of masculine characteristics occurring at puberty, including lowering of the voice and growth of body hair. Testosterone stimulates and maintains the male sex organs, promotes the growth of bone, muscle, skin, and hair, and influences emotional responses characteristic of the adult male.

When anabolic steroids are taken to build muscles, users commonly engage in what is called "megadosing"—that is, taking much larger amounts than those prescribed for therapeutic purposes. They may also "stack" them, or take a combination of brands, each in large quantity, daily. Because the brain does not discriminate between the steroids and natural testosterone, it responds to a high level of steroids in the bloodstream by sending messages to shut down the body's natural production of testosterone. One dangerous result of this process in children is that the long bones stop growing and fuse prematurely, thus preventing the child from reaching normal height. Steroids can also push a child into early puberty.

Side Effects

More than 70 side effects have been attributed to anabolic steroids, ranging in severity from liver cancer to acne, and encompassing psychological as well as physical reactions. The parts of the body most seriously affected are the liver and the cardiovascular and reproductive systems. Although steroids themselves may not cause liver cancer, they appear to promote tumor development caused by other factors. They also raise levels of blood fats, leading to increased risk of heart disease.

In women, who normally produce little testosterone, the use of anabolic steroids can lead to such masculine traits as male-pattern balding, facial hair, and a deepened voice. Most of these changes are reversible; some (such as deepening of the voice) may be permanent. Other problems in women include menstrual irregularities, breast reduction, and sterility.

Ironically, taking steroids may not even produce the quick gain in muscle mass that their abusers seek.

In males, too, stopping steroid abuse does not always mean that the processes that have gone awry will return to normal. Most side effects, such as feminization of the breasts (which become enlarged and may even produce milk) and withered testicles, are reversible when steroid use is stopped, but others, such as sterility and impotence, can be permanent.

Most of what is known about side effects has been gathered from patients receiving therapeutic doses. But because abusers frequently take as much as ten times the recommended dose and indulge in stacking, no one really knows how bad the damage can be or, in the case of long-term abuse, what additional effects are yet to be discovered.

Not only will some side effects—such as heart attacks and strokes—probably not show up for years, but some—such as an adolescent's stunted growth—may not even be recognized as a result of steroid abuse. Others can cause immediate difficulties, among them uncontrollable aggressive and combative behavior, known as "roid rages."

Withdrawal from the drugs can be especially difficult for some athletes and bodybuilders because weight and muscle mass are quickly lost, although evidence suggests that this is actually water loss, since steroids cause water retention. Depression can also result from ceasing to take steroids, prompting some former abusers to turn to amphetamines for a psychological lift. Generally, there is little risk associated with stopping steroid use abruptly, but a parent who discovers a child using them should have the withdrawal process monitored by a physician.

Signs of Steroid Abuse

- **Aggressive behavior ("roid rages")**
- **Moodiness**
- **Blurred vision**
- **Headaches**
- **Lightheadedness**
- **Trembling**
- **Chills and fever**
- **Hives**
- **Jaundice (yellowing of the skin)**
- **Darkening of the skin**
- **Purple or red spots on the body**
- **Abdominal pains**
- **Muscle cramps**
- **Swelling of the feet or lower legs**
- **Bad breath**

Signs of Abuse

Unlike the signs of abuse of other substances, indications of anabolic steroid use can be subtle and therefore difficult to detect. Telltale signs for parents to watch for in their children include rapid growth and sexual development, as well as muscle and weight gain beyond what can be accounted for by any sort of weight-training program.

Besides roid rages, behavioral changes may include moodiness. Other signs that can signal use are abdominal pains, blurred vision, chills, fever, hives, headaches, lightheadedness, and muscle cramps. Still others are jaundice (yellowing of the skin), small purple or red spots on the body, swelling of the feet or lower legs, trembling, unexplained darkening of the skin, and continual bad breath.

Ironically, there is evidence to suggest that anabolic steroids may not even produce the quick gain in muscle mass that the youngsters taking them so desperately seek. Current thinking is that only persons who are already weight training and who continue intensive training and high-protein, high-calorie diets will benefit. Thus, the youngest abusers—preteens looking for more mature bodies—are in for a disappointment, as well as more serious troubles.

Seeking a Magic Elixir

Particularly for athletes, trying to get the body to perform better by taking a potion is nothing new. The ancient Greeks used certain herbs and mushrooms to enhance performance at their Olympiads. Around 1900, a mixture of coca leaf extract and wine called Vin Muriani was advertised as the drink for athletes.

Steroids first entered the American athletic scene in 1964 when Dr. John B. Ziegler, team physician for the U.S. weight lifters at the world championships in Vienna, found out that the Soviets were giving testosterone to their weight lifters and to some women athletes to improve their performance. Wishing to give American athletes an equal boost, Ziegler developed a synthetic form of testosterone which he tested on himself and a few athletes. However, he soon found that some of the athletes were taking up to 20 times the recommended dose and developing liver problems. Ziegler stopped his experiments, but the die was cast.

Steroid use can cause children's long bones to stop growing, preventing them from reaching normal height.

Obtaining Steroids Illegally

Because of their powerful, often dangerous side effects, anabolic steroids are infrequently prescribed for medical purposes today. Their uses are limited, for the most part, to certain types of inoperable breast cancer, severe anemia, and a few other conditions. But while relatively small quantities are being manufactured by pharmaceutical companies, underground laboratories have flourished, and a lucrative black market trade has sprung up. In the United States federal authorities place the size of this market in the neighborhood of $300 million a year. Large quantities of black market steroids come into the United States from Mexico, Canada, and Europe.

The small amount of steroids made by pharmaceutical companies is dwarfed by the amount made for the black market.

Beyond the obvious dangers of taking anabolic steroids, however, buyers dealing on the black market should beware of substances produced in underground laboratories. Such steroids may be of questionable quality and purity and, in fact, may not even be steroids at all. Black market sales also extend to other prescription drugs that are used to counter the side effects of the steroids.

Although the only legal means of obtaining steroids is by prescription, they are readily available through ads in muscle magazines, unscrupulous doctors and pharmacists, and even dealers who sell from cars parked outside neighborhood weight lifting gyms.

Since steroids do not fall under the U.S. Controlled Substances Act, the federal government cannot impose quotas on their production. However, in an attempt to reduce their availability, the U.S. Food and Drug Administration (FDA) has limited the number of different steroids approved for medical application. Still, whether the substances are banned or not, athletes and abusing youngsters seem to be able to get their hands on what they want.

Controlling Sales

Arrests for selling black market anabolic steroids are on the rise in the United States, thanks to the combined efforts of four federal agencies—the Department of Justice, FBI, Customs Service, and FDA. The FDA has also undertaken an education campaign aimed primarily at high school and college students.

Some state legislatures have passed bills that put anabolic steroids on controlled substances lists or otherwise increase penalties for their illicit distribution. Both the print and broadcast media have raised interest and consciousness with expanded reporting of the problem. Responsible members of the athletic community, in high schools and elsewhere, are also conveying the message that steroids have no place in sports competition.

Despite government efforts to control the availability of anabolic steroids, athletes and abusing youngsters seem to be able to get all they want.

However, in the face of unethical coaches and others who continue to push the use of anabolic steroids, it is the youngsters themselves who must be convinced of how harmful the drugs really can be and how important it is to respect and take good care of their bodies. □

INCONTINENCE
A Treatable Problem

Paul Russo, M.D.

Urinary incontinence is the involuntary loss of urine severe enough to create social or personal hygiene problems. It is not itself a disease, but rather a symptom of an underlying disorder, and it can have many causes. Although incontinence is most common among older individuals, it can occur in people of all ages.

A Common Problem

It is estimated that as many as 30 percent of Americans over the age of 65 and living at home suffer from incontinence. As many as 50 percent of patients living in nursing homes are affected. However, incontinence should not be considered a normal part of the aging process. With precise diagnosis and proper treatment, most cases of urinary incontinence can be cured or markedly improved.

For many years, people often suffered in silence, too embarrassed to seek medical attention. Over the past decade, however, patients have become more inclined to report the problem to their doctors, and the medical profession is increasingly able to help.

Urinary Control

To comprehend urinary incontinence, it is necessary to understand the mechanisms of urine storage and elimination. Urine is produced when waste products in the blood are filtered out by the kidneys. The urine is transported from the kidneys, via the ureters, to the urinary bladder, where it is stored until it is passed out of the body through the urethra.

When a sufficient amount of urine has collected—in the average adult about 10 to 14 ounces—the desire to urinate is felt. Until an appropriate place to urinate is reached, the muscles that surround the urethra, called the sphincter, remain contracted and do not allow the urine to escape the bladder. When an individual strains or exercises to the point where pressure within the abdomen is raised, that pressure is transmitted to the area of the sphincter and serves to assist it in maintaining continence.

When it is the proper time to urinate, the brain sends nerve signals to the bladder to contract its muscular wall and to the sphincter to relax. The bladder then empties.

The Urinary System

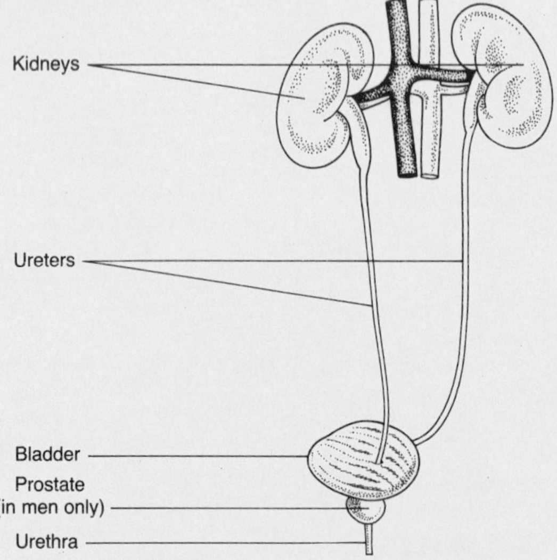

Types of Incontinence

Any disease or physical condition that allows the pressure inside the bladder to exceed the ability of the sphincter to withstand that pressure can lead to incontinence. The most commonly encountered forms of incontinence in adults are called stress incontinence, urge incontinence, and overflow incontinence.

Stress Incontinence. This occurs when a person leaks urine during activities such as coughing, lifting, or laughing. Stress incontinence is most common in women who have delivered several children and have developed weakened pelvic floor muscles, allowing the sphincter to fall out of the abdominal cavity and sag against the vagina. Then, when exertion causes the intra-abdominal pressure to increase, the pressure can no longer be transmitted to the area of the sphincter. Instead, the pressure within the bladder increases beyond what the sphincter muscles can control, and urine leaks. The mainstay of treatment for this type of stress incontinence is surgery to resuspend the urethra inside the abdominal cavity. These operations are more than

90 percent effective in correcting stress incontinence in women.

Stress incontinence can also occur following injury to the sphincter muscles as a result of pelvic trauma or pelvic surgery, such as removal of the prostate gland in a man. In these cases, the damaged sphincter does not have the power to hold the urine in the bladder. Special exercises, popularized by Dr. Arnold Kegel in the 1940s, can increase the muscle mass of the sphincter and gradually improve or completely restore urinary continence. (The exercises consist of contracting the muscle that controls the opening and closing of the urethral opening.) Minor degrees of stress incontinence can be managed by wearing protective pads and by urinating frequently. In certain severe cases, an artificial, inflatable sphincter device can be surgically placed to restore continence.

Urge Incontinence. In this form of incontinence the individual, when sensing the urge to void, is unable to keep from urinating long enough to get to the toilet. Special diagnostic studies called urodynamics have demonstrated that urge incontinence often happens as a result of uncontrollable contractions of the bladder muscle. A variety of disorders can cause these contractions, including bladder infections, stones, or tumors. A urine culture or cystoscopy can usually identify the source of the problem. (In cystoscopy a telescope-like instrument, or cystoscope, inserted through the urethra, enables the physician to look inside the bladder.) Treatment may include the use of antibiotics to combat an infection or the removal of a bladder tumor or stone (done through the cystoscope).

Diseases that affect the central nervous system, such as stroke, senile dementia, or multiple sclerosis, can disrupt coordination between the brain and the nerves that transmit and receive signals from the bladder. In these conditions, signals that the bladder is full may go unrecognized, or signals for the bladder to empty may occur inappropriately.

In some cases of urge incontinence, abnormal bladder contractions are observed by urodynamics but a cause cannot be identified. These cases are usually treated with medications called antispasmodics, which relax the bladder muscle, or with drugs called anticholinergics, which reduce the bladder contractions.

Overflow Incontinence. This occurs when the bladder muscle has lost its muscular tone, becomes enlarged and floppy, and no longer has the capacity to contract normally. As a result, the bladder is always full, leading to frequent and small-quantity urination or to constant urine loss. A common cause of overflow incontinence is the presence of an obstruction to urine outflow. In older men, such obstructions are commonly produced by diseases of the urethra or the prostate gland—an enlarged prostate can press against the urethra and impede urine flow. Surgery to eliminate the obstruction can alleviate the problem, allowing improved bladder emptying and urine flow. However, if the blockage is longstanding, bladder dysfunction may persist despite surgery.

An injury to the spinal cord or other nerves that interferes with nerve signals to and from the bladder can result in an understimulated bladder muscle, which becomes enlarged and floppy. Certain diseases, such as diabetes, that cause nerve degeneration can lead to a flaccid bladder which fills passively but cannot contract. Often the only effective treatment in such cases is the use of a catheter, a flexible tube that is briefly inserted through the urethra into the bladder every four to six hours to drain the urine.

Other Cases. Not all cases of urinary incontinence are easily classified. In some patients, especially the elderly, an infection, immobility following a hip fracture, or narcotic medications can upset the delicate physiologic balance that controls normal urinary function. With treatment of the primary problem, the incontinence usually disappears. Even seemingly simple problems, such as an elderly person's restricted mobility, may impair the ability to reach a bathroom in time. Portable commodes or assistance to and from a rest room often is the only treatment required.

Seeking Help

It is important for a person suffering from urinary incontinence to seek medical attention, both to alleviate the troublesome symptoms and to identify any underlying disease which may be causing them. The doctor will begin with questions about the duration and frequency of the incontinence, its impact on the individual's daily life, and the manner in which the patient is coping with the problem. Often, the physician will ask the patient to keep a voiding diary to more precisely describe the nature of the incontinence. In addition, the doctor will want to know about any past urologic, gynecologic, or neurologic problems, any previous operations, injuries, or illnesses, and any medications currently being taken. From this information alone, the physician frequently will be able to determine which type of incontinence the patient probably has and formulate a tentative treatment plan.

The doctor will then perform a physical exam with special emphasis on mental status, mobility and dexterity, neurologic testing, and examination of the abdominal and pelvic regions and, in a man, the prostate. Urinalysis will be performed to look for signs of infection or minute amounts of blood. Occasionally, the physician may order blood tests to assess kidney function or to rule out diabetes. If a reasonable cause for the incontinence still cannot be found, cystoscopy or urodynamics can be performed. □

Congestive Heart Failure

Michael J. Koren, M.D., and Jeffrey Fisher, M.D.

Congestive heart failure is a major health problem affecting approximately 2.5 million people and accounting for over 1 million hospitalizations annually in the United States. About 400,000 Americans are diagnosed with the condition each year. Despite new drugs and improved surgery, about 25 percent of those initially diagnosed with the condition will die within one year, and fewer than half will survive for five.

In its broadest sense, heart failure is the inability of the heart to pump blood at a rate that meets the body's metabolic needs. The term congestive heart failure refers to the condition that results when the pressures in an ailing heart are elevated, subsequently causing the blood to back up into the lungs and veins.

The onset and progression of heart failure, and the prognosis for patients, vary considerably. Although it occurs most frequently in the elderly, it can affect people of any age. It may progress so gradually it is not noticed until it has become a very serious problem, or it may strike with frightening rapidity. It is sometimes completely reversible or curable, but in most instances it is progressive and fatal. Underlying this variability is the fact that inadequate heart function has numerous causes, many of them not fully understood. In a significant number of patients, the cause of heart failure is never found.

Causes

Congestive heart failure usually, but not always, occurs when there is impaired contraction of the left ventricle, the main pumping chamber of the heart that sends out oxygen-rich blood to all parts of the body. In some medical conditions, such as hyperthyroidism, anemia, or beriberi (thiamine deficiency), heart failure may occur because of increased metabolic demands that cannot be met, despite normal or even above-normal cardiac contraction. In other conditions, heart function impairment is limited to the right ventricle, the cardiac chamber that pumps blood to the lungs for oxygenation. However, these last two causes of heart failure, termed high output heart failure and primary right heart failure, are relatively uncommon. To most physicians congestive heart failure and impaired function of the left ventricle are synonymous.

The condition may progress so gradually that it is not noticed until it has become very serious. Or it may strike with frightening rapidity.

Heart Attack. In the United States and Canada, heart attack is by far the most common cause of impaired left ventricular function. A heart attack usually occurs when a blood clot blocks a coronary artery that has been previously narrowed by atherosclerosis (hardening of the arteries), thus cutting off part of the blood supply of the heart muscle. Heart attacks destroy cardiac muscle cells, which may lead to inadequate pumping ability and thus to congestive heart failure. Heart failure can occur immediately following a heart attack, as a result of massive loss of muscle function, or over days, weeks, or months because of progressive stretching of the scar which develops at the site of the heart attack. Alternatively, a series of small heart attacks may result in a scarred, ineffective left ventricle.

Valve Disease. Disease of the heart valves can also cause heart failure. The heart valves regulate the flow of blood between the chambers of the heart, and damage to either of the valves (the mitral and the aortic) on the left side of the heart can lead to heart failure. For example, the mitral valve, which prevents blood from flowing back into the lungs, may suddenly rupture, causing acute congestive heart failure and usually necessitating surgery to repair or replace the valve. Slowly developing leaks (backflow of blood) of the mitral or aortic valve or restricted blood flow through an aortic valve that has become thickened and immobile can also lead to heart failure by overwhelming the heart's ability to pump blood efficiently.

Hypertension and Alcohol. High blood pressure (hypertension) and alcohol abuse are two other important causes of congestive heart failure. Hypertension damages the heart by forcing it to work harder over time against increased resistance. It responds by becoming enlarged and weakened. Hypertension was once a leading cause of heart failure, especially in blacks, but it is becoming a less common cause in the United States, probably because of better detection and treatment of high blood pressure.

Alcohol, in large quantities, depresses heart function by a mechanism that is not well understood. Cardiac dysfunction due to alcohol, especially in its early stages, is reversible, but only with abstinence from drinking.

Infections. Viral, parasitic, and bacterial infections are important causes of congestive heart failure. Viruses that cause heart dysfunction sometimes damage it permanently. Viral infections of the heart appear to be particularly virulent in infants and pregnant women. Many types of viruses have been associated with heart failure. Recently, viral particles have been isolated from the hearts of patients with AIDS who had heart failure.

Parasitic and bacterial infections of the heart occur more frequently in less-developed regions of the world. In South America, for example, a leading cause of cardiac failure is Chagas' disease, a parasitic disease transmitted to humans by an insect bite. Rheumatic fever, once common in the United States, is caused by streptococcal bacteria and can lead to valve disease and heart failure. This condition has become far less common in areas of the world with access to modern medicine, largely because of the widespread use of antibiotics for strep throat, a common cause of sore throat in children.

Rare Causes. The list of rare causes of heart failure is long. Some unusual causes discovered over the years include exposure to or ingestion of cobalt, a metallic element once used as a foam stabilizer in a particular brand of beer, and the venom of some insect bites. Certain medications can also lead to heart failure as a side effect, such as the anticancer drug doxorubicin (brand name, Adriamycin).

Stiff Ventricles. In recent years physicians have come to realize that not only impaired contraction but also impaired relaxation of the heart can lead to symptoms of congestive heart failure. Normally the ventricles fill with blood during a relaxation phase of the cardiac cycle called diastole. In some patients with high blood pressure, diabetes, and other conditions, the ventricles are stiffer than they should be during diastole, preventing adequate filling of the pumping chamber. The result can be congestion in the lungs caused by the backup of blood. It is important for physicians to ascertain whether congestive heart failure is due to impaired contraction or impaired relaxation since the treatments needed are quite different—enhanced contraction of the heart in one case, enhanced relaxation in the other.

Symptoms

The first symptom of congestive heart failure is usually increased breathlessness during physical activity. As the condition progresses, individuals may experience chronic coughing, accumulation of fluid in the feet and ankles, fatigue, and shortness of breath when lying down. In severe cases continual breathlessness and confusion can occur. Especially in their early stages, the symptoms may be difficult for a physician to distinguish from those of other illnesses, such as pneumonia, asthma, or blood clots in the lungs. However, a dramatic symptom highly characteristic of congestive heart failure is sudden episodes of breathlessness at night, a condition that specialists call paroxysmal nocturnal dyspnea. These episodes usually awaken sufferers and may cause them to sit bolt upright or rush to an open window seeking relief. Symptoms of heart failure progress at very different rates in different people. Life-threatening complications may develop over hours or over years.

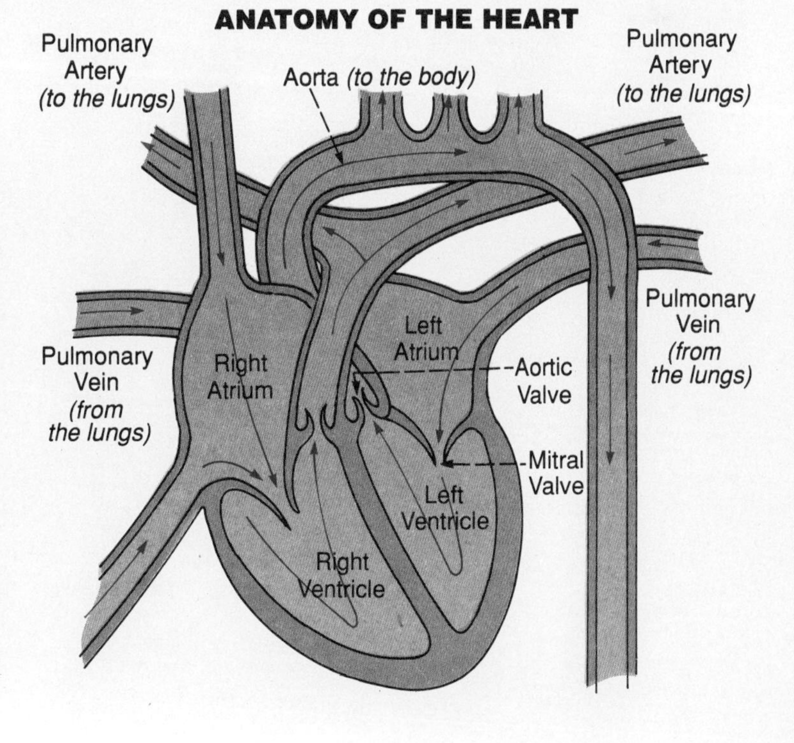

Diagnosis

Physicians usually diagnose congestive heart failure by taking a patient's medical history, conducting a physical examination, and confirming the findings with a chest X ray, echocardiogram, or nuclear scan of the heart. Upon physical examination the physician will frequently hear a crackling noise in the lungs (caused by excess fluid) and an extra heart sound. Swelling of the lower extremities and engorged veins in the neck are also characteristic findings. The chest X ray typically shows an enlarged heart and signs of abnormal accumulation of fluid in the lungs.

Echocardiography, or sound wave imaging of the heart, and scans of the heart using a radioactive isotope (harmless to the patient) are important adjuncts to the diagnosis of congestive heart failure. These techniques help in determining the severity of the problem and in establishing the cause of heart failure. Echocardiography is the best way to assess the heart valves, and nuclear scans are usually used to find out whether blockages in the coronary arteries are the source of trouble. Either technique is capable of establishing a quantitative value for the strength of the left ventricle's contraction, something called the ejection fraction, which is a measure of the proportion of blood volume in the ventricle being propelled into the body. Numerous studies have now shown that the lower the ejection fraction, the worse the prognosis.

When examining the patient, the doctor will often hear a crackling sound in the lungs along with an extra heart beat sound.

On occasion, cardiologists may perform a biopsy of the heart in order to obtain a small tissue sample for microscopic analysis. This procedure may help in the diagnosis of some unusual causes of heart failure.

Treatment

Standard medical treatment for congestive heart failure includes several classes of medications—some very old and some very new. The oldest effective medication was described over 200 years ago by the English physician Sir William Withering, who announced that a remedy called digitalis, suggested to him by an old woman in Shropshire, was useful in the management of edema, the swelling of limbs or tissues. This drug, prepared from the foxglove plant and now known as digoxin or digitoxin, causes the heart to beat with greater force. Compounds such as digitalis that enhance cardiac contraction are called positive inotropic agents. Although there are several newer intravenous positive inotropic agents for hospitalized and very ill patients, digitalis remains the standard therapy for congestive heart failure. A highly touted drug with similar properties, called milrinone, is now being studied but appears to be no more effective than digitalis.

Another way to treat heart failure is to reduce the resistance against which the heart must pump by lowering the blood pressure. A new class of medications called angiotensin-converting enzyme inhibitors, or ACE inhibitors, works in this manner and has proven to be dramatically effective in reducing symptoms of congestive heart failure and in improving the prognosis for patients with the disease. In fact, a study comparing the ACE inhibitor enalapril (brand name, Vasotec) to a placebo showed a 40 percent reduction in one-year death rates in patients taking enalapril.

Other tried and true medications are diuretics (water pills), which help remove excess fluid from the body, and nitroglycerin preparations, which reduce pressures in the heart by dilating the veins and arteries carrying blood into and out of the heart. Nondrug treatments are also important and include a low-salt diet, maintenance of ideal body weight, modest restriction of activity, and stress reduction.

In some cases, surgery is needed. If the underlying cause of heart failure is valvular disease or coronary artery obstruction, a valve replacement or repair or a coronary artery bypass operation may alleviate the symptoms. In extreme cases, transplantation of the heart may be the only effective treatment. However, the scarcity of donor hearts and the tremendous cost make heart transplantation feasible for relatively few individuals. Artificial hearts and left ventricular assist devices, which take over all or some of the work of the failing heart, have been successful in the hospital setting but have not been adequately developed for routine use at home.

The oldest treatment for congestive heart failure was suggested by a Shropshire woman to an English physician over 200 years ago.

In cases of congestive heart failure caused by insufficient relaxation of the ventricles, medications designed to slow the heart rate and help the heart muscle relax are administered. However, these drugs can aggravate heart failure attributable to impaired contraction. As a result, they are used with great care because impaired contraction and impaired relaxation often coexist. □

CIRCUMCISION
Pros and Cons

Martin L. Finkelman, M.D.

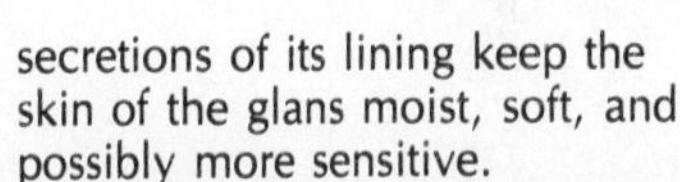

Circumcision is the surgical removal of the foreskin of the penis, usually done within a few hours or days of a boy's birth. It is the oldest known operation, having been performed since ancient times for religious or cultural reasons. In the United States it is by far the most common of all surgical procedures, most often performed because the parents believe it will help prevent future medical problems. But in recent years a number of parents and pediatricians have questioned whether routine circumcision really has substantial benefits or is unnecessary surgery that just inflicts pain on a newborn. An American Academy of Pediatrics task force appointed to study the issue reported in 1989: "Newborn circumcision has potential medical benefits and advantages, as well as disadvantages and risks." The AAP concluded that the decision on circumcision was best left to parents in consultation with individual physicians.

A Long-standing Debate

Nonritual circumcision of newborns became particularly widespread in the United States in the 19th century when improved surgical techniques made any operation less dangerous. In addition, many people at that time considered the uncircumcised penis overly erotic in appearance and thought the foreskin was an irritant that would lead to excessive masturbation.

For much of the 19th and 20th centuries, as many as 85 percent of American newborn males underwent circumcision. Among some immigrant groups circumcision was a hallmark of assimilation and enlightenment. As studies revealed possible risks of noncircumcision, such as sexually transmitted diseases and cancers of the penis and of the cervix (in partners of uncircumcised men), the medical community wholeheartedly supported the procedure.

In the 1970s, many new parents reexamined childbirth methods, returned to breast-feeding, and generally explored more "natural" ways to raise children. Routine circumcision was questioned as part of this reassessment. Consumer groups such as INTACT and NO-CIRC actively—and effectively—opposed the practice, and many pediatricians supported their efforts, maintaining that proper penile hygiene could minimize any risks. Insurance plans, which used to routinely pay for circumcision, have increasingly been refusing to cover it. It is estimated that by 1990 only 60 percent of newborn males were being circumcised in the United States.

The Operation

The foreskin, or prepuce, is a tubular fold of skin which completely covers the head of the penis (or glans penis) except for an opening for urine flow. Although in most boys the foreskin is completely retractable by three to four years of age, in infancy it is adherent to the glans, a normal condition called phimosis. The foreskin is perhaps a protective sheath in infancy, and it may also serve a function in later life. The secretions of its lining keep the skin of the glans moist, soft, and possibly more sensitive.

Material called smegma collects under the foreskin. It consists of perspiration, dead skin cells, and microorganisms such as viruses and bacteria. If the penis is not kept clean, this material becomes foul-smelling and is potentially infective, especially after the onset of puberty, and it may cause medical complications.

The foreskin is nonerectile but is supplied with nerves. Its role in sexual function is debatable.

In the United States circumcision is almost always done in the hospital, within a few hours of a boy's birth, by the obstetrician who performed the delivery. The infant is restrained on a "papoose" board with Velcro straps. After an initial incision along the length of the glans penis, the adherent foreskin is separated from the glans, perhaps the bloodiest and most painful part of the procedure. A plastic or metal bell-shaped apparatus is then placed over the head of the penis, and the foreskin is clamped and cut away.

Possible complications of circumcision are excessive bleeding, infection, and surgical mishap (all of which are risks in any operation). Complications are rare, occurring in only 0.2-0.6 percent of cases. Death from circumcision is virtually unheard of, despite reports on television talk shows by representatives of anticircumcision groups. Late complications of circumcision include meatal stenosis, or narrowing of the urethral opening. This condition can occur years after the operation but is quite uncommon. It results in painful or bloody urination and requires a surgical procedure to dilate the urethra.

Circumcision is typically performed without anesthesia. Attempts to anesthetize the penis by injection have been largely abandoned because of possible complications from the anesthesia itself. Irritability, poor feeding, excessive crying, and measurable physiological changes are common immediately following the procedure. After 24 hours visible signs of distress have disappeared. Postoperative care is relatively simple; the head of the penis is protected with vaseline and gauze until the wound has healed. Complete healing occurs in about one week. Any psychological effects on the infant can only be the subject of speculation.

Why Circumcise?

Advocates of routine circumcision of newborns say it protects against a variety of possible problems. Up to 5 percent of males not circumcised as newborns may need the operation later in life because phimosis persists. Phimosis can make it impossible to clean under the foreskin, with the attendant risk of infection, and can also lead to sexual dysfunction. Circumcision of an adult (or older child) is more complicated, requiring anesthesia and stitches, and postoperative recovery takes longer.

Several studies have been undertaken since the 1970s to determine whether circumcision offers protection against certain diseases. In formulating its 1989 recommendations, the AAP task force reviewed new evidence on a variety of topics.

Penile Cancer. Cancer of the penis is a fairly rare condition that can be fatal in up to 25 percent of cases. In the United States its estimated annual incidence is 0.7-0.9 cases per 100,000 men. It afflicts only uncircumcised men, among whom the estimated incidence is 2.2 per 100,000. In Western Europe, where circumcision is rarely practiced, the annual incidence is still low, only 0.3-1.1 new cases a year per 100,000 men. However, in areas of the world with low standards of hygiene and in tropical countries, the incidence can rise to 3-6 per 100,000. Some viruses present in smegma, but which have not been found on the penises of circumcised men, have been implicated in cancer of the penis.

The AAP report emphasized the importance of proper hygiene in preventing penile cancer in uncircumcised men. To maintain proper penile hygiene once the child's foreskin has become retractable, it should be retracted as part of the normal bathing routine, and the head of the penis should be cleaned and rinsed as would any other part of the body.

Cervical Cancer. The viruses implicated in cancer of the penis have also been found in women with cervical cancer, and some studies have reported a higher incidence of cancer of the cervix in the sexual partners of uncircumcised men in the United States. (This cancer is virtually unknown in Israel, where circumcision is essentially universal.) However, recent studies have implied that there is no greater incidence in American women whose uncircumcised partners practice optimal penile hygiene.

STDs and AIDS. Perhaps because of the moist environment of the foreskin, which may allow bacteria and viruses to survive longer, some sexually transmitted diseases (STDs)—including syphilis and genital herpes—occur more often in uncircumcised men. It has been proposed that the human immunodeficiency virus (HIV), the virus that causes AIDS, can enter the body through lesions caused by these diseases, and hence that uncircumcised men are at increased risk of HIV infection. The most important study of HIV infection rates in circumcised and uncircumcised men, carried out in Kenya, found that the rate was five to eight times higher in the uncircumcised group. However, U.S. studies did not bear out this association, and differences in sexual practices, levels of hygiene, and climate, as well as public education, have to be considered in assessing the implications of the African study for the United States. The incidence of STDs and AIDS can be drastically reduced with the use of condoms and increased attention to penile hygiene.

Urinary Tract Infections. Uncircumcised male infants may be more susceptible to urinary tract infections. A 1987 study of the records of 220,000 boys born in U.S. Army hospitals found the incidence of such infections in the first month of life to be ten times higher in the uncircumcised boys, although still only 0.24 percent. Other studies have found similar incidences. Advocates of circumcision are concerned about the risk of urinary tract infections. Opponents question the studies' methodology. The AAP report found the evidence inconclusive.

Parents Must Decide

For most parents, if religious observance is not an issue, whether to have a son circumcised is a choice to be made with the same care as other decisions on child rearing. Once performed, circumcision cannot be undone easily. If a child is not circumcised, it is important that he be instructed in penile hygiene. Ridicule of an uncircumcised boy by his peers, once a matter of concern, should not be an issue for American parents in the 1990s, since 40 percent of boys his age will also be uncircumcised. In any case, circumcision is no longer a mark of enlightenment or an indication of socioeconomic status. □

PREVENTING GUM DISEASE

Irwin D. Mandel, D.D.S.

Gum disease, the popular label for what dentists call periodontal disease, is the inflammation or degeneration of the tissues that surround and support the teeth. (Periodontal means, literally, around the teeth.) The condition can affect not just the gums, but the fibrous tissue that connects the teeth to the bony sockets in which they are housed, as well as the bone itself. Because periodontal disease usually causes little discomfort in its earlier stages, it is often ignored, but if left untreated, it can cause teeth to loosen and eventually fall out. If caught early, however, it is reversible.

Periodontal disease (which used to be known as pyorrhea) is more common in older people, and in the United States it is a major cause of tooth loss in adults. While the disease is not new, it has received more attention in recent years because of both a decline in tooth decay and the aging of the U.S. population.

Stages of the Disease

Periodontal disease most commonly begins as gingivitis, a completely reversible inflammation of the gums, or gingiva. In gingivitis the gums are red, swollen, and tender and tend to bleed easily on brushing or touching with a toothpick or dental instrument. The symptoms, however, are often mild and overlooked by the patient.

Gingivitis can remain unchanged for many years, affecting only the gums, or it can develop into a more advanced form of periodontal disease known as periodontitis, which involves loss of fibrous connective tissue and supporting bone.

Periodontitis is characterized by the formation of pockets, or spaces, between the teeth and supporting tissue or by recession of the gums. The pocket areas become infected and bleed readily, and they can cause bad breath and a bad taste in the mouth. In time, if untreated, the loss of connective tissue and then bone causes teeth to loosen and fall out.

In adults periodontitis is usually a chronic, generalized, slowly progressive disease. A small percentage of adults suffer from a rapidly progressing severe type which is very difficult to treat.

Children and adolescents are also susceptible to periodontal disease. Gingivitis, especially, is common. A very rare form of severe periodontitis can begin as soon as the baby teeth erupt into the mouth. More frequently encountered but still uncommon is localized juvenile periodontitis, a destructive disease that occurs in adolescents and that results in severe bone loss around the lower front teeth and the four first molars (those that come in behind the baby teeth at around age 6).

A Widespread Problem

The most recent information on the prevalence of periodontal disease in the United States comes from a national survey on adult dental health conducted in 1985 and early 1986 by a team of dentists trained by the National Institute of Dental Research. Working adults aged 18 to 65 and people over 65 attending senior citizens centers were given very thorough oral exams which included measurement of gingivitis and periodontitis. The determination of gingivitis was made by gently probing 28 sites in the mouth of each subject to see if bleeding occurred. In the group aged 18 to 65 bleeding was found in 43 percent of those examined; in the over-65 group it was found in 47 percent.

Periodontitis was evaluated by the use of a special probe that measured "loss of attachment," or the amount of gum, connective tissue, and bone that had been lost to disease over the years. In general, the prevalence of periodontal loss was high: 77 percent of the working adults and 95 percent of the seniors had at least one site with loss of attachment. But the actual amount of supporting tissue lost was modest; the depth of periodontal pockets averaged about 2 millimeters in the employed adults and 3.2 in the over-65 group. More severe destruction (4 millimeters or greater) was noted in 24 percent of the below-65 group and 68 percent of the senior group.

When compared with surveys done in the 1960s and 1970s, this national study indicated an improvement in the periodontal health of the adult population. Rates of both gingivitis and advanced periodontitis were lower. Only 8 to 10 percent of the people surveyed in the 1980s had very advanced disease. However, many population groups, such as the unemployed, homemakers, and institutionalized patients, were not included in the survey, and the state of their dental health is not known.

The Cause of Gum Disease

Periodontal disease is caused by certain species of bacteria (a small percentage of the more than 300 species the mouth is host to). The bacteria that produce gum disease form what is called bacterial plaque, gel-like mats made up of millions of microorganisms that closely adhere to tooth surfaces. Other bacterial communities are involved in tooth decay, but the plaque associated with periodontal disease is concentrated, initially, along the gum line.

The periodontally related bacteria produce within the plaque a variety of destructive agents such as toxins, irritating chemicals, and enzymes that break down the normal structure of the tissues that support the teeth. These products and the alterations they cause in the tissues produce inflammation, which leads to still further tissue destruction.

Although the early disease is confined to the gums, in time the bacteria begin to grow along the root surfaces that become exposed as the gums separate from the teeth or recede. The bacteria then start to detach and destroy the fibrous connective tissue. The resultant periodontal pocket between teeth and supporting tissue below the gum line provides optimal conditions for further growth of the bacterial plaque. The environment here also promotes the hardening, or mineralization, of the plaque to form tartar, also known as calculus. The tartar, which is covered by a layer of unmineralized plaque, acts as an accelerating factor in the progression of the disease. The eventual result can be destruction of the teeth's bony support.

Careful clinical studies over the past few years have shown that in the most common form of periodontitis in adults, the disease does not progress in a gradual, uniform manner. On the contrary, there are long periods during which there is no progression and then sudden bursts of activity. In some instances there may also be periods of repair, in which the body replaces destroyed tissue. Researchers are currently working to develop simple office procedures that will identify the times of active disease, so that proper treatment can be given when it is needed most.

THE STAGES OF GUM DISEASE

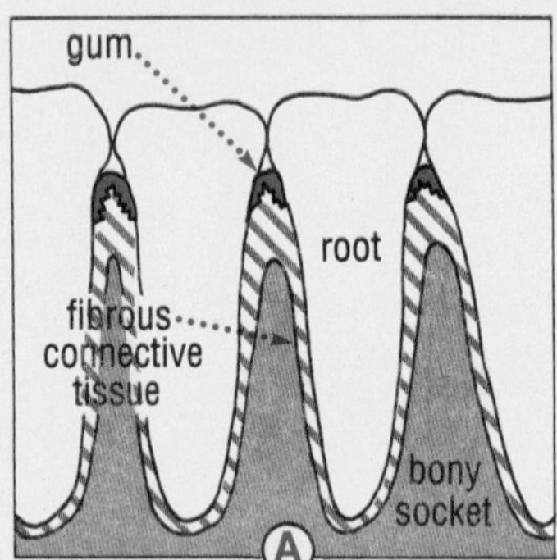

When gums are healthy they fit snugly around the teeth.

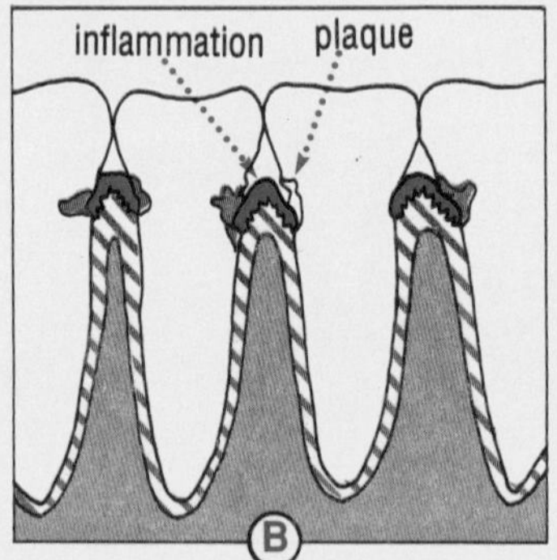

As plaque builds up, gingivitis develops—the gums become inflamed and begin to detach from the teeth.

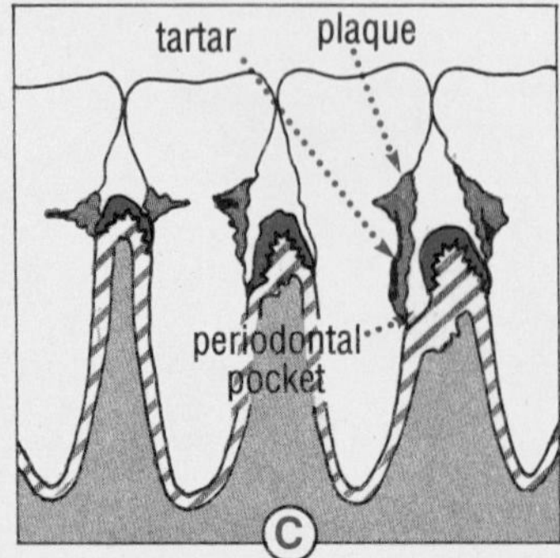

With the formation of peridontal pockets, periodontitis develops, and plaque and tartar begin destroying fibrous connective tissue and bone.

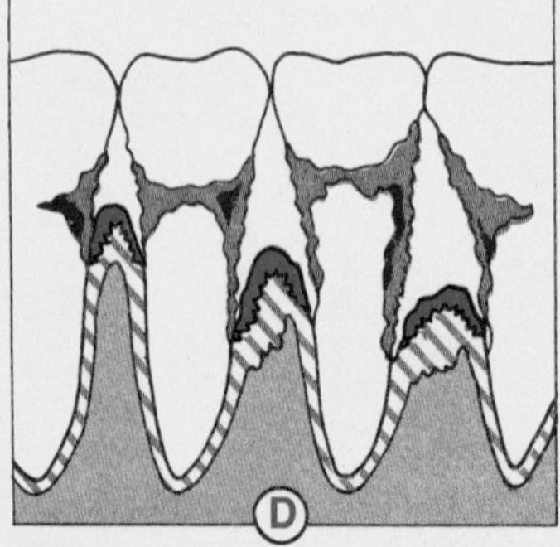

Eventually, if enough supporting tissue and bone are destroyed, teeth may loosen and fall out.

Contributing Factors

People vary in their susceptibility to periodontal disease. Some people, about 10 percent of the U.S. population, go through life with virtually no disease, while others can have rapid breakdown at a relatively young age of the tissues supporting the teeth. Why some people are resistant and others are not is unknown, but several factors seem to contribute to more rapid progression of the disease (or to a slower response to treatment). These factors include smoking and the use of chewing tobacco; systemic diseases such as diabetes; pregnancy and the use of oral contraceptives, both of which increase the hormone levels in the gum tissue and thus make them more sensitive to the effects of plaque bacteria; and various medications, including steroids, some of the drugs used in the treatment of epilepsy, and drugs used to combat cancer.

When the diet is grossly inadequate—especially in cases of extreme vitamin deficiency or protein malnutrition—tissue resistance in general is compromised and susceptibility to periodontal disease increases. For people with an adequate diet, however, there is no evidence that vitamin, mineral, or special supplements offer extra benefits.

Anything that increases plaque retention and makes plaque removal more difficult will complicate periodontal disease. Overhanging fillings, for example, can create areas in which plaque can accumulate, and some rear molars may be nearly impossible to keep clean. Also, if some teeth are missing, there may be spaces in which food particles accumulate, irritating the gum and aggravating gum disease.

Problems such as badly aligned teeth, malocclusion (an abnormal bite), or badly fitting bridges can cause excessive biting forces during chewing and aggravate periodontal disease. They do not cause disease, but they can make things worse.

Heredity plays a role in adult periodontal disease, although the genes involved have not been identified and how they increase susceptibility is not known. Recent studies have shown that identical twins exhibit much greater similarity in the various clinical measures of periodontal disease than fraternal twins. Localized juvenile periodontitis often affects multiple members of a family, especially females.

Prevention

The most effective way to prevent gingivitis and periodontitis is regular, thorough oral hygiene. This means brushing twice a day, preferably with a multi-tufted, soft-bristle brush, and using dental floss daily to remove plaque from between the teeth, areas not reached by conventional toothbrushes. A dentist or dental hygienist can provide instruction on how best to brush and floss.

Some of the new high-tech brushes—such as Interplak, an electric device with rotating tufts of bristles—are more effective between the teeth than hand brushing, but they are not superior to flossing. There are also a variety of supplementary aids for cleaning between the teeth and around bridges and other hard-to-reach areas. These include special brushes small enough to fit between some teeth and a number of variations on toothpicks. Water irrigating devices can also be of benefit when used appropriately.

The American Dental Association recognizes several mouthrinses as effective in preventing and reducing plaque and gingivitis when used twice daily in addition to brushing and flossing. One of them, Peridex, is available only by prescription. The others, such as Listerine, are over-the-counter products and can be recognized by the ADA seal of acceptance on the bottle.

Even with good oral hygiene, professional tooth cleaning at regular intervals, which can be done by a dentist or dental hygienist, is necessary to remove plaque remnants and tartar that brushing cannot dislodge. Antitartar toothpastes and rinses are only partially effective and work only against tartar on the tooth surface above the gums; they have no effect on deposits on the root surfaces below the gums.

Treatment

Some general dentists treat periodontal diseases themselves, while others refer patients to a periodontist, a specialist in the diagnosis, prevention, and treatment of gum disease. The steps taken to treat periodontal disease are an extension of those used to prevent it. Treatment includes regular professional cleaning to remove all the deposits above the gum and scaling, which is a scraping below the gum line to remove plaque and tartar deposits in the pockets. The dentist or periodontist may also plane the roots, that is, scrape and smooth root surfaces to remove infected material and allow gum tissue to heal and reattach itself to the teeth. In some instances, where considerable infection is present, antibiotics may be prescribed. Special antibiotic-coated fibers designed to deliver antibiotics directly into periodontal pockets are currently being developed.

When the pockets are deep and cannot be kept clean by regular brushing and flossing or are shaped so that they cannot be adequately treated professionally, periodontal surgery is required. The goals of surgery are thorough removal of all deposits and infected material and recontouring of the gum to eliminate the pockets and allow for optimal home care. In advanced periodontal disease the bony tissue has to be recontoured before the gum tissue can be repositioned. Periodontal surgery is generally an office procedure, performed under a local anesthetic.

Experimental Treatments

Several experimental procedures are now beginning to be used to treat patients in special situations; their aim is to generate new connective tissue and even, through bone grafts, to replace bone. There is also a strong possibility of stimulating new bone formation in some sites.

The most advanced of the new procedures is guided tissue regeneration. After periodontal surgery a special membrane is placed on the root surface which promotes reattachment of the fibrous connective tissue to the root. Use of other special materials on the root surface can further aid the regenerative process (these materials are synthetic equivalents of substances normally found in the body that are involved in the natural attachment of connective tissue). Some day the combination of connective tissue and bone regeneration could actually restore the supporting tissues lost because of periodontal disease. □

The New Medical Education

Janis A. Work, Ph.D.

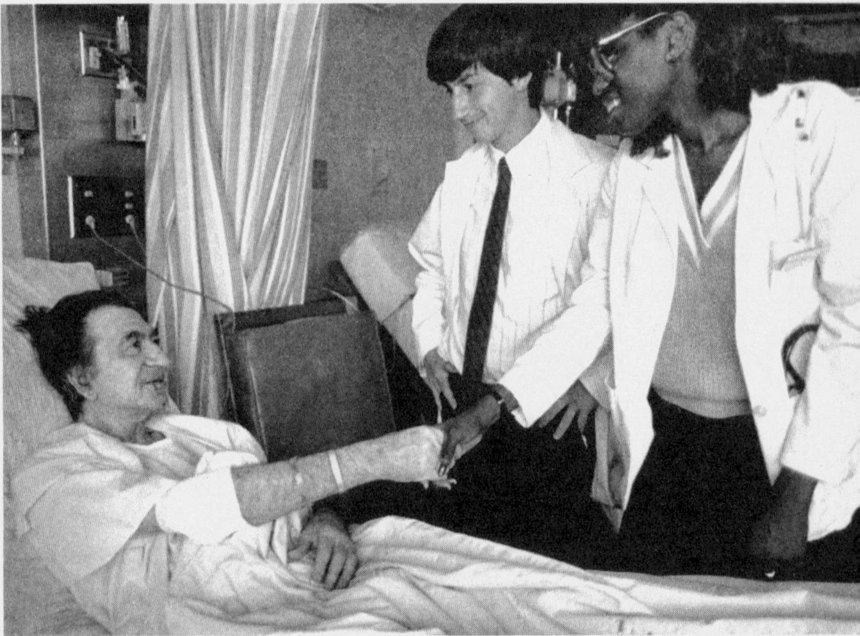

Medical students in Harvard's New Pathway curriculum bone up on their bedside manner.

STICK IT TO YA said large orange letters on the back of the T-shirt worn by the person in front of me. I was sitting in on a first-year clinical medicine lecture at the University of Minnesota, surrounded by young men and women about half my age, almost all of whom wore shorts, T-shirts, and tennis shoes.

Attire isn't the only thing that has changed since my husband attended medical school over 30 years ago; now almost half of the students are female. And the lecture topic—the medical ethics of the sexual history and examination—illustrates how much the curriculum has evolved. The speaker reported:

"A 65-year-old man from California was seen by three squads of specialists, who made the diagnosis of multiple sclerosis. MS is an astonishing diagnosis for a 65-year-old. No previous doctor had thought to ask him his sexual orientation. It turned out that he was gay and had AIDS. The whole doctor-patient relationship had been desexualized, and relevant information was missed."

The lecturer, Steven Miles, M.D., who is affiliated with the Bioethics Institute at the University of Minnesota, related this story to illustrate how the doctors' preconceived attitudes toward the patient's sexuality, or assumed lack of it, affected medical treatment.

Challenging the Tradition

What's going on here? Have the traditional basic science courses been abandoned? Are faculty members having to resort to topics like sex to attract students?

Of course not. The basic sciences are still there, but in many American medical schools they have been supplemented with medical ethics and other humanities courses or courses have been totally reorganized. A number of schools are responding to what they see as public demand for a physician who is more caring, more in tune with the patient.

In a traditional curriculum medical students may spend up to seven hours a day in lectures the first two years, studying basic sciences, followed by two years of clinical medicine. Students usually have little patient contact in the first two years. In recent years this tradition has been challenged. Among other things, medical educators say that students should be enjoying their educational experience rather than being turned off by the traditional curriculum and should be having patient contact earlier. Memorizing everything is no longer an option—there is too much material and not enough time. Students need to learn to think about problems in new ways, not just depend on memorized facts.

Problem Solving

A few years ago, Harvard Medical School instituted a curriculum called the New Pathway. The human aspect was one of the reasons for establishing this type of program. Students begin interacting with patients in their first year. They spend less time in lectures but a great deal of time studying on their own. They participate in small group tutorials with a faculty facilitator, using a problem-solving approach to analyze carefully selected cases that tie into other facets of the curriculum. Not only the medical aspects of the problem are discussed but also the social and psychological. Students study the problem for several days, pursuing independent research in anatomy, histology, and other relevant areas.

Over 20 years ago the University of New Mexico started a somewhat similar case-based tutorial program, the Primary Care Curriculum (PCC), for a limited number of first-year and second-year students. According to one PCC student, "What's really important to me is the feeling I get from figuring something out. When I would sit in lectures in college, there would never be any thrill of discovery for me. The scientists had experienced all that excitement 20 years before, and now I was just memorizing their findings. But in the PCC the student makes the discoveries and says, 'Look what I figured out'!" First-year students also spend four months off campus in rural settings under the guidance of physician preceptors, learning from real patients.

Northwestern University Medical School recently incorporated formal instruction in the medical humanities into the existing curriculum. "We have a lot of physicians—clinicians—who teach medical humanities, and this has a wonderful effect on students," says Kathryn Montgomery Hunter, Ph.D., associate professor of medicine and codirector of Northwestern's Ethics and Human Values Program. "The actual techniques of bedside manners, such as interviewing, are taught by physicians [including psychiatrists] and psychologists." In the medical humanities, she continues, "We take a larger view. We teach the general ethical principles that students can later apply to actual cases."

Other schools have experimented with innovative ways of using the humanities. Third-year medical students at Virginia Commonwealth University's Medical College of Virginia were asked to draw on their own experiences to prepare a case study involving ethical issues; some of the studies were used for discussion during student-faculty workshops. Internal medicine residents at Oregon Health Sciences University learn, through role playing, how to interact with families after a patient's death. Students at Columbia University's College of Physicians and Surgeons have learned about doctor-patient relationships and the patient's perspective through literature and writing courses.

Medical schools also teach doctor-patient relationships by means of large-group lectures, interactive video programs, simulations, and audiovisual aids. Some schools use professional simulators—people who are paid to memorize a case history and act as a patient. Most students, however, probably still learn their "bedside manner" from that the old standby, the doctor role model.

Role Models

Morris Davidman, M.D., winner of the 1990 Outstanding Medical Teacher Award at the University of Minnesota Medical School, is an excellent example of a role model. I joined his Clinical Medicine tutorial on the afternoon his four students performed their first physical examinations—on each other. Davidman says, "These students don't have the content yet—we teach human skills. This is where we begin patient contact, at the end of the first year. These students are so young in their careers and the subject matter so fundamental that many faculty don't enjoy this part of it." But Davidman obviously does.

The two women students, Monica Myklebust and Sue Barden Johnson, are a bit older than the average first-year student, having worked for several years before entering medical school, but both still show discomfort with their new role. "This is a nerve-wracking experience, thinking you're going to have to know all this stuff at some point," says Monica, the examiner.

Davidman suggests, "Plan your exam so there is a minimum of lying down and sitting up. We don't want a jack-in-the-box routine." He continually offers advice and reinforcement. "Great. Get the patient used to your hands. Ask the patient to point her toes toward her nose instead of asking her to flex her foot."

When asked how students learn the techniques and etiquette of physical examination, Monica replies, "We have lectures, videos, books, but we actually learn it from Dr. Davidman, from his demonstrations."

"Some schools don't do as much role modeling of the doctor-patient relationship," says Ilene Harris, Ph.D., associate professor medical education at the University of Minnesota. "We have it taught by family practitioners and internists. Other schools may not feel that this is a good use of the faculty, but we feel they make good role models."

A Better Doctor?

Is the new curriculum making better doctors? It's probably too early to tell—and maybe not even an answerable question. A better doctor means different things to different people. Dr. Miles of the University of Minnesota says that studies show middle-class patients want their autonomy respected, a peer relationship with their physician, informed consent—and don't want their doctor to interrupt them. Little work has been done on what minority or poor patients want, aside from access to medical care. Gay patients are unhappy with the amount of homophobia they may encounter in the doctor-patient relationship. Dying patients tend to feel that chronic pain is not taken seriously enough by their doctors.

But if the goal is to produce young caregivers who, as Montgomery Hunter explains it, are knowledgeable in their field and can apply that knowledge to patients' needs, who are interested enough in the human condition that they are not discouraged by death or defeat, and who go on learning throughout life, then today's medical schools may be on the right track. □

CHRONIC FATIGUE SYNDROME

James F. Jones, M.D.

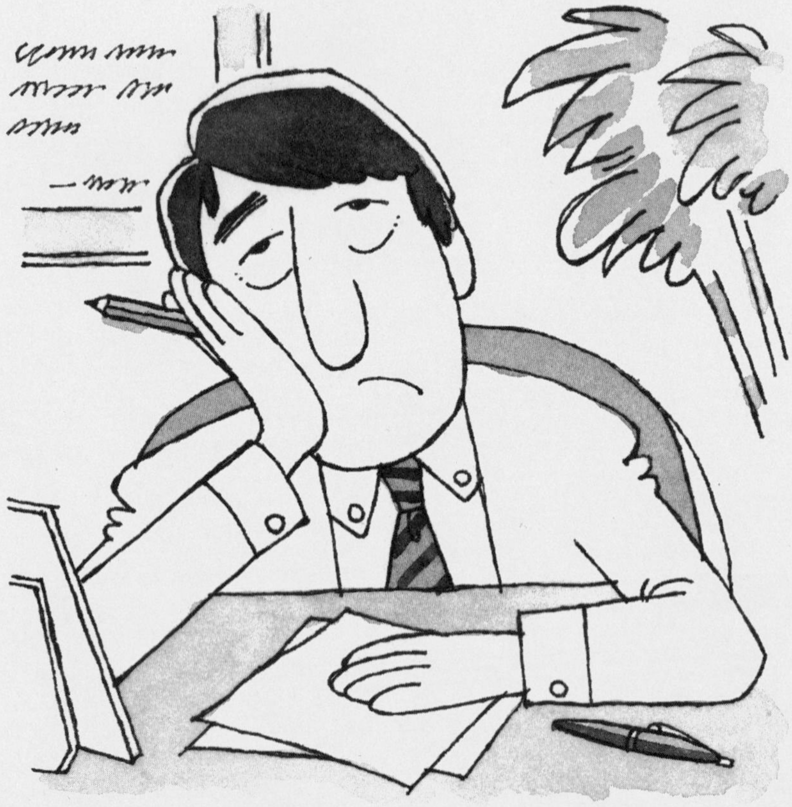

Chronic fatigue syndrome (CFS) has been described in the medical literature for at least a hundred years, and perhaps for as long as five hundred, but it remains poorly understood. Its myriad symptoms range from persistent fatigue severe enough to interfere with daily activities to muscle aches and depression. There are no laboratory tests that identify the syndrome, and it was long considered to be primarily a psychiatric complaint. But attitudes toward CFS have begun to change in recent years, and today more and more physicians recognize it as a physical disorder. Whether it is a unique illness with a single cause has not yet been determined.

Defining CFS

A hundred years ago what was probably CFS was diagnosed as neurasthenia, literally, sluggish nerves. In this century, many illnesses labeled as headache-tension fatigue syndrome, environmental allergy, hypoglycemia, myalgic encephalomyelitis, fibromyalgia, postviral fatigue syndrome, and somatization disorder (a form of depression) were probably really cases of CFS. None of these illnesses can be diagnosed with available laboratory tests, and all have common, often vague, symptoms.

The different names probably arose from the different viewpoints of the specialists seeing the patients. Rheumatologists might base their diagnosis on muscle pain and call the illness fibromyalgia, while psychiatrists might concentrate on the psychological effects and consider it somatization disorder. Because CFS affects so many systems in the body, patients today continue to seek help from a wide variety of specialists, from internists and allergists to infectious disease specialists.

In 1988 the U.S. Centers for Disease Control sponsored a working definition of CFS in an attempt to standardize the diagnosis. Diagnosis according to the CDC definition is based on fulfillment of two major criteria and one of two sets of minor criteria. The major criteria are: (1) the new onset of debilitating fatigue in a person with no history of similar symptoms such that the patient's activity level is diminished by 50 percent during a period of at least six months and (2) the exclusion of other conditions capable of producing the same symptoms. The two sets of minor criteria consist of either 6 of 11 symptoms and 2 of 3 physical criteria, or 8 of 11 symptoms. The symptom list includes mild fever, sore throat, painful neck or armpit

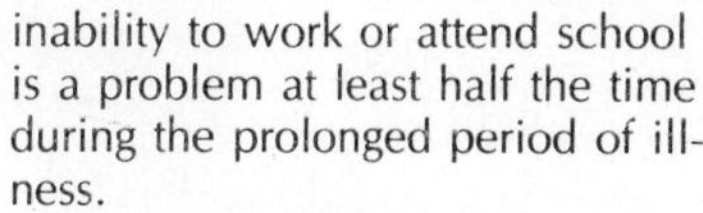

It has not yet been determined whether chronic fatigue syndrome is a unique illness with a single cause.

lymph nodes, muscle weakness, muscle pains, fatigue lasting more than 24 hours after activity, headache, joint pains, difficulty concentrating, sleep disturbance, and abrupt development of the symptoms over a few hours or days. The physical criteria include an oral temperature between 99.7°F and 101.5°F, an inflamed throat, and easily detectable or tender lymph nodes.

Labeling the syndrome as a distinct illness has been criticized on the grounds that the symptoms described by patients are nonspecific. But the same can be said for many illnesses. The human body has a limited means of initial responses to injury, particularly when the immune system is involved, as in the case of infection. The immune system's reaction produces a similar set of symptoms for any acute infection, regardless of its cause. Since the same symptoms are seen in chronic fatigue syndrome as in acute infections, although in different distribution and perhaps intensity, it is logical to consider that they are produced by the same immune mechanism, but it cannot be assumed that the same infectious agents are to blame.

CFS and Psychiatry

Historically, medical schools have taught that if no biological basis can be found for a person's symptoms, a psychological disorder must be considered. It is not surprising, then, that CFS, with no definitive laboratory test to identify it, has been at times labeled a psychiatric problem. In addition, some studies have suggested that unrecognized psychiatric conditions were present in patients with CFS before the onset of the syndrome. But these studies assumed that symptoms such as fatigue, weight gain or loss, trouble concentrating, and difficulty sleeping were caused by psychiatric disorders. Readers need only remember their last episode of the flu to recognize that these symptoms are not limited to psychiatric disease alone. Some patients complaining of chronic fatigue are still referred to mental health professionals, but today most psychiatrists readily recognize CFS patients as being different from the bulk of their psychiatric cases.

Searching for a Cause

Epstein-Barr Virus. At one time researchers believed that CFS patients were suffering from a chronic form of mononucleosis or from chronic active Epstein-Barr virus (EBV) infection. (The Epstein-Barr virus is a type of herpesvirus and causes a number of infections, including mononucleosis.) Mononucleosis has many of the same symptoms as CFS, including fatigue, fever, sore throat, lymph node swelling, muscle aches, joint aches, headaches, trouble concentrating, and difficulty sleeping. However, mononucleosis is usually an acute illness—the symptoms peak after a few days and reverse slowly over a few days or weeks. CFS patients experience symptoms for at least six months. In acute illness, the loss of time from work or school is usually limited to the duration of active symptoms, if time is lost at all. In CFS, the inability to work or attend school is a problem at least half the time during the prolonged period of illness.

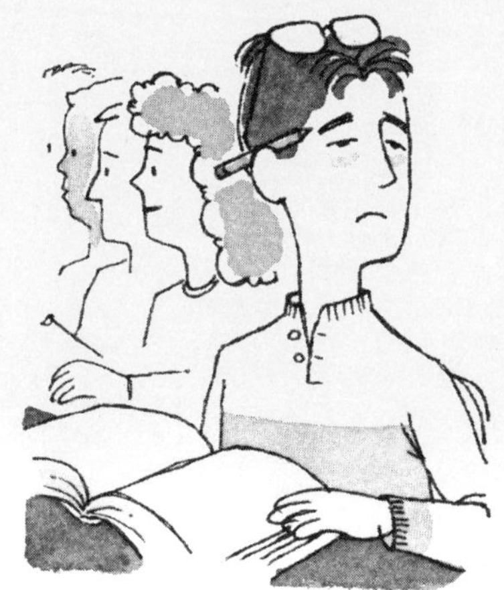

The medical literature has discussed the possibility of long-term illness due to EBV ever since the virus was discovered to cause mononucleosis in the late 1960s. Unlike most other viruses, EBV and its five cousins within the herpesvirus family—cytomegalovirus, herpes simplex 1 and 2, varicella-zoster virus, and human herpesvirus-6—remain in the body in a latent state once the original infection is contained. The latent viruses may be reactivated and produce disease symptoms: for example, herpes simplex 1 may reactivate as fever blisters, while the varicella-zoster virus (the cause of chicken pox) can reactivate in the form of shingles. One reason EBV was thought to be the origin of chronic fatigue syndrome was that high levels of antibodies against certain parts of EBV were found in patients with the syndrome. Healthy subjects did not have such levels of anti-EBV antibodies. However, 90 percent of Americans over 30 have some antibodies to EBV, and if levels are measured only once, it is impossible to determine if they are high or normal for the patient in question. In addition, differences among laboratories that perform the test are such that a "high" value in one laboratory may be "normal" in another.

For now the recommendation in the Centers for Disease Control definition is for physicians to exclude specific infectious agents before reaching a diagnosis of chronic fatigue syndrome. However, researchers continue to ask many questions about possible roles not only for EBV but also for human herpesvirus-6 and other viruses. The current state of these studies does not allow the pinpointing of a specific infectious agent as the cause of all cases. But some researchers hypothesize that a single, as yet unknown agent may be responsible.

Nonspecific Agents. Because, according to the working definition of CFS, the syndrome begins abruptly (and because it usually follows an apparent infectious illness), some investigators now think that mediators of inflammation—products of cells involved in the body's immune response to foreign organisms—may be ultimately responsible for the illness. According to this theory, no single infectious agent is to blame, but many such microorganisms can

Some researchers believe that an overreaction or a mistaken reaction of the immune system may play an important part in the disorder.

trigger the disease in people predisposed to developing it. This predisposition is probably caused by an unusually active immune system. Some researchers theorize that the overreaction of the immune system that produces allergic reactions (to ragweed, dust, and so on) also produces a continuing response to microorganisms that cause acute illnesses. In most studies that have examined the link between allergies and CFS, up to 80 percent of CFS sufferers have had preexisting allergies.

Another possibility is that the infectious agents remain in the body and continue to aggravate the immune system, thus causing illness. Still another possibility is that the body rids itself of the infecting agent, but because the microorganism resembles normal cells, the immune system mistakes "self" for "other" and continues to attack what it thinks is foreign. This type of mixed-up identification is called an autoimmune reaction.

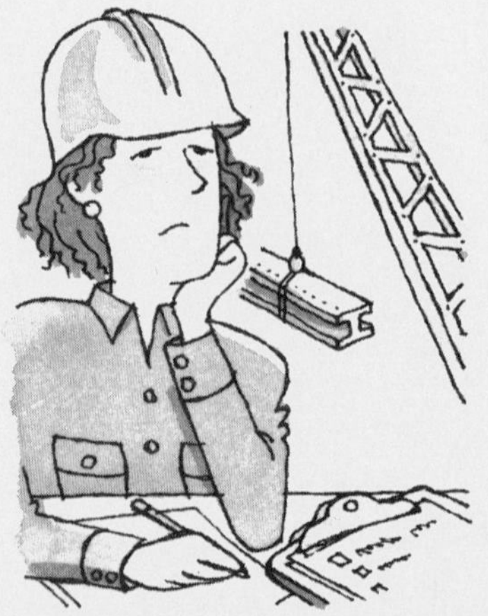

Course of the Illness

The intensity of the illness varies over time and from person to person. Usually, however, throughout the illness patients feel less well than is normal for them. By and large the illness does not progress rapidly, nor is it fatal. Some patients feel so ill they have to stop going to work or school altogether, while others are able to continue part-time. There is no way to predict in any patient when or if the symptoms will decrease or increase. The persistent symptoms, however, prevent patients from doing what they need and want to do, a situation that can be devastating, personally, socially, and financially.

Treatment

Although many patients recover spontaneously, there is no known cure for CFS. There is not even a proven way of alleviating a patient's fatigue. Treatment can improve CFS victims' quality of life. Treatment includes counseling, regular exercise, and medications to relieve physical symptoms. Other diseases must also be ruled out. Every patient need not undergo an expensive laboratory evaluation to exclude all known diseases, however. A patient evaluation should be directed at the complaints that are interfering the most with that patient's daily life.

Information about the illness can help many patients come to terms with having a chronic disorder. Most patients are frustrated because they can't do what they know they are capable of doing. Learning how to reorder priorities, accepting assistance, using notepads or tape recorders to keep track of daily routines, resting before and after scheduled activities, and never exercising or working to the point of tiredness are ways for patients to improve their state of well-being.

Treatment for chronic fatigue syndrome includes counseling, regular exercise, and medications to relieve physical symptoms.

Some patients have reported that taking certain medications or food supplements or following particular diets has made them feel better, but these claims are anecdotal and have not been tested in carefully controlled scientific studies. Antiviral drugs have been used but have not been helpful. Medications that *are* useful include those that increase the effectiveness of sleep, relieve aches and pains, and lessen anxiety or depression. □

Sources of Further Information

In the United States there are three national organizations that offer patient support and education and information about local support groups.

Chronic Fatigue Syndrome Society, P.O. Box 230108, Portland, OR 97223. Tel.: 503-684-5261.

National Chronic Fatigue Syndrome Association, 3521 Broadway, Suite 222, Kansas City, MO 64111. Tel.: 816-931-4777.

Chronic Fatigue and Immune Dysfunction Syndrome Association, P.O. Box 220398, Charlotte, N.C. 28222-0398. Tel.: 704-362-2343.

TUBERCULOSIS

Michael D. Iseman, M.D.

Labeled the "Captain of all these Men of Death" by John Bunyan in 1680, tuberculosis, or TB, has been found on all continents and in all civilizations throughout history. It afflicted the early Egyptians, ancient Andean tribes in South America, and early Indian tribes of North America.

While always present to some degree, the disease has at times caused prolonged epidemics, some stretching over many centuries. Europe and North America are at the end of a 300-400 year epidemic cycle which at its peak resulted in the deaths of 10 to 15 percent of the population. Due presumably to the acquisition of herd immunity (group resistance to an infection), to incidental improvements in living conditions in terms of crowding, hygiene, and nutrition, and to deliberate human intervention (including isolation of infectious cases and the development of effective drug therapy), the incidence of the disease waned steadily in these regions over the past 100 years.

By contrast, tuberculosis is epidemic now in most of Africa and Asia, with attack rates in some populations 100 times higher than rates in the United States or Europe. However, beginning in 1986, public health officials became aware of a distinct resurgence of tuberculosis in the United States, particularly in the nation's inner cities.

In general, the epidemic cycles of tuberculosis have resulted from the introduction of the infecting organism into a population that is relatively more vulnerable because of genetically determined aspects of immunity as well as aggravating environmental factors, such as poor housing and overcrowding, malnutrition, and poor sanitation. Unlike the influenza virus, which can cause recurring global epidemics by means of viral mutations that circumvent previously acquired immunity, the tuberculosis microorganism does not appear to have undergone significant biological modifications to promote its prevalence.

However, the appearance of the AIDS epidemic threatens to have a massive impact on the prevalence of tuberculosis throughout the world. The reasons for the potentially disastrous interaction of these two diseases are discussed below.

Masked to prevent the spread of infection, a man ill with both TB and AIDS confers with doctors.

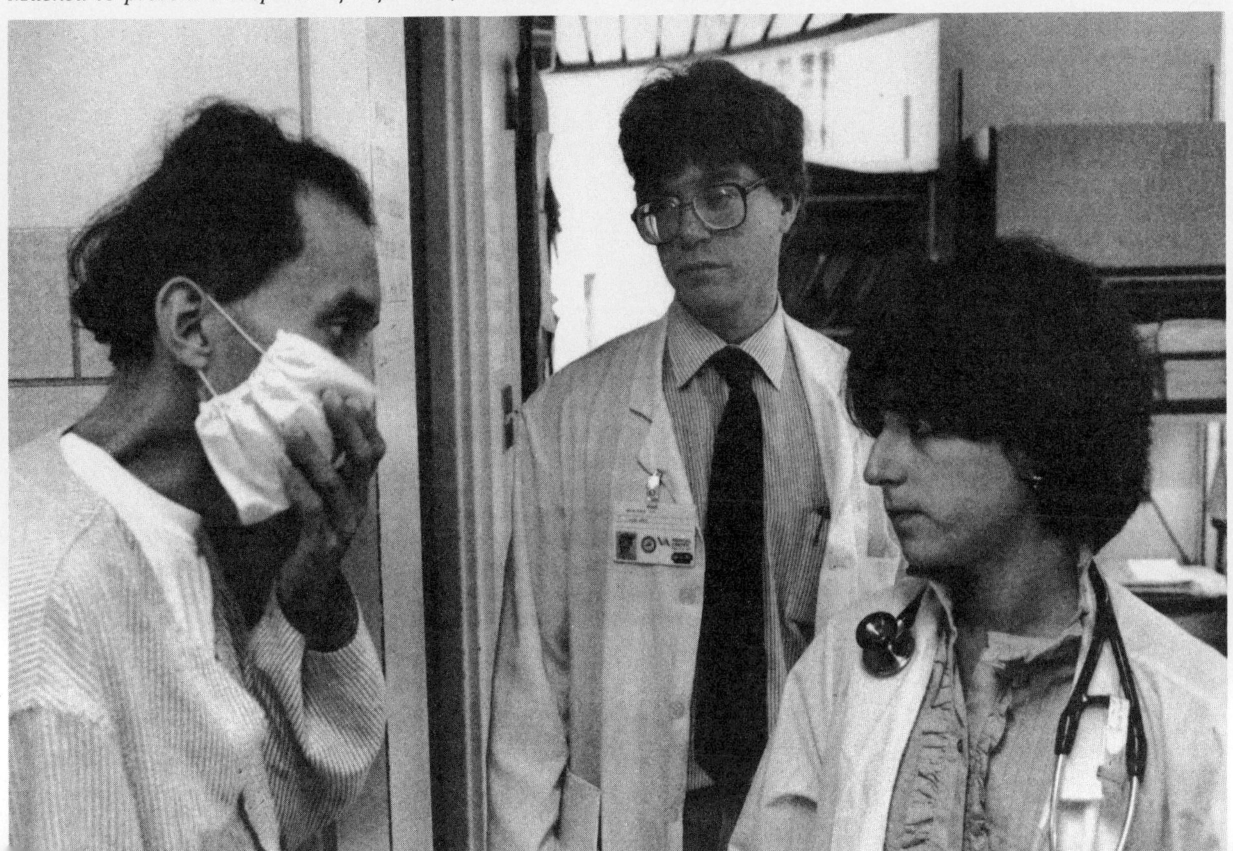

The Germ

Tuberculosis is a chronic wasting disease that primarily attacks the lungs, although it can also affect other parts of the body. It can be fatal if not treated. Tuberculosis is caused by a type of bacterium (a bacillus) that belongs to a highly unusual family of microbes, the mycobacteria. The cell walls of mycobacteria are substantially different from those of most other disease-causing bacteria, such as staphylococci or streptococci. Instead of being composed largely of carbohydrates and proteins, mycobacterial cell walls are composed largely of lipids, or waxes. And in contrast to most bacteria, which multiply under suitable circumstances in as little as 12 to 20 minutes, *Mycobacterium tuberculosis* requires roughly 24 hours to replicate. These basic attributes play prominent roles in the transmission and course of the disease.

The chemical structure of the cell walls of *M. tuberculosis* means that the body's usual mechanisms of defense against bacterial infections—antibodies and polymorphonuclear leukocytes, the type of white blood cells that fight off acute infectious agents—are largely ineffective. The barrier provided by its cell wall also makes the tubercle bacillus resistant to most standard antibiotics.

In most cases TB attacks the lungs, although sometimes it affects other parts of the body, including the bones and kidneys.

The slow replication rate means that there is a substantial incubation time between the primary infection and the manifestations of illness—a few months at minimum and commonly many years. Further complicating the control of tuberculosis is the extraordinarily long period required for a cure: 6 to 18 months of continuous medication. This is due both to the relative resistance of *M. tuberculosis* to standard antibiotics and to its indolent metabolism and replication rate. (Bacteria are most vulnerable to antibiotics while they multiply.)

Transmission and Immunity

Tuberculosis is spread almost exclusively by human-to-human aerosol transmission of the bacilli. A patient with pulmonary tuberculosis (tuberculosis of the lungs), the most common form of the disease, coughs the bacilli into the air to be inhaled by someone else. Unlike some of the virulent, aggressive respiratory infections that may invade the body through the lining of the upper airways, tuberculosis can take hold only if the bacilli are inhaled deep into the lungs, into the microscopic air sacs called alveoli. Once the bacilli reach the alveoli, the battle between host and parasite commences.

Even though the classic antibody defense system does not offer significant protection against tuberculosis, humans have evolved a modestly successful defense: cell-mediated immunity, in which a team of specialized cells of the immune system, macrophages and T-lymphocytes, combine to inhibit replication of the bacilli.

Macrophages (literally, "large eaters") may reasonably be compared to the figures in the electronic game Pac-Man. Macrophages patrol many of the tissues of the body, alert to the presence of foreign material, both organic and inorganic. Their response on encountering a tubercle bacillus is to engulf it. However, the macrophage by itself does not fare well in its battle with the mycobacterium. In order to exert a significant inhibitory effect on the organism's survival and replication, the macrophage requires assistance from two types of T-lymphocytes, "helper" and "killer" T-cells. Once activated by chemical interaction with these T-cells, macrophages can curtail the growth and spread of the bacilli.

In most immunologically normal people, tuberculosis never takes hold: Of 100 people infected with the bacilli, only 10 will come down with the disease during their lifetime. In the others, the bacilli will lie dormant in the lungs and other tissues, producing no symptoms. This is called latent tuberculosis. Sometimes, however, the cell-mediated immunity system fails, and the bacilli multiply and spread throughout the body. They lodge in a variety of organs and ultimately may cause progressive infection and destruction of vital tissues. Although the great preponderance of tuberculosis cases involve the lungs, 5 to 20 percent of cases involve other parts of the body, such as the lymph nodes, kidneys, bones, or central nervous system. Among AIDS patients the percentage of cases in which organs or tissues outside the lungs are affected is much higher, ranging up to 65 percent.

Specialized cells of the immune system in most people are able to curtail the growth and spread of the tubercle bacilli.

AIDS and Tuberculosis

Unfortunately, the human immunodeficiency virus (HIV), the virus that causes AIDS, destroys "helper" T-cells. Thus, patients with HIV infection are rendered incapable of mounting or sustaining an effective defense against tuberculosis (and many other infections against which the major defense is cell-mediated immunity). Most cases of tuberculosis seen among HIV-infected individuals represent reactivation of a latent tuberculosis infection which antedated the HIV infection, often by decades.

Tragically, the epidemiological patterns of HIV and tuberculosis infections demonstrate considerable overlap. In many of the nations of sub-Saharan Africa, the march of HIV through the population has been shadowed by burgeoning rates of tuberculosis. Similar parallel epidemics are being witnessed among the inner city population of the United States, where high rates of HIV infection coincide with other factors that increase the risk of getting TB, including homelessness, drug use, alcoholism, malnutrition, and the presence of immigrants from countries where TB rates are high.

Medical authorities anticipate that as HIV infection spreads, the incidence of tuberculosis worldwide will rise substantially. In recent years there have been roughly 10 million new cases of TB and 2-3 million deaths from the disease annually worldwide—without a major contribution from HIV. While rising HIV infection rates in Africa, the United States, and Brazil are ominous, the biggest disaster could occur if AIDS becomes widespread in Asia, where, in addition to a very high prevalence of latent tuberculosis, there is severe crowding, which could promote rapid spread of tuberculosis even to those without HIV infection.

Treatment and Prevention

After centuries of frantic searching, a truly effective treatment for tuberculosis was discovered in the 1940s: the antibiotic streptomycin. This discovery was soon followed by the development of two other drugs: para-aminosalicylic acid and isoniazid. By the early 1950s it was recognized that the combination of these three drugs, given for 24 months, would cure more than 95 percent of patients with tuberculosis of the lungs. A combination of drugs was necessary to prevent the bacillus from developing resistance to any one of the antimicrobial agents being used against it.

Subsequently, other effective drugs were discovered, such as pyrazinamide, ethambutol, and rifampin. Combinations of these and the early medications need to be taken for a much shorter period of time—as little as six months—and they can be taken as infrequently as two or three times a week without losing their effectiveness. This reduces the problem of patient noncompliance—that is, the tendency of patients whose symptoms have cleared up fairly quickly with treatment to discontinue their medication or take it erratically before they are completely free of the disease.

Medical authorities predict that as HIV infection spreads, the incidence of tuberculosis worldwide will rise substantially.

Despite these advances, there has been a steady erosion in the success rates of treatment programs. Failure to take medication consistently has led to steadily escalating rates of drug resistance. (If a patient's TB germs are exposed to doses of medicine that are not high enough to cure the disease, the germs can develop resistance to those drugs.) Noncompliance has resulted in cure rates as low as 25 percent among patients enrolled in urban clinics in the United States. Facilitated by the confluence of AIDS, drug resistance, noncompliance, and very limited public health resources, tuberculosis has made a distinct resurgence in the United States, and the prospects for its control are not good. So far, there has been little success in broad efforts to develop new drugs that will shorten further the required duration of treatment or replace drugs the bacillus has developed resistance to. Thus, the 1990s may be seen as a critical juncture in the historic struggle with tuberculosis. Ironically, 50 years after the discovery of drugs that raised hopes of eliminating this ancient scourge, tuberculosis appears poised to earn all over again its old reputation as the White Plague. □

SYMPTOMS OF PULMONARY TUBERCULOSIS

- **persistent cough**
- **fever**
- **night sweats**
- **weight loss**
- **extreme fatigue**
- **chest pain**
- **hemoptysis (coughing blood)**

Athletic Shoes
Not Just Sneakers Anymore

Ingrid J. Strauch

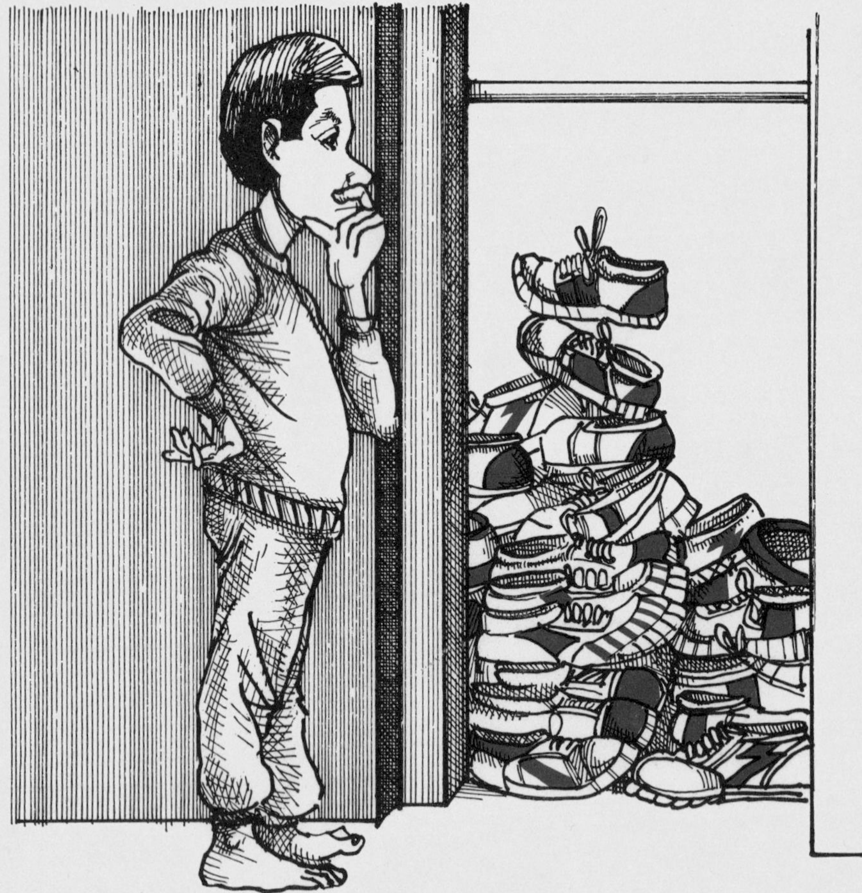

Buying athletic shoes used to be simple. They were called sneakers, and they came in limited styles and colors. Today it's a different story. There are more than a dozen major brands, hundreds of models, a continually changing array of colors (although plain white and black remain popular), and so many claims made for the latest technology it's hard to know where good design ends and hype begins.

There are specially designed shoes for just about any sport: breathable nylon and leather shoes for running, hiking, and volleyball, supportive high tops for aerobics and basketball, and cleated shoes for baseball and softball. There are stiff leather shoes for bicycling and similar, slightly more flexible shoes for biathletes and triathletes. There are waterproof shoes for golf with "shawl tongues" to protect the laces from spattering mud; shoes with extra lateral support for tennis, handball, and squash (to hold the foot steady and prevent blisters during quick changes of direction); sturdy, cushioned shoes for walking; and shoes promoted specifically for cheerleading and coaching. There are colorful nylon mesh slippers with rubber soles for windsurfing. There are cross-trainers, a fairly new addition to the market, for people who like to do a little of several sports—they are light enough for running but have lateral support for sports such as aerobics or basketball. There are even plain old canvas sneakers, sometimes called "casual" shoes, for people who just want something to scuff around in. And for those with fashion foremost in mind, there are sneakers made trendy with neon colors, plaids, polka dots, sequins, seed pearls, and beads.

Manufacturers promise to add spring to the step with high-tech features such as the "energy return system"—a row of plastic cylinders set in the heel that are said to act like mini-trampolines. Other shoes have "dynamic reaction plates," "torsion rigidity bars," "energy waves," or "HydroFlow"—two-chambered units in the heels filled with silicone fluid. Some shoes come with cushioning pockets of compressed air or nitrogen microballoons in the sole, some with inflatable tongues (for a custom fit that cushions and supports the foot), "kinetic" wedges under the forefoot, or "variable impact soles." Others have supportive molded ankle collars, outrigger soles, adjustable straps, "Y-bar" ankle braces, or "stabilizing pillars." Even the materials used to make the shoes sound impressive: Hytrel, Durathane, Hexalite, Stytherm, Surlyn, Purolite, and Phylon.

Evolution of the Shoe

The evolution of athletic shoes from canvas and rubber clunkers to space-age masterpieces of technology began as early as 1900, spurred on by runners' complaints that their shoes were uncomfortable. But few substantial advances were made until the 1960s. First, rubber wedges were inserted into the heels of running shoes to absorb shocks and relieve stress on the Achilles tendon. Then heavy leather and canvas uppers were replaced with lightweight nylon, and leather soles were redesigned in rubber and urethane to provide more cushioning and traction. Another important development was the midsole, a shock-absorbing layer in the sole that was first made of rubber and now is usually polyurethane or a plastic foam called ethylene vinyl acetate (EVA). As the jogging craze took hold in the United States in the 1970s, sales of the lighter, more comfortable running shoes boomed, as did the number of athletic shoe manufacturers.

But jogging wasn't for everyone. In the mid-1980s aerobics was in, and the shoe to wear was a white or black leather aerobics shoe with plenty of ankle and lateral support for quick, varied movements. Then fitness walking became the national pastime, and stores stocked up on walking shoes, rather sedate-looking footwear, available mostly in white, black, or tan. Walking shoes have more toe room than running shoes, to allow for the toes' natural splaying during walking, and provide more cushioning and shock absorption than dress shoes, although some are designed to look very much like men's dress shoes. All the while basketball shoes were advancing from canvas high tops to extravagantly cushioned wonders, and tennis shoes were being reengineered to absorb the shocks from quick stops and pivots.

Today, with all the competition and emphasis on technology, designing athletic footwear has become a laboratory science. Manufacturers hire podiatrists and experts in sports medicine, biomechanics, and locomotion studies to develop new products. Their equipment includes electronic monitors that attach to the legs and feet of those they are studying, computer sensors that measure the force of motion on a shoe, plaster casts of athletes' feet, cameras that record the motions of feet during exercise, and machines that bend and twist shoes to test their durability.

Is It All Necessary?

Are so many kinds of shoes and so much high technology really necessary? After all, people ran, cycled, and played volleyball and tennis before there were tri-density midsoles, stability straps, and special shoes for each sport. Some people still walk in aerobics shoes, do aerobics in running shoes, or run in basketball shoes with no ill effects. But good athletic shoes do provide much more shock absorption, comfort, and foot support than old-fashioned sneakers, and wearing a shoe designed especially for a sport increases the likelihood that the extra padding and support will be where it's most needed. If exercising in a certain pair of shoes is causing pain in the feet or legs, the shoes are either too old or not designed for what they're being used for, and it's time to replace them.

Whether one advanced technology is better than another is more a question of personal preference and need. (Shoe company executives, of course, might disagree.) Many of the nuances of sports shoes—for example, the difference between air capsules in the soles and tubes of gel—may be important only for serious competitive athletes for whom every second on a race clock counts, although recreational athletes, too, may feel they perform better or are more comfortable in shoes with certain technologies. But no one has proven that all runners run faster or all basketball players jump higher with a particular shoe. The person who intends to wear the shoes mainly for fashion or casual walking probably doesn't need the fancier features and won't notice the less visible ones.

Finding the Right Pair

In spite of all the technical language used to promote athletic shoes, it is not necessary to understand engineering in order to find the right pair. The most important criteria in choosing a shoe are that it fits well, feels comfortable, and is appropriate to the sport for which the buyer will use it. Athletic equipment stores generally group shoes by sport, and often a label attached to the shoe lists its special features and uses.

A prospective buyer may wish to consult one of several sport magazines that publish seasonal ratings of athletic shoes with comments on construction and the shoes' ability to live up to their manufacturers' promises. Many ratings guides also give tips on which shoes to use for different purposes, for example, training versus racing or high-impact versus low-impact activities.

But all the recommendations and good designs in the world don't mean a thing if the shoe doesn't fit the foot, and the only way to find the shoe that fits best is to try on several styles while wearing the type of socks that will be worn during exercise. The best time to try on shoes is in the

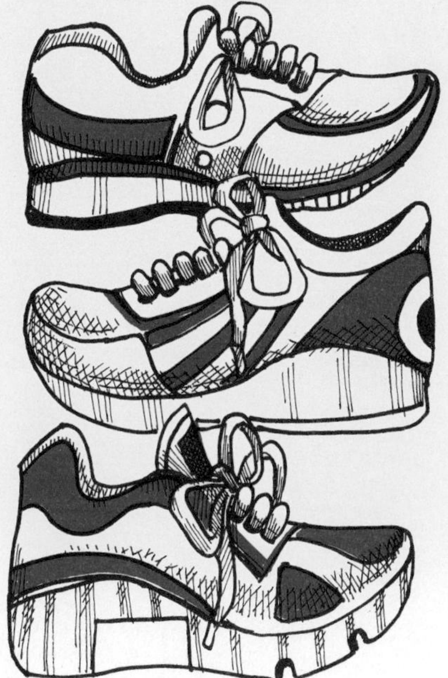

afternoon or evening, when the feet are bigger (feet tend to swell slightly as the day goes on). Athletic shoe sizes may be slightly different from street shoe sizes.

It's important that the toe box, the front area of the shoe where the toes are, be roomy enough. All five toes should lie flat, and there should be one-quarter of an inch to one-half inch of space between the big toe and the tip of the shoe.

A padded tongue and a padded collar around the ankle add to comfort, but too much padding can make the foot overheat. In ankle-height shoes a notch in the back of the ankle collar may relieve pressure on the Achilles tendon. Shoes with a hard plastic strip where the upper heel meets the sole, called a heel stabilizer or motion control device, will provide more heel support than shoes without such a strip. (Which is more desirable is a matter of personal preference.) Some athletic shoes need a little breaking in, but they should feel comfortable even when new. Shoes that are uncomfortable in the store almost never become comfortable later, no matter how much they are worn.

How the shoe is lasted affects its relative stability and flexibility. The last is the foot-shaped form around which the shoe is built. In a board-lasted shoe the upper part of the shoe is first sewn to a stiff piece of cardboard to add stability, then is attached to the sole. A more stable shoe is also more durable and will stand up better to repeated practices or workouts or to wear by heavy athletes. In a slip-lasted shoe the upper material is sewn together at the bottom to form a sort of moccasin, then glued to the sole, allowing more flexibility. Such shoes would most likely be used for competitions because their lighter weight and increased flexibility can help quicken the pace. A combination last means that the shoe is board-lasted in the rear and slip-lasted in front. Reading the labels attached to the shoe or asking a salesperson are good ways to find out about a shoe's construction.

Other features found in some athletic shoes include:

- Air vents: Small round vents in the sides or tops of leather shoes help keep feet cooler.
- Speed-lacing eyelets: Getting shoes on and off quickly is made easier with large, plastic eyelets. There should be a smaller eyelet at the top to keep laces secure.
- Sockliners: Removable insoles can be aired, cleaned, or replaced to keep shoes fresher longer.
- Tongue anchor: Two parallel slits in the tongue allow the laces to pass through so that the tongue won't slip to one side.
- Heel reflectors: Reflective material can be important for joggers who run on public streets after dark.

Any runner whose shoes show abnormal wear or whose feet feel sore or uncomfortable after running should consider seeing a podiatrist.

Some athletes know they have special needs that will influence their shoe choices. Many running-related injuries are caused by overpronation (the feet roll too far inward) or supination (the feet roll outward). The wear patterns on running shoes are often the first sign that there is a problem, with heavy wear on the outside of the heel and the inside of the ball of the foot indicating overpronation, wear along the entire outside edge of the shoe indicating supination. It is possible to walk into a good athletic store and buy shoes designed to compensate for these problems. But any runner whose shoes show abnormal wear or whose feet are sore or uncomfortable as a result of running should consider getting the expert advice of a podiatrist. The podiatrist can not only recommend which shoes would be best for a particular runner but can also supply any shoe implants needed to correct the foot's rotation.

Beginning athletes may not know whether their feet require extra cushioning or support in some areas, and a trot around the shoe store can't possibly substitute for a 30-minute workout. Still, costly mistakes can usually be avoided by enlisting the help of a knowledgeable salesperson and comparing several models to find the one that feels best. While purchasing the most expensive shoe is generally not necessary, it is rarely advisable to buy cheap athletic shoes.

There's a Price to Pay

With manufacturers racing to develop new technologies and spending anywhere from $25 million to $70 million each year on advertising alone, and more on public relations and special promotions, it's no surprise that most of today's souped-up sneakers don't come cheap. Most running shoes cost more than $50, and some of the fancier basketball shoes go for more than $150. (The most expensive shoes, a status symbol among some inner-city teenagers, have been blamed as the source of muggings and even some murders.)

In 1990, Americans bought more than 390 million pairs of athletic shoes, paying about $11.7 billion. Although advertisements for athletic shoes generally show physically fit people, often celebrities, engaged in vigorous activity, muscles bulging and sweat dripping, some 80 percent of the sports shoes purchased in the United States are actually used for nothing more athletic than cleaning the garage or shopping at the mall. For most, apparently, looking as though they just came from the gym is as good as actually having gone. □

LEG CRAMPS

Jeffrey P. Cohn

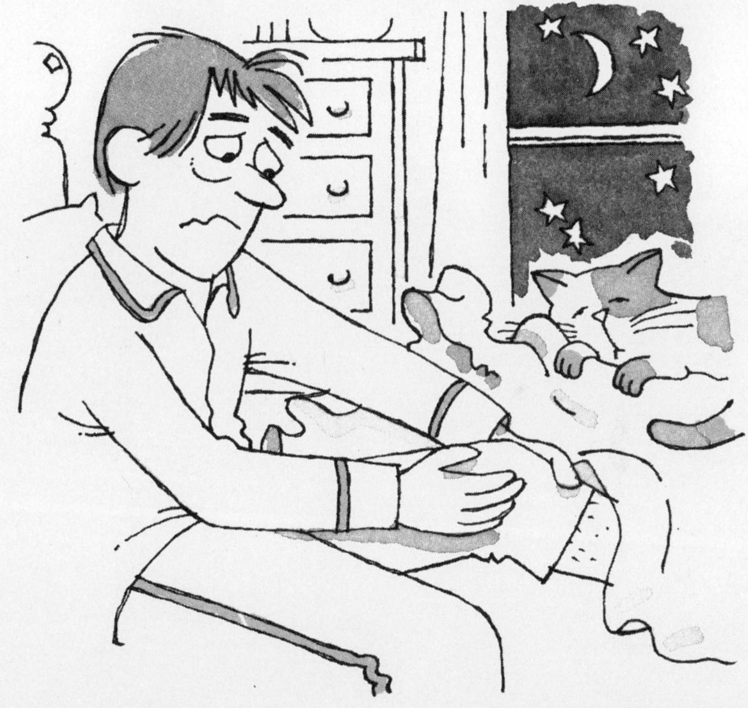

Three A.M. I was awakened from what had been a typically uneventful sleep by a sharp, shooting, and excruciating pain in my lower leg. My calf muscle had suddenly cramped, apparently when I stretched my leg while asleep. The muscle was pulled into a hard, tight cramp that refused to relax or ease on its own. It was as if I had lost all control over the muscle.

I rolled over, writhing in pain. I tried to rub the muscle, but the pain prevented my doing much except cussing and moaning. Even massaging the muscle did little right away to stop the spasm. Finally, all else having failed, I sat up, put my feet on the floor, and stood up, placing my weight on the cramped leg and foot.

Almost immediately the muscle began to relax. Taking a few steps further relieved the cramp. Within seconds, the pain that only moments before had virtually crippled me was gone. My disposition markedly improved, and within a few minutes I was asleep.

Common but Mysterious

Occasional leg cramps afflict millions of Americans, although no one knows exactly how often they occur or why. They may result from overexertion, certain medical conditions such as diabetes, or a reaction to medication, among other causes. Because leg cramps are not usually symptoms of a disease or medical condition and rarely lead to more serious problems, little research has been done on them.

Thus, physicians do not know the precise physiological causes of muscle cramps, why they seem to occur more often in the leg than other muscles, or why particular medications, most used primarily for other medical conditions, and home remedies seem to relieve them.

Perhaps the biggest unknown is why cramped muscles fail to relax. "Why someone who lifts weights and keeps the muscles contracted for a sustained time doesn't suffer a cramp or pain is beyond me," says Dr. Raymond Lipicky, director of the U.S. Food and Drug Administration's division of cardiorenal drugs. "A contraction is a contraction," he says, adding: "There is apparently something different about contractions that cause cramps, but nobody knows what."

What is known is that leg cramps seem to occur most commonly in athletes and others who exercise strenuously, in people who have reached middle age and beyond, and in those who suffer circulatory problems. They occur most often at night or when resting. Also, people who stand for long periods can suffer leg cramps. However painful at the moment, most leg cramps last no more than a few minutes, and they do not interfere with daily functioning.

In a few cases, however, leg cramps can cause a persistent, severe pain that may prevent sleeping, walking, or other activities. Dr. Vincent Karusaitis, a medical review officer in the FDA's division of oncology, says such cramps are "a sign that you should seek medical attention."

How Do Muscles Cramp?

Most leg cramps seem to occur for no apparent reason. "No physician can tell you why they happen," says Dr. Stanley Silverberg, a Chevy Chase, Md., cardiologist and vascular specialist. Silverberg explains the general process of how muscles cramp by likening the body's cells to electrical batteries. Both function, he says, by passing electrical charges across their surfaces.

Muscles contract when electrical impulses travel from the brain along the nerves and are transferred to muscle cells by special transmitters operating at the nerve-muscle junction. Most muscle contractions are voluntary, organized, and controllable. A cramp or spasm occurs when the electrical impulses from the brain occur very rapidly, causing the muscle to contract in a sudden, disorganized, and uncontrollable fashion.

In these cases, muscular activity is somehow related to changes in the balance of various body chemicals called electrolytes. Of these, calcium, potassium, and sodium have the most effect on muscle and nerve activity. Sweating a lot can alter the body's chemistry by decreasing sodium and potassium levels and total body fluids. An altered chemical balance can prevent the transmitters from functioning properly, perhaps preventing the muscle from relaxing after contracting.

Some cramps may be an aftermath of overexercising or failing to properly stretch muscles before exerting them. Athletes have to prepare their muscles before running or playing a vigorous game, Karusaitis says, encouraging all who exercise to do the same. Cramps are particularly common among older or "weekend" athletes, who are less active and less likely to warm up first.

But athletes are not the only ones who overexert muscles. It can happen to other people, too, especially normally inactive individuals. People who spend more time than usual in the garden, for example, may exercise their muscles more than they are used to and suffer leg cramps later. Again, those who are middle-aged or older are more likely to experience such cramps.

Weight can be a complicating factor, Karusaitis says. Being overweight can change body posture in ways that put extra pressure on leg muscles, leading to cramps. Also, the enlarging uterus in the late months of pregnancy can interfere with blood flow from the lower legs. Swelling of the legs, varicose veins, and frequent leg cramps are not uncommon. Pregnant women are often advised to wear elastic stockings to reduce swelling and cramps.

Drugs and Cramps

Some medications can alter chemical (and fluid) balances in the body, causing leg cramps. Patients taking diuretic drugs to control heart, blood pressure, and kidney disorders can suffer cramps. The reason is that diuretics remove electrolytes from the body, taking with them fluids, both needed for proper muscle function. "The only way to really stop these kinds of leg cramps is to reduce the dosage [of electrolyte-affecting drugs]," says Dr. Frederick Smith, a Washington, D.C., physician. "But I prefer to prevent cramps with other medications."

One prescription drug that helps is diphenhydramine hydrochloride (brand name, Benadryl), a widely prescribed medication. The FDA has approved it as an antihistamine, for motion sickness, as a sleep aid, and for Parkinson's disease, but not for leg cramps. Physicians may prescribe a drug for uses beyond those approved by the FDA, but on their own responsibility. Why Benadryl works for leg cramps is unknown, Smith says, but it does.

Another prescription drug is the popular tranquilizer diazepam (commonly sold as Valium). Yet a third is cyclobenzaprine hydrochloride (brand name, Flexeril). In all, Karusaitis says, about half a dozen prescription drugs are used to relax cramp-prone muscles.

There are also several over-the-counter medications sold for leg cramps. Most are quinine-derived (as are some prescription drugs, such as quinine sulfate), and some contain vitamin E as well. Patients on diuretics or with other chemical-balance problems can take sodium or calcium supplements, or eat foods rich in these nutrients.

Like most drugs, the quinine-based medications have side effects, such as nausea, vomiting, ringing in the ears, and skin rashes. Pregnant women are advised not to take these medications, nor should anyone take them for more than five days unless under the supervision of a physician.

Home Remedies

There are many simple home remedies that relieve leg cramps. Standing on the cramped leg and foot and walking around works by forcing the muscle in the direction against the cramp, which relaxes it. Home health guides often advise people to pull their toes forcefully yet smoothly up toward the knee, which similarly forces the muscle against the cramp.

Other home remedies include massaging the cramped muscle, applying heat to it, and wearing loose-fitting clothing to bed. Heating the muscle with a hot-water bottle or electric blanket, for example, increases blood flow to the leg, thus improving the electrolyte and other chemical balances needed for muscles to function properly, Silverberg says.

For people who stand in the same position for much of the day, such as cashiers, Karusaitis recommends putting a spongy mat on the floor to cushion the legs. He also advises flexing the muscles periodically by moving about.

When It Gets Serious

Unfortunately, not all leg cramps are occasional or so easily treated. Some, in fact, result from serious medical conditions and can themselves make normal functioning difficult. In some cases, medical attention and treatment, beyond medications and home remedies, are required.

One Israeli study linked muscle cramps with liver disorders. By comparing healthy people with patients who had cirrhosis of the liver, researchers found that 88 percent of the latter had painful muscle cramps compared with 21 percent of healthy subjects. Dr. Fred Konikoff and Emanuel Theodor, the authors, concluded that "painful muscle cramps might be regarded as a symptom of liver cirrhosis."

A more common cause of leg cramps is varicose veins, Silverberg says. Varicose, or abnormally swollen, veins affect the interchange of fluids between the veins and muscles. Also, damaged valves in the veins can let blood leak back down the leg and into the muscles, causing cramps.

Other circulatory ailments, such as arteriosclerosis and arteritis, can likewise cause leg cramps. They result in narrowed leg arteries, thereby preventing an adequate supply of blood from reaching the muscles. People with these conditions often cannot walk long distances or for sustained periods without suffering pain or a cramp or both. Such symptoms, known collectively as intermittent claudication, are usually associated with cigarette smoking and high blood cholesterol levels.

To prevent or treat these cramps, physicians often advise patients to rest or sit with their legs elevated. Some also prescribe pentoxifylline (brand name, Trental), a drug that can postpone or sometimes prevent the need for surgery, the FDA's Lipicky says. Trental changes the outer layer of red blood cells so they can better squeeze through narrower openings in arteries, thus improving the flow of blood to muscles. Studies show that people with arterial diseases can walk up to 50 percent longer after taking Trental.

Surgical Treatment

Often, however, such circulatory disorders require surgical treatment. In recent years, that has meant bypass surgery (in which the clogged artery is replaced by another blood vessel), amputation (in the most severe cases), or balloon angioplasty.

In the last, surgeons make an incision in the patient's leg and insert a probe into the blocked artery. The probe is then threaded through the artery to the site of the obstruction. There a tiny balloon is gently inflated to open the blocked vessel. Once the job is done, the balloon is collapsed and withdrawn.

While a significant advance over amputation or bypass surgery, balloon angioplasty is costly and cannot always be done. It cannot unclog totally blocked arteries, for example, nor can it be done on some older patients or those who have other health problems. And balloon angioplasty is reported to be only 56 percent to 84 percent successful.

A newer surgical technique is thermal angioplasty. Similar in some respects to balloon angioplasty, it may one day supplement or replace it. The technique uses a specifically designed metal-tipped, fiber-optic probe that allows surgeons to aim a laser beam directly at the blockage within an artery, says Dr. Timothy Sanborn, a cardiologist at Mt. Sinai Hospital in New York City and one of the technique's pioneers. The laser vaporizes the blockage, thereby opening the clogged artery. Once the blockage is at least partially destroyed, surgeons can insert the balloon into the artery to open it more. Sanborn reports that thermal angioplasty is successful 80 to 90 percent of the time, depending on the degree of the blockage, how long the artery has been blocked, and how much calcium is present. When the procedure is successful, patients are usually able to walk immediately with no pain or cramps.

Other Causes

While intermittent claudication involves only large arteries, leg cramps can be caused by blockages in smaller ones, too. Diabetes, for example, can cause small arteries to become constricted, thereby cutting the blood flow through them, Lipicky says, but Trental can be prescribed.

Yet other medical conditions can cause leg cramps. Patients suffering from low calcium levels, which can be diagnosed easily by blood tests, can get leg cramps, as can patients on hemodialysis for end-stage renal disease. Patients with chronic kidney disorders who undergo dialysis may have leg cramps near the end of the dialysis session. This has been shown by medical studies to be related to fluid and salt depletion occurring during dialysis and can be relieved by giving the patient intravenous salt and sugar solutions.

It should be pointed out that most people who suffer from arterial disorders, diabetes, or other medical conditions linked to leg cramps do not get cramps, or get them only occasionally. Similarly, only about 1 or 2 percent of those on diuretics get leg cramps. But since millions of people take the drugs, that can add up.

Because of their unpredictable nature and the fact that so little is known about them, leg cramps are a disconcerting problem. "As a doctor, I get frustrated by being unable to prevent leg cramps in my patients despite their frequency," says Smith. Those of us who experience occasional leg cramps get frustrated, too. □

An earlier version of this article appeared in *FDA Consumer*, March 1988.

THE RESURGENCE OF SYPHILIS

Robert C. Noble, M.D.

Syphilis is a sexually transmitted disease for which highly effective treatments have existed for almost half a century. It was thought to be nearly eradicated in the United States in the 1950s, but in recent years syphilis has made a strong comeback, with the number of reported cases rising 61 percent between 1985 and 1989, to reach a 40-year high.

Unfortunately, the disease is easy for patients to ignore. Unlike some other venereal diseases—such as genital herpes, which produces painful ulcers, and gonorrhea, which causes pain on urination—syphilis may not cause pain at first, and many of the signs and symptoms disappear spontaneously without treatment. But syphilis left untreated can be readily transmitted to sexual partners and can cause irreversible, life-threatening damage to the infected individual's internal organs. When passed from a pregnant woman to her fetus, syphilis can cause birth defects, stillbirth, or infant death.

Syphilis was thought to be nearly eradicated in the United States, but in recent years it has made an unwelcome comeback.

Transmitting the Bacteria

Syphilis is caused by a microscopic spirochete (a type of bacteria) called *Treponema pallidum*. The spirochete, which has the shape of a thin corkscrew, does not exist on its own in the environment but must be passed from one person to another by direct contact. Humans are its only hosts.

The majority of cases of syphilis are acquired in sexual intercourse. Spirochetes from an open sore or rash on the already infected individual enter the partner's body through a mucous membrane or break in the skin. The use of a condom can provide substantial protection against syphilis infection.

Occasionally, the syphilis spirochete may be picked up through touching or kissing an infected lesion. During what is known as the latent phase of syphilis, when no open sores or rashes are present, the disease is generally not contagious—although pregnant women can still infect their unborn children. Fetuses are especially susceptible to infection and can acquire the spirochete from the mother either through the placenta or during the passage through the birth canal. (Syphilis contracted in this way is called congenital syphilis.) In rare cases syphilis has been transmitted by blood transfusion.

When left untreated, syphilis can be readily transmitted to sexual partners and can cause irreversible damage to internal organs.

Cases on the Rise

In the United States the incidence of syphilis was highest (approximately 70 new cases a year per 100,000 people) during World War II, before the antibiotic penicillin, shown to be effective against syphilis in 1943, was generally available. By the mid-1950s, thanks to penicillin, syphilis was believed to be conquered; the number of new cases annually had fallen to approximately 4 per 100,000 population. However, with social mores loosening and sexual promiscuity on the rise, the incidence of syphilis began to increase again. By the mid-1960s there were 10 to 12 new cases a year per 100,000 population, a rate that remained fairly stable throughout the 1970s.

For many years males accounted for almost twice as many cases as females. The imbalance grew in the 1970s as homosexual life-styles became more accepted and more widely practiced; by the early 1980s new cases of males with syphilis outnumbered female cases three to one. In many large U.S. cities prior to the AIDS epidemic, over 50 percent of cases of infectious syphilis occurred in homosexual men. But the advent of AIDS motivated substantial behavioral changes among homosexual males, and the incidence of syphilis has dropped sharply in this population.

In recent years, there has been another increase in syphilis, and in 1989 there were more than 18 new cases per 100,000 people, higher than any year since 1949. Prostitution associated with crack cocaine abuse is thought to be a reason for this rise. Between 1985 and 1989 the incidence of syphilis doubled among blacks. In 1990 an estimated 137,400 cases of syphilis were reported in the United States.

The Stages of Syphilis

Syphilis has several stages, called incubating, primary, secondary, latent, and late syphilis. After the spirochete enters the body, the incubation period, during which there are no symptoms, lasts from 3 to 90 days (the mean is 3 weeks). Then, in the primary stage, a chancre develops at the site where the spirochete entered the body. The chancre is a painless, round ulcer less than one-half inch in diameter that heals in two to eight weeks. Chancres usually appear at sites of sexual contact—the genitals, mouth, or rectum.

The primary stage is followed by the secondary, or disseminated, stage of syphilis, which begins 2 to 12 weeks (mean, 6 weeks) after infection. In this stage, spirochetes disseminate to all parts of the body, and the response of the body's immune system produces a myriad of symptoms, including fever, enlarged lymph nodes, a variety of skin rashes, headache, weight loss, and sometimes hair loss.

Even without treatment, secondary syphilis subsides. If untreated, the patient then enters the latent

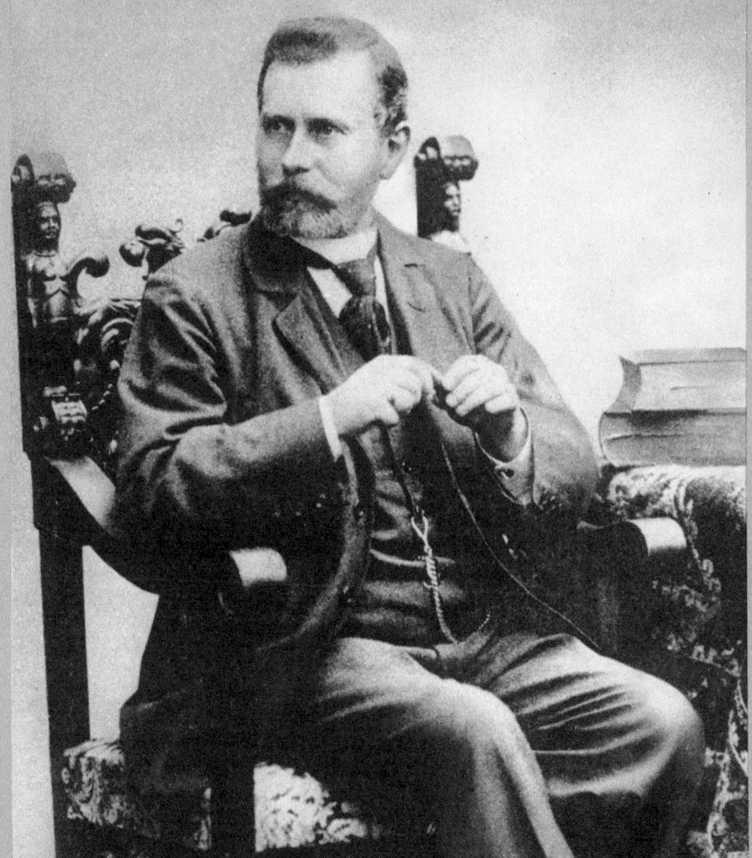

Paul Ehrlich, the discoverer of Salvarsan, an effective syphilis drug.

SYPHILIS THROUGH THE AGES

The true origins of syphilis are unknown, but that hasn't stopped people throughout history from placing the blame. It has been hypothesized that Columbus's sailors brought the disease back from the New World, setting off a pandemic of "great pox" that spread through Europe and Asia at the time of the explorer's return. In France during the pandemic, syphilis was known as the disease from Naples, in Naples as the French disease, and in England as the Spanish disease.

In 1530, Girolamo Fracastoro, an Italian pathologist, named the disease in a mythical poem he wrote, *Syphilis sive Morbus Gallicus*, telling of a shepherd boy named Syphilis who suffered from the French disease as a result of angering the gods.

Although recognizable descriptions of syphilis had appeared by 1500 and its mode of transmission was known, there was some confusion for centuries between the symptoms of syphilis and gonorrhea. The two afflictions were long thought to be different stages of the same disease. It wasn't until the early 19th century that the diseases (caused by two different types of bacteria) were clearly differentiated by Philippe Ricord, a French physician.

Early treatments for syphilis included preparations containing iodine, bismuth, and heavy metals such as mercury. These treatments were not very effective and were potentially toxic. In the early 1900s, Paul Ehrlich, a German physician, was searching for a drug to cure trypanosomiasis, a tropical parasitic disease. The 606th chemical that he tested was found to be effective both for the tropical parasite and for the syphilis spirochete. This chemical was an arsenic compound, a yellow powder that he called Salvarsan. Commonly referred to by the Germans as "606," it was superior to the earlier treatments.

A Viennese psychiatrist, Julius Wagner von Jauregg, treated syphilitic patients by inducing fever—through inoculating them with the malaria parasite; for this he received the Nobel Prize in medicine in 1927. In 1943 penicillin was shown to be a highly effective, nontoxic therapy, and it remains the mainstay of treatment.

Syphilis has counted among its victims some of the world's most famous and infamous people, including rulers Ivan the Terrible, Henry VIII, Peter the Great, and Charles V; the writers Flaubert and Oscar Wilde; the poet Goethe; the painters Gauguin and Toulouse-Lautrec; the violinist Paganini; the explorer Captain James Cook; and the gangster Al Capone.

stage. By definition, patients with latent syphilis have no apparent signs or symptoms of the disease, although a blood test for the spirochete would be positive. In the first four years of the latent stage, patients may have relapses of secondary syphilis. Latency may last a lifetime or be followed, after a period of years (usually no more than 20), by late syphilis.

Two-thirds of people with untreated syphilis never develop the devastating, potentially fatal complications of late syphilis. In the unlucky third who do, the syphilis spirochete may damage the walls of blood vessels, the heart, or the brain, resulting in cardiovascular syphilis or neurosyphilis.

Patients with latent syphilis have no apparent symptoms of the disease, but a blood test for the spirochete would be positive.

In cardiovascular syphilis, there may be irreversible damage to heart valves, causing the heart to malfunction. Damage to the aorta (the principal artery carrying blood from the heart) can cause it to balloon and perhaps rupture. Untreated neurosyphilis can cause irreversible damage to the brain and spinal cord. This may result in strokes, blindness, deafness, loss of bladder control, personality changes, impairment of balance, impotence, and severe pains in the extremities. There may be a loss of deep pain sensation in the feet and toes, as a result of which injuries may go undetected and develop into nonhealing ulcers.

A fortunately uncommon lesion that occurs in late syphilis is called a gumma. Gummas are round lesions found most commonly in the skin (sometimes breaking through the surface of the skin to form ulcers), in the bones, and in the liver. As they expand and then eventually heal and form scars, they damage surrounding tissue.

Congenital Syphilis

Syphilis is highly dangerous to the fetuses of infected pregnant women. Approximately half of such fetuses will become infected. Many are stillborn or die very shortly after birth. Others may be born blind, deaf, or with deformed teeth and bones, nerve damage, or arthritis. Sometimes, however, there are no overt symptoms at birth. There were more than 850 cases of congenital syphilis in the United States in 1989. In areas where syphilis is prevalent, blood tests for syphilis should be performed on infants who are ill with fever.

Babies born with syphilis can be successfully treated with penicillin, but this therapy may not reverse all the damage caused by the spirochete, particularly damage to the eyes and ears. However, if the mother is treated during the first four months of pregnancy, the fetus usually escapes harm. This is one of many compelling reasons for pregnant women to have adequate prenatal medical care.

When passed from a pregnant woman to her unborn child, syphilis can cause stillbirth, early death, or damage to eyes, bones, and other body parts.

Diagnosis and Treatment

The method used to diagnose syphilis depends on the stage of the disease. In primary syphilis and in some cases of secondary syphilis, the spirochetes may be seen by examining under a microscope a sample of discharge from a lesion. However, syphilis is routinely diagnosed by means of one of many available blood tests.

If diagnosed before permanent damage has taken place, syphilis can be completely cured by adequate treatment with any of a number of antibiotics. Unlike the bacteria responsible for many cases of gonorrhea, the syphilis spirochete has not developed resistance to antibiotics. It has remained sensitive to the type of penicillin called penicillin G, which is the mainstay of therapy. For patients allergic to penicillin, other antibiotics are effective, including doxycycline, tetracycline, erythromycin, and ceftriaxone. Patients who require treatment must be periodically reexamined by their physicians for six months to a year to ensure that the therapy has been effective. Antibiotic therapy given late in the course of the disease will arrest the damage from the spirochete but may not restore the function of damaged organs and tissue.

If diagnosed before permanent damage has taken place, syphilis can be completely cured by any of a number of antibiotics.

Syphilis and AIDS

Patients with genital ulcers such as those caused by syphilis may be more susceptible to infection with the human immunodeficiency virus (HIV), the virus that causes AIDS. The ulcer disrupts the natural defenses of the skin and allows the virus to enter the body. Thus, more effective control of syphilis may contribute to controlling the spread of HIV infection as well. □

SCOLIOSIS

Jesse H. Dickson, M.D.

Scoliosis is a medical term for a condition that most people would call curvature of the spine. All patients with scoliosis have curvatures of the spine, but not all people with curvatures of the spine have scoliosis.

A diagnosis of scoliosis is made when two conditions are present. The first is a fixed lateral, or sideways, curving of the spine; that is, the curve does not disappear when the individual bends in the direction opposite to the curve. The second is rotated, or twisted, vertebrae (the bones that form the spine) in the area where the spine is curved.

Causes

Cases of scoliosis can be put into five basic classes depending on their cause. Metabolic scoliosis is caused by underlying problems of the metabolism such as those seen in serious bone diseases like osteogenesis imperfecta and juvenile osteoporosis. (The metabolism is the sum of all physical and chemical processes within the body.) Myopathic scoliosis results from muscle disorders like muscular dystrophy or arthrogryposis. Neuropathic scoliosis occurs in association with neurological disorders like poliomyelitis, spinal muscular atrophy, or cerebral palsy. Osteogenic scoliosis, the only form that is present at birth, results when the bones of the back do not form normally in the fetus. Idiopathic scoliosis, by far the most common type, is so called because it has no known cause. From 85 to 90 percent of all scoliosis cases are idiopathic.

Approximately 3 to 4 percent of Americans have true scoliosis. Another 40 to 45 percent have a curvature of the spine that will show up on X rays, but because there is no rotation of the vertebrae, they do not have scoliosis.

Lateral curvature of the spine is measured in degrees. If straight, the spine has a zero degree curve; if the spine forms a right angle, it has a 90 degree curve. A curve of greater than 20 degrees is considered significant. Most cases of scoliosis do not involve significant curves and are neither disfiguring nor disabling.

Scoliosis can develop in the upper part of the spine (thoracic scoliosis), the lower part (lumbar scoliosis), and halfway between the two (thoracolumbar scoliosis). Where there is only one curve, it can be called C-shaped. Sometimes the curve is double, or S-shaped, as both the thoracic and lumbar regions are affected. Thoracic curves are usually to the right, looking at the back, lumbar curves to the left.

Onset and Progression

Most cases of scoliosis develop after birth, and, as noted earlier, most of these have no known cause. Depending on the age of onset, doctors divide these cases into three separate types.

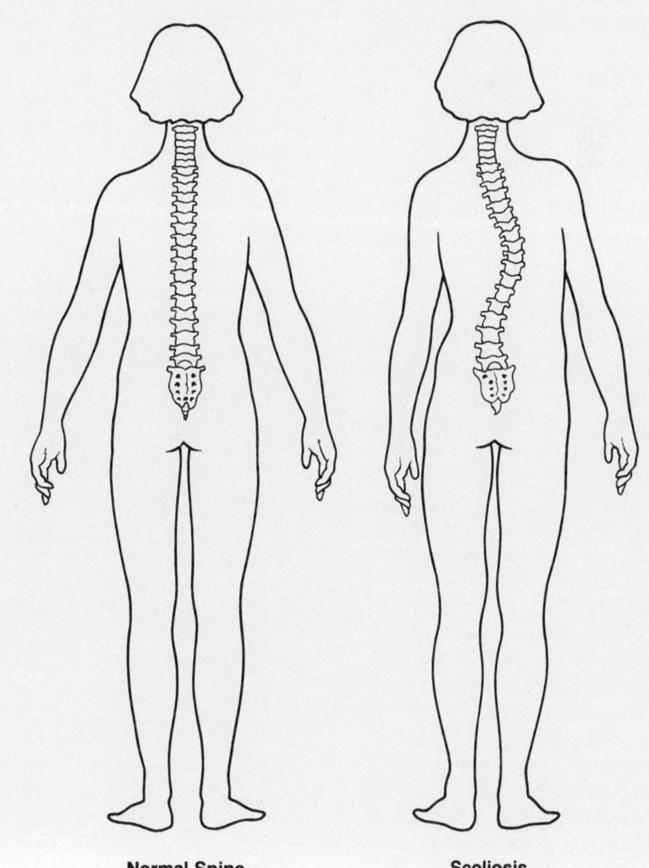

Infantile idiopathic scoliosis develops between birth and three years of age. It is seen primarily in boys, the curve is usually left thoracic, and it spontaneously disappears in 95 percent of cases. In the other 5 percent, if left untreated, it becomes quite severe.

Juvenile idiopathic scoliosis develops between the ages of three and ten. In children younger than seven, this type of scoliosis appears with equal frequency in boys and girls; after age seven, it is more common in girls.

The course juvenile idiopathic scoliosis takes varies: the spinal curvature may spontaneously disappear, it may remain the same throughout the child's growing life, it may remain stable for a time and then begin to progress as the child grows older, or it may progress at a steady constant rate.

Adolescent idiopathic scoliosis begins after age ten. Girls are five times as likely as boys to have curves greater than 20 degrees.

Girls are most susceptible to the onset and the progression of scoliosis between the time they start breast budding and the time they start menstruating. During this time, scoliosis can progress rapidly. Once the menstrual periods have started, the spine, for some reason, becomes less and less vulnerable to scoliosis, and there is not as great a chance of progression. If a girl who has just started breast budding is found to have a curve of 20 degrees or greater, the chance of this curve's becoming greater is about 90 percent. However, the same curve in a girl who has already started menstruating has a less than 10 percent chance of progressing.

Once an individual has stopped growing, the risk of progression in a curve of less than 30 degrees is almost zero. However, in almost 100 percent of fully grown individuals with curves of 50 degrees, their scoliosis gets worse as they age. The outcome varies for individuals with curves of between 30 and 50 degrees. In these individuals curves in the lower back have a greater tendency to progress than those in the upper, or thoracic, spine. Curves that are very flexible have a greater chance of progression than those that are stiff. Curves that have left the spine unbalanced, so that the head, shoulders, and upper trunk are offset to one side relative to the middle of the pelvis, are at greater risk of progressing than curves that have left the spine well balanced.

Symptoms and Effects

When first developing in the growing child, scoliosis generally does not cause pain. More likely signs of the condition are a shoulder that appears higher than the other, clothes that don't hang straight, or one hip that is higher than the other.

It is rare that scoliosis has any effect on other organs of the body. Scoliosis in a pregnant woman does not adversely affect the pregnancy or delivery.

In the adult severe scoliosis, even if untreated, will not in the vast majority of cases shorten life expectancy, nor will it necessitate the use of crutches, a wheelchair, or a cane. It will, however, cause back pain, fatigue, arthritis, and decreasing activity levels. As adults with severe scoliosis age, they have increasing problems to the point where they cannot participate to any degree in normal daily activities.

Treatment

Many forms of treatment have been tried, such as exercises, manipulations, electrical stimulation, shoelifts, special diets, rest periods, and vitamin supplements. None of these has ever been shown scientifically to be of any value. The two forms of treatment that *will* alter the course of scoliosis are braces and surgery.

Braces. A back brace cannot correct or lessen a curve, but it can prevent a curve from progressing in a growing child. Some braces extend from the hips to the neck while others reach only as high as the midback and can be concealed by clothing.

The brace is applied when the child has a mild curve that seems likely to progress and is worn until growth is completed. In 80 to 85 percent of cases, when the brace is removed the curve is the same as when the brace was initially applied. The brace is of no value in an individual whose growth is complete, in a growing individual with minimal scoliosis that is not progressing, or in someone who already has a severe curve. People with severe scoliosis require surgery.

Surgery. Surgery cannot cure an individual of scoliosis, but it can partially straighten the spinal curvature, usually reducing the curve by half or more, and then permanently stabilize the spine in the corrected position. First, metal rods and hooks are attached to the spine to straighten it and temporarily hold it in place. Permanent stabilization is achieved through what is called a bone fusion. Small pieces of bone, usually taken from the pelvis, are packed between the vertebrae, causing them to grow together and form a solid bar of rigid bone. The fusion is performed only on vertebrae in the abnormally curved portion of the spine. Once fusion is complete, the metal rods and hooks do not need to be there, but they are usually left in place since they rarely cause any problems and would require further surgery to remove.

Individuals who have had surgery for scoliosis can lead a normal life and are free to engage in such activities as tennis, golf, horseback riding, skiing, dancing, and bowling. They should not do manual labor or repeated bending on a regular basis. Their real limitation of activity is not what they do but how much they do. It is permissible to plant trees and shrubs as well as take care of one's yard but not to work for a landscape company and perform these tasks every day. □

ATHLETE'S FOOT

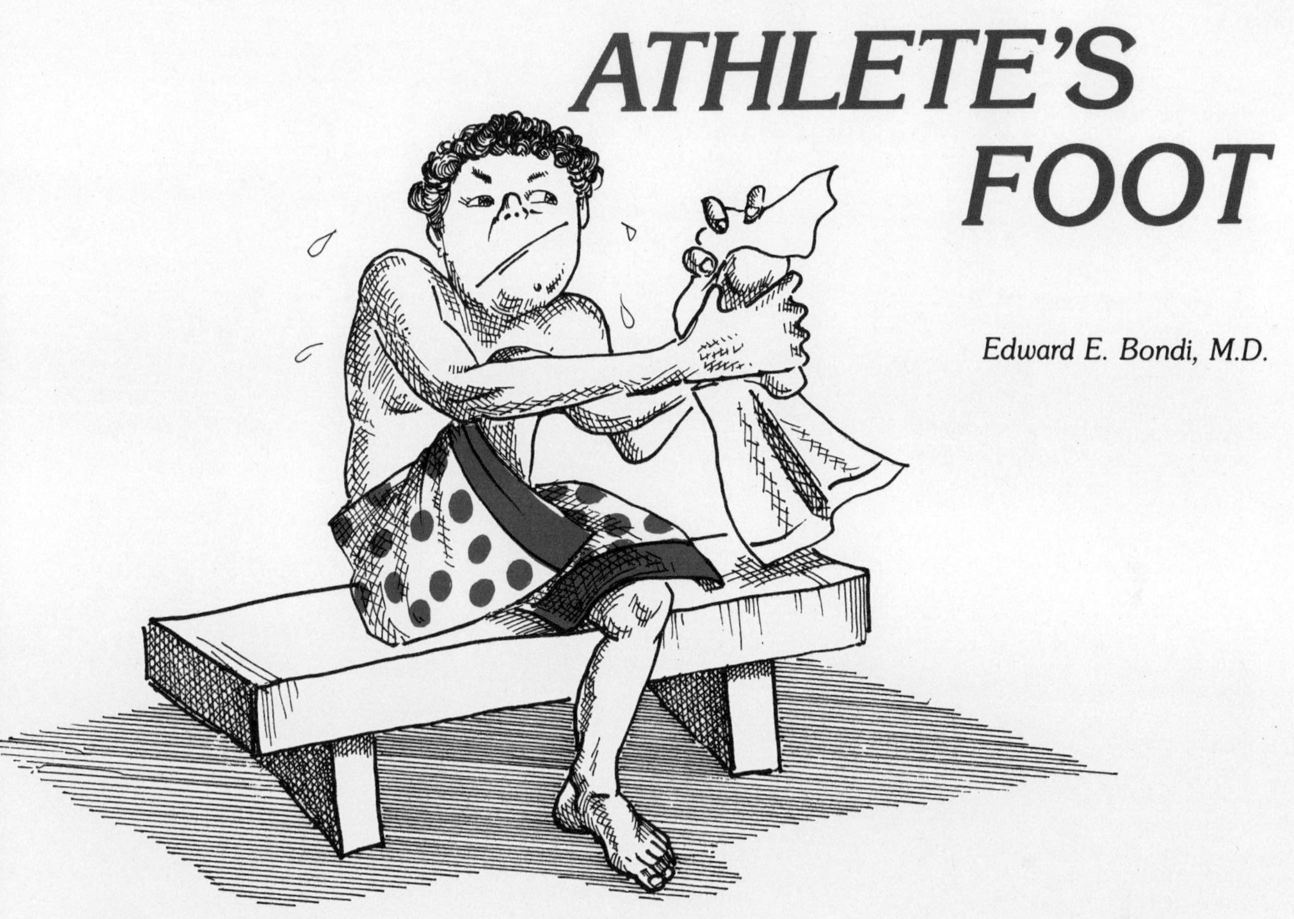

Edward E. Bondi, M.D.

The catchy phrase "athlete's foot" is used to describe an extremely common skin disease that affects all shoe-wearing populations throughout the world. It has been estimated that up to 40 percent of Americans will suffer at some time from this infection of the outer horny layer of the skin.

Physicians have historically considered athlete's foot to be a simple fungal infection. However, recent studies have shown that bacteria can also play a key role. It is now clear that bacteria, moisture, and fungi participate in a complex interaction that leads to development of the severe forms of athlete's foot.

Athlete's foot is characterized in its mild form by minor scaling and itching in the spaces between the toes. This mildly itchy annoyance can evolve into an incapacitating disease characterized by foul-smelling, soggy, cracked, and ulcerated skin. The spaces between the third, fourth, and fifth toes are most commonly involved, although the infection can spread to the soles of the feet and to the toenails.

Causes

Moisture. It has long been established that moisture plays an important role in producing athlete's foot. While the condition is almost nonexistent among primitive peoples who do not wear shoes, it is a common problem of all shoe-wearing populations. It is particularly common among athletes, whose feet are continually moist from perspiration, and in warm climates, where people sweat more. It is believed that by enclosing the feet so that sweat cannot evaporate, shoes produce the ideal moist environment for athlete's foot. Furthermore, because the third, fourth, and fifth toes are so close together, sweat is trapped in the spaces between them. Individuals whose toes are naturally fat and thus especially close together are particularly prone to athlete's foot.

Athlete's foot is an extremely common skin disease that affects not only athletes but also all shoe-wearing populations around the world.

Fungi. It has been estimated that 10 to 20 percent of the world's population harbor fungi between their toes at any given time. These are dermatophytes, skin-loving fungi that thrive in warm, moist environments and feed on keratin, a protein in the layer of dead cells on the surface of the skin. For years, dermatophytes were thought to be solely responsible for causing athlete's foot because they could be recovered more frequently from the spaces between the toes of diseased feet than from normal healthy feet. However, the fungi were sometimes present on normal, healthy feet without any evidence of the disease. And in approximately 70 percent of cases of severe athlete's foot, scientists could not find any fungi. This fact was frequently de-emphasized. New medications were routinely tested only on patients afflicted with the mildest forms of athlete's foot, concealing the fact that treatment of the severe form with antifungal products was frequently ineffective.

Bacteria. Studies at the University of Pennsylvania focused on why fungi are not always present in athlete's foot and investigated the factors that transformed mild athlete's foot into the severe forms of the disease.

Wearing sandals is recommended for both treatment and prevention of athlete's foot.

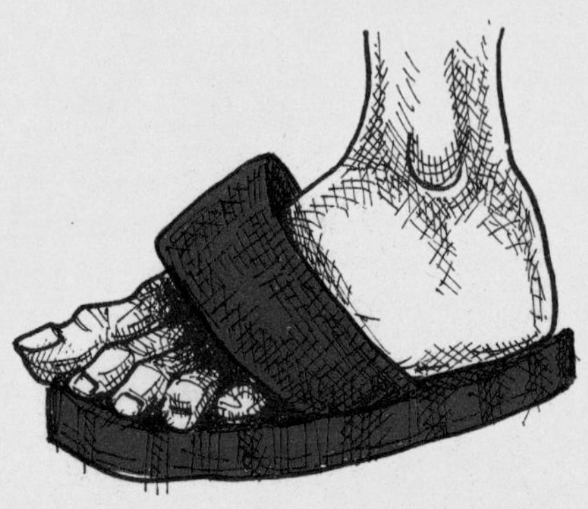

It seem that in mild cases of athlete's foot, if the amount of moisture trapped between the toes increases, the number of dermatophytes also increases. As the fungi increase in numbers, they damage the skin, thus weakening its ability to act as a barrier against infection. They also produce antibiotics, including penicillin and streptomycin, locally in the skin. This has an important effect on the bacteria that are normally present on the skin. It kills many of them off and encourages the growth of more dangerous antibiotic-resistant bacteria. Like the fungi, the harmful bacteria thrive in moisture. And as the numbers of these bacteria increase in the spaces between the toes, they release substances that further damage the skin. Ironically, these substances also eventually kill the local fungi, which is why cultures from patients with severe athlete's foot routinely show no fungi.

Treatment

Once the origin and development of athlete's foot are understood, it is not surprising to find dermatologists promoting dryness as the most effective treatment. Keeping the feet dry not only reduces fungal overgrowth, but it also limits the bacterial growth seen in severe cases of the disease.

Removing shoes when possible, changing socks frequently, avoiding footwear that promotes sweating and instead wearing sandals or other well-ventilated and loose-fitting shoes, dusting the feet and inside the shoes with talcum powder, and using gauze to separate the toes are all highly effective in promoting dryness. In most patients these practices clear up athlete's foot.

In addition, in severe cases dermatologists frequently apply aluminum chloride solutions or aqueous dye solutions such as gentian violet to the affected skin. These agents produce an additional drying effect, but they also have a potent antibacterial effect. The newest generation of antifungal agents for treating athlete's foot, the imidazole compounds, are also useful. The imidazole compounds are actually highly effective even for severe athlete's foot, partly because they also have an antibacterial effect. They are available both as over-the-counter products (for example, Micatin, Lotrimin) and as prescription medications (brand names, Mycelex, Spectazoke, and Nizoral). In recurrent cases, particularly when the toenails are infected with fungi, a systemic antifungal such as griseofulvin or ketoconazole may be prescribed.

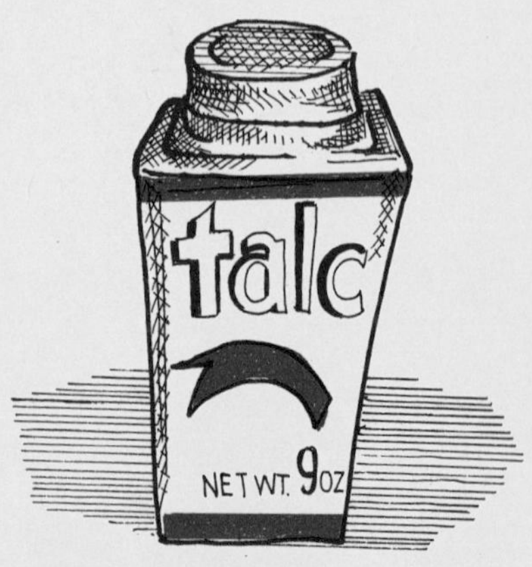

Talcum powder absorbs the moisture that helps cause athlete's foot.

Steps Toward Prevention

Not surprisingly, keeping the feet clean and dry is of primary importance in preventing athlete's foot. After bathing, the feet should be thoroughly dried, particularly between the toes. A light sprinkling of powder on the feet and in the shoes to absorb moisture will help keep them that way. Shoes should be allowed to air out and dry between wearings. Sandals, open-toed shoes, or thongs, should be worn as much as possible, weather permitting. □

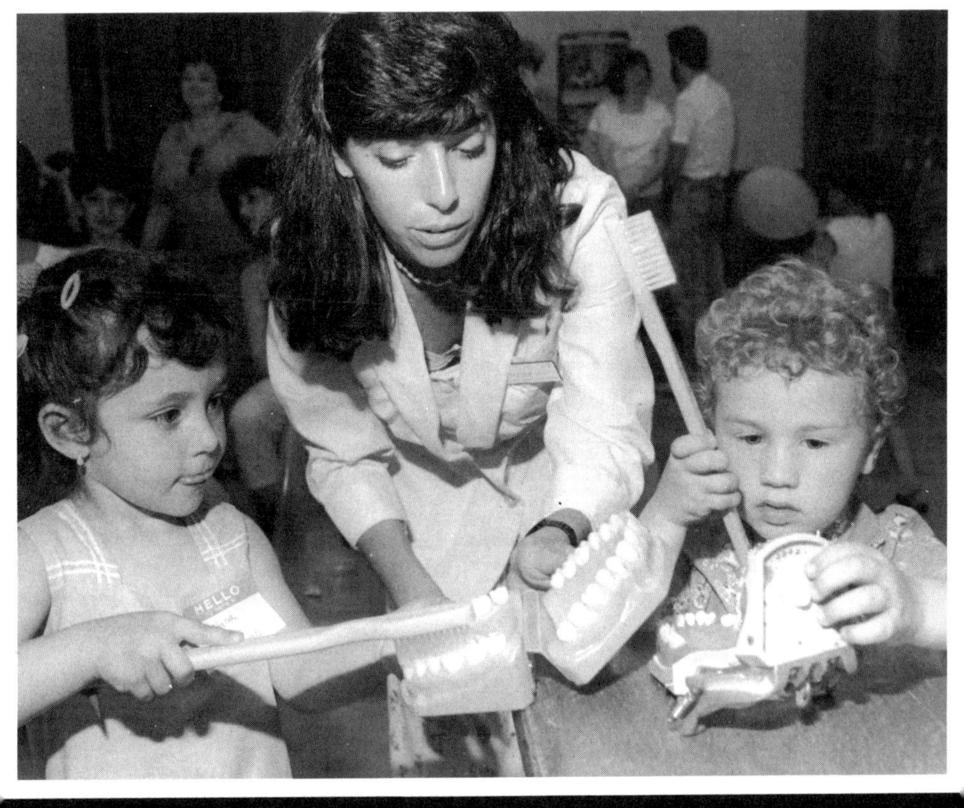

HEALTH AND MEDICAL NEWS

Contributors

Authors of articles in the Health and Medical News section

Boettcher, Iris F., M.D. Assistant Professor, Department of Medicine, Michigan State University; Director of Geriatrics, Butterworth Hospital; Medical Director, Grand Valley Health Center, Grand Rapids, Mich. AGING AND THE AGED.

Bondi, Edward E., M.D. Associate Professor, Department of Dermatology, University of Pennsylvania. SKIN.

Casey, Patrick H., M.D. Associate Professor and Chief, Division of Child Development and Behavior, Department of Pediatrics, University of Arkansas for Medical Sciences; Medical Director, James L. Dennis Developmental Center, Arkansas Childrens's Hospital, Little Rock, Ark. CHILD DEVELOPMENT AND PSYCHOLOGY.

Cohen, Lynne. Ottawa-based medical writer. Instructor in magazine writing, Carleton University School of Journalism. GOVERNMENT POLICIES AND PROGRAMS: CANADA.

Comerci, George D., M.D. Professor, Departments of Pediatrics and of Family and Community Medicine, University of Arizona Medical Center; Director, Pediatrics and Adolescent Medicine, Desert Hills Center for Youth and Families, Tucson, Ariz. PEDIATRICS.

Cowart, Virginia S. Principal, Medical Information Service; Contributing Editor, *Physician and Sports Medicine.* MEDICAL TECHNOLOGY.

Davis, Sharon Watkins, M.P.A. Director, Cancer Information Service, Project Coordinator, Community Clinical Oncology Program, Fox Chase Cancer Center, Philadelphia. CANCER (coauthor).

Engstrom, Paul F., M.D. Vice President for Population Science, Fox Chase Cancer Center, Philadelphia; Professor of Medicine, Temple University Medical School. CANCER (coauthor).

Fisher, Jeffrey, M.D. Associate Professor of Clinical Medicine, Division of Cardiology, New York Hospital-Cornell Medical Center, New York City. HEART AND CIRCULATORY SYSTEM (coauthor).

Hager, Mary. Correspondent, Washington Bureau Staff, *Newsweek.* HEALTHCARE COSTS AND INSURANCE.

Holt, Linda Hughey, M.D. Chairman, Department of Obstetrics and Gynecology, Rush North Shore Medical Center, Skokie, Ill.; Assistant Professor, Rush-Presbyterian-St. Luke's Medical Center, Chicago. OBSTETRICS AND GYNECOLOGY.

Hume, Eric L., M.D. Assistant Professor, Department of Orthopaedic Surgery, Thomas Jefferson University, Philadelphia. BONES, MUSCLES, AND JOINTS.

Hurko, Orest, M.D. Associate Professor of Neurology, The Johns Hopkins Hospital; Scientifc Advisory Board, National Ataxia Foundation and Charcot-Marie-Tooth International; Medical Advisory Board, Little People of America. BRAIN AND NERVOUS SYSTEM.

Jekel, James F., M.D., M.P.H. Professor of Epidemiology and Public Health, Yale University School of Medicine. AIDS; PUBLIC HEALTH; WORLD HEALTH NEWS.

Koenigsberg, Harold W., M.D. Associate Professor of Clinical Psychiatry, Cornell University Medical College; Associate Director of Education, New York Hospital-Westchester Division. MENTAL HEALTH.

Koren, Michael J., M.D. Assistant Attending Physician, New York Hospital-Cornell Medical Center; Fellow in Cardiology, Cornell University Medical College. HEART AND CIRCULATORY SYSTEM (coauthor).

Mandel, Irwin D., D.D.S. Professor of Dentistry and Director, Center for Clinical Research in Dentistry, Columbia University School of Dental and Oral Surgery. TEETH AND GUMS.

Maugh, Thomas H., II, Ph.D. Science Writer, Los Angeles *Times.* GENETICS AND GENETIC ENGINEERING.

McLellan, A. Thomas, Ph.D. Director of Clinical Research, Psychiatry Service, Philadelphia Veterans Administration Medical Center; Associate Professor, Department of Psychiatry, University of Pennsylvania. DRUG ABUSE (coauthor).

Minter, Stephen G. Editor, *Occupational Hazards* magazine. OCCUPATIONAL HEALTH.

Noble, Robert C., M.D. Professor of Medicine, Division of Infectious Diseases, University of Kentucky College of Medicine. SEXUALLY TRANSMITTED DISEASES.

O'Brien, Charles P., M.D., Ph.D. Chief, Psychiatry Service, Philadelphia Veterans Administration Medical Center; Professor and Vice Chairman, Department of Psychiatry, University of Pennsylvania. DRUG ABUSE (coauthor).

Pelot, Daniel, M.D. Associate Clinical Professor, Division of Gastroenterology, Department of Medicine, University of California, Irvine. DIGESTIVE SYSTEM.

Repka, Michael X., M.D. Assistant Professor, The Johns Hopkins University; Consultant, Howard University, Washington, D.C.; Consultant, Sinai Hospital, Veterans Administration Medical Center, Baltimore. EYES.

Rodman, Morton J., Ph.D. Professor Emeritus of Pharmacology, Rutgers University, New Brunswick, N.J. MEDICATIONS AND DRUGS.

Rotherham, James A. Consultant on the federal budget and public policy issues, Reston, Va. GOVERNMENT POLICIES AND PROGRAMS: UNITED STATES.

Spivak, Jerry L., M.D. Professor of Medicine and Director, Division of Hematology, The Johns Hopkins University School of Medicine. BLOOD AND LYMPHATIC SYSTEM.

Thro, Ellen. Science writer specializing in environmental and medical topics. ENVIRONMENT AND HEALTH.

Trenk, Barbara Scherr. Writer specializing in health issues. SMOKING.

Williams, Eleanor R., Ph.D. Former Associate Professor, Department of Human Nutrition and Food Systems, University of Maryland. NUTRITION AND DIET.

Woody, George E., M.D. Chief, Substance Abuse Treatment Unit, Philadelphia Veterans Administration Medical Center; Clinical Professor, Department of Psychiatry, University of Pennsylvania. DRUG ABUSE (coauthor).

Zuckerman, Connie, J.D. Assistant Professor of Humanities in Medicine and Coordinator of Legal Studies, State University of New York Health Science Center, Brooklyn, N.Y. BIOETHICS.

AGING AND THE AGED

High Cholesterol in the Elderly • Setback in Alzheimer's Treatment • Human Growth Hormone and Aging

Treating High Cholesterol

A review published in 1990 discussed the problem of treating high cholesterol in men and women over the age of 60. High cholesterol is a risk factor for coronary heart disease, the cause of death for almost half the U.S. population over 65. Unfortunately, no research has yet been carried out involving exclusively those over 60 to determine if lowering cholesterol levels at that age appreciably reduces the incidence of heart disease or prolongs life.

Since cholesterol levels in the United States tend to increase with age until about age 55 in men and age 60 in women, high cholesterol is most prevalent among the elderly. Low-density lipoprotein (LDL) cholesterol, the component of total cholesterol that is most likely to cause heart disease, also rises with age. The LDL level is better in predicting health problems than is the total cholesterol level, but it is a less powerful predictor in this age group than it is in younger people. That is because as people grow older they have an increased risk of other conditions associated with heart disease and blood vessel problems, such as high blood pressure and diabetes. These conditions appear to be unrelated to higher cholesterol levels. If high blood pressure and diabetes occur in combination, which they often do in the elderly, merely lowering an elevated cholesterol level will not have much impact on preventing heart problems or prolonging life. In these patients it is more important to seek medical treatment for high blood pressure and diabetes, to quit smoking, and to maintain ideal body weight than to lower cholesterol.

Because the term "elderly" covers a broad span of ages, other considerations should be made when deciding to treat high cholesterol. The elderly who should be considered for treatment are those who appear to be in good health and have many years of high-quality life remaining which might be severely impaired by the development of heart disease. Those who do not fit these criteria will receive little benefit from treatment, because studies show that although cholesterol-lowering treatment helps to reduce heart disease and strokes, it takes seven to ten years of treatment before a benefit is seen.

Those eligible for treatment should have a cholesterol profile, which includes LDL, performed on at least two occasions. If on both profiles the LDL is above 160 (160 milligrams of LDL cholesterol per deciliter of blood), treatment should be considered. Careful evaluation and control of other heart disease

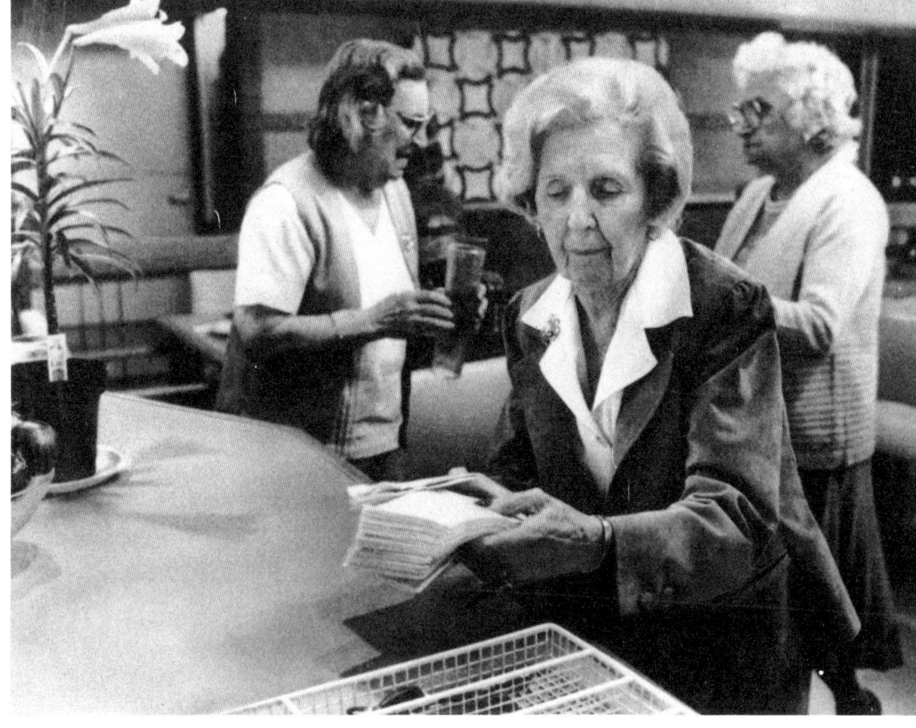

Great disappointment followed the publication of a study reporting that Hydergine, the only drug approved by the U.S. Food and Drug Administration for Alzheimer's disease, may actually not help. These residents of an Ohio Alzheimer's Center, because they are in the illness's early stages, are still able to assist with the chores.

risk factors should be done prior to the treatment of high cholesterol.

Diet modification is the first step in reducing high cholesterol. However, caution should be used in restricting diet too much in older people as their diets are often already inadequate. The diet must provide adequate carbohydrates, protein, minerals, and vitamins. A low cholesterol diet should be followed for at least six months before any further treatment is considered. If after six months the LDL is still above 160, drug therapy may be added to the dietary regimen. Since all of the drugs available to reduce cholesterol have higher toxicity risks in the elderly, they must be given in lower doses and the side effects carefully monitored.

Thus, the review concluded, cholesterol-lowering treatment to prevent heart disease may do more harm than good in some older people. The risk/benefit ratio must be carefully weighed for each older adult (especially for those with declining or fixed incomes for whom the cost of treating high cholesterol may be an unnecessary burden) before considering cholesterol-lowering treatment.

Alzheimer's Drug Ineffective

A study published in 1990 demonstrated the ineffectiveness, and possible harm, of treating Alzheimer's disease patients with the drug Hydergine (a combination of ergoloid mesylates). Hydergine, the 11th most prescribed drug in the world, is currently the only drug approved by the U.S. Food and Drug Administration for treating Alzheimer's disease, a debilitating brain disease that affects one in seven Americans over age 65. Hydergine was thought to improve the brain's ability to transmit messages and reduce memory loss.

For the study, researchers followed for 24 weeks 80 people who had been diagnosed with Alzheimer's disease. Hydergine was given to roughly half of the group, while the other half received a placebo. Standardized tests of behavior and cognitive function were given periodically throughout the study period. Surprisingly, those who had received Hydergine failed to improve or even maintain their cognitive function. In fact, the Hydergine group had more of a decline in cognitive function than the placebo group.

These findings contradicted previous studies in which patients given Hydergine had shown improvement in cognitive function when compared to those given a placebo. A possible explanation is that the recent study was more thorough than any previous Hydergine study. A larger group of people were studied, and they were treated almost twice as long as in any previous study. In addition, each received a complete examination before entering the study in an attempt to include only those who had Alzheimer's disease and no other type of dementia or depression.

Based on this study, Hydergine does not help and may actually harm Alzheimer's patients.

Possible Use of Growth Hormone

A much heralded study published in 1990 showed the possible benefits of human growth hormone in reversing some physical signs of aging. It is believed that a reduction of this hormone causes signs of aging such as increased body fat, atrophied muscles, and wrinkled skin in some older people. Researchers synthetically created the hormone, which is produced naturally by the pituitary gland, and instructed 12 men aged 61 to 81 to inject it at regular intervals. The other nine men in the study received no treatment. At the end of the six-month study period, the men given the hormone treatment showed a significant increase in lean body mass and skin thickness compared to the men given no treatment.

These results were considered highly preliminary, however. While human growth hormone seems to benefit physical appearance, its effects on longevity and health have not been proven, and prolonged use may even be harmful. The long-term effects of synthetic human growth hormone are not known, but large doses are known to cause diabetes, high blood pressure, arthritis, and possibly heart disease or cancer. In addition, this study was performed only on men with an unusually low production of human growth hormone. Although other studies have shown that human growth hormone production decreases with age, the majority of people over age 60 do not have levels low enough to be considered abnormal. The $14,000 yearly cost would also deter most people. At present, the hormone is approved only for very short children who produce none of the natural human growth hormone. Further study is needed before conclusions can be drawn about its benefits for older people.

Iris F. Boettcher, M.D.

AIDS

Medical Personnel With AIDS • A Case From 1959 • The Epidemic Grows • Vaccines and Drugs

Transmission From Infected Doctors

One of the most worrisome events of 1990 was the development of AIDS in a 22-year-old woman who had had no known exposures to the disease except for two tooth extractions in 1987 by a Florida dentist who, unknown to her, had AIDS. She said that the dentist wore gloves and a mask—in accordance with guidelines set down by the U.S. Centers for Disease Control (CDC)—and she did not recall anything that would explain how any of his blood could have gotten into her system. Before his death the dentist wrote that he had consulted experts for advice on how to carry on his practice and had followed the CDC guidelines completely. However, the strain of human immunodeficiency virus (HIV) infecting the patient was similar to the dentist's strain (HIV is the virus that causes AIDS), and experts considered it very likely that he was the source of her infection.

Their conclusion received further support when two other patients of the same dentist also developed HIV infection with strains of the virus similar to the dentist's but different from other strains identified in the community. Neither of the two other patients were in high-risk groups (on the basis of sexual activity, intravenous drug use, or receipt of blood or blood products). One possibility that was considered is that the dentist did some work on himself or others who were infected, and the instruments were not adequately sterilized. However, just how the dentist managed to infect three patients remained a mystery. The infections are apparently the first incidents of AIDS transmission from a healthcare provider to patients.

In two related cases, surgeons with AIDS were discovered to have practiced while carrying HIV. After a careful follow-up of patients of an infected Nashville, Tenn., surgeon, only one was found to be infected with HIV, an intravenous drug user and therefore someone at high risk because of this activity. The patients of a Baltimore surgeon who died from AIDS in November 1990 were being followed up to see if any had been infected and, if so, what other possible exposures might have caused their infections.

The implications of these events for medical and dental care may be far-reaching. The CDC began revising its guidelines for medical and dental practice by doctors with HIV infection, and the possibility of screening medical personnel for HIV was raised. In January 1991 both the American Medical Association and the American Dental Association recommended that practitioners infected with HIV inform their patients about their condition or refrain from performing any surgical procedures.

Earliest AIDS Case

In 1990 doctors in Manchester, England, diagnosed a case of AIDS in a 25-year-old sailor who had died in 1959—the earliest case of AIDS identified to that point. When the patient was first seen, the case puzzled one of the most prominent physicians in England, who wondered if it might represent a new viral disease. The sailor had *Pneumocystis carinii* pneumonia and cytomegalovirus infection, both of which are frequently found in AIDS patients. Fortunately, some of the sailor's tissue was stored, and by applying a new technique of cell analysis called polymerase chain reaction, scientists found evidence of HIV in the sailor's kidneys, spleen, and bone marrow. It was theo-

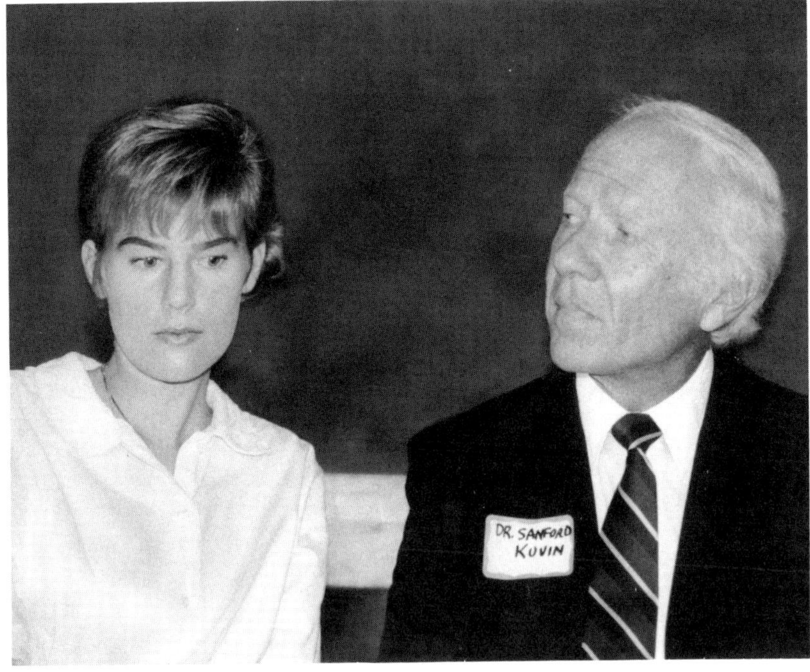

AIDS victim Kimberly Bergalis, left, became the focus of national attention when it was determined that she had apparently contracted the disease from her dentist during a tooth extraction, thus becoming the first documented case of AIDS transmission from a healthcare provider to a patient. With her is Dr. Sanford F. Kuvin of the National Foundation for Infectious Diseases.

rized that he may have acquired his infection from sexual activity in some port.

Size of the Epidemic

By the end of 1990 about 30,000 new AIDS cases had been reported in the United States for that year, although delayed reports were expected to increase the final figure to around 60,000. The total number of Americans who had died from AIDS passed the 100,000 mark in 1990, and the total number of cases reported since June 1981 passed 160,000.

There was uncertainty about how many people in the United States were infected with HIV but as yet had no symptoms of AIDS; estimates were about a million. This meant that even if no more people were to be infected, the epidemic would take decades to wind down unless a cure were to be discovered, because 3 to 5 percent of those infected with HIV develop AIDS each year. For the foreseeable future the CDC estimated continual yearly increases in the number of new AIDS cases, so that unless a cure were to be found soon, AIDS would be a major health problem well into the 21st century.

Improved methods of treating AIDS, which prolong life but do not cure the disease, continued to allow more persons to live longer with AIDS. This, in turn, was pushing up the cost of patient care. Increasing numbers of AIDS patients in the United States were receiving Social Security disability payments. This also meant they were eligible for Medicare coverage, an extra burden on the Medicare system which caused some to fear for its long-term financial solvency.

Mycoplasma and HIV

HIV has become so well accepted by the scientific community as the cause of AIDS that any alternative explanation would face an uphill battle. In 1989 a research team at the Armed Forces Institute of Pathology in Washington, D.C., stated that it believed it had found a mycoplasma (a type of microorganism which is smaller than a bacterium but larger than a virus) that contributes to the development of AIDS. Skepticism greeted this report, but scientists began listening much harder when, in May 1990, Dr. Luc Montagnier, the French scientist who first discovered the AIDS virus, reported the same thing. A continuing puzzle about AIDS is why the virus causes so much damage when there seems to be so little of it in the body. Montagnier suggested that the mycoplasma can stimulate the virus to become much more active and dangerous. Should this theory prove correct, treatment focusing on the mycoplasma cofactor might be an easier way to prolong life than the current medications aimed at the virus itself, which are expensive and toxic. At the very least, physicians' ideas about the ways in which the disease spreads and does its damage would have to be reconsidered.

Because some mycoplasma strains are spread by sexual activity, the mycoplasma theory might explain why AIDS spreads readily and is very severe in geographic areas (such as Africa) and population groups (such as male homosexuals) where transmission is mostly through sexual contact (as opposed to, for example, infected needles). The sexual activity may spread both HIV and the necessary mycoplasma cofactor.

The newly discovered mycoplasma apparently can cause fatal disease on its own. The Armed Forces Institute of Pathology team recovered it from six persons who died quickly from a disease that appeared initially to be influenza. No other infectious organisms known to be capable of causing such a disease were found at autopsy. The mycoplasma is now being studied actively, both as a possible cofactor in AIDS and as an independent cause of disease.

Kaposi's Sarcoma

Kaposi's sarcoma, which starts as a brown or purple skin cancer, is one of the most common killers of homosexual men with AIDS, yet it is rare among hemophiliacs with AIDS, who got the virus from blood products rather than from sexual activity. A study published in January 1990 revealed that Kaposi's sarcoma had been found in homosexual men who did not carry HIV, suggesting that it may be caused by a different, also sexually transmitted, microbe and is merely made worse by AIDS.

Vaccines and Drugs

A number of reports appeared on the development of "promising" vaccines, but while the Food and Drug Administration approved several vaccines for limited testing on humans in the United States, no vaccine was yet ready for the major trials in human populations which must be conducted before a vaccine can be released for general use. Most encouraging were reports that a new vaccine can protect rhesus monkeys from infection by a retrovirus closely related to HIV and that a vaccine from China protects horses from an equine retrovirus. These studies, plus a few others, increased optimism among scientists that an effective vaccine could be developed, but one was not expected to be ready for public use soon.

The first drug to prove effective in delaying the progression of AIDS was zidovudine (sold as Retrovir and formerly known as AZT). After an experimental antiviral drug called DDI showed good results when combined with zidovudine in a clinical trial, AIDS activists mounted a campaign for release of DDI to a wider population before the ongoing clinical trials required by the Food and Drug Administration were completed. The FDA reluctantly agreed in 1989 to cooperate in this "expanded access" program, with the effects on patients being closely monitored. In March 1990, DDI's manufacturer announced that the death rate among patients taking the drug in the expanded access program was more than ten times as high as among those taking it in clinical trials. In addition, six of those taking DDI in the expanded access program died of pancreatitis (an inflammation of the pancreas), and other patients had nonfatal complications, such as diarrhea and painful damage to the nerves of the hands and feet. Some scientists claimed these results meant that the expanded access program of DDI distribution should be stopped. Supporters of the distribution system countered that the patients in the expanded access program (about 8,000) were much sicker than the 700 taking DDI in the clinical trials, so a greater death rate was to be expected.

A closely related drug that also received much attention was DDC (dideoxycytidine), which was being given to a small number of people on an experimental basis. Under pressure from gay activists, the FDA agreed in June 1990 that it too would be offered in an expanded access program, at first involving some 1,000 to 2,000 patients who had failed to respond to, or were unable to tolerate, either zidovudine or DDI.

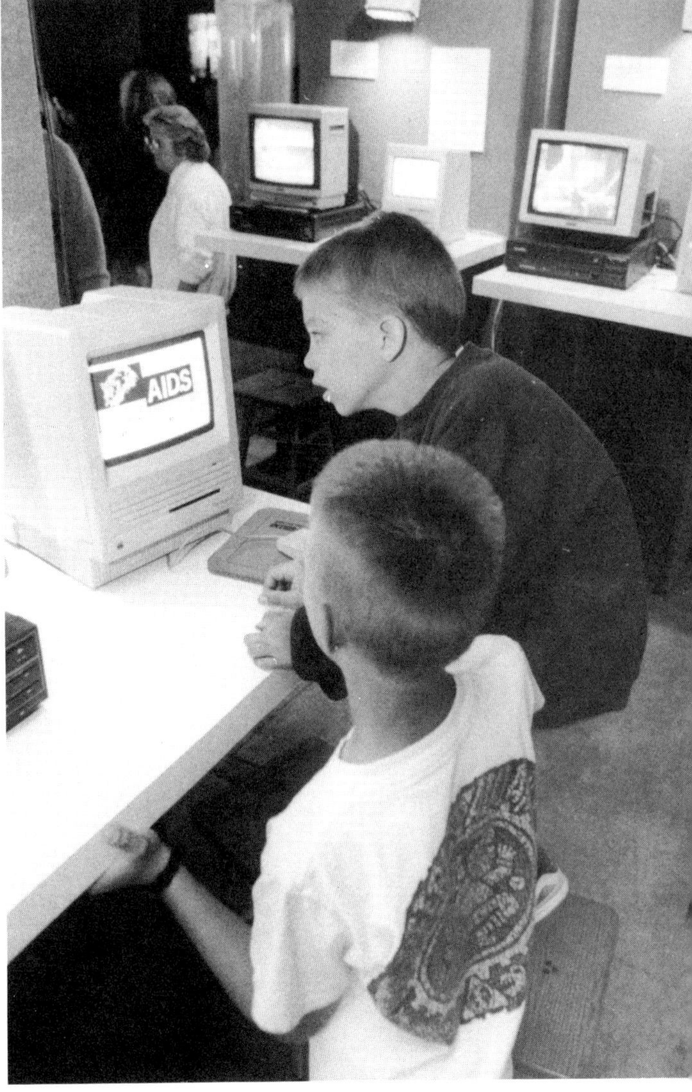

Computers have become pressed into service in the campaign to publicize the facts about AIDS. Here, two youngsters in San Francisco's Exploratorium investigate an exhibit mounted as part of the Sixth International Conference on AIDS.

Tuberculosis

The incidence of tuberculosis was increasing rapidly among Americans infected with HIV, which produced many calls for tough new public health measures to halt the spread of TB. In 1989 some 20,000 new cases of tuberculosis were reported in the United States, which was about equal to the number of new tuberculosis cases in 1960—and much higher than the number reported in the early 1980s. At least half the increase in tuberculosis cases was considered to be due to AIDS, which decreases the body's ability to resist *Mycobacterium tuberculosis*, the microorganism that causes TB. New York City had the largest number of cases of any city in the United States.

International AIDS Conference

The Sixth International Conference on AIDS was held in San Francisco in June 1990. The speakers reported some gains but no real breakthroughs in the battle against AIDS.

One study reported at the conference focused on prostitutes in Nevada, where prostitution is legal in some areas. The researchers found that since 1986, when condoms were required for all sexual activities between prostitutes and clients, there had been no cases of HIV or syphilis infection and only two cases of gonorrhea among prostitutes—a sharp drop in incidence. Another paper reported that HIV-infected men who smoked became ill more quickly with AIDS than those who did not.

Other experts reported that many homosexual men were reverting to high-risk behaviors, despite the major efforts made in the 1980s to warn against those sexual practices most likely to transmit HIV. Younger male homosexuals, many of whom were children when the AIDS epidemic first struck and have not yet seen AIDS among people of their own generation, appeared to be most likely to engage in such risky sexual practices. The reasons men reported for engaging in high-risk sex included partner pressure, drugs or alcohol, not having condoms, or stress. A San Francisco study found that 41 percent of young (age 20-24) male homosexuals studied were infected with HIV. The youthfulness of the group suggested that they were infected recently—during a time when many older homosexuals were engaging in safer practices.

Before 1990 the United States prohibited some persons infected with HIV from entering the country and used a stamp signifying HIV positive on the passports of those infected persons allowed in. In January 1990 these rules were relaxed but not dropped. The San Francisco conference on AIDS was boycotted by some people to protest these rules, and when Dr. Louis Sullivan, U.S. secretary of health and human services, gave an address at the conference, he was drowned out by AIDS activists as a protest against the regulations. In October 1990, Congress passed a revision of the immigration law which removed AIDS from the list of diseases for which a visitor may be excluded from the United States.

On the international front, it was reported in San Francisco that the second known virus to cause AIDS, called HIV-II, which originally was found only in West Africa, had become endemic in an area of Portugal and was spreading, mostly through heterosexual contact. When this virus was first discovered in 1988, researchers were unsure it had the potential to spread globally, as HIV-I had done.

AIDS Hospitals?

Many people proposed the building of AIDS hospitals in the United States—facilities with special equipment and specially trained physicians and nurses to deal with the characteristic problems of AIDS patients. Others, however, remembering that one-disease hospitals, such as those for tuberculosis and mental illness, stigmatized patients while failing to give the best of care, opposed the idea.

New York City created a Task Force on Single-Disease Hospitals which concluded in a 1990 report that AIDS patients should be treated in general hospitals and get care on special AIDS wards or floors, if necessary. The task force reasoned that since AIDS patients have a wide range of complications, they need a broader array of specialists and equipment than an AIDS hospital could afford.

See also the Spotlight on Health article TUBERCULOSIS.

JAMES F. JEKEL, M.D., M.P.H.

BIOETHICS

Bone Marrow Donor Controversy • Rationing Healthcare • The Right to Die • Surrogate Mother Case • Religion and Medicine

Baby Marrow Donor

For two years, the parents of Anissa Ayala, who was dying from leukemia, searched for a compatible bone marrow donor for their daughter. Frustrated by their lack of success, the suburban Los Angeles couple decided to conceive a child to create a potential donor for Anissa. Doctors estimated that Anissa, in her late teens, had a 70 to 80 percent chance of survival with a successful marrow transplant—but no chance of survival without one.

Many experts in the field of bioethics publicly expressed concern over the Ayalas' course of action and questioned the morality of creating one human being to be used for the treatment of another. Critics suggested that the Ayalas' decision violated the fundamental ethical principle that all individuals are ends in and of themselves and that it is unacceptable to use one person to benefit another.

The Ayalas' choice reflected the desperate circumstances often created by the lack of suitable donors. However, it did yield a marrow donor. In defiance of difficult odds, the baby girl that was born in April 1990 had marrow compatible to Anissa's. Because the amount of marrow that can be extracted from a child is much less than from an adult, doctors saved the umbilical cord in order to use its cells as a supplement (recent advances in transplant technology have made it possible to use umbilical cord cells for transplant purposes). At first it was thought that the transplant would have to occur when the baby was six months old, but Anissa's leukemia temporarily stabilized, allowing doctors to postpone the procedure until the baby was about a year old, which would enable them to extract a larger amount of bone marrow. The doctors said that the marrow extraction would pose little risk to the child, who would be put under general anesthesia during the procedure.

Oregon Healthcare Rationing Plan

In recognition of the limited availability of public funds at a time when healthcare costs are escalating, Oregon took steps to limit the availability of certain medical procedures under its Medicaid program. (Medicaid is the federally and state financed health insurance program for the poor.) An Oregon Health

Services Commission developed a computerized listing of 1,600 medical procedures ranked to balance the cost of each procedure against the number of patients who would benefit from it. In drawing up the list the commission took into consideration public debates held around the state to ascertain attitudes toward a variety of healthcare concerns and options. The ranking was intended to be the basis for decisions on which procedures Medicaid would pay for and which it would not.

Oregon first began to place limits on its Medicaid program in 1987, when it denied Medicaid reimbursement for organ transplants. At that time the state defended its policy by explaining that the money saved would provide more Medicaid funding for prenatal care. The new rationing plan was intended to increase basic Medicaid coverage for the poor and to emphasize preventive medicine rather than highly sophisticated procedures that benefit only a few. The plan would not, however, apply to Medicaid recipients who are elderly, blind, or disabled.

Response to the Oregon plan, the first of its kind in the United States, was mixed. There was support for the idea of placing limits on healthcare expenditures and praise for the plan's attention to preventive and primary care. Yet critics questioned the justice of developing a rationing plan which would affect only the poor—and which some considered flawed in its categorization of procedures. Routine treatments for headaches and toothaches, for example, ranked much higher than life-saving interventions in cases of chronic ulcers and advanced AIDS. As a result, a revised plan was released in February 1991. Many well-known diseases, such as pneumonia and tuberculosis, moved up in the rankings, ahead of less familiar or less threatening ones.

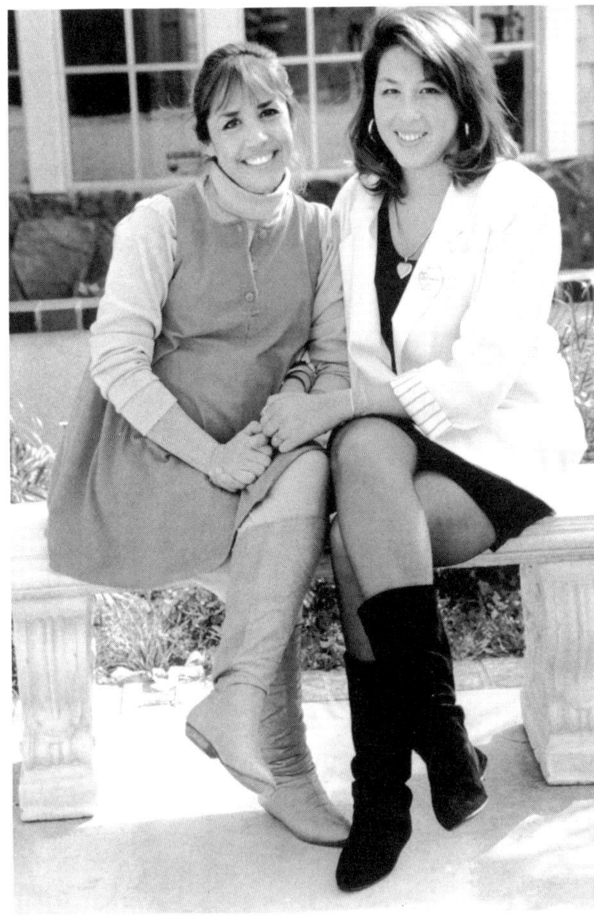

Anissa Ayala, right, appeared to be doomed to die from leukemia for lack of a compatible bone marrow donor until her mother, Mary, left, determined to become pregnant in the hopes of creating a donor—a decision which provoked substantial controversy. Despite long odds, the baby turned out to have compatible marrow.

Suicide and Euthanasia

The right of people suffering from chronic, critical, or terminal illnesses to end their lives—and the role of caregivers in such decisions—figured prominently in the news in 1990.

Suicide Device. Shortly after Dr. Jack Kevorkian, a suburban Detroit pathologist and proponent of active euthanasia (mercy killing), announced his invention of a "suicide device" which permits individuals to inject themselves with lethal medication, he was contacted by Janet Adkins, 54, an Oregon woman suffering from the early stages of Alzheimer's disease. A member of the Hemlock Society, an organization supportive of suicide and euthanasia, she wished to end her life before the disease progressed further. Following a dinner meeting at which Kevorkian decided that Adkins understood the implications of her request, he agreed to allow her to use his device.

After being refused permission to carry out the procedure in various hospitals and funeral homes, on June 4, 1990, Kevorkian set up his machine in the rear of his van. He hooked Adkins to the machine through intravenous tubing, and she was able to push a button that caused her to be injected first with thiopental, which induced unconsciousness, and then with potassium chloride, which quickly stopped her heart. Having assisted in and witnessed the suicide, Kevorkian contacted local officials to inform them of the circumstances of Adkins's death.

In December 1990, Kevorkian was indicted on charges of first degree murder; the charges, however, were later dismissed. In February 1991 a Michigan judge banned him from using the machine again, but

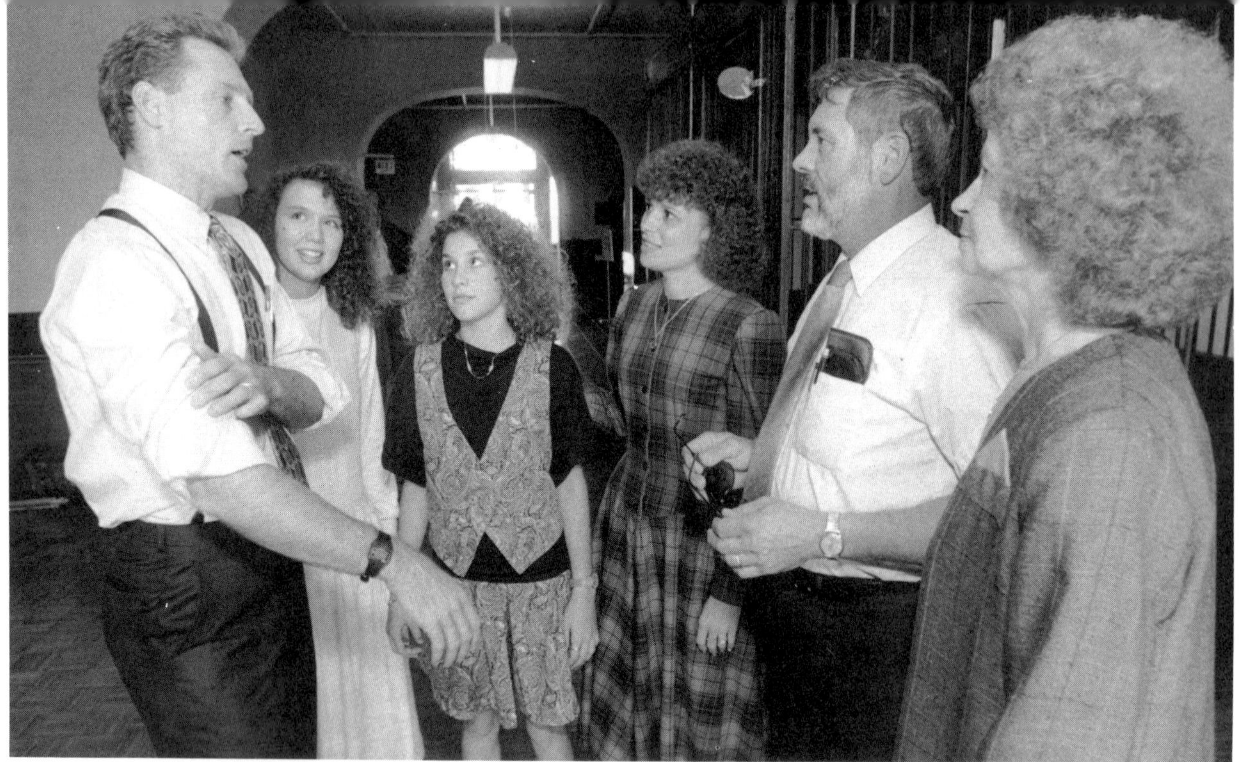

The family of Nancy Cruzan won a bittersweet victory when they finally gained legal approval to have the comatose woman detached from the feeding tube that had been keeping her alive for seven years. Seen in the Carthage, Mo., courthouse are (right) Nancy's parents, Joe and Joyce Cruzan, along with, from left, their lawyer William Colby, their granddaughters Angie and Miranda White, and their daughter Chris White.

he said he would appeal the ruling. Kevorkian also disclosed that he had been advising a cancer-stricken dentist who had built a similar device that he was considering using on himself.

It had been expected that Kevorkian's actions would be viewed by law enforcement officials as assisting a suicide. Michigan law is particularly unclear as to criminal liability for assisting suicide, although most other U.S. states clearly prohibit such help as criminal.

In a related case, three months after Adkins's death, 72-year-old Californian Bertram Harper was indicted in Michigan for murder and conspiracy to commit murder after he told local officials that he had helped his cancer-stricken wife kill herself by asphyxiating her with a plastic bag after she took what she believed was a fatal dose of painkillers. The couple had traveled to Michigan in the belief that the ambiguity of state law on assisting suicide would work in their favor.

The availability and use of Kevorkian's device aroused tremendous public response. Following the news of Adkins's death, a New York *Times*/CBS News poll found that 53 percent of the respondents favored physician assistance for suicide in cases of serious illness, but almost as many (42 percent) opposed it. Many ethicists publicly expressed concern that physician involvement in suicide and euthanasia would undermine the trust patients have in their physicians and would send a mixed message about the doctor's role in caring for seriously ill patients. Yet other commentators noted that the institutionalization and use of sophisticated technology that accompany the majority of deaths in the United States (estimates are that 80 percent of all Americans now die in hospitals) frighten people and may lead them to take their own lives or ask for assistance rather than risk an agonizing death prolonged by technology.

The Cruzan Right-to-Die Case. In 1983, Missouri resident Nancy Cruzan was involved in a critical car accident that left her in what physicians describe as a "permanent vegetative state"—she would never regain consciousness, be able to recognize or relate to others, or in any way care for any of her bodily needs. She could breathe without assistance, but she had to be fed by means of a tube. She was placed in a state institution, and doctors estimated she could live for decades.

Her parents sought legal permission to have Nancy's feeding tube removed, which would necessarily lead to her death. They believed, based on comments Nancy had made prior to her accident, that she would not have wanted to live out her life in a vegetative state. In 1988 the Missouri Supreme Court denied the parents' request and stated that despite Nancy's prior comments, there was no "clear and convincing" evidence that she would have wanted termination of her treatment under her current circumstances. Missouri state law demanded such explicit evidence of a patient's prior wishes before life-sustaining treatment could be withdrawn.

Cruzan's parents appealed this decision to the U.S. Supreme Court, and in June 1990 the Court issued its opinion in *Cruzan* v. *Director, Missouri Department of Health*. In its first consideration of a "right-to-die" case, the Court ruled, 5-4, that Missouri had the right to employ such a rigorous evidentiary standard (and thus deny the Cruzans' request), though no state is required to use this standard. The Court also said there is a 14th Amendment "constitutionally protected liberty interest" which ensures the right of competent patients to refuse life-sustaining treatment and to leave clear evidence of their wishes. Treatment that may be refused includes artificial nutrition and hydration, which the Court considered no different from any other "medical" intervention.

Cruzan's parents continued their efforts to have her feeding tube removed, by renewing litigation on the state court level. Citing additional evidence of their daughter's wishes, they ultimately prevailed. The state of Missouri chose not to oppose their efforts in this new litigation, and Probate Judge Charles E. Teel, Jr., held that there was indeed clear and convincing evidence that Nancy Cruzan would not want her life continued in this way. Following this ruling, Nancy Cruzan's feeding tube was withdrawn, leading to her death 12 days later on December 26, 1990.

Most courts that have ruled in cases involving the withholding or withdrawal of life-sustaining medical interventions have distinguished them from other cases involving what is more traditionally thought of as suicide. While public policy remains against supporting intentional self-destruction, courts and commentators have supported the right of individuals to be free of undesired bodily "invasion," even if such refusals of care lead to serious harm or death.

The Cruzan decision sparked public interest in documents generally known as "advance directives." Through these documents, also known as living wills or durable powers of attorney, competent patients can clearly articulate in advance what types of care they would not want in the event of injury or illness that causes them to lose decision-making capacity. Individuals may also designate someone to make decisions for them in case of unforeseen developments. Depending upon the jurisdiction and the circumstances, these previously expressed wishes of a now-incompetent patient could be respected as though the patient were still capable of making decisions.

In 1990 the U.S. Congress passed the Patient Self-Determination Act, which mandates that all hospitals, nursing homes, health maintenance organizations, hospices, home healthcare companies, and other health-related organizations which receive federal funds must inform patients, upon admission or initiation of service, about that state's laws on refusing, withholding, and withdrawing life-prolonging care. The legislation, scheduled to take effect in late 1991, will most likely lead to increased use of advance directives.

Postmenopausal Pregnancy

Doctors at the University of Southern California reported the occurrence of pregnancy in six postmenopausal women who utilized eggs donated by younger women. Published in the *New England Journal of Medicine*, the report makes clear that biological age, per se, is no longer a barrier to bearing a child. Through the process of in vitro fertilization (in which eggs removed from a woman's ovaries are fertilized in the laboratory), and using a husband's sperm and donor eggs, it is possible for a woman well into her 40s, or even beyond, to become pregnant, although the child will carry no genetic link to her.

As in the case of many other developments relying on sophisticated technology, however, the question remains whether because something is possible it *ought* to be done. This new pregnancy opportunity could extend the enormous financial and emotional burden many infertile couples (and by extension, society at large) already bear in their efforts to conceive a child. The prospect of giving birth at an age when the body may not be as physically capable of withstanding pregnancy raises questions of risk to the woman and potential harm to the fetus. Also, whether society is willing to accept older women with young children could become a perplexing social issue.

Surrogate Motherhood

An unusual instance of surrogate motherhood resulted in litigation in 1990. The case involved Crispina and Mark Calvert, who contracted with Anna Johnson in a surrogate mother arrangement. Unlike other surrogate motherhood cases, in which the sperm of the contracting father is used to fertilize the egg of the surrogate mother, Johnson was implanted with an embryo created through in vitro fertilization using Mark Calvert's sperm and his wife's egg. In essence, Johnson was paid $10,000 to serve as a "gestational mother," carrying to term a fetus with whom she shared no genetic link.

After giving birth to a boy, Johnson sought custody of the child. Orange County (California) Superior Court Judge Richard Parslow, however, denied Johnson's request and awarded sole legal custody of the

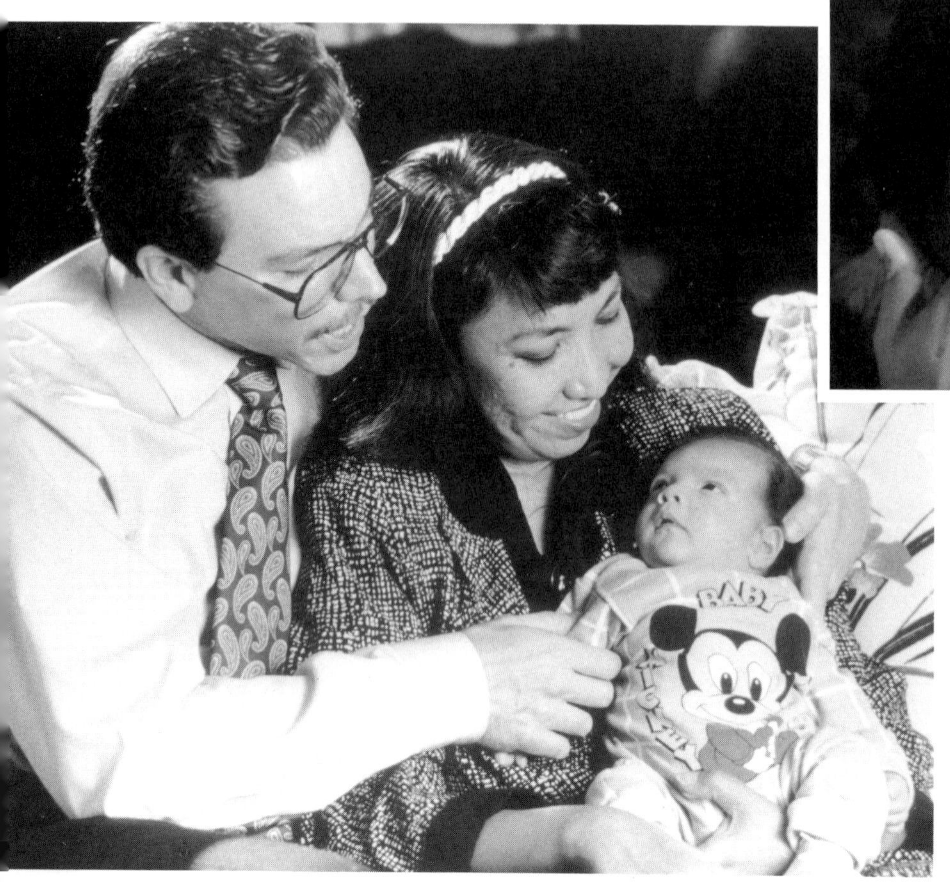

After bearing a baby boy for Mark and Crispina Calvert, left, in a surrogate mother arrangement, Anna Johnson, seen above reacting to her loss in court, unsuccessfully sought legal custody of the child. Since both of the Calverts were the actual genetic parents, the judge compared Johnson's role to that of a foster parent who provides a child a temporary "home."

child to the Calverts. Frustrated by a lack of guidance from judicial precedents or legislation, Parslow emphasized in his decision the importance of the genetic link between the Calverts and the child, and he compared Johnson's role to that of a transitory foster parent who provided a temporary "home" for the child. Parslow questioned the relevance of the "gestational environment" provided by Johnson and looked to the customarily employed legal standard of "the best interest of the child" when he declared, "A three-parent, two natural-mom situation is ripe for crazy making." He continued, "I decline to split the child emotionally between two mothers."

The case served to reemphasize significant public policy concerns about the appropriateness of surrogate motherhood. Questions concerning the exploitation of poor women who may be recruited to serve as surrogate mothers, the lack of consensus on the definition of a "parent," and the similarities of surrogate mother contracts to "baby selling" all influence the public's perception and acceptance of surrogate mother arrangements. Yet many experts view such choices as private reproductive decisions over which government should have no control.

Decisions on Children's Healthcare

Increasingly, public attention has been drawn to cases of severely ill children whose parents use religious counsel and faith healing, rather than conventional medical assistance, to treat the child's health problems. A number of religious groups, including Christian Scientists and Jehovah's Witnesses, shun traditional medical procedures, at least under certain circumstances, as being inconsistent with the tenets of their faith. In several U.S. states in 1990, parents were charged with negligent homicide or manslaughter after a child died without having received traditional medical care.

Perhaps the most prominent case of this kind was the Boston case of David and Ginger Twitchell, devout Christian Scientists, whose two-year-old son died of bowel obstruction after the Twitchells relied on prayer, rather than conventional medical treatment, to cure him. The Twitchells were found guilty of involuntary manslaughter and were sentenced to ten years' probation.

The Twitchells' case and others like it raised many legal and ethical issues. While the majority of states had "exemption" laws—statutes exempting parents from legal charges of child neglect when they rely on treatment through spiritual means—such laws have been increasingly put aside when children die as a result of the course chosen by their religiously devout parents. The religious groups opposing medical intervention consider the prosecutions a fundamental attack on their constitutionally protected right of freedom of religion. Prosecutors and law enforcement officials see their actions as justified under the *parens patriae* doctrine, which empowers the government to act on behalf of those powerless to help themselves (such as children). Prosecutors also seem to be following the guidance of the U.S. Supreme Court when it stated in *Prince* v. *Massachusetts* (1944), "The right to practice religion freely does not include the liberty to expose the child . . . to ill health or death." While it is generally acknowledged that parents in such cases truly believe they are acting in their child's best interest, a societal consensus appears to be emerging to place limits on parental decision-making when a child's life is at stake.

CONNIE ZUCKERMAN, J.D.

BLOOD AND LYMPHATIC SYSTEM

Hormone Fights Cancer-Related Anemia • "Designer Molecule" Treatment for Lymphatic Cancer • Umbilical-Cord Blood Rebuilds Bone Marrow

Erythropoietin Update

Researchers are finding new evidence that anemia can sometimes be successfully treated with a genetically engineered, or "recombinant," form of the hormone erythropoietin, a protein that stimulates production of red blood cells. Anemia is a reduction in the number of red blood cells, resulting in fatigue, weakness, and shortness of breath, among other symptoms.

Two studies published in June 1990, for example, dealt with cancer-related anemia. According to one, the low levels of erythropoietin seen in the blood of anemic patients with malignant tumors may lead to the development of the anemia; the researchers suggested that treatment with recombinant erythropoietin might be beneficial. The other study found that treatment with recombinant erythropoietin helped correct anemia in patients with multiple myeloma, a cancer of the bone marrow.

Thanks to today's biotechnology, scientists can often isolate the genes for specific protein molecules such as erythropoietin and can harness these genes inside cells growing in test tubes to produce large quantities of the protein. (The human body normally makes only minute amounts of most proteins.) The recent availability of such recombinant proteins has permitted the development of sensitive tests to measure the presence of the proteins' normal counterparts in the body. It was through such measurements that scientists learned that anemia is often due to a deficiency of erythropoietin.

Since erythropoietin is produced in the kidneys, it was not surprising that people with severe kidney disease have low levels of it. But scientists soon found that some anemic individuals suffering from certain other disorders also have low levels of erythropoietin even though their kidneys are normal. Studies have suggested that treatment with recombinant erythropoietin can correct anemia associated not only with kidney disease and certain forms of cancer but also with rheumatoid arthritis and AIDS. (A 1990 study showed that it may help counteract the anemia that develops in some AIDS patients as a side effect of taking the drug zidovudine, or Retrovir.) Not only do many anemic patients with these disorders have an increased sense of well-being, but many no longer require blood transfusions. While occasionally lifesaving in cases of anemia, blood transfusions can be hazardous, since they may reduce the body's ability to resist infection or cancer and they carry the risk of an allergic reaction to the transfused blood.

In persons scheduled to undergo elective surgery, erythropoietin therapy has been successfully employed to improve their capability to donate their own blood for any transfusions they may need. A person's own blood is safer than other people's, but the amount of blood that an individual can donate is normally limited. However, pretreating a patient with recombinant erythropoietin can increase the amount of blood the person can donate while avoiding the development of anemia.

"Designer Molecules" Versus Lymphatic Cancer

Drugs used in treating cancer tend not to distinguish between cancerous cells and normal cells—a fact that limits the amount of drug that can be safely given to cancer patients. In some cases, however, scientists can now design molecules that attack only a specific type of cell. This approach has recently been employed to treat several types of lymphatic cancer.

The white blood cells known as lymphocytes, in contrast to other cells, are rich in an enzyme called adenosine deaminase. This enzyme prevents the accumulation within lymphocytes of adenosine-contain-

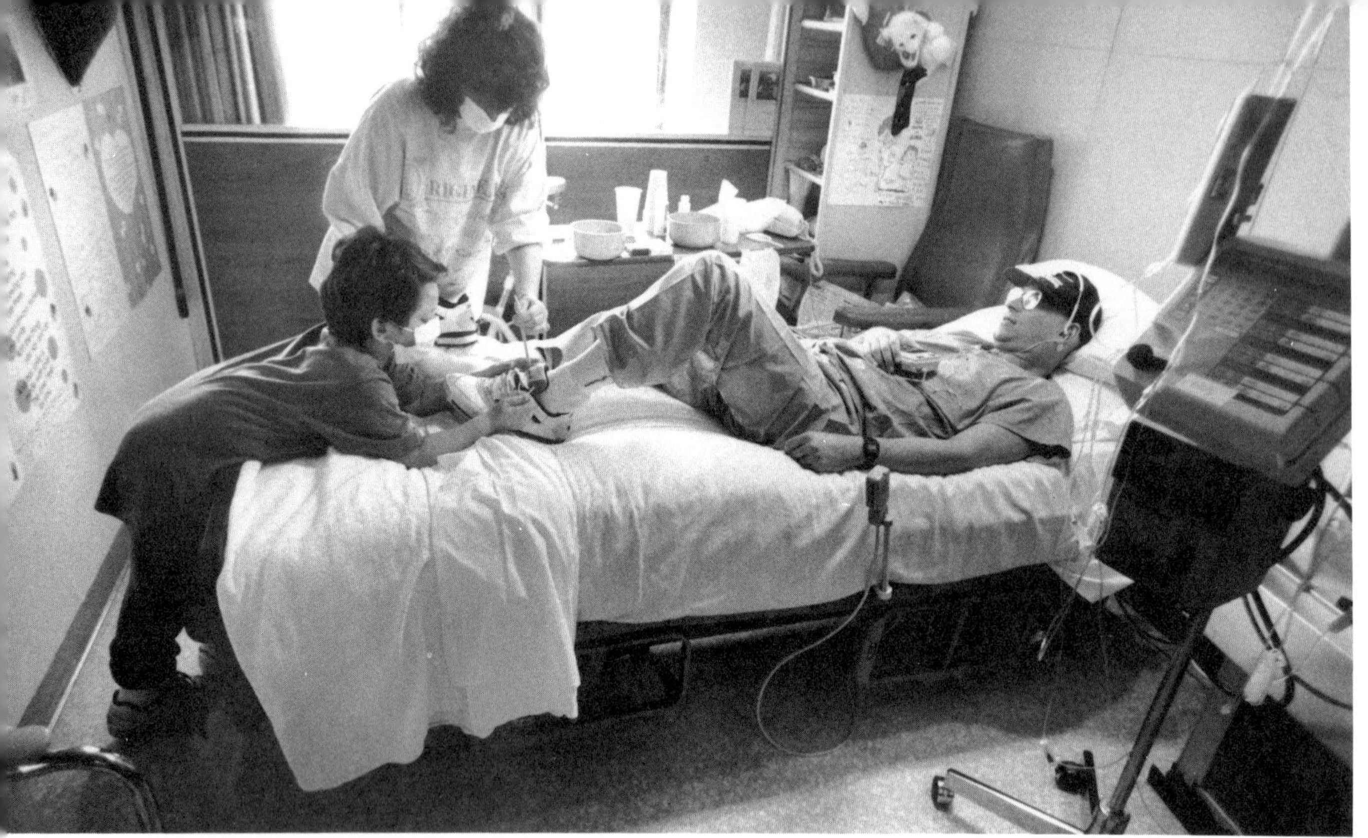

Faced with the prospect of death from leukemia, a cancer of the blood, California lawyer Marc Smith underwent an "autologous" bone marrow transplant—with himself as the donor—in a Seattle hospital in March 1990. The marrow, which produces blood cells, was removed from his hipbone and treated with chemotherapy before being returned to his body. After a period of complete isolation, Smith was visited by his wife and youngest son, above. Later, Smith was free to resume a normal life at home, right, taking weekly blood tests as a precautionary measure.

ing molecules, which are building blocks for DNA. Accumulation of such molecules causes lymphocytes to die, but other types of cells are not sensitive to adenosine and its derivatives. By designing an analogue of adenosine that cannot be broken down by adenosine deaminase, medical scientists have created a method of killing cancerous lymphocytes while sparing other types of cells. One such "designer molecule," 2-chlorodeoxyadenosine, has been successful in substantially reducing the extent of several types of lymphatic cancer in patients, with few side effects. A 1990 study of hairy-cell leukemia, in fact, found that a high percentage of patients had complete remission of the cancer.

Drug Therapy for Sickle-Cell Anemia

Research published in 1990 suggested that hydroxyurea, a drug used for certain types of leukemia, might prove an effective treatment for sickle-cell anemia.

In sickle-cell anemia, which is an inherited lifelong condition most common among black families, the hemoglobin in red blood cells has a slightly different structure from that of normal hemoglobin. (Hemoglobin carries oxygen to tissues.) The sickle-cell hemoglobin molecule, known as hemoglobin S, differs by a single amino acid from normal adult hemoglobin, or hemoglobin A. As a result, hemoglobin S molecules aggregate, or clump together, with each other. This usually happens when the amount of oxygen in the blood is reduced, as occurs in the veins. The aggregation not only damages red blood cells but causes them to become rigid and sickle-shaped, so that they obstruct small blood vessels, producing pain and leading to tissue damage through oxygen deprivation.

To date, there has been no effective preventive therapy for the periodic painful crises that occur in sickle-cell anemia patients. In the 1980s, however, partly by means of studies in monkeys, scientists discovered that hydroxyurea and other drugs used to treat certain forms of leukemia can stimulate the production in red blood cells of a form of hemoglobin usually present in large quantities only before birth. This fetal hemoglobin, or hemoglobin F, will not form aggregates with hemoglobin S and thus prevents the red cell changes caused by the genetic defect responsible for sickle-cell disease. The extent to which treatment with hydroxyurea or similar drugs will improve the lives of sickle-cell anemia patients continues to be studied. The hydroxyurea treatment is mild and does not interfere with daily activities.

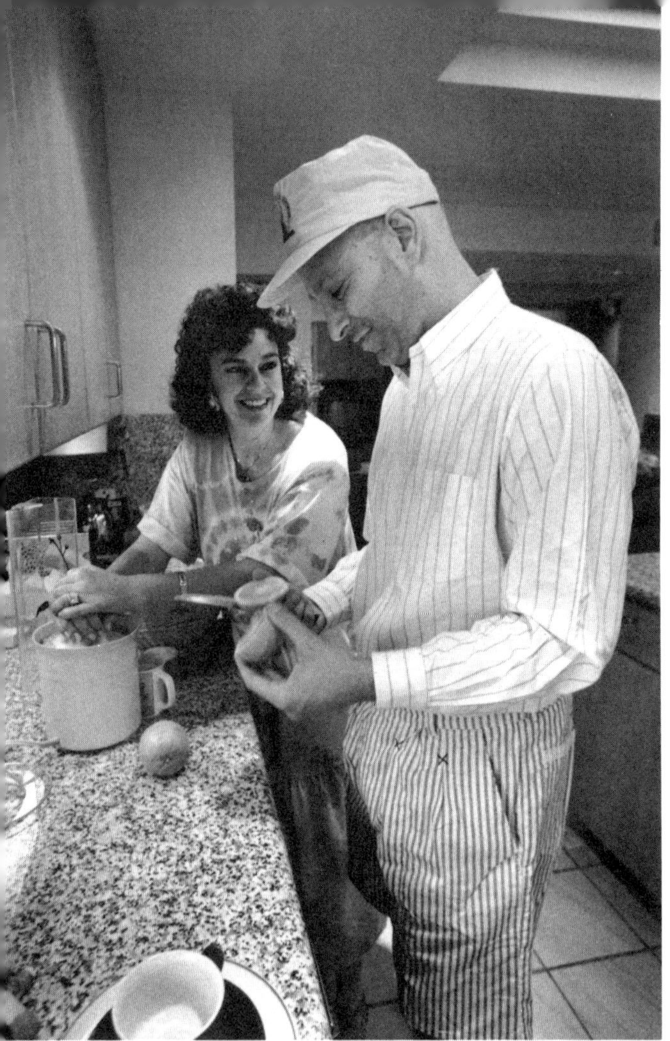

Bone Marrow Failure

The 1990 Nobel Prize in medicine or physiology was awarded in part for the development of bone marrow transplantation as a practical treatment. In children and adults with bone marrow failure, transplantation of healthy bone marrow from a suitable donor can be not only lifesaving but also curative. Finding a suitable donor, however, can be a major problem. The donor must have an immune system compatible with that of the patient requiring the transplant and must also be able to donate the quantity of bone marrow cells necessary for a successful transplant. It now appears that an alternative treatment may be able to help some patients who have a newly born brother or sister. Researchers have found that umbilical-cord blood from newborn infants contains enough blood-forming "stem" cells to restore bone marrow function to normal in some cases. The first successful use of umbilical-cord blood to correct bone marrow failure was reported in 1989. It was used to cure an inherited form of this problem called Fanconi's anemia. The technique is currently being applied to other forms of marrow failure in patients for whom no marrow donor is available. JERRY L. SPIVAK, M.D.

BONES, MUSCLES, AND JOINTS

Correcting Uneven Limbs • Preventing Blood Clots After Orthopedic Surgery • Lowering the Risk of Bone Infection

Surgery for Uneven Limbs

Surgeons continue to expand the methods available to correct limb length inequalities. While uneven arms tend to present mainly cosmetic problems, in the legs inequalities of more than an inch can cause functional disorders such as back pain and difficulty walking.

Problems that can lead to unequal leg lengths include congenital abnormalities, neuromuscular disorders, and injuries to the growth centers in a child's leg from a fracture or an infection. In younger children, who are still growing, the inequality can sometimes be treated by destroying selected growth centers in the longer, unaffected leg. When the child's growth is completed the legs will be equal in length but shorter than they normally would have been. Another approach to treating a growth center injury is to try to remove the bony scar from the growth center with the hope that the injured leg will then be able to grow more nearly to its potential.

If the leg length discrepancy exceeds the remaining growth potential of the shorter leg or occurs in an adult with no growth potential, a surgeon may elect to shorten the longer leg by removing a portion of bone. This can be done using instruments inserted through a small incision in the buttock region. In general, for technical reasons related to the muscles, nerves, arteries, and veins, shortening is better tolerated in the thigh bone than in the shin bones, although excessive amounts of shortening in either region will cause muscle weakness. Also, a short lower leg compensated by a shortened thigh on the other leg will give the patient uneven knees, despite even hips.

An important treatment method still being evaluated is bone lengthening. In a technique that has been used successfully for several years, the limb is immobilized in an external fixator, or frame, with connecting pins that are inserted through the skin and into the bone. The bone is then cut between the sets of pins, and the limb is gradually stretched. Sometimes the gap created by the cut fills spontaneously with new bone, but frequently a bone graft must be performed. The fixator is then removed and a plate is applied to the bone to stabilize it while bonding of the graft takes place. The plate is removed one or two years after its installation.

A newer technique, developed by Gavriil Ilizarov, a Soviet surgeon, is more complex technically, using multiple fine wires rather than pins, a more careful method of cutting the bone, and a slower rate of elongation of the limb. The bone is cut in such a way as to avoid injuring the blood vessel that goes through the center of the fatty marrow or cutting the membrane (the periosteum) around the bone's surface, both of which are very important to new bone formation. The slower rate of elongation allows the blood vessel and periosteum more time to fill in the gap with new bone as the gap is widened. Once the desired length is attained, only a short period of further immobilization in a fixator is required. In comparison with the older technique, which frequently required three operations—the pin placement and bone cut, pin removal and grafting, and plate removal—the Ilizarov technique frequently requires only the initial operation for pin placement. Both techniques, however, have a high complication rate. They are uncomfortable, require much daily care, and present a constant risk of infection, bone malalignment, and joint, muscle, nerve, and blood vessel complications. Still, for major limb length discrepancies in a person for whom shortening would be impractical, these techniques at least offer the hope of enough limb length to correct deformity.

The Ilizarov technique can also be used when there is significant bone loss from trauma or infection. In these cases the limb length is appropriate but a gap exists in the bone. The Ilizarov equipment essentially pulls the gap closed by moving the entire bone segment on one side of the gap to meet the other. This creates another gap at the other end of the bone being moved, but the slow rate of movement allows new bone to form in this second—healthier, unscarred—region. This procedure carries with it a significant rate of complication but also offers the potential benefits of salvaging an extremity that may be difficult to salvage by the more traditional techniques.

Blood Clots and Surgery

Orthopedists are studying ways to prevent an important surgical complication, pulmonary embolism, the medical term for blood clots that form in the large veins of the legs and travel to the lungs. If a blood clot lodges in the arteries supplying blood to the lungs, it can cause shortness of breath, chest pain, coughing up blood, rapid heartbeat, and, in some cases, death. Three conditions that contribute to the likelihood of a blood clot developing in the leg veins are inactivity, blood that is prone to clotting excessively, and injury to a vein in the leg. Orthopedic surgery often creates

Flat Feet Boot Bad Reputation

The flat foot has long been regarded, by grandmothers and doctors alike, as a defective model, sure to cause pain and suffering somewhere along the line. Over the years children with flat feet have been made to do foot exercises and wear inserts in their shoes in attempts (usually futile) to create gracefully arched insteps. Some have even undergone surgery. During World War II, recruits with flat feet were categorically turned down by the U.S. military, on the grounds that flat feet are more prone to injury.

The military later changed its policy, and recently the U.S. Army published a study that may forever change the flat foot's bad reputation. The study found that flat feet are not only functionally normal but might be better suited to rigorous physical activities than arched feet. The study evaluated the number of foot injuries among some 300 Army infantry trainees and discovered that flat-footed soldiers had far fewer injuries than those with moderate to high arches. In fact, trainees with high arches had twice as many injuries as the flat-footed, including sprains and stress fractures. The flat foot, it seems, is more flexible than an arched foot and thus better able to absorb stress.

Although not all orthopedists agree that flat feet are advantageous, most have seen enough problem-free flat feet that they no longer automatically view them as a liability.

Normal, healthy flat feet should not be confused with flattened feet or fallen arches. When a foot is placed under too much stress, from prolonged marching, for example, the ligaments supporting the arches collapse, and the foot develops a flattened appearance. And sometimes a very painful flat foot in a child or young adult is a sign that some of the bones have fused. In both cases, a doctor's care is needed.

What's important is not how a foot looks, but how it functions and feels.

all three of these conditions because it generally necessitates bed rest, the tendency of blood to clot increases in the period immediately after surgery, and veins are injured during an operation. In early hip replacements, the rate of fatal embolism was 1 to 2 percent—an unacceptably high rate of fatal complication for an elective procedure. Theoretically, the clots could be prevented if the blood could be thinned adequately, but a patient after surgery whose blood has been thinned excessively may end up with potentially fatal bleeding at the surgical site.

Over the years a variety of blood-thinning drugs, including aspirin, heparin, and warfarin, have been used to combat clot formation. For elective hip replacement surgery, many medical centers use warfarin at half the dosage normally used to treat an established blood clot in the leg. Several new large studies have shown that this lower dosage appears to be very effective in preventing fatal embolism or blood clots traveling to the lung, but the same studies show a 20 to 30 percent rate of blood clot formation in the calf. Such clots can cause calf pain and swelling and, more seriously, long-term swelling and impairment in the leg. Because warfarin's blood-thinning effects are very difficult to reverse, its use is limited in situations where the patient may require further surgery.

Heparin continues to be an important anticoagulant. When administered at carefully adjusted doses, it is effective at preventing blood clots from forming in the deep veins and traveling to the lungs. Researchers are currently investigating combinations of heparin, warfarin, and bootlike devices that intermittently compress the calf to keep the blood from pooling in the lower legs.

Bone Infections

A second dreaded complication of orthopedic reconstructive surgery is bone infection. The very low blood flow and dense structure of bone make it difficult to treat with antibiotics and inhibit the ability of the natural immune defenses to fight infection. The presence of a surgical implant further interferes with the blood supply; several types of bacteria are known to adhere to such implants.

In the past decade progress has been made toward lowering the risk of bone infection following surgery. The use of preventive antibiotics before and after the operation has significantly decreased the rate of infection. Many hospitals that do a significant amount of joint reconstruction have begun installing special air filters and air circulating equipment in their operating rooms to cut down on airborne bacteria. Clean air is directed toward the patient's wound; it then circulates through the room before being sucked back into the filtering device. The air pressure in the operating room is kept slightly higher than normal to prevent the air outside the room from coming in. In addition, surgical teams wear space helmet-like devices with air filtration systems so that the normal bacteria they exhale don't contaminate the surgical wound. As much of the patient's skin as possible is covered with a variety of synthetic fiber and plastic drapes and wraps to prevent bacteria from the patient's sweat and oil glands from entering the surgical wound. Finally, the patient is kept in isolation during the recovery period.

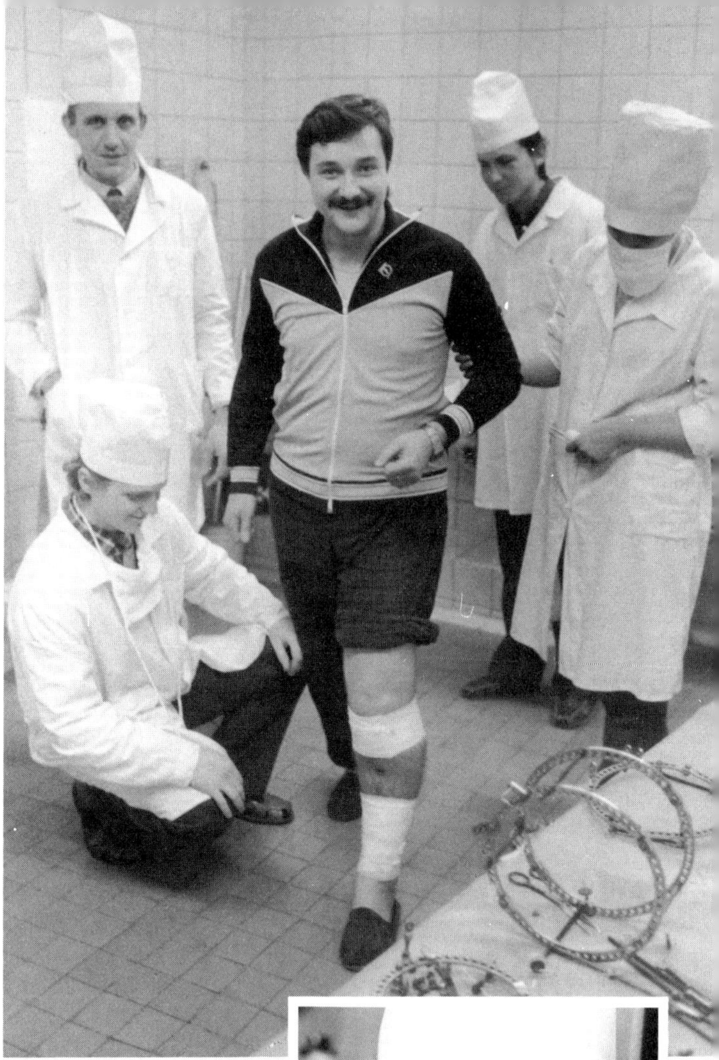

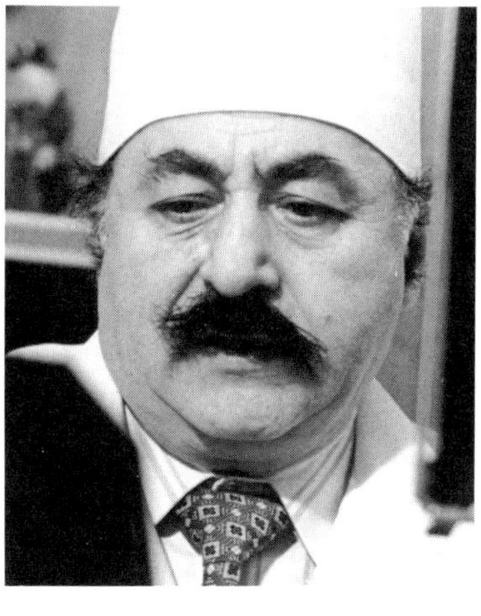

A man whose shin bone was shattered by a rubber bullet tests out his newly repaired leg. The framelike device on his left allowed the uninjured portions of his shin bone, plus new bone growth, to fill in the gap left by the wound. The technique was developed by Soviet orthopedist Gavriil Ilizarov (right).

These precautions have lowered the infection rate of total hip and total knee replacement to approximately 1 in 400, down from 3 to 4 percent in early operations. ERIC L. HUME, M.D.

BRAIN AND NERVOUS SYSTEM

Genetic Diseases of the Nervous System • AIDS and the Brain

Genetic Diseases

Neurofibromatosis Discovery. In July 1990 researchers in Michigan and in Utah used a process called positional cloning (formerly known as reverse genetics) to determine the gene responsible for von Recklinghausen neurofibromatosis, commonly called Elephant Man disease. Neurofibromatosis is the most common nervous system defect caused by a single gene; it affects one out of roughly every 3,500 people. The gene responsible for the disease was found to be a tumor suppressor, which normally holds cell growth in check. A defect or mutation in the gene predisposes individuals to the formation of multiple tumors of peripheral nerves and the brain. To date, the only available treatment has been surgical removal of accessible tumors. Knowledge of the responsible gene will now guide the development of medical treatment.

Locating Other Genes. Von Recklinghausen neurofibromatosis is only one of many degenerative diseases of the nervous system on which a worldwide explosion of genetic research has shed valuable light in recent years. Most of these disorders, which have long baffled the medical profession, are uncommon, but collectively they pose significant hardship to a large number of individuals.

Each kind of these diseases targets a particular part of the nervous system and results in characteristic disabilities. Hereditary ataxias, such as Friedreich's ataxia, selectively involve the cerebellum, progressively impairing coordination. Peripheral nerve diseases, such as Charcot-Marie-Tooth disease, and muscular dystrophies, such as Duchenne muscular dystrophy, result in progressive weakness of the arms and legs. Other disorders, such as Huntington's disease, cause deterioration of higher brain centers, progressively impairing movement, mood, and intellectual ability.

It has long been suspected that each of the complex neurological diseases mentioned above stems from a single biochemical error or mutation. Knowledge of what this is would permit more accurate diagnosis of a disease, ideally before it takes its toll on the nervous system. In some circumstances, knowledge of the mutation may permit design of more effective treatment.

Until recently, the mutations responsible for these diseases have been maddeningly elusive. Normal functioning of the nervous system depends on a complex cascade of thousands of individual chemical reactions, each influencing many of the others. Neuropathologists analyzing brain specimens from affected patients by traditional biochemical and microscopic techniques encounter a confusing myriad of deviations from normal. In only a small handful of diseases has it been possible to determine which biochemical alteration is the primary culprit, which merely a secondary change.

The power of molecular genetics lies in its ability to identify the location of a gene underlying a disorder, even if there are no biochemical clues. In humans, there are 100,000 individual genes, each encoding either an enzyme that catalyzes a particular chemical reaction or a structural protein that serves as a scaffold on which cells and tissues are erected. The vast majority of these genes are in the cell nucleus, arranged like beads on 23 pairs of string-like chromosomes. Except for those on X and Y sex chromosomes, each gene is represented twice—once on a chromosome inherited from the father and once on a chromosome inherited from the mother.

Certain diseases, such as Charcot-Marie-Tooth disease, are dominant—that is, a person is born with the disease even if only one of the two copies of the relevant gene is mutant. Others, like Friedreich's ataxia, are recessive, that is, a person is born with the disease only if both copies of the relevant gene are mutant. Parents randomly transmit either member of a chromosome pair to each of their children. Individuals affected with a dominant disorder have a 50 percent chance of transmitting the same disorder to each of their children. Parents who each have one copy of the mutant gene responsible for a recessive disease have a 25 percent chance of transmitting the disorder to each of their children.

If the location of the gene responsible for a neurological disease is known, it is possible to determine if the chromosomes inherited by a particular individual contain normal or mutant genes. In the last five years, the chromosomal locations of genes responsible for Charcot-Marie-Tooth disease and Friedreich's ataxia—and dozens of other neurological disorders—have been determined. This has been accomplished through a process known as linkage analysis. In linkage analysis, investigators analyze DNA specimens, usually obtained from small blood samples, to keep track of which chromosome segments an affected individual has received from each parent. A chromosome segment consistently present in affected individuals, but absent in normal relatives, must contain the responsible gene.

In addition to providing information for genetic counseling, identification of the chromosomal segment responsible for a given disorder has in several instances already allowed identification of the offending gene itself, as was the case with the gene responsible for von Recklinghausen neurofibromatosis.

Investigators are now working on tracking down the genes suspected of underlying more common neurological and psychiatric disorders. Many of these disorders, such as Alzheimer's disease, schizophrenia, and even alcoholism, have long been suspected of running in families, although it has been difficult to pin down a simple inheritance pattern. In February 1991 researchers discovered that a mutation in a single gene is associated with some cases of Alzheimer's. Other research has suggested that two different genes can each cause some cases of the disease. It is possible that diseases other than Alzheimer's may also be caused by more than one gene. And research is continuing into whether some cases of Alzheimer's and other disorders are caused by physical or psychological stresses in the environment.

AIDS and the Nervous System

In 1990 the broader medical community became more aware of what AIDS specialists regard as a rather surprising finding—that the most common form of nervous system disease encountered in AIDS patients, AIDS-related dementia, does not appear to involve the immune system but instead appears to result from direct invasion of brain cells by the AIDS virus itself. Indeed, autopsy studies aimed at quantifying the number of AIDS virus particles present in different organs have found more particles in the brain than in the lymph nodes and spleen, both organs associated with the immune system. AIDS-related dementia causes loss of intellectual function and shrinkage of the brain.

It has long been known that the AIDS virus selectively targets certain cells of the immune system called T4 helper-inducer cells. The normal function of these cells is to combat infection and prevent the development of certain tumors. Impairment of these cells in AIDS patients predisposes them to infection with microorganisms that rarely cause disease in individuals with normal immune systems. Many of these so-called opportunistic infections affect the nervous system. Chief among them is cerebral toxoplasmosis—the formation of multiple solid pockets of infection, or abscesses, within the brain—which causes paralysis, incoordination, or changes in personality over the course of several days. Others include encephalitis (generalized brain inflammation) and meningitis (inflammation of the membranes covering the brain).

Occasionally, the immune system affected by AIDS turns on the nervous system directly, attacking it as if

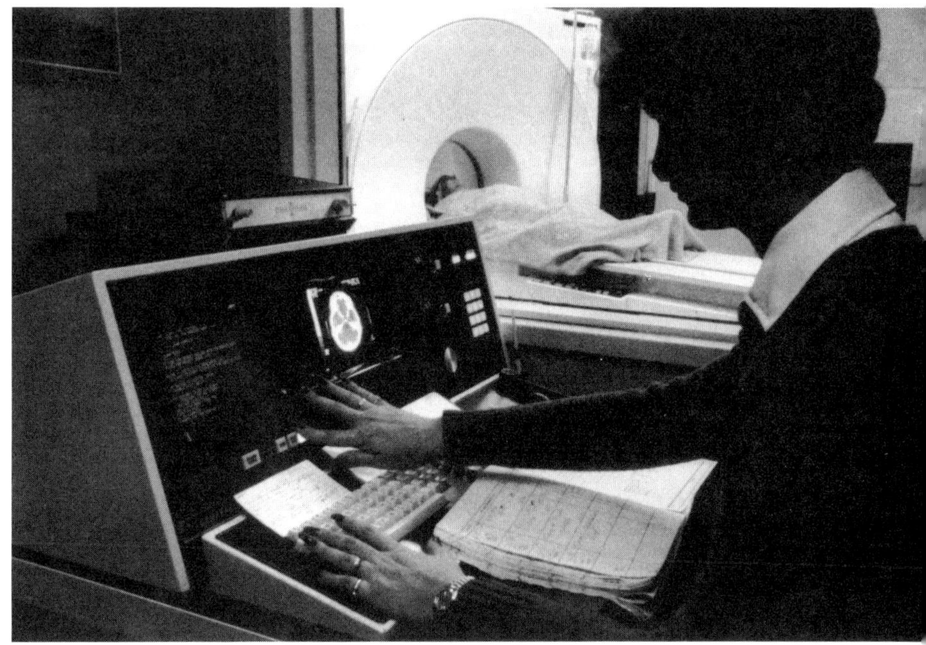

Chief among the many opportunistic infections that can affect the nervous systems of AIDS patients is cerebral toxoplasmosis, which creates pockets of infection in the brain. These abscesses can now be detected by computed tomography, or CT scans, of the brain, such as the one being administered here.

it were a foreign invader. This is most clearly seen in the development of Guillain-Barré syndrome—a rapidly progressive paralysis of arms and legs that results from an immune attack on the Schwann cells, specialized cells that insulate the peripheral nerves. This syndrome commonly occurs in individuals not infected by the AIDS virus but it appears that AIDS patients are more susceptible. Other forms of immune-mediated attack on the nervous system include inflammation of muscles (myositis), the spinal cord (inflammatory myelopathy), and individual nerve bundles (mononeuritis). OREST HURKO, M.D.

CANCER

Genetic Link for Lung Cancer • Fatty Diet Tied to Breast and Colon Cancer • New Therapies for Malignant Melanoma

Cancer Death Rates

The death rate from cancer in the United States has steadily increased over the years. The number of cancer deaths per 100,000 people rose from 143 in 1930 to 171 in 1987. Lung cancer, caused primarily by smoking, was the major cause of this increase. Age-adjusted cancer death rates for many other major types of cancer, such as uterine and stomach cancer, have declined over the past 50 years. There are over six million Americans alive today who are cancer survivors.

Prevention and Early Detection

New diagnostic techniques have enabled medical researchers to develop new tests for cancer, while improvements in old tests have increased their accuracy. Studies continue to confirm the dangers of cigarette smoke and smoking and the benefits of a low-fat, high-fiber diet.

Doppler Vibration Imaging. Efforts to detect prostate tumors using conventional ultrasound, where sound waves are bounced off tissues to produce an image, have not been very successful. A new ultrasound technique, called doppler vibration imaging, uses a speakerlike horn to generate very low frequency sound waves that cause tissue to vibrate. Cancerous tumors are more rigid and vibrate less rapidly than healthy tissues, and a doppler device can detect this difference in tissue motion and display a color image of it. Researchers are testing the technique on prostate and breast tumors.

Pap Test Improvement. New standards for reporting results improved the Pap test, which has helped to reduce illness and death from cervical cancer over the past 40 years. When women get regular Pap tests, abnormalities are more likely to be found early when they can be cured. The test's developer, George Papanicolou, originally devised a system of reporting test results based on five classes: Class I smears were normal, Class II smears showed minor cell abnormalities, Class III smears showed suspicious cell abnormalities, and Class IV and V smears showed definite cancer cells. This reporting system was used by most U.S. laboratories, but many labs modified the interpretation of the classes. Tissue pathologists then came up with additional classifications based on how likely it was that abnormal cells would turn into cancer. Because of this confusion in reporting, doctors were not able to compare results from different labs.

In December 1988 a group of experts met under the auspices of the U.S. National Cancer Institute and developed a new, uniform reporting system for cervical smears. The new system requires the lab report to include information about whether the smear was adequate (had enough cells and was taken correctly), a primary assessment of whether the smear was normal or not, and a descriptive diagnosis of any abnormalities.

Mammography. In October 1990 the U.S. Congress added mammography benefits to Medicare. Coverage for breast cancer screening for women 65 and older and the disabled began in January 1991. Mammograms, X rays of the breast using specialized equipment, are the best method of detecting breast cancer at its earliest, most curable stage. The National Cancer Institute recommends that every woman over 40 get a mammogram every two years and annually after age 50.

In spite of these recommendations, less than a third of American women over 40 have regular mammograms. The main reasons appear to be that physicians often fail to advise their patients to have mammograms and that many insurance plans do not cover the procedure, making it unaffordable for poor women. Confounding the issue further, the quality and accuracy of mammograms is unequal from one screening center to the next, and not all U.S. states have licensing procedures for the technicians who operate mammography machines. Anger over these conditions and over the lack of attention and funds given to breast cancer has spurred activists and lobbying groups in recent years to push for better regulation of mammography standards, mandatory insurance coverage of mammograms, and more federal money for research into the causes and prevention of breast cancer.

Genetics. Researchers continue to make advances in locating certain genes, called oncogenes,

ALL WOMEN ARE
ARE AT RISK FROM
BREAST CANCER!
MORE FEDERAL
FUNDS TO
FIGHT CANCER
END THE EPIDEMICS
IGNORED
EPIDEMIC!
LET'S
GET RID
OF
CANCER
We Do Not Accept
the FACT that:

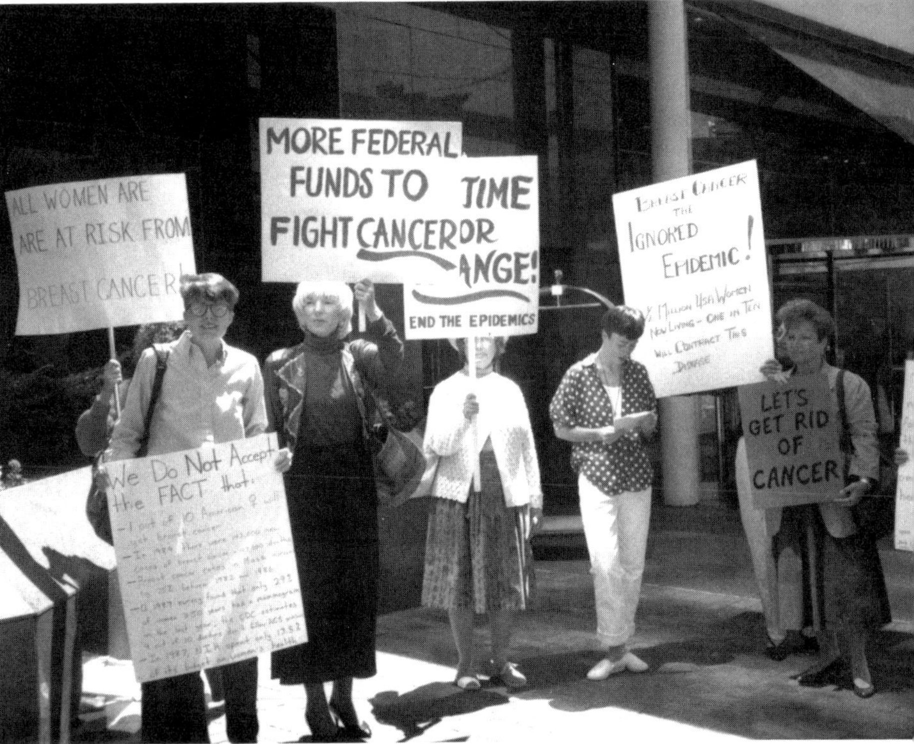

"The Ignored Epidemic" is what many have begun to call breast cancer. Frustrated by the lack of insurance coverage, the government's failure to regulate mammography standards, and what they perceive as the sluggish pace of research, activists have begun to take to the streets in protest.

that seem to have a role in initiating or promoting cancer. In August 1990 it was reported that patients with a certain type of lung cancer were more likely to suffer a relapse or to die sooner after surgery if they had a mutation in what is called the K-ras oncogene.

A genetic factor is also suspected in susceptibility to lung cancer. One study showed that cigarette smokers who inherit the ability to quickly metabolize the high blood pressure drug debrisoquine (not approved for marketing in the United States but sold under the brand name Declinax in Canada) are six times more likely to develop lung cancer. The smokers who keep the drug in their bodies for longer periods of time are less likely to get cancer. A separate study also found a pattern of lung cancer incidence in the families of lung cancer patients that suggested certain family members had inherited a gene that raised their chances of developing the disease.

Smoking. Smoking is still the biggest factor in getting lung cancer. Researchers have known for over 25 years that people who smoke cigarettes are significantly more likely to develop lung cancer than nonsmokers. New studies show that being exposed to other people's smoke can also increase the chances for lung cancer. Results of one study showed that household exposure to 25 or more "smoker-years"—calculated by multiplying the number of years in each residence by the number of smokers in the household—during childhood and adolescence doubled the risk of lung cancer. The findings suggest that about 17 percent of lung cancers among nonsmokers can be attributed to high levels of exposure to cigarette smoke during childhood and adolescence.

The good news about smoking was presented in the Surgeon General's 1990 report, *The Health Benefits of Smoking Cessation*. The report concluded that quitting smoking results in longer life and better health for people of all ages, even those in older age groups. Benefits apply both to healthy people and to those already suffering from smoking-related diseases. Quitting smoking decreases the risk of lung cancer, many other cancers, and other heart and lung diseases.

Nuclear Power Plants. A study initiated in 1987 by the National Cancer Institute and reported on in 1990 found that residents of counties containing or adjacent to nuclear facilities do not have a higher risk of dying from cancer than residents of similar counties without nuclear facilities. Researchers used county mortality records dating from 1950 to 1984 to compare cancer death rates from 16 kinds of cancer before and after the nuclear plants started operating. They also compared the rates with counties with similar populations that are not near nuclear facilities. Despite their conclusions, the study's authors cautioned that the study had limitations and did not necessarily prove that nuclear facilities are harmless.

Diet and Cancer. Research results continued to confirm the role of fat and fiber in breast and colon cancer. Colorectal cancer survivors and people whose rectal surface cells proliferate at an abnormally rapid rate have a high risk of developing or having a recurrence of colon cancer. A recent study of colorectal cancer survivors showed that eating two-thirds of a cup of high fiber cereal daily induced a dramatic reduction in cell proliferation among patients with a rapid baseline rate. The study helped researchers understand how fiber works to prevent colon cancer and also demonstrated that changing one's diet can have a big effect within a short time.

A large-scale study of Western diets published in December 1990 found a strong link between colon cancer and consumption of animal fat. Researchers followed the diets of nearly 89,000 women in the United States for six years. It was found that women who ate a daily main dish of beef, pork, or lamb had 2½ times the risk of developing colon cancer of women who ate red meat less than once a month. On the other hand, women who ate skinless chicken two or more times a week had half the risk of those who ate it less than once a month. No association was found between high-fat dairy products, which also contain animal fats, and colon cancer. The researchers said the cancer rate might be related to a high total intake of animal fat but did not rule out the possibility that red meat itself contains cancer-causing chemicals.

Reducing dietary fat intake could decrease the risk of breast cancer, concluded two studies published in April 1990. A study of American women found an increased incidence of invasive breast cancer from 1960

"Left out" and "confused" are two of the terms that describe the feelings of children who have brothers or sisters with cancer, which is why Memorial Sloan-Kettering Cancer Center in New York City has established workshops to answer some of their questions. Here, doctors and a make-believe patient shed some light on what is, to the kids, one of the center's biggest mysteries—the operating room.

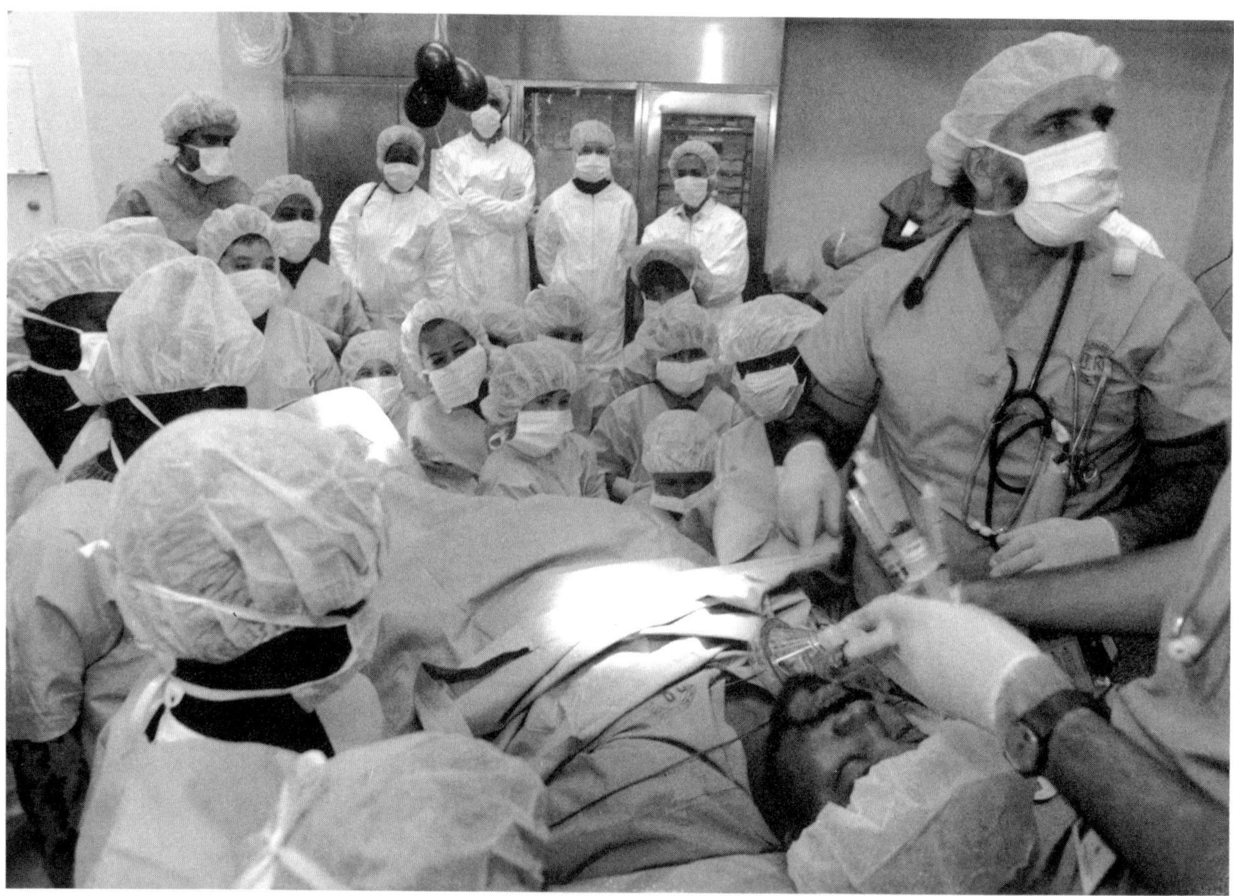

to 1985 among women age 45 and over. The study also found that the incidence of breast cancers that are stimulated by the hormone estrogen increased much faster than the incidence of those that are not. The researchers believe that fatty diets could be a major contributor to these increases. Obesity can elevate circulating estrogen levels in older women, possibly making them more prone to estrogen-stimulated breast cancer. An analysis of data from 12 studies of diet and breast cancer indicated that if North American women were to lower their daily saturated fat consumption to 9 percent of total calories, down 30 percent from the current average level, the breast cancer rate among postmenopausal women would fall 10 percent.

A study of cruciferous vegetables such as broccoli, cabbage, and bok choy found that they contain a chemical that assists the body in converting more estrogen into an inactive form. Thus, eating more crucifers might lower the risk of developing estrogen-fueled breast cancer.

Treating Breast Cancer

As the incidence of breast cancer in the United States continued to rise, researchers studied how to tell which patients would benefit from additional treatment after surgery and whether bone marrow transplants were beneficial in the treatment of breast cancer. From 1973 to 1987 breast cancer increased by 25.1 percent in whites and 27.2 percent in blacks. Much of this increase can be attributed to the growing use of mammography screening. Through mammography, women are finding breast cancers earlier. Indeed, the proportion of early breast cancers rose in the 1980s, especially in women 50 and older. Some scientists think that changing risk factors may also play a major role in the increasing breast cancer incidence. These risk factors include changes in diet, delayed childbearing and longer usage of oral contraceptives, and increased alcohol consumption.

Women whose breast cancer is detected early, when the tumor is small and is confined to the breast, have the best long-term survival rates. To see if the cancer has spread outside the breast, doctors look for cancer cells in the lymph nodes under the arms. Lymph nodes, also called lymph glands, are small, bean-shaped structures that act as filters, collecting bacteria or cancer cells that may travel through the network of channels that carry lymph fluid. If the lymph nodes contain cancer, the patient is a candidate for postsurgery chemotherapy or hormonal therapy. Even if the lymph nodes have no cancer cells, some women will benefit from additional treatment after surgery. Researchers looking for factors that can help predict which women would benefit the most from the extra treatment found that the cancer cells in these women have one or more of the following characteristics: a high percentage of cells that are dividing at any one time; an increased chromosome number; more signs of activity by a specific oncogene; or cells that are not stimulated by estrogen.

The National Cancer Institute is evaluating bone marrow transplantation as a treatment for advanced breast cancer. Bone marrow transplantation has traditionally been a last-ditch treatment for cancers that involve the entire lymph or blood system, such as lymphoma or leukemia. Its use has increased with recent improvements in the technique, especially the development of genetically engineered colony stimulating factors, hormones that increase the production of blood cells to help replenish the transplanted bone marrow.

The type of bone marrow transplantation being used experimentally for breast cancer is called autologous, because bone marrow is taken from the patient, stored, treated, and reinfused. After the bone marrow is removed, the patient is treated with whole-body radiation or high doses of chemotherapy to wipe out hidden cancer cells. The stored bone marrow is examined for cancer cells, and if any appear, they are killed with drugs. The marrow is then reinfused into the patient. Researchers have discovered that by growing marrow cells in a culture medium, they can detect small numbers of cancer cells that might have been missed using conventional cell staining techniques. Women whose breast cancer has metastasized, or spread throughout the body, can call the NCI's Cancer Information Service at 1-800-4-CANCER to get information about the bone marrow studies. For the first time ever, 15 Blue Cross and Blue Shield plans and a major health maintenance organization, US Healthcare, have agreed to participate in the funding of these clinical trials.

New Treatment Methods

A new testing process to discover anticancer drugs and three experimental therapies for malignant melanoma are expanding the treatment options for cancers that do not respond to existing chemotherapy or radiation.

Drug Discovery Screen. The National Cancer Institute developed a new method of testing 300 to 400 chemicals weekly to see if they kill a broad array of human tumors. Each new chemical is placed along with cancer cells from seven types of cancer in tiny wells on a plate and incubated for two days. Then the cells are stained and checked by computer to see if they grew normally or died. Researchers hope the new drug screen will help them identify new chemotherapy agents more quickly.

Malignant Melanoma. A new trial is underway to test a vaccine against malignant melanoma, a potentially deadly form of skin cancer. Melanoma is the most serious type of skin cancer, killing an estimated 6,000 Americans per year. Although the vaccine cannot prevent cancer, it has shown success in keeping the cancer from coming back after surgery. It works by stimulating the patient's immune system to destroy melanoma cells. Side effects of the vaccine have been minimal.

Another approach in treating melanoma deploys human monoclonal antibodies. These specialized proteins, which are similar to the antibodies normally produced by the immune system to fight disease, are made from specially cultured human cells in a laboratory. Monoclonal antibodies bind only to particular target cells and so can be used to attack tumors directly or deliver poisons selectively to cancer cells. In the past, scientists made monoclonal antibodies from mouse cells, but this sometimes triggered life-threatening allergic reactions in human patients. Human monoclonal antibodies offer a solution but have so far been grown only in small quantities. In a recent procedure, researchers cultured three kinds of infection-fighting cells from melanoma patients. These cells make antibodies directed against molecular markers found only on cancer cells. Tiny amounts of the antibodies were injected directly into the cancerous growths of patients with recurrent melanoma. Results of the experimental therapy were very promising: many tumors disappeared after injection, and some patients began producing their own antibodies in response to the injections.

Gene Therapy. In November 1990 scientists at the National Institutes of Health received final approval from the U.S. Food and Drug Administration to begin the first study using human gene therapy to treat cancer. In January 1991 two patients with advanced melanoma that had not responded to conventional treatments received transfusions of specialized, tumor-fighting white blood cells that had been taken from their own bodies and altered in the laboratory by inserting the human gene for a natural toxin called tumor necrosis factor (TNF). The gene-spliced cells were then cultured in growth factors until they multiplied to several hundred billion cells, and some of the cells were reinfused in the patient. It was hoped that the altered cells would seek out tumors and infiltrate them with enough of the toxin to kill the cancer. The patients were to receive increasingly larger doses of cells for about a month.

In the past the same type of white blood cells have been used unaltered to treat cancer, but only about half of patients showed any improvement. TNF alone has been shown to kill cancer cells by shutting off the blood supply, but humans cannot tolerate large enough doses to make it effective. By targeting the TNF directly to the cancer tumors using the white blood cells as vehicles, the researchers hoped to achieve the potency of TNF without toxic side effects.

Basic Research

Basic researchers continue to try to discover how cells grow and behave under different conditions. Ultimately, they seek to understand how cancer occurs in the first place and how treatments can be improved to combat it more effectively.

Preventing Hair Loss. One treatment that has proven effective against many different kinds of cancer is chemotherapy, or treatment with cancer-killing drugs. Most chemotherapy works by interfering with cells that are dividing rapidly. This works to kill cancer cells, since one characteristic of cancer is uncontrolled growth. Unfortunately, many chemotherapy agents also kill healthy cells that divide rapidly, such as the cells that produce hair. As a result, a common side effect of chemotherapy is hair loss. A new drug being developed for use against leukemia unexpectedly prevented hair loss when tested on mice. When used in combination with standard chemotherapy, the drug, ImuVert, blocked the leukemia more effectively than chemotherapy alone and additionally blocked the hair loss induced by other anticancer drugs. ImuVert is also being studied in humans to combat brain cancer.

Drug Resistance. Another problem with chemotherapy is that some cancer cells become resistant to the drugs being used and continue to grow in spite of increasing dosages. Researchers have used laboratory techniques for many years to try to understand what allows cancer cells to survive the onslaught of normally toxic drugs. New studies indicate that the test-tube studies of the past may not be telling the whole story. In vivo studies (studies done inside a living animal or human) show that resistant tumor cells in the body appear to rely in part on interactions with noncancerous tissues. Chemotherapy-resistant breast cancer tumor cells were first grown in mice and then transferred to a laboratory dish. When exposed to chemotherapy in the dish, the cells showed no resistance, but when they were reinjected into other mice, their resistance returned almost immediately. This study may help doctors to give chemotherapy on more effective schedules, allowing chemotherapy resistance to fade between treatments.

Oxygen and Cancer. Oxygen deprivation followed by reoxygenation seems to enhance cancer aggressiveness. When researchers shut off oxygen to cancer cells, then flooded them with oxygen, the reoxygenated cells developed aggressive qualities and increased ability to survive anticancer drugs. Other studies found that cancer cells located far from blood vessels—and thus from the oxygen supply—showed a greater tendency to metastasize, or spread, to distant parts of the body after being exposed to oxygen. This work brings into question new cancer therapies that work by cutting off the blood supply to tumors.

See also the feature article LIFE AFTER CANCER.

PAUL F. ENGSTROM, M.D.
SHARON WATKINS DAVIS, M.P.A.

CHILD DEVELOPMENT AND PSYCHOLOGY

Mother-Child Attachment • Quality of Child Care and Success in School • Low Standards of Math Achievement • New Hope for Premature Infants

The Attachment Relationship

Two studies published in 1990 advanced understanding of the relationship between a mother and her child during infancy, the attachment relationship. This relationship affects how well children function intellectually, behaviorally, and socially in later years.

The Role of Physical Closeness. Research has shown that the amount of early physical contact between a mother and her infant improves the security of attachment. In a study published in October 1990, researchers investigated whether the increased physical contact between a mother and her child resulting from use of the kind of soft baby carrier that holds the baby securely against the mother's body during infancy would result in more secure emotional attachment later on. Forty-nine mothers from similar backgrounds took part in the study. They were assigned randomly either a soft baby carrier or a plastic infant seat for the newborn children. When the children were 13 months old, the 23 mothers who received the soft baby carriers were found to be more sensitive to and more likely to respond to their infants' vocalizations than the other mothers. Of the infants who used the soft carriers, 83 percent were securely attached to their mothers, compared to only 38 percent for those carried in the plastic seats. This study shows that a simple measure such as using a soft carrier, taken early in the child's life, can foster a healthier mother-child relationship.

Attachment and Success in School. A study of the association between mother-child attachment and social competence in first grade was published in February 1990. Security of attachment as assessed in infants has been found to be positively associated with peer and teacher reports of behavior in the first five years of life. Researchers wanted to determine if this remains true for older children. The study included 89 six-year-old children (42 boys, 47 girls) and their mothers. All were from white middle-class backgrounds. The quality of attachment was measured in a laboratory setting during the summer before the children entered the first grade, with researchers assessing the children's behavior when they were reunited with their mothers after a one-hour separation. In the fall, ratings of behavior and liking were collected from peers and teachers. Boys who were insecurely attached to their mothers were less well liked by peers and teachers than were securely attached boys; the insecurely attached boys were also seen by their classmates as being more aggressive and were rated by teachers as having more behavior problems and being less competent. There were no such associations with girls; the researchers were not able to pinpoint any definite reason for this finding. The findings showed that, for boys, quality of attachment at six

Snuggling up to baby with one of these soft infant carriers brings real psychological benefit, a new study reported. Researchers found that such close physical contact fostered a greater degree of attachment between mother and child.

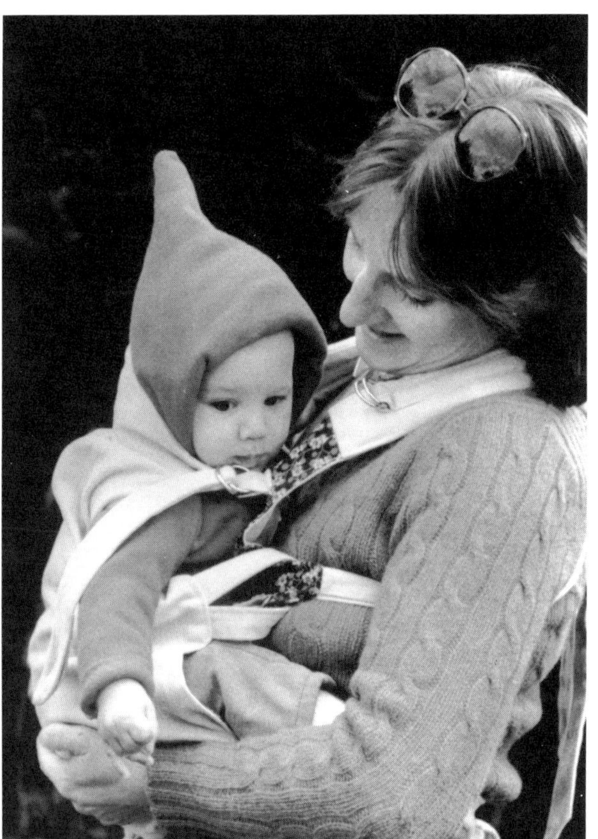

years of age is associated with social competence in the classroom.

Child Care and Social Adjustment

A 1990 study from Los Angeles clarified the complex relationship between behavioral adjustment of children in kindergarten, the age they were placed in child care, the quality of the child care, and family characteristics.

The study included 80 middle-class children, their families, and their child care centers and continued until the children were in kindergarten, where the children were given behavior ratings by their teachers. The children were classified according to whether they entered child care as infants (12 months of age or less) or toddlers and according to the quality of the child care they received. The parents who enrolled their children in low quality child care were found to be less involved and invested in their children's behavior, reported their lives to be more complex, and were less well integrated into social networks, such as friends or community groups, than parents who enrolled their children in high quality care. Children who entered low quality child care as infants had the most difficulty with peers and received the poorest behavior ratings in kindergarten. Children who entered low quality care as toddlers fared better on behavior ratings but were rated more hostile and less competent in peer play than were the children enrolled in high quality care at any age. There were no differences in behavioral adjustment between children who entered high quality care as infants and those who entered as toddlers. Family socialization practices were the primary influences on adjustment to kindergarten for children enrolled in child care during the toddler years. However, the quality of child care was the most powerful predictor of adjustment to kindergarten for children who were enrolled in child care during infancy.

The findings show that placement in low quality child care is more likely to result in adjustment problems in school, but that the placement itself is influenced by family characteristics that independently affect children's behavior.

See also the feature article HOW TO CHOOSE CHILD CARE.

Poor Math Achievement

A study published in August 1990 by Chinese and American researchers demonstrated that first and fifth grade Chinese children scored consistently higher on mathematics tests than their American peers.

Chinese and U.S. researchers evaluated 1,630 first and fifth graders from 11 schools in Beijing and 1,975 children from 20 schools in Chicago. All children were given a test involving computation and a subgroup were tested on their application of mathematical concepts. In addition to the mathematics tests, interviews regarding attitude toward mathematics were administered to the children, their teachers, and some of the Chinese and American mothers.

The scores of American children were significantly below those of the Chinese children on nearly all the tests. Chinese children solved problems more rapidly as well. However, when interviewed, only 8 percent of American children found mathematics to be "hard" or "very hard" compared to 20 percent of the Chinese children, and 52 percent of the American children judged their mathematics achievement to be "above average" or "among the best" compared to only 29 percent of the Chinese children. More American children than Chinese children thought their parents were pleased with their mathematics performance and, indeed, most of the American mothers were satisfied with their children's performance while less than half of the Chinese mothers were satisfied. In general, mathematics held a lower status in the eyes of the American than the Chinese teachers. The researchers concluded that American children have widespread deficiencies in the area of mathematics. The American children's positive self-evaluation in spite of this reflects the low standards held for their performance by American parents and the relative de-emphasis on mathematics by American teachers.

New Hope for Premature Infants

According to a report published in June 1990, the developmental and behavioral status of some low-birth-weight (LBW) premature infants can be improved by the time they are three by participation in an early intervention program. LBW premature infants, who comprise around 7 percent of all U.S. births, are considered more likely than normal-sized newborns to have developmental, behavioral, and health difficulties in later childhood. While intervention programs such as Head Start that target children from low income families have yielded successful results, there has been little adequate research into whether early intervention would work for LBW infants. One persistent problem has been concern that placing young LBW infants in group settings, which might expose them to more infectious conditions, could endanger the health of this vulnerable population.

Researchers in eight U.S. cities recruited a total of 985 premature infants from families of varying economic and educational backgrounds. All had weighed less than 5.5 pounds at birth and two-thirds had weighed less than 4.4 pounds. From the time the infants left the hospital until they reached three years of age, they were monitored in a medical follow-up clinic according to standard procedure and were referred for medical and other services as needed. In addition, one-third of the infants (including some from both the heavier and the lighter groups) were assigned randomly to the intervention program. This included routine home visits until the child reached age three, during which health information, educational activities, and parental support were provided; child attendance from the ages of one to three at a child development center, which used an educational program tailored to each child's needs in a small group setting; and bimonthly parent group meetings.

At the age of three, all of the children in the study were given intelligence, behavioral, and health tests. The average IQ score was significantly higher in children who had participated in the intervention program (93.5) than in those in the comparison group (84.5). The latter were nearly three times more likely to have IQ scores below 70, which is in the range of mental retardation. The mothers of the intervention group reported significantly fewer behavior problems. The mothers of the lighter birth weight infants in the intervention group reported more minor illnesses than did the comparison group's mothers, but there was no difference in the frequency of serious illnesses, and there were no serious accidents or epidemics at any child development center. The study showed that a comprehensive early intervention program has substantial promise of decreasing the number of LBW premature infants at risk for later developmental disabilities, and that such an intervention can be performed safely with this biologically vulnerable group.

PATRICK H. CASEY, M.D.

DIGESTIVE SYSTEM

Drugs Affect Alcohol Metabolism • Help for Slow Stomach Emptying in Diabetes • New Colon Cancer Treatment

Medications Affect Alcohol Metabolism

How fast a person gets drunk is influenced by a number of factors including the type of alcoholic beverage being consumed, the speed with which it is ingested, and the presence of food in the stomach. Researchers now say that the use of certain antiulcer medications and aspirin also influence how much alcohol is digested in the stomach and how much is absorbed into the bloodstream.

Antiulcer Medications. Some antiulcer medications may inhibit the action of a stomach enzyme, alcohol dehydrogenase (ADH), that metabolizes, or breaks down, some alcohol before it enters the bloodstream, researchers reported in May 1990. As a result, those taking the medications, called H-receptor antagonists, attain higher blood alcohol levels for a given amount of alcohol ingested. About 10 percent of the American population suffers from peptic ulcer disease (sores in the lining of the stomach or upper small intestine) for which these drugs are used.

Investigators found that H-receptor antagonists such as cimetidine (Tagamet), ranitidine (Zantac), and nizatidine (Axid) may inhibit the activity of ADH in the stomach. However, another of these agents, famotidine (Pepcid), was not shown to have this effect. Further studies are needed to establish how great an influence these medications have on blood alcohol levels. In the meantime, doctors warn people taking these drugs to consider avoiding alcohol.

Aspirin. Researchers also have linked higher blood alcohol concentrations with aspirin consumption. In a study involving five healthy men between 30 and 45 years of age, all ate the same breakfast then some took two aspirin tablets and some took no aspirin. One hour after breakfast all five drank an ounce of alcohol. The subjects ingesting two aspirins following breakfast had higher blood alcohol levels than those who did not take aspirin.

Although the increase in the blood alcohol level caused by aspirin consumption was small, the researchers concluded that it might be significant if driving a motor vehicle or engaging in any activity requiring mental alertness was necessary.

Drugs Improve Stomach Emptying

A team of researchers reported in April 1990 that erythromycin, a common antibiotic, improves stomach emptying in patients with severe diabetic gastroparesis—delayed emptying of the stomach following a meal. The condition is associated with a type of diabetes called insulin-dependent, or Type I, diabetes. The impaired stomach emptying results in difficulty controlling the blood sugar level, and in some patients erratic blood sugar levels can be life-threatening.

In the study, involving ten men and women with severe diabetic gastroparesis and ten healthy control subjects, the rate at which the stomach emptied following a solid or liquid meal was determined using a nuclear medicine technique called scintigraphy. The study subjects ingested a small amount of a radiation-emitting material with the meal. A machine that measures radiation could then be used to clock the rate at which the meal passed through the stomach.

The diabetics were initially given either erythromycin or a placebo intravenously, and stomach emptying was measured. Healthy controls received neither placebo nor the drug. Two hours after ingesting the solid meal, diabetics who had been given the placebo had 63 percent of the meal still present in the stomach, whereas those who took erythromycin retained 4 percent of the meal and the healthy controls retained 9 percent. Following a liquid meal, diabetics who had the placebo retained 32 percent in their stomachs, diabetics given erythromycin retained 9 percent, and untreated healthy controls retained 4 percent. In subsequent tests erythromycin was given orally three times a day for four weeks. Stomach emptying measured at the end of this period also revealed improved emptying with the drug but to a lesser degree than when it was given intravenously. No significant side effects were reported as a result of taking the drug.

The drug currently used to treat diabetic gastroparesis, metoclopramide (Reglan), is limited in that its effectiveness may last only for a few months. In addition, the drug can cause serious side effects including various types of movement disorders.

Cisapride (Prepulsid), a new drug shown to be effective in the treatment of diabetic gastroparesis, has fewer side effects than metoclopramide, but it is still undergoing clinical testing in the United States and is not yet approved for marketing. The drug is available commercially in Europe.

New Drug for Colon Cancer

The U.S. Food and Drug Administration in June 1990 approved the use of levamisole (Ergamisole) in combination with the established anticancer drug 5-fluorouracil (5-FU) for the prevention of cancer recurrences and death following surgery in patients with colon cancer that has spread beyond the bowel wall to involve nearby lymph nodes. Neither drug used alone is effective against this type of cancer, but in combination they have been shown more effective than other treatments. It is not known why this combination is so effective.

Colon cancer, the second most common cause of cancer deaths in the United States, results in over 53,000 deaths annually. Detected early, it may be cured surgically. But when the cancer has spread beyond the colon wall to involve nearby lymph nodes or more distant sites in the body, additional therapy is required.

In February 1990 researchers published the results of a multiyear study, sponsored by the National Cancer Institute, involving nearly 1,000 patients who had had surgery for colon cancer that had spread to nearby lymph nodes. Beginning three to five weeks after surgery and continuing for one year, some patients were treated with a combination of levamisole and 5-FU, some with levamisole alone, and some were not given drug therapy. In the combination drug therapy group, levamisole tablets were taken orally on three consecutive days every other week, and 5-FU was given by vein once a week. The most common side effects included nausea, vomiting, headache, diarrhea, mouth sores, loss of appetite, and low white blood cell count. The treatment itself caused one death, which was associated with a low white blood cell count and infection. Therapy with the two drugs resulted in a 41 percent reduction in cancer recurrence and a 33 percent decrease in the death rate.

This form of combination therapy is not recommended for other stages of colon cancer. Patients with the least advanced stage of colon cancer have a very low risk for cancer recurrence following surgery and therefore this therapy is not indicated. Patients whose cancer is confined to the colon wall have been treated with the drug combination but the results are inconclusive and no recommendation has been made. The therapy is also not recommended for colon cancer that has spread beyond nearby lymph nodes to distant sites.

DANIEL PELOT, M.D.

DRUG ABUSE

Bennett Steps Down • Drug Abuse Treatment Efforts Stepped Up • More Young People Spurn Drugs • The "Ice" Menace Grows

Drug Czar Resigns

William Bennett, the first director of the U.S. Office of National Drug Control Policy, stepped down in November 1990. Bob Martinez, defeated in his reelection bid for the Florida governorship on November 6, was nominated to be Bennett's successor on November 30 and confirmed in March 1991.

During his 20 months as drug czar, Bennett developed a national strategy aimed at reducing the supply of illicit substances by more vigorous law enforcement and cutting down on the demand through treatment and prevention. Although police action was stepped up relatively quickly, the major aspects of the demand reduction strategy were slow in being implemented. Nonetheless, during Bennett's regime federal money for drug treatment nearly doubled (to $1.5 billion in fiscal 1991), and in January 1990 the Office of Treatment Improvement (OTI) was established.

Headed by Beny J. Primm, a New York City physician who has long specialized in addiction research and treatment, OTI set in motion a number of changes designed to improve the quality and administration of drug treatment programs. OTI targeted several large cities—including New York, Chicago, and Los Angeles—where the need for drug treatment was greatest, and it was trying to develop a centralized system of referrals to treatment centers. The agency was also concerned with upgrading drug treatment facilities, hiring more highly trained staff, and improving the skills of existing personnel.

Scientists generally agreed that the overall quality of treatment for substance abuse had been declining since the early 1980s, when the federal government slashed funds for treatment and stipulated that the remaining monies be allocated to the states rather than to specific areas of greatest need. Recent increases in funding, along with the programs launched by OTI, have been directed toward reversing the effects of this so-called "block-grant" program.

Prevention Is Working

The use of cocaine by high school students showed a decline, even though the supply remained relatively constant, suggesting that prevention efforts aimed at emphasizing the serious health hazards associated with even occasional cocaine use were at least partially successful. (This finding is similar to a trend that was observed in cigarette smoking, another area in which prevention efforts appeared to be having a significant impact on decreasing overall use.) Unfortunately, however, among a smaller, hard-core group of drug abusers, cocaine use was increasing.

An organization that was taking a leading role in the campaign to decrease drug use through increased public awareness of the often devastating effects of illicit substances was the Partnership for a Drug-Free America (PDFA). A coalition of concerned citizens representing the advertising and communications industries, PDFA persuaded advertising agencies and the media to contribute almost $1 million daily toward an effort to "denormalize" drug use by turning public opinion against it. PDFA's nationwide antidrug advertising campaign, aimed primarily at young people, included a widely seen television spot in which an egg being fried was said to represent "your brain on drugs."

Measuring Outcome

The new emphasis on treatment led to a call for more cost-effective treatment plans. Many programs were being built around a 28-day inpatient treatment model that delivers a therapeutic "package" consisting of education; individual and group therapy; orientation to and participation in the 12-step method of combating substance abuse originated by Alcoholics Anonymous; exercise; stress reduction; planning for leisure-time activities; and relapse prevention strategies. The choice of a four-week inpatient regime was determined largely by the reimbursement policies of

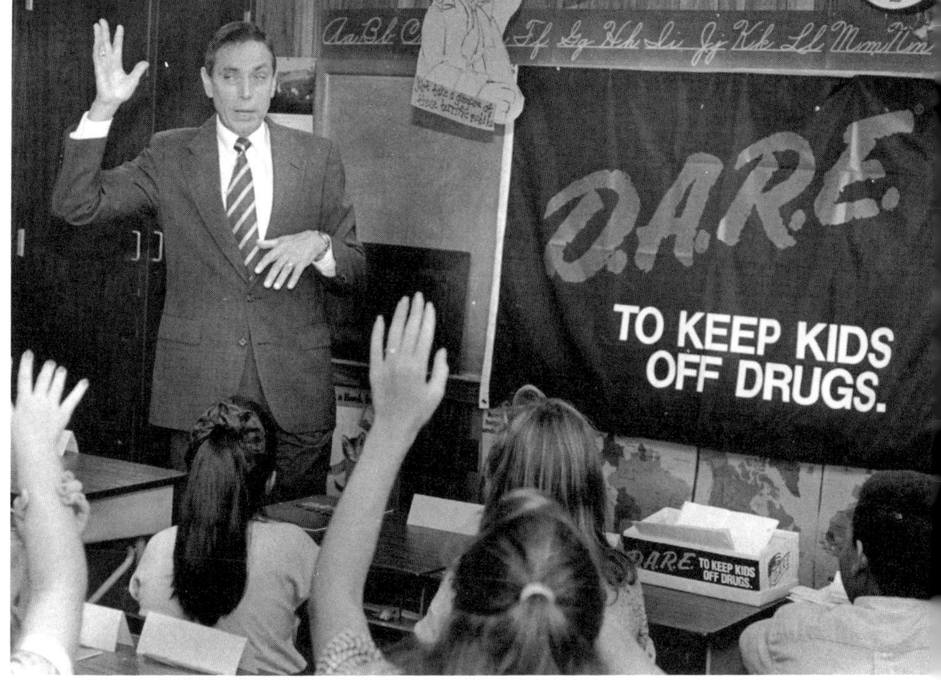

Bob Martinez, who lost his reelection bid for governor of Florida, was chosen by President Bush to become the new director of U.S. drug policy, replacing William Bennett, who stepped down in November 1990.

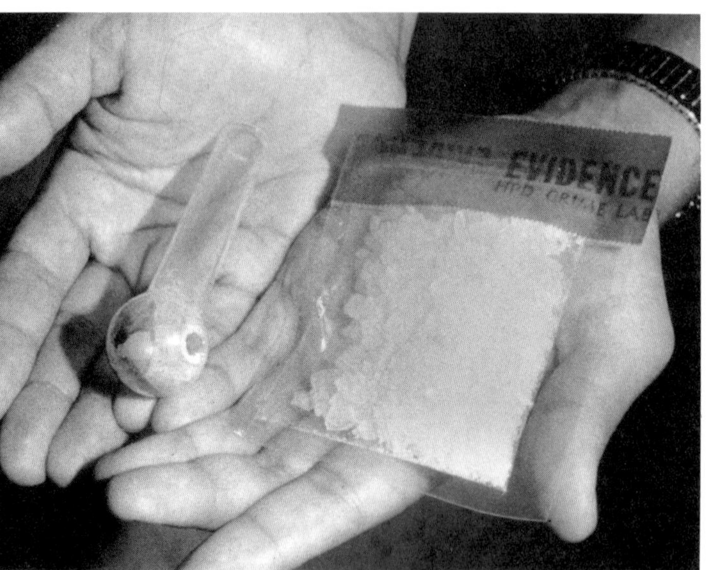

"Ice," a smokable form of methamphetamine, has begun to appear in Hawaii and on the West Coast of the United States. With effects lasting much longer than crack, the new drug has caused paranoid psychotic reactions in users.

insurance carriers rather than scientific studies. With the increasing demand for cost-effective treatments, both insurance companies and government agencies, such as the Department of Veterans Affairs, showed considerable interest in exploring other, less expensive therapeutic models, such as outpatient hospital programs for rehabilitation and detoxification.

"Ice"

Ice, a pure crystalline form of methamphetamine that can be smoked, became the number one drug problem in Hawaii, surpassing cocaine, and an ice laboratory was seized in Northern California in January 1990, giving rise to fears that this very dangerous substance would become the "recreational drug of the 1990s."

Like crack cocaine, ice produces an intense "high," but unlike cocaine, whose effects last only 10 to 30 minutes, the euphoria from methamphetamine lasts for hours. This long exposure of the central nervous system to ice is thought to be the main reason why psychotic reactions requiring emergency treatment are seen more commonly with ice than with cocaine.

Medications Development Program

The Medications Development Program of the National Institute on Drug Abuse (NIDA) was established by Congress in 1989 to encourage pharmaceutical companies to develop new medicines to fight drug and alcohol dependence. Although these research efforts continued throughout 1990, the only drugs that had so far been found to be effective for treatment of substance-abuse disorders were methadone, used as substitution therapy for opiate dependence; naltrexone (sold as Trexan), a narcotic-blocking agent also used to counter opiate dependence; disulfiram (sold as Antabuse), used to induce aversion to alcohol; desipramine (sold as Norpramin and Pertofrane), used to fight cocaine addiction; benzodiazepines, tranquilizers used to ease the withdrawal symptoms associated with alcohol detoxification; and nicotine polacrilex gum for nicotine dependence. Efforts were also underway to streamline the drug approval process so that promising new agents can be identified and tested quickly. Several pharmaceutical companies expressed an interest in the Medications Development Program, and more than a dozen drugs were under consideration for testing. A special focus of this program is on drugs for cocaine use disorders, an area that is especially lacking in effective drug therapies.

GEORGE E. WOODY, M.D.
A. THOMAS MCLELLAN, PH.D.
CHARLES P. O'BRIEN, M.D., PH.D.

ENVIRONMENT AND HEALTH

Lead Poisoning in Children • Lower Radiation Limits • Radon in the Home • Atomic Bomb Survivors • Environmental Carcinogens

Eradicating Lead Poisoning

In early 1991 the U.S. government unveiled a strategy aimed at eradicating lead posioning in American children over the next 20 years. The strategy involves major efforts from three federal agencies—the cabinet departments of Health and Human Services (HHS) and Housing and Urban Development (HUD), along with the Environmental Protection Agency (EPA). HHS Secretary Louis W. Sullivan, M.D., described lead poisoning as the number one environmental hazard facing children. The government believes that lead poisoning in children is entirely preventable.

The major source of lead poisoning in children is lead-based paint. Even though the use of lead-based paint in homes was banned by the U.S. Consumer Product Safety Commission in 1978, an estimated 57 million private homes built before 1980 have lead paint in them, and 10 million of these homes are estimated to have children under 7 years old living in them. (An estimated 900,000 units of public housing still contain lead-based paint.) The second major source of elevated blood lead is urban soil and dust contaminated by lead-based paint and by lead in gasoline. Lead in drinking water, the third major source, comes mainly from lead solder used in water pipes (though banned in 1986, EPA enforcement of the ban has been extremely limited) and lead used in brass plumbing fixtures.

In December 1990, John Rosen, M.D., a pediatrician at Montefiore Medical Center in New York City, presented the following description of the effects of lead poisoning on young children: "It causes impairments in reading, writing, mathematics, abstract thinking, concentration span—all the skills necessary for academic success. We don't know if it is ever possible to reverse the effects later in life, but once success in those key years is gone, it's gone forever."

James O. Mason, M.D., chief of the U.S. Public Health Service, said in February 1991 that a recent study had shown that "young people exposed to moderate levels of lead as preschoolers were seven times more likely to drop out of high school and six times as likely to have a significant reading disability."

As harmful effects from elevated blood-lead levels have been observed at lower and lower levels over the past 15 years, the CDC lowered the level at which children are diagnosed as being at risk from 40 micrograms per deciliter in 1978 to 25 currently, and it is expected to lower it further to 10 or 15 in 1991. (A microgram is one millionth of a gram; a deciliter is one-tenth of a liter, about 3.4 ounces.) In 1990, HHS estimated that 250,000 children had blood-lead levels greater than 25, a level at which damage to the child's nervous system has already begun. An estimated minimum of 3 million children had levels greater than 10, where nervous-system damage is thought to be imminent.

A major thrust of the HHS strategy is increased monitoring by local health departments of children who are at greatest risk of lead poisoning. Health officials will make home visits when deemed necessary to advise on lead paint removal and on dietary changes. The plan projected that for each child saved from reaching a blood-lead level of 25, society would in the long run save $1,300 in medical expenses and $3,331 in the cost of special education. In addition, the child would most likely have a higher income in adulthood and thus pay more in income taxes.

The Department of Housing and Urban Development is directly responsible for the control and removal of lead-based paint in public housing and has established programs to assist private homeowners. In 1990, HUD estimated that the total cost of testing and removal for private homes with young children judged to have serious lead-paint hazards would be between $1.9 billion and $2.4 billion. The cost of cleanup is about $3,000 to $5,000 per dwelling. The most expensive method involves stripping all the paint. A less expensive, and less effective, method involves covering the lead-based paint with a protective layer of plastic, paneling, or wallboard.

The EPA is conducting policy reviews of standards for lead in the air, in drinking water, and in plumbing fixtures and for the disposal of waste products containing lead. It also serves in an advisory capacity to the other agencies.

In December 1990 a coalition of child advocacy, environmental, and civil rights groups filed a class-action lawsuit against the California Department of Health Services charging that the state was not conducting the mandatory testing of Medicaid-eligible children under the age of 6 for lead poisoning. The suit claimed that California had failed to test at least 570,000 of these young children. (In 1989 Congress had added a specific provision to the Medicaid statutes requiring that states test all eligible children under age 6 for lead and monitor those Medicaid-eligible young people between ages 6 and 21 who have already shown elevated blood-lead levels.)

Another source of lead poisoning for children is school drinking water. A 1990 study by the EPA found that more than 250,000 children are affected by the failure of school districts to test drinking water, use adequate monitoring methods, or comply with updated lead-concentration recommendations. The EPA found that half of U.S. school districts had not tested their water supplies. The lead can enter the water from lead solder in pipes or from lead-lined storage tanks. Despite a 1988 federal law that directed states to require schools to test their drinking water and remove problem water fountains, the EPA found that only Minnesota and the Virgin Islands had thus far required their school districts to comply. The EPA recommends that school drinking water have no more than 20 parts of lead per billion.

An unexpected environmental source of lead is the outside of bread wrappers, which often have colored lettering containing lead. If the wrapper is turned inside out and used to heat food in a microwave oven—a not uncommon practice—the lead can flake off into the food.

Children are not the only victims of lead poisoning. The traditional view has been that after lead is inhaled or taken in by mouth, it is stored in the bone, where it stays permanently. But recent research has shown that lead can be more dynamic. In healthy bodies it does remain in the bone, but researchers have discovered that in some people the bones can release lead at the same time they release calcium and that the lead then circulates in the blood. This effect can occur when a person consumes too little calcium for the body's needs or during osteoporosis, a disease often found in post-menopausal women which is characterized by rapid loss of bone calcium. Scientists have found that women with osteoporosis may show as much as a 25 percent increase in blood-lead levels.

Johns Hopkins University scientists reported in 1990 that traditional methods of removing lead-based paint from homes where children have elevated blood-lead levels, such as sanding and the haphazard removal of debris, have caused large short-term increases in the amount of lead dust in the air and in the blood-lead levels of the children. Modified removal methods, such as using heat guns for paint removal and the careful disposal of debris, resulted in modest short-term decrease in blood-lead levels. But six months later, although lower than it had been, the amount of lead in the blood of the children in both groups of homes remained unacceptably high.

Lower Radiation Limits

In December 1990, for the first time in 30 years, the U.S. Nuclear Regulatory Commission (NRC) completely revised the recommended limits on the amount of radiation to which a person should be exposed in a year. For a member of the general public, the new level was set at 100 millirem per year of whole-body radiation, down from the previously recommended limit of 500. (A rem is a unit of radiation exposure; a millirem is one-thousandth of a rem.) This limit refers to sources other than those occurring naturally (such as from radon or cosmic rays) or in the course of medical examination. The U.S. National Council on Radiation Protection and Measurement has estimated that a typical American is exposed to 300 millirem per year from natural sources, 200 of which come from radon. Some examples of radiation exposure that should be included in calculating the 100 millirem yearly limit: from watching a television set, between 0.3 and 1.0 millirem; from ordinary construction materials such as bricks, mortar, and wood, about 7 millirem; from a typical luminous-dial watch, approximately 1-3 millirem per year.

New standards were also set for workers in radiation industries, which must be licensed by the NRC. The maximum total dose was lowered to 5,000 millirem per year, down from 12,000. The 5,000 is a total of both external and internal radiation. The internal radiation can come from the worker inhaling or ingesting radioactive material. And for the first time a limit was set for exposure of the unborn child of a pregnant radiation worker: 500 millirem over the entire pregnancy.

Radon in the Home

In February 1991 the National Research Council of the U.S. National Academy of Sciences reassessed the risk of lung cancer resulting from buildups of the naturally occurring radioactive gas radon in homes and found that it may be less than was previously thought. Several studies have found that in many parts of the country radon seeps into houses from the underlying soil and rocks. The concentrations can build up, especially in wintertime, in poorly ventilated houses that are heavily insulated or tightly sealed against cold weather.

The colorless, odorless gas radon-222 is produced by the naturally occurring radioactive decay of radium-226, which in turn, is the decay product of uranium-238. The concentrations of naturally occurring uranium and radon vary in different geographical areas. After it is inhaled, radon in the lungs decays into products that emit alpha radiation, heavy nuclear particles that can damage normal lung cells, sometimes turning them into cancer cells.

Scientists had previously estimated the risk of lung cancer due to radon inhalation in the general U.S. population by comparing earlier studies of lung cancer among miners, for whom there is long-term data on radon exposure. The new National Research Council study concluded that the previous estimates of cancer risk may be as much as 30 percent too high, mainly because at the same radon levels, the miners' greater physical exertion causes them to breathe more deeply and inhale larger amounts of radon.

The EPA may now reduce from 21,000 its estimate of the number of deaths from lung cancer each year that it attributes to radon in the home. Nevertheless, the report stressed that radon in the home is still a potent carcinogen (cancer-causing agent). It is described by the EPA as the second leading cause of lung cancer after smoking.

Two British studies published in *The Lancet* in 1990 linked radon in the home to cancers other than lung cancer. The first found that in 15 countries, including the United States, radon in the home is correlated with several cancers in adults and children, including myeloid leukemia, melanoma (skin cancer), prostate cancer, and kidney cancer. The overall concentration of indoor radon in the countries studied varied greatly, with Sweden reporting the highest level and Poland the lowest. The U.S. average was just about in the middle, allowing, of course, for wide regional variations.

Atomic Bomb Survivors

The survivors of the atomic bombs dropped on Hiroshima and Nagasaki, Japan, in August 1945 have been studied intensively for clues to the aftereffects of exposure to intense whole-body radiation. The results of several studies of both survivors and their children, conducted under the auspices of the Radiation Effects Research Foundation in Hiroshima, were made public in 1990.

The major health problem faced by the survivors of the bombings was an increased risk for several types of cancer. Cancers that were conclusively linked to radiation among atomic bomb survivors are those of the thyroid, breast, bone marrow, lung, stomach, colon, bladder, and esophagus. While links to some other forms of cancer (such as kidney and ovarian) were tentatively established, there were some cancers (such as liver and testicular) for which no connection was found. In addition, those survivors who were young children at the time of the bombings tended to experience impaired growth.

There were several effects reported on in studies of the children of bomb survivors. Most surprising was the conclusion that atomic bomb radiation exposure did not cause the inherited genetic damage it had been expected to. However, children of mothers who were pregnant at the time of the bombings were found vulnerable to mental retardation, small head size, seizures, and poor performance on conventional intelligence tests and in school. Bomb exposure in weeks 8 through 15 of pregnancy, when the central nervous system is especially sensitive to radiation, were the most critical period for the creation of these problems.

A study that looked specifically at cancer risk among the children of atom bomb survivors considered separately those who had been exposed while their mothers were pregnant and those who were conceived after the bombings (for whom one or both parents had experienced the bomb radiation). Although between 1950 and 1984 only 18 cancer cases were identified in the first group, cancer risk did appear to rise significantly as the dose reportedly received by the mother increased. The results for the second group remained inconclusive and follow-up studies were being planned.

Studies of atomic bomb survivors and their children are of importance because they provide the framework for scientists attempting to understand the biological effects of radiation exposure in humans in general.

Environmental Carcinogens

In a study published in 1990, University of South Carolina psychologists found that for some people the fear of cancer combined with living near a source of environmental pollution created symptoms of anxiety and depression that they mistook for cancer warning signs. The report stated that such fears and their expression may be widespread and offered several reasons for them. The cancer-causing properties of some toxic substances have been widely publicized. This is the case, for example, with the PCBs, or polychlorinated biphenyls, which are major soil and water pollutants and are found in fish and elsewhere in the food web. There is also psychological pressure from simply knowing that toxic substances are near by, often without being able to see them or otherwise detect them.

In a study reported in January 1991, the EPA found that members of the public tended to be preoccupied with environmental hazards that scientists considered of lesser importance, while neglecting those about which scientists are much more seriously concerned. Hazardous waste sites, judged to be most risky by the public, are considered by scientists to be of relatively low risk, mainly because they are limited in area and in the number of people they affect. On the other hand, the public ranked the EPA's high-risk problems, such as global warming and the hole in the ozone layer, far down on the list.

In an article published in the fall of 1990, Lawrence Garfinkel, an epidemiological consultant for the American Cancer Society, pointed out that any statement about the risk of cancer should emphasize two things. First, no single study, whether of humans or laboratory animals, tells the whole story, and studies that seem to show significant relationships between substances and disease may later be proved wrong. Also, the relationship between substance and disease should make sense biologically. That is, the substance should be able to cause changes in cells; there must be a long interval between first exposure and detection of cancer; and the greater the amount or the longer the exposure to the substance, the greater the risk of the cancer should be.

The question of which potential carcinogens should be given the most attention was addressed by a multinational study of cancer rates published in 1990 in *The Lancet*. Devra Lee Davis of the Mt. Sinai Medical Center in New York City and colleagues found that rates of some cancers for people over the age of 55 in the United States and four other industrial nations—Italy, Japan, the United Kingdom, and West Germany—are rising. For many years, scientists have debated the significance of increased cancer rates. Do they reflect greater actual numbers of cases or are they the result of improved diagnosis and greater access to care? (The study noted that increases in the rate of lung cancer during the 1940s were at first explained this way.) Could the rise in number of cases be a reflection of unwillingness in many societies until recently to name cancer as a cause of death? The report concluded that the increases require further study.

Some possible factors affecting the cancer rate in people now over the age of 55 are: long-term smoking of high-tar cigarettes; workplace exposure to numerous chemicals; eating smaller amounts of fresh vegetables and fruits; and poorly controlled exposure to new household chemicals and pesticides, especially during the 1940s and 1950s. The researchers stressed that since the populations of the industrialized countries are aging, a clear understanding of the increasing incidences of some cancers in the over-55 age group can be of considerable use in assessing future demands for health care.

Two questions debated in 1990 in the evaluation of possible carcinogens were: Which of the multitude of chemicals in existence should be placed on the list for study? How should risk be evaluated? The traditional original view of "cancer development" involves a change in a cell's genetic material. New research has shown that a second mechanism—rapid cell reproduction—may also be a cause of cancer. The traditional definition of a carcinogen is a substance that is toxic to genetic material, so that the cells it produces are cancerous mutations.

Determining the cancer risk of a substance is a multi-stage process. Laboratory animals are exposed to high doses of the material and the cancer effects are measured. Scientists then make mathematical models to translate the animal test results into risk to humans from low doses. Cancer researchers at the University of Nebraska pointed out in 1990 that some chemicals that cause cancer in animals, especially at high doses, don't act that way in humans. Sodium saccharin, for example, administered to rats in high doses leads to a significant increase in bladder cancer, but a similar effect has not been found in humans. And in 1990 scientists at the University of California at Berkeley discussed the often overlooked fact that many natural substances found in common foods can be shown to cause cancer at high doses; yet people have eaten them, apparently safely, at much lower doses for many generations. (They give the example that an average cup of coffee contains about 40 parts per million of substances that have been shown to cause cancer in mice in high doses.) They called into question the regulation of very low doses (in concentrations of a few parts per billion) of synthetic chemicals that cause cancer in animals at high doses, considering it a misallocation of money and effort and seeing it as a separate issue from the regulation of these substances for the protection of the natural environment.

See also the feature article YOUR AIR, YOUR HEALTH.

ELLEN THRO

EYES

New Treatments for Diabetes Complication • How Common Are Vision Problems?

Controlling Diabetic Retinopathy

Researchers in 1990 reported on several treatments to prevent the progression of diabetic retinopathy, a leading cause of blindness in the United States. Retinopathy is a condition characterized by abnormalities of the blood vessels of the retina, the light-sensitive membrane that lines the eye and sends visual images to the brain via the optic nerve.

In diabetes, the body either cannot produce or cannot properly utilize the hormone insulin, necessary for metabolism of carbohydrates. As a result, excessive amounts of sugar circulate in the blood. The disease can damage all the tissues of the body, including those in the eyes. People with diabetes tend to develop cataracts (a progressive clouding of the lens of the eye) at a younger age than those without the disease, and they are prone to severe retinal disease. Most cataracts can be successfully treated with surgery to replace the natural lens of the eye with an artificial one. Retinal disease, which may include swelling of the retina caused by excessive fluid leakage from retinal blood vessels and growth of abnormal new blood vessels, is more difficult than cataracts to correct. It can be treated in its early stages with laser therapy. Carefully aimed laser light destroys a portion of the retina, reducing the amount of leakage and halting abnormal vessel growth. This technique has been shown in numerous clinical studies to reduce the visual impairment associated with retinopathy—but it does not eliminate the problem.

In the absence of a completely successful treatment for retinopathy, physicians have tried to prevent this complication of diabetes by rigidly controlling patients' blood sugar levels. Trials using frequent injections of insulin or continuous infusion of insulin through a pump implanted under the skin have not, however, dramatically reduced the frequency of retinal damage.

Drug Treatments and Transplants. The search for a more promising treatment strategy has led physicians to test a variety of drugs that might delay or prevent diabetic retinopathy. In September 1990 researchers released the results of a seven-year evaluation of the drug sorbinil, conducted under the joint sponsorship of the U.S. National Eye Institute and the pharmaceutical company Pfizer Incorporated. (Sorbinil is thought to block the production of sorbitol, a sugar alcohol that circulates in the bloodstream and has been linked to diabetic complications.) Some 500 patients age 18 to 56 with Type I, or insulin-dependent, diabetes (the most severe form of the disease, in which the pancreas loses the ability to produce insulin) took either sorbinil or a placebo (a pill with no medicinal value) for 3½ years. Sorbinil appeared to slow the progression of diabetic retinopathy, but it did not stop the disease process. Moreover, nearly 7 percent of patients treated with sorbinil suffered allergic reactions to it, an unacceptably high level. As a result, sorbinil was not likely to gain widespread use as a treatment for diabetic retinopathy, and researchers were testing other medicines that did not appear to cause as high a rate of allergic reactions and might even be more effective in retarding the advancement of retinopathy.

Another potential method of staving off the complications of diabetes—transplanting a human pancreas to restore normal insulin production—was the focus of a University of Michigan research project that was completed in 1990. Investigators, who charted the progress of 12 of the approximately 1,500 people worldwide who had undergone pancreas transplants, found the procedure ineffective in halting the progression of diabetic retinopathy. However, because transplants are used as a treatment of last resort, the patients studied had severe retinal disease at the time of their transplant surgery. Restoration of insulin production was apparently not enough to reverse the abnormal changes that had already occurred.

Puberty and Retinopathy. The longer a person has diabetes, the greater the likelihood that he or she will develop diabetic retinopathy. However, in a study of 70 children and young adults with diabetes, physicians at the Wilmer Eye Institute of The Johns Hopkins University discovered that prepubescent children had far less severe retinopathy than young people who had reached puberty, even when the youngsters in both groups had had diabetes for the same periods of time. These findings suggest that the hormones associated with puberty—including growth hormone and insulin-like growth factor—may play a role in accelerating the abnormal changes diabetes causes in the eye. This information will allow physicians to test drugs known to inhibit the effects of the hormones involved, to see whether these drugs can prevent retinal damage.

Visual Impairment in America

Accurate data on the causes and prevalence of visual impairment and blindness in the United States have been unavailable until February 1990, when investigators at the Wilmer Eye Institute published the results of a four-year study in which they examined the eyes of over 5,300 residents of east Baltimore, Md. The research subjects were all over the age of 40; about 45 percent were black, and 55 percent were white. A wide range of socioeconomic classes were represented. The rates of visual loss varied widely: less than 1 percent of whites age 40 to 49 had significant vision problems, but this figure jumped to 26 percent among blacks age 80 and older. The most striking finding was that the overall rate of blindness and visual impairment among blacks was twice that of whites. There was no difference detected based on sex. Extrapolating from their findings, the investigators estimated that more than 3 million people in the United States have impaired vision. Almost 1 million people are legally blind, with distance vision of 20/200 or less in both eyes with corrective lenses.

The researchers were especially troubled to find that more than half of the patients examined could not see as well as they should solely because of inadequate eyeglasses. These patients lived in an area well served by both optometrists and opthalmologists, leading the researchers to speculate that an even higher percentage of people in areas where eye care is less accessible suffer needlessly from easily correctable vision problems.

MICHAEL X. REPKA, M.D.

Professional examination is necessary in order to obtain proper eyeglasses. A 1990 survey on visual impairment in the United States found that a surprisingly large number of Americans had trouble seeing solely because their glasses were inadequate.

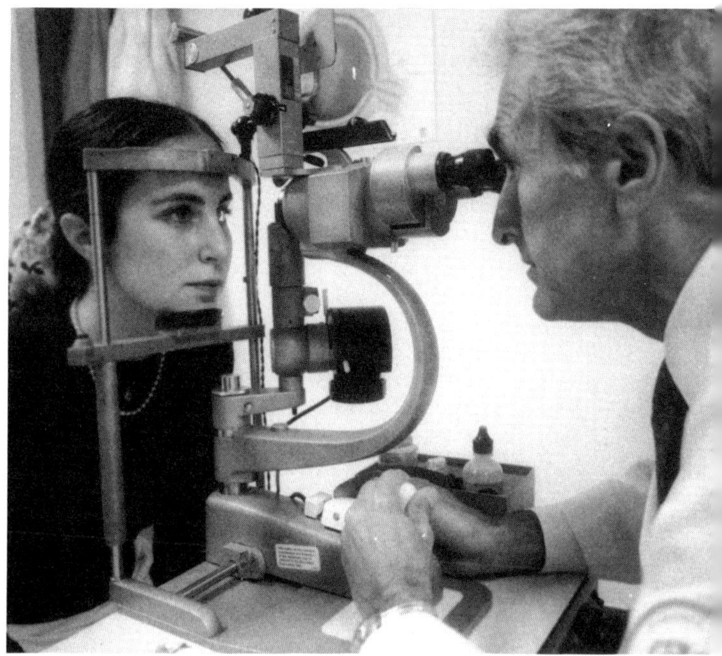

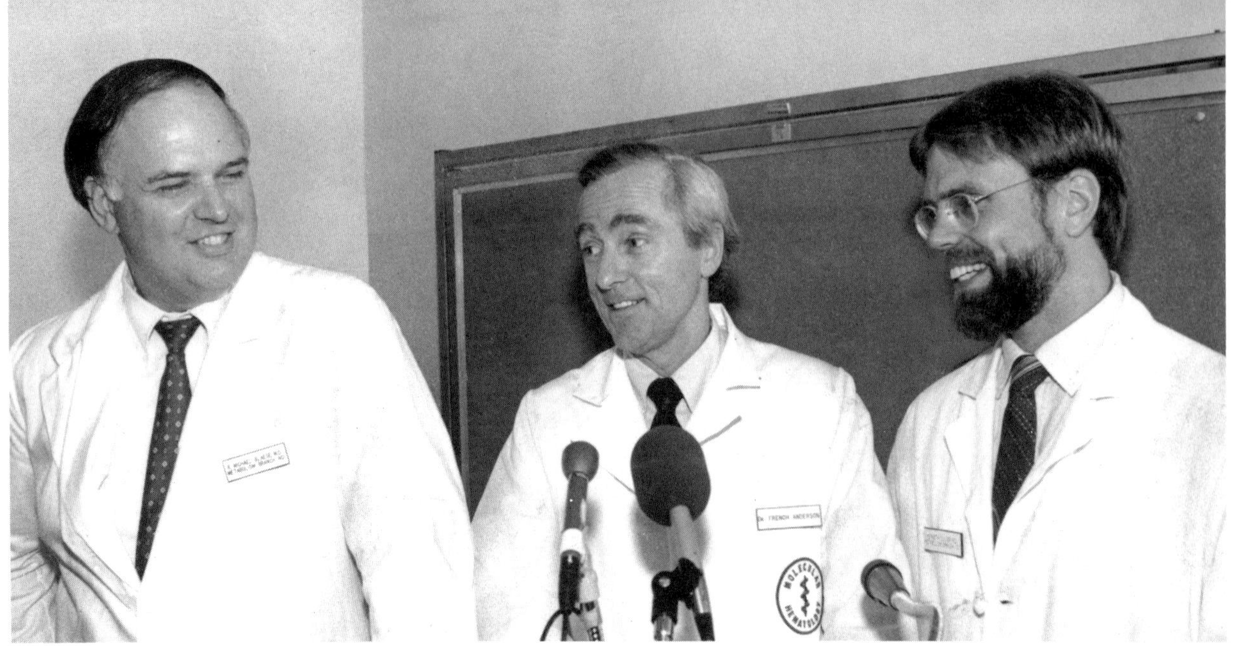

The first approved treatment of disease with gene therapy was undertaken in September 1990 by researchers at the U.S. National Institutes of Health. The landmark experiment, performed on a four-year-old girl with a rare immune system disorder, was led by (left to right) Drs. R. Michael Blaese, W. French Anderson, and Kenneth Culver.

GENETICS AND GENETIC ENGINEERING

Human Gene Therapy • New Disease Findings • Screening Embryos • Heredity More Important Than Environment? • Drug Revolution

Gene Therapy's First Trial

After years of study, legal wrangling, and ethical debate, the first approved use of gene therapy in humans began on September 14, 1990, when researchers at the U.S. National Institutes of Health (NIH) injected genetically altered white blood cells into a four-year-old girl with an inherited disease of the immune system. The disorder, called ADA deficiency, prevents a person's immune system from mounting an attack against infections. (The most famous case was that of the "bubble boy" in Houston who spent most of his life in a sterile plastic chamber until his death in 1984.)

In the therapy, some of the girl's own white blood cells were extracted and genetically altered so that they would produce a crucial enzyme (adenosine deaminase, or ADA) that doctors hoped would restore immune function. The altered cells were then reproduced by the billions and injected into the patient. In December the researchers reported that the altered cells seemed to be stimulating the growth of the girl's own white blood cells, causing them to proliferate and improve her immune system's functioning. The altered cells were also producing ADA as hoped. The researchers were continuing monthly infusions of the genetically altered cells and had received approval to treat nine more patients suffering from the same disease.

In January 1991 a second group of NIH researchers began using genetically engineered cells to treat patients with malignant melanoma, an often fatal form of cancer. The researchers removed white blood cells from the patients, added the gene for a protein that would increase the cells' ability to kill cancer cells, and infused them back into the patients. The researchers said it would take several months to judge the effectiveness of the highly experimental technique.

Genetic Diseases

Scientists accelerated the pace of research on genetic diseases in 1990, discovering genes that cause or play a role in several types of illness.

Aneurysms. The discovery of a genetic defect that predisposes its bearer to aortic aneurysms was announced in November 1990 by Pennsylvania researchers. These aneurysms are swellings of the aorta (the main artery that carries blood from the heart) that can rupture fatally. They kill more than 15,000 Americans each year, and more than 2 million people in the United States are thought to be at risk.

The researchers discovered the genetic defect by studying a family with a history of aneurysms. The defective gene is the blueprint for a protein called collagen III that is a primary structural material of the wall of the aorta. The researchers developed a saliva test for the defect and identified five other members of the family who were at risk of developing aneurysms.

The ability to identify individuals at risk may enable physicians to possibly prevent aneurysms with blood pressure lowering drugs or to surgically repair them before they burst. It is not yet known whether other families with a history of aortic aneurysms share the same collagen III gene defect.

Arthritis. In September 1990 researchers in Pennsylvania and Ohio reported that they had found a defective gene that causes some cases of osteoarthritis, the most common form of arthritis. In this disorder, the protective cartilage in joints frays, wears, ulcerates, and, in extreme cases, disappears entirely, leaving a bone-on-bone joint. Individuals with the disease suffer pain, stiffness, and, often, limitations in mobility that get worse over time. Osteoarthritis is the major reason for the more than 150,000 total joint replacement procedures performed each year in the United States. The gene that was discovered is the blueprint for a protein called collagen II, which strengthens the protective cartilage.

Myoclonic Epilepsy. Georgia researchers reported in July 1990 that they had discovered a genetic defect that causes myoclonic epilepsy. The symptoms of this form of epilepsy range from mild aberrations in brain electrical patterns to uncontrolled jerking, hearing loss, muscle disease, mental impairment, and heart problems.

Surprisingly, the defect was not located in the deoxyribonucleic acid (DNA, the blueprint of life) found in the nucleus of cells, but in the small amount of DNA found in mitochondria, specialized parts of cells that provide energy. Because of the defect, the mitochondria were not able to produce enough energy to power the cells, especially those in the brain and nervous system. The discovery marked the fourth genetic disorder that had been linked to mitochondrial DNA in two years. Some researchers now believe that other diseases, particularly those related to aging, may also have their roots in mitochondria.

Neurofibromatosis. Also in July, researchers in Utah and Michigan independently announced the discovery of the defective gene that causes von Recklinghausen neurofibromatosis, commonly—and incorrectly—known as Elephant Man's disease. Neurofibromatosis is the most common nervous system disorder caused by a single gene. It affects one out of roughly every 3,500 Americans, causing symptoms ranging from brownish-colored lesions on the skin to large, deforming growths similar to those exhibited by the Elephant Man (although researchers now believe that Joseph Merrick, the horribly disfigured 19th-century Englishman, actually suffered from an unrelated disorder called Proteus syndrome). In the most severe cases, neurofibromatosis causes fatal tumors of the nervous system.

The gene that was discovered provides the blueprint for a protein that acts as a tumor suppressor, holding the growth of cells in check. When the gene is defective, or inactivated by exposure to radiation or carcinogenic chemicals, cells grow without restraint, resulting in the growth of tumors. The discovery should thus shed light not only on neurofibromatosis, but also on the mechanisms of tumor formation.

Alport Syndrome. In June 1990 researchers in Utah and Finland reported the discovery of the genetic defect that causes Alport syndrome, a form of inherited kidney disease that affects one person in 5,000. The disorder leads to loss of the kidneys' ability to function, necessitating dialysis or a kidney transplant. Although Alport syndrome accounts for only about 2 percent of the 100,000 Americans now on dialysis, the discovery should make possible genetic counseling for families with a history of the disease, and it may provide clues to the cause of other types of kidney disease.

Cancer. Massachusetts researchers reported in November 1990 that they had found a common genetic defect in cancer-stricken members of families with Li-Fraumeni syndrome (a rare condition that predisposes people to develop various types of cancer in adulthood) and that this defect might be common among the population at large. In the Li-Fraumeni families at least three close relatives suffer from cancer and many have more than one type of malignancy. Only about 100 such families have been identified, but more may exist.

The researchers found that the stricken individuals have a defect in a gene called p53, which is known to control cell division and prevent tumor formation. Among women, the most common manifestation of Li-Fraumeni syndrome is breast cancer, but those with the mutation are also at risk for tumors of the brain, muscles, bones, and adrenal glands, as well as leukemia. The p53 gene had previously been linked to cancer in other individuals, and researchers hope that a close study of it may lead to new ways to fight tumor formation.

In December, French researchers reported discovering a gene that is linked to the progression of breast cancer. The gene is the blueprint for a protein, called stromelysin-3, that is capable of destroying the breast tissue that surrounds a tumor and hinders the spread of cancer cells. Researchers now think that such destruction may play a critical role in allowing the cancer to spread to other sites in the body.

Alcoholism. Considerable excitement greeted the publication of a study in April 1990 announcing that researchers had found a gene called the D2 receptor that was linked to alcoholism. This gene, it was reported, affected the brain's handling of dopamine, a chemical that plays a key role in pleasure-seeking behavior such as alcohol consumption. The excitement turned to disappointment, however, the following December when a follow-up study done at the U.S. National Institute on Alcohol Abuse and Alcoholism (NIAAA) failed to confirm the finding. Nevertheless, scientists remained confident that alcoholism would eventually be found to have a genetic component, and the NIAAA launched a massive five-year, $25 million project to investigate the issue.

Prenatal Screening

In July 1990 a 29-year-old British woman named Debbie Edwards gave birth to healthy twins that had been subjected to an unprecedented form of prenatal screening. London physicians removed eggs from her ovaries, fertilized them in the laboratory, using her husband's sperm, and grew them until they had reached the eight-cell stage—the smallest size from which a single cell can be removed without risk to the embryo. The physicians removed one cell from each embryo and determined the embryo's sex. Male embryos were discarded, and two female embryos were implanted in Edwards's womb, where they grew to maturity.

By becoming the mother of healthy twin girls in July 1990, Debbie Edwards (right) became the first beneficiary of a revolutionary form of prenatal screening pioneered by British geneticist Robert Winston (center). With them is Christine Mundy, another recipient of the technique, which allows doctors through in vitro fertilization to implant only female embryos, which are not subject to a sex-linked disorder carried by the mother.

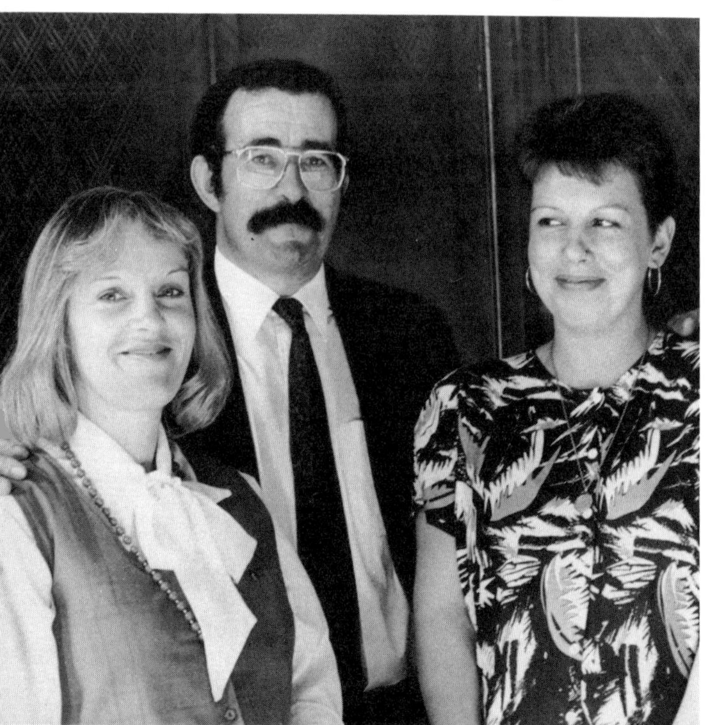

The procedure was not used simply because the couple wanted girls. Debbie Edwards carries the gene for a birth defect called adrenoleukodystrophy, which strikes only boys, leaving them blind and totally disabled. The unique procedure allowed her to become pregnant without taking the risk that the embryo would be male.

Although the procedure can so far be used only to determine the embryo's sex, the researchers said that within a year or two, it could also be used to screen for specific birth defects. Later in 1990, three other women also gave birth to healthy daughters conceived through the new procedure, and the physicians expected to work with dozens of additional couples to refine the technology.

Maleness Gene

For decades geneticists have known that two X chromosomes (one from the mother and one from the father) produce a female offspring and that the combination of an X chromosome from the mother and a Y from the father creates a male. But the specific gene on the Y chromosome that is responsible for maleness remained unknown until British scientists announced in July 1990 that they had identified it. By comparing DNA segments from a variety of mammals, including humans, they isolated a segment that was present in all males and absent in all females. The gene, named SRY (sex-determining region Y) becomes active in the seventh week of pregnancy and is responsible for turning the fetus's budding sex organs into testes rather than ovaries.

Twins Study

In a landmark study of identical twins reared apart, Minnesota researchers concluded that genes almost always play a more important role in shaping behavior than does the family environment. Identical twins occur when a fertilized egg splits shortly after conception, so that the twins have exactly the same genetic complement. Studying identical twins who are reared apart enables researchers to separate the effects of heredity (nature) from those of the family environment (nurture).

The study, in progress since 1979, is the largest in the world, with more than 100 sets of twins enrolled, and its results were eagerly awaited. In a series of 1990 reports culminating in a paper in the journal *Sci-*

ence in October, the researchers concluded, "For almost every behavioral trait so far investigated, from reaction time to religiosity, an important fraction of the variation among people turns out to be associated with genetic variation." The study, they wrote, "does not show that parents cannot influence those traits, but simply that this does not tend to happen in most families."

The Minnesota researchers concluded that a person's IQ (intelligence quotient) is strongly genetic in origin, with heredity accounting for nearly 70 percent of the variability found among individuals. Heredity, they said, also accounts for about 50 percent of personality differences, including whether someone is outgoing or not; 50 percent of religiosity, including how often someone attends religious services; and about 40 percent of variations in job interest.

Genetics of Native Americans

More than 95 percent of all North and South American Indians are descended from a small band of pioneers that crossed the Bering Strait from Asia to Alaska between 15,000 and 30,000 years ago, Georgia researchers reported in July 1990. The researchers arrived at their conclusion by studying mitochondria. The DNA in mitochondria is passed directly from mothers to progeny and thus does not undergo genetic mixing like the DNA in the nucleus of a cell. Mitochondria, therefore, provide a way to establish genetic relationships among various groups of people. Previous studies of mitochondria have shown, for example, that everyone living today is descended from a single woman who lived in Africa 200,000 years ago, the so-called "mother of us all."

The Georgia researchers used the same techniques on blood samples from various native American groups and determined that most must be descended from a small number of ancestors—the original migrating group, in fact, could have contained as few as four women. The remaining 5 percent—including natives of Northwestern Canada and the Apache, Navajo, and Eskimo-Aleut nations—arrived in subsequent immigration waves about 6,000 and 4,000 years ago. The new results provided strong support for a small controversial group of linguists who have been arguing that as many as 600 different Indian languages may have all evolved from one mother tongue.

Genetically Engineered Drugs

The U.S. pharmaceutical industry was on the verge of a revolution engendered by the use of genetic engineering techniques to produce new drugs and other biologically active products. By the end of 1990, 11 drugs and vaccines produced by such techniques had been approved by the U.S. Food and Drug Administration (FDA) for use by physicians. Those products included human insulin to treat diabetes; erythropoietin to combat anemia; two forms of human growth hormone to combat growth deficiencies in children; tissue plasminogen activator to dissolve blood clots that cause heart attacks; two forms of interferon to combat hairy cell leukemia, AIDS-related Kaposi's sarcoma, and genital warts; two forms of a hepatitis vaccine; a vaccine against *Haemophilus influenzae* type B (an organism which causes meningitis and other infections); and a monoclonal antibody, called OKT3, to combat kidney transplant rejection.

Many more were in the works. According to the annual survey taken by the Pharmaceutical Manufacturers Association, as of mid-1990, 18 genetically engineered medicines had completed clinical trials and were awaiting approval by the FDA. Another 14 medicines and one vaccine were in the final stage of clinical testing. Finally, another 71 medicines were in earlier stages of clinical testing.

See also the feature article PRENATAL SCREENING.

THOMAS H. MAUGH II, PH.D.

GOVERNMENT POLICIES AND PROGRAMS

UNITED STATES

New Efforts to Control Costs and Provide Access to Healthcare • Generic Drug Scandal Continues • Abortion Controversy Update

Cost Crisis

Turmoil has recently marked federal government health policy, but quiet progress has been made on the state level in developing ways to deliver adequate healthcare to Americans despite escalating costs. In 1990 about 12 percent of the gross national product was devoted to healthcare—the largest proportion for any developed nation. Americans did not, however, enjoy the best health status in the industrialized world. The U.S. infant mortality rate was higher than that of many other developed countries. (In 1987, the most recent year for which data are generally available, the U.S. rate stood at 10.1 deaths for every 1,000 live births—more than twice the rate for Japan. Canada had 7.3 infant deaths per 1,000 live births.) The pernicious combination of the highest spending for healthcare and a mediocre record on health status is attributable to an incredibly complex medical delivery system, the American emphasis on high technol-

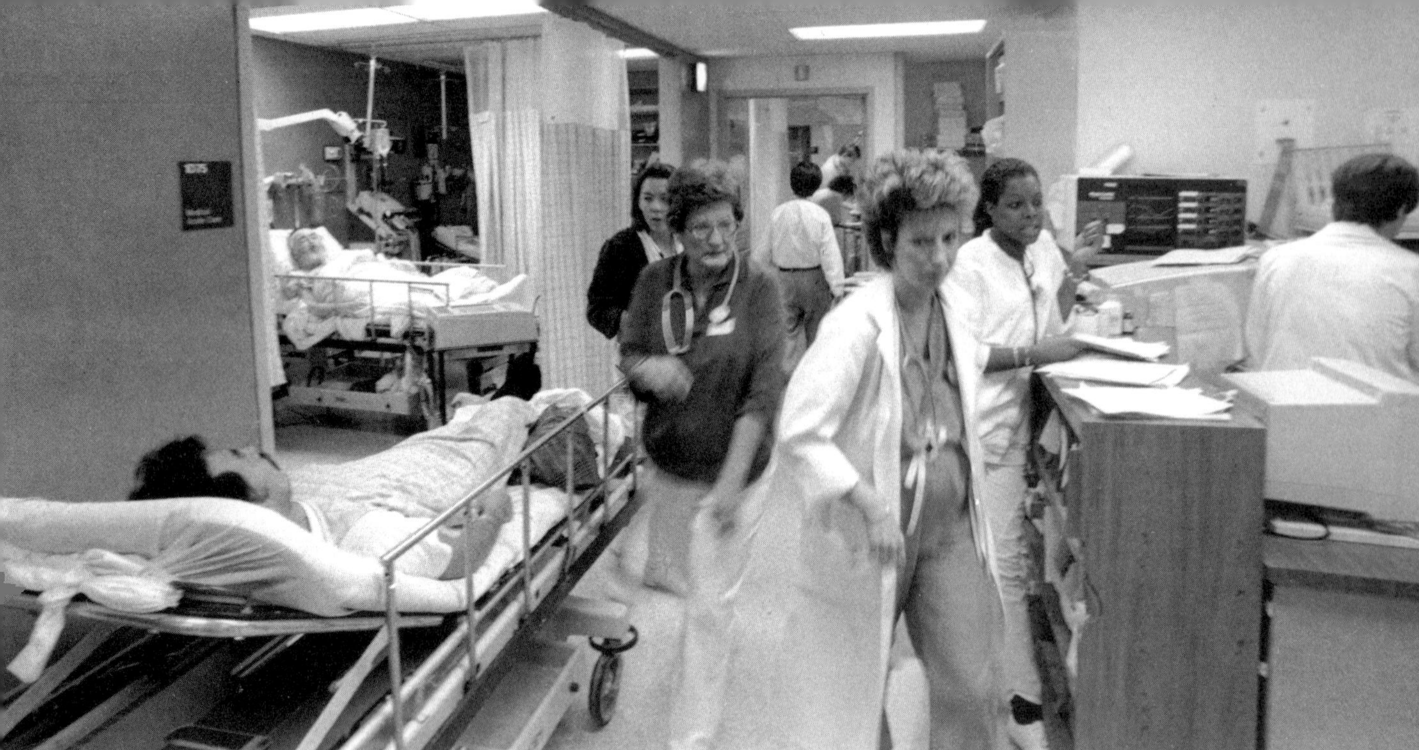

Emergency rooms, such as this one in New York City's Beth Israel Medical Center, have found themselves overloaded as poor and medically uninsured patients increasingly used them for all kinds of medical care.

ogy healthcare, significant gaps in insurance coverage, and insufficient attention to preventive care.

Federal Reform Proposal. In March 1990 the Pepper Commission, a 15-member bipartisan congressional commission named in honor of the late Democratic Congressman Claude Pepper, recommended a far-reaching program to (1) provide health insurance for the more than 30 million Americans who lack coverage and (2) greatly expand coverage for long-term nursing care for the elderly and disabled. The annual cost of the program to the government was estimated at $66.5 billion. Businesses were also expected to provide an additional $20 billion a year to bankroll the initiative. The high price tag and the preoccupation of government officials with the massive federal budget deficit precluded action on the recommendations in 1990.

Crisis in Public Healthcare. With immediate federal action unlikely, state and local governments attempted to deal with the seemingly intractable problems of the medically uninsured and rising healthcare costs. The public hospitals in much of the country faced a crisis that threatened to overwhelm their emergency rooms. Lacking any alternative, the poor, many AIDS victims, and the medically uninsured used emergency rooms for all kinds of medical care. In New York City, it was not uncommon for a patient to spend three or four days in the emergency room before a hospital bed could be found. California health examiners cited as unacceptable routine waits of 18 hours in emergency rooms in a public hospital in Oakland. At a public hospital in Los Angeles, the emergency room was so backed up that ambulances were turned away at least 25 percent of the time. While the problem was most acute in the Northeast and on the West Coast, the American College of Emergency Services reported serious overcrowding in emergency rooms in at least 41 states.

Many state administrators have complained that in the area of healthcare the state becomes, in effect, the "payer of last resort," since it must foot bills that the federal government and private insurers do not pay. States have long been struggling with the problem of how to finance their share of the Medicaid program, which provides health coverage to low-income persons. The federal government assists in financing the program and establishes minimum benefit and coverage levels. Medicaid reportedly accounted for 14 percent of state budgets in 1990, up from 9 percent in 1980. In December 1990, Arkansas Governor Bill Clinton, a Democrat, told a congressional committee that expansions of the Medicaid program mandated by Congress represented a "back-door approach to universal health care" that used "the states' credit cards as a financing mechanism."

Medicaid Benefits Expansion. Clinton's remarks were in response to the massive deficit-reduction package enacted by Congress in October 1990, which included a major expansion in the Medicaid program. Under the old law, children from families with incomes below the federal poverty level received Medicaid benefits through age 5. The new legislation raised the top age of eligibility to 8 in 1991, with the age to be increased by one each year thereafter until the eligibility pool includes all poor children through age 18. The combined federal-state cost for the first five years was estimated at over $1 billion, with the states picking up about 45 percent of this amount.

State Healthcare Initiatives. In March 1990, California Governor George Deukmejian, a Republican, unveiled a radical universal health plan for his state that would mandate private employers to provide health insurance for their employees. Faced with considerable business opposition, Deukmejian quickly distanced himself from the proposal, which had been drafted by two of his cabinet agencies. Nevertheless, the California Legislature drew up a compromise bill in 1990 to require private employers to provide minimum health insurance to the state's 4 million uninsured workers. The Democratic speaker of the California Assembly, Willie Brown, made the enactment of this plan his top priority for 1991.

Among states considering major restructuring of the financing of the healthcare delivery system in 1990, Washington was studying a universal comprehensive health plan modeled on the Canadian system. Oregon and Massachusetts have set target dates for employers to either provide health insurance or pay a tax to enable the state to provide coverage. (Because of the depleted Massachusetts coffers, however, state administrators have expressed doubts that the plan can meet its target date of April 1992.) For the poor covered under Medicaid, Oregon officials have devised an innovative plan to ration medical care. Under this proposal, which requires federal approval, medical conditions are ranked based on the costs and benefits of treating them. Higher ratings are given to treatable life-threatening conditions affecting large numbers of people than to minor conditions or to fatal incurable diseases. The poor would receive greater access to basic medical care, but Medicaid coverage would be limited to procedures in the upper part of the ratings list. In the version of the plan adopted by the Oregon Health Services Commission in February 1991, for example, appendicitis and certain types of pneumonia are near the top of the list, and superficial wounds and terminal AIDS near the bottom.

Prescription Drugs in Medicaid. The federal government took action in 1990 to reduce the heavy burden of prescription drug costs borne by Medicaid—estimated at nearly $5 billion—but the results were not entirely successful.

Democratic Senator David Pryor, chairman of the Special Committee on Aging, in May introduced a bill to require competitive bids on therapeutically equivalent prescription drugs in the Medicaid program. This approach was broader than requiring the use of low-cost generic drugs, which are chemically equivalent to their brand-name counterparts. Therapeutically equivalent drugs can be prescribed to treat the same symptom or disease even though they may be chemically different. Pryor's measure was based on findings that the U.S. Department of Veterans Affairs and other large-volume drug customers were paying significantly less than Medicaid for prescription drugs. While the Department of Veterans Affairs used competitive bids to purchase drugs, the federal government established upper limits on allowable costs for Medicaid drugs, permitting states to set the cost of dispensing the drug.

Hoping to head off restrictions on the lucrative Medicaid market, some drug companies began offering states discounts on the list prices of drugs used in the Medicaid program. The Bush administration and Congress made the discount approach a mandatory national policy for Medicaid by including it in the deficit reduction package approved in October 1990. The discounts were to be phased in, and by October 1992 drug manufacturers would have to give Medicaid the best price they offer to any customer. Savings over five years were expected to total $1.9 billion for the federal government and $1.4 billion for the states. Doubts soon arose that these savings would be achieved, as many drug companies began raising the prices they charged their big customers.

See also the Health and Medical News article HEALTHCARE COSTS AND INSURANCE.

FDA News

Generic Drugs. New developments emerged in the scandal involving the licensing of generic drugs by the U.S. Food and Drug Administration. In October 1990, American Therapeutics Inc. of Long Island, New York, was fined $1 million for making illegal cash payoffs to FDA drug reviewers and other law violations. In the same month federal prosecutors charged that Bolar Pharmaceutical Company, also of Long Island, had used Dyazide in FDA equivalence tests of Bolar's generic version of that hypertension drug. By early 1991 several former Bolar employees had pleaded guilty to criminal charges connected with this substitution or other activities in the unfolding scandal. Federal prosecutors filed criminal charges against Bolar in February 1991, charging the company with distributing misbranded or adulterated drugs, making false statements to the FDA, and obstructing federal investigations. Bolar pleaded guilty and was ordered to pay $10 million in fines.

In December 1990, Democratic Congressman John D. Dingell, chairman of the House Subcommittee on Oversight and Investigations, issued a damning indictment of the generic drug industry, calling it "the most pervasively corrupt this subcommittee has ever uncovered." Of the 36 generic drug companies investigated by federal prosecutors and the FDA by December, subcommittee sources estimated that only about a half dozen were free of criminal or regulatory violations. The U.S. attorney leading the investigation condemned the industry for showing a "reckless disregard for the health and safety of the consuming public" but also noted that he had found no evidence of harm to anyone from taking improperly tested generic drugs.

New Agency Head. Dr. David Kessler was confirmed by the Senate as FDA commissioner in late 1990 and took office in February 1991. Kessler, a lawyer as well as a physician, had been medical director of a New York hospital and a lecturer on food and drug law at Columbia University. On taking up his new post, he promised to work to strengthen the agency's enforcement powers and to streamline procedures for approval of drugs and medical devices. The previous permanent commissioner, Dr. Frank E. Young, had resigned in 1989 amid the controversy set off by the generic drug scandal.

Abortion Controversy Continues

Since July 1989, when the U.S. Supreme Court voted in the case of *Webster* v. *Reproductive Health Services* to expand states' power to limit the right to abortion, the combatants in the abortion controversy have fought several battles in the courts and state legislatures.

In August 1990 a federal district judge declared unconstitutional a statute enacted a few months before in the U.S. territory of Guam that forbade all abortions except in situations in which the mother's life was threatened. Shortly thereafter, in Pennsylvania, a federal district judge struck down parts of that state's restrictive abortion law, which had been adopted in November 1989. A provision requiring a

Making TV Better for the Deaf and Blind

Many people are surprised to learn that deaf and blind people watch television. But they do. On average people who are deaf or hard of hearing and people who are blind or visually impaired watch as much as viewers with normal hearing and vision. Unfortunately, they miss much or all of either the dialogue or the action. Two recent developments should change this situation for the better.

In October 1990, President George Bush signed a bill requiring that by July 1993 all new television sets sold in the United States, regardless of where they were made, must contain a computer chip that makes closed captioning available at the touch of a button. For more than a decade TV channels have broadcast captions, similar to subtitles, so that deaf people can "hear" the dialogue and other sounds. The captions are encoded, or closed, so they don't appear on the screen unless a decoding device is used. Currently, all prime time TV and some cable and home video shows offer closed captioning, but studies have shown that fewer than 10 percent of the 25 million Americans with hearing problems have decoders, which cost around $200. The computer chip is expected to raise the price of a television set by only a few dollars.

A new service developed for blind and visually impaired TV audiences is called descriptive video (DSV). DSV is an additional sound track that describes between segments of dialogue a show's scenery, character movements, and body language. The technology for DSV was originally developed by a blind woman and her husband for use in theaters in the Washington, D.C., area. It was first used on TV by Boston's public television station, WGBH, which remains at the forefront of the effort to expand its usage. DSV made its national debut on public television in January 1990, and it has begun to be used by some cable networks.

Visually impaired people who have experienced DSV say their TV sets have never seemed clearer. One woman reported being moved to tears as a whole new element of the story was opened up to her. The sound track is broadcast on an additional audio channel that can be received by stereo television sets and videocassette recorders; it is accessed by pressing the multichannel stereo button. Viewers who don't want the sound track simply don't press the button. Some 15 million stereo TV sets already have the feature, as do about 45 percent of all new television sets being sold today.

married woman to notify her husband before getting an abortion was declared unconstitutional, as were requirements that women listen to a state-prepared talk from a doctor about the risks of abortion and the benefits of childbirth and then wait 24 hours between the talk and the actual abortion. Also declared unconstitutional was a stipulation that minors seeking an abortion get permission from at least one parent or a court order. Appeals were filed in both the Pennsylvania and Guam cases.

In June 1990 the Supreme Court held, by a 5-4 vote, that a Minnesota law requiring minors to inform both parents before obtaining an abortion was unconstitutional. In another 5-4 vote, however, the Court ruled that such a law would be constitutional if minors had the option to request that a judge waive the parental notification requirement.

The parental notification issue flared up in Michigan as well. After Democratic Governor James J. Blanchard vetoed a law requiring girls 17 and younger to obtain a parent's or a judge's consent before getting an abortion, Right to Life of Michigan gathered more than 330,000 signatures to put the bill on the ballot as a voter initiative. As was permitted in such a situation by the state constitution, the legislature then enacted the bill into law without submitting it to the electorate or the governor. A state ban on Medicaid-financial abortions for poor women was struck down by the Michigan Court of Appeals in February 1991. According to the court, the ban violated the rights of women to privacy and to equal protection under the Michigan constitution, which, the court noted, protects the right to abortion.

In Louisiana, a colorful drama was played out in the summer of 1990 between Democratic Governor Buddy Roemer and the legislature. Shortly before adjourning, the legislature sent the governor a restrictive abortion law that, like the law adopted in Guam, would have allowed abortion only to protect the mother's life. Roemer vetoed that measure on the ground that it made no exception for pregnancies that resulted from rape or incest, and his veto was narrowly sustained by the legislature. The legislature then redrafted the bill, allowing abortions in cases of rape reported to the police within seven days, as well as in cases of incest or to save the mother's life. To expedite consideration of this second bill, the lawmakers tacked it onto legislation that would have made an assault on flag burners a misdemeanor. After deliberating for several weeks, Roemer vetoed the new bill, noting that he objected to the legislative procedure, the failure to allow consideration of the mother's mental health as a factor, and the requirement that a rape be reported within seven days.

A relatively liberal abortion law was enacted in Maryland in February 1991. Aimed at guarding the right to an abortion if it should ever be restricted by the Supreme Court, the law guaranteed to adult woman access to abortion during the period the fetus is unable to survive out of the womb. After that period an abortion would be allowed in order to protect the woman's health or if the fetus is deformed. The law required notification of a parent if an underage girl sought an abortion, but allowed doctors to ignore the requirement.

AIDS Initiatives

In March 1990, in his first address on AIDS since taking office, President George Bush called for ending discrimination against those infected with the disease. Speaking before the National Leadership Commission on AIDS, the president voiced support for the Americans with Disabilities Act, legislation that would prohibit discrimination against people with a mental or physical disability, including persons infected with the AIDS virus, chiefly in regard to employment and access to public services. (He signed the bill into law in July.) Bush also defended the federal effort to finance research on the cause and treatment of AIDS. JAMES A. ROTHERHAM

CANADA

Abortion Bill Fails • Quebec Proposes User Fee • Federal AIDS Strategy • Doctors and Nurses Strike

Abortion

Canada remained without an abortion law following the defeat of a new bill by an unusual tie vote in the Senate on January 31, 1991. Bill C-43 was killed by a 43-to-43 tally in Parliament's upper chamber, where a tie is considered a defeat. Federal Justice Minister Kim Campbell quickly announced that there would be no further efforts to draft abortion legislation during the government's remaining two or three year mandate.

The country had been without an abortion law since the Supreme Court of Canada struck down the old one in 1988. The former statute stipulated that abortions could be performed only at accredited hospitals and only after approval by a hospital committee. The proposed Bill C-43, which would have allowed the operation in clinics as well as hospitals, would have prohibited abortions except when a doctor determined that a woman's physical or mental health was threatened by a continued pregnancy. Doctors who violated the law would have faced up to two years in prison.

From its inception, Bill C-43, pieced together by the House of Commons under pressure from both pro-choice and anti-abortion factions, seemed to satisfy no one. It aroused intense, sometimes agonizing, debate in the House of Commons, where one effort to pass it failed before it finally carried in May 1990 by a mere nine votes.

Meanwhile, the Ontario government committed itself to increasing access to abortion by fully funding freestanding abortion clinics and by covering the costs of flying residents from remote areas in northern Ontario to cities to receive the operation.

Quebec's Proposed User Fees

In November the Quebec government announced sweeping reforms of its healthcare system, designed to streamline the program that consumes about one-third of the provincial budget. Among the anticipated changes was a controversial, and perhaps illegal, proposal to charge a $5 deterrent fee (Canadian dollars used throughout) for some users of Quebec's overcrowded hospital emergency wards. The fee, which was denounced by federal opposition Liberals and New Democrats as a threat to universal access to healthcare, would be charged to people who use emergency wards for nonemergencies such as sore throats and colds.

Federal Health Minister Perrin Beatty said that the fee may violate the Canada Health Act (CHA), which bans both extra billing of patients and hospital user fees. "The provisions of the Canada Health Act stand," he said. "We do not believe in taxing the sick." Beatty refused to say what the federal government would do if it determined that the fee violate the CHA, which stipulates that medicare payments to provinces can be withheld if they charge user fees.

Other proposed changes to Quebec's healthcare system included a service tax on eyeglasses, prescription drugs, and hearing aids; extending patients' rights in the area of decisions about their care; and expanding home health services.

Breast Implant Controversy

Canadian scientists announced in June that the controversial Meme breast implant, used to increase breast size or for reconstruction following surgery, decomposes quickly at body temperature, producing highly toxic carcinogens. Already known to decompose at extremely high temperatures, the device's polyurethane foam coating was found by a Laval University research team to break down within two weeks of implantation.

The federal government, which fired a top researcher in 1989 for publicly criticizing the American-made implant as "unfit" for human use, refused to remove it from the market, but leaked documents revealed there was concern among Department of National Health and Welfare officials about the device's safety. A spokesman said the government was conducting its own research into what happens when polyurethane breaks down and mixes with human tissue.

Since 1984 some 13,000 Canadian women have received the Meme implant. Doctors in Ottawa, the nation's capital, were not using it, but plastic surgeons from Vancouver, Calgary, Montreal, and Quebec City continued to.

Federal AIDS Strategy

The long-awaited federal AIDS strategy was finally introduced in June by Health Minister Beatty, but its reception was anything but positive. "HIV and AIDS: Canada's Blueprint" was criticized for everything from its failure to commit more funds to fight the deadly disease (the $112 million proposed in the paper is already included in the $168 million the government tagged in 1988 for AIDS programs) to its virtual silence in giving credit to the doctors who are on the front lines treating AIDS victims.

Critics attacked the federal government for the paper's ignoring of a number of issues, including immigration policies, AIDS in prisons, and the rising prejudice against homosexuals. The strategy was also condemned for being vague—but here, the federal government had a defense. Because the Canadian constitution assigns healthcare to the provinces, not the federal government, it is up to the provinces to design and implement specific AIDS projects. The report placed strong emphasis on "education and prevention programs [as] the most effective tools in preventing the spread of the disease" and discussed involving community groups, including AIDS sufferers and caregivers, in AIDS programs.

Two months after the strategy was released, the federal government's Canadian International Development Agency announced it would commit $11 million over five years to four national health groups—including the Canadian Public Health Association and the Canadian Society for International Health—to aid them in their work fighting AIDS in Africa.

Reproductive Technology

A royal commission examining the ethics, economics, and legal implications of reproductive technologies completed 2½ months of hearings in December 1990. The $11.8 million effort included 350 presentations in more than 15 cities which were to be incorporated into a report slated to be released around October 1991. The report was designed to recommend limits, standards, and guidelines in the use of such techniques as in vitro fertilization, prenatal screening, surrogate motherhood, and embryo research. The goal, said commission chairman Dr. Patricia Baird, was to make sure "we don't have a laissez-faire and commercial situation as many feel occurs in the U.S. And there is a concern . . . to make sure that the use of these technologies doesn't dehumanize our society."

See also the feature article PRENATAL SCREENING.

Manitoba Labor Strife

Manitoba's 2,000 doctors came to a four-year agreement on fees with the provincial government in late August 1990, following a weekend strike which lasted almost two full days. Like all provincial governments in Canada, Manitoba pays most of its doctors on a fee-for-service basis through public health insurance. Under the new contract doctors were to receive a 3 percent raise in fees the first year, followed by three years of binding arbitration, under which the doctors' fee levels would be assessed annually by an independent appraiser whose determination will be mandatory. The doctors forfeited their right to strike until 1994.

Manitoba's nurses' union battled frigid temperatures and hospital management in a strike for higher wages that began on January 1, 1991. After rejecting an earlier offer, on January 31, 61 percent of the union membership ratified a new contract that gave them a 13 percent increase over two years. (Most nurses were making about $37,000 a year when they went out on strike.)

LYNNE COHEN

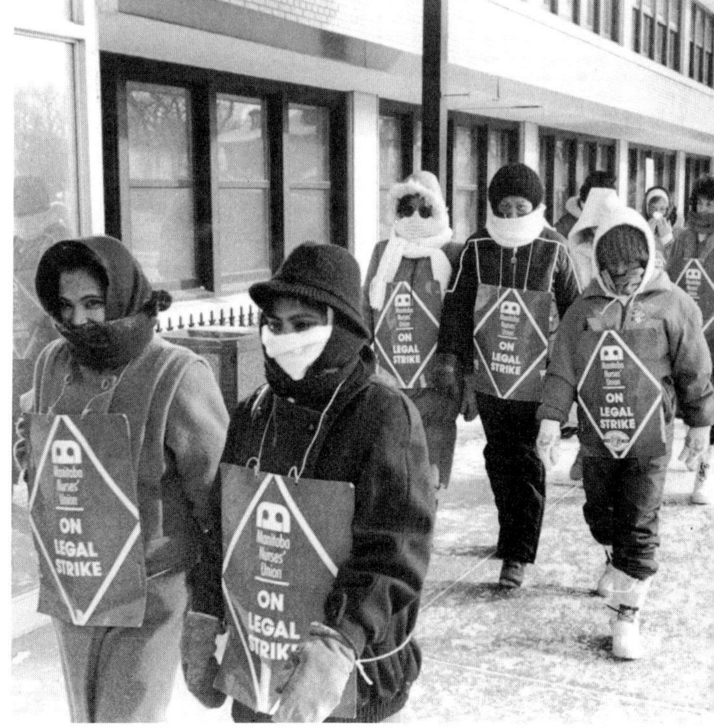

Manitoba nurses walked a chilly picket line in January 1991 when they went on strike in a wage dispute. The provincial government threatened to intervene, but an agreement was reached by the end of the month.

HEALTHCARE COSTS AND INSURANCE

Cost Increases Continue • Private and Public Cost-cutting Efforts • Healthcare Rationing Gains Support

Cost Increases Continue

Healthcare costs in the United States continued their relentless upward surge in 1990, defying once again all attempts at fiscal restraint. The total U.S. healthcare bill was expected to reach around $650 billion, or 12 percent of the gross national product. That compares with about 5.2 percent in 1960, 7.4 percent in 1970, and 9 percent in 1980. Within a decade, annual costs are expected to top the $1.5 trillion mark.

Health analysts attribute the rampant growth to many factors, among them advances in technology and the growing number of older and sicker Americans. But in a speech in the fall, Health and Human Services Secretary Dr. Louis Sullivan set a new tone for the growing national debate over how to control costs and at the same time assure quality healthcare for all Americans.

Dr. Sullivan identified three major factors fueling the growth of costs. First, consumers have been "desensitized" to the costs of their healthcare by insurance. Second, doctors, hospitals, and other providers of care have "focused on curing and caring" with little attention to the costs of their decisions. And finally, Americans choose life-styles and behaviors that are harmful to health, then turn to the healthcare system as a "fix-it shop."

Proposed Solutions

Growing costs, coupled with a number of other factors, spurred new efforts to restructure the nation's healthcare system. These other factors were concerns about meeting the health needs of the over 30 million Americans with no health insurance, the need to find a mechanism to cover the expense of long-term care, a new emphasis on assuring quality, and growing talk of rationing healthcare.

Over the years, numerous groups have suggested possible reforms, including a comprehensive national healthcare system based on the Canadian model and mandatory insurance coverage by employers for all workers. None of these groups, however, had the offi-

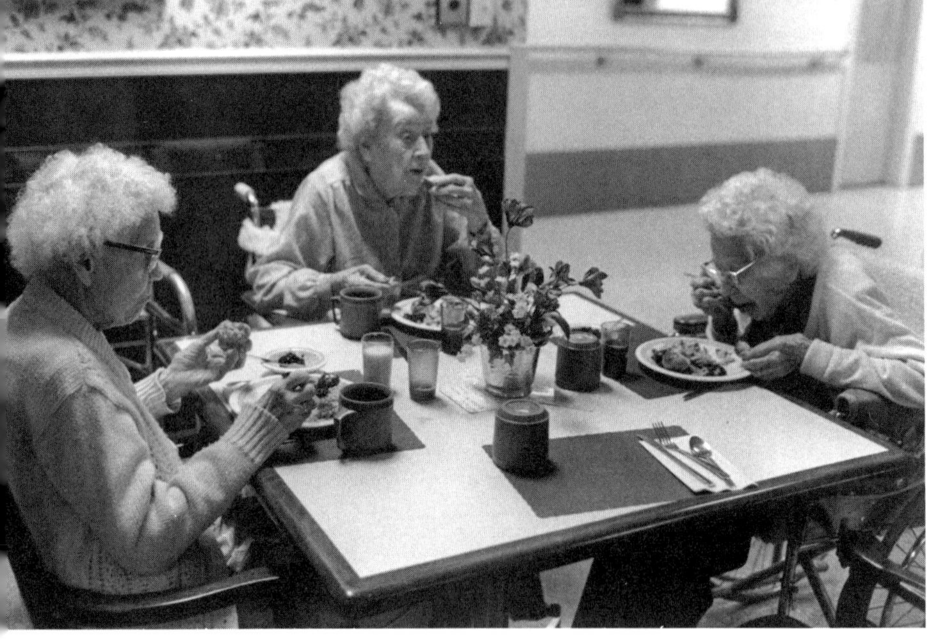

The difficult issue of how to pay for long-term nursing home care, such as that being received by these residents, was addressed in a report issued by a U.S. federal panel known as the Pepper Commission. It recommended a system under which costs would be shared three ways—by families and by federal and state governments.

cial clout of the three federal panels addressing the issues during 1990.

Only one of the three completed its work and issued a final report. Members of the Bipartisan Commission on Comprehensive Health Care, renamed the Pepper Commission in honor of the late Congressman Claude Pepper, unanimously agreed that "all Americans should have access to affordable health and long-term care coverage in an efficient and effective system."

To that end the commission recommended that employers and the government together should provide a minimum package of healthcare benefits for all. The minimum package would cover preventive and primary care and hospital and physician bills. Employers would continue to operate through the private insurance market and the government through an expanded federal Medicaid program for the poor that would replace the current state-federal system.

To meet the long-term care needs of the nation's disabled, many of them elderly, the commission proposed a new social insurance program, fully financed by the federal government, to cover the costs of home and community-based long-term care and the first three months of nursing home care. All the elderly and disabled, regardless of income, would be eligible.

After the first three months, nursing home costs would be shared by families, to the degree possible, and the federal and state governments. To protect families from becoming impoverished because of the high costs of long-term nursing home care, the commission proposed to protect $30,000 in assets for individuals and $60,000 for couples. People would not be eligible for assistance until assets were depleted to those levels; income and assets above those levels would be applied toward the costs of nursing home care.

To qualify for long-term care benefits, individuals would need to meet strict criteria. An individual would need either help with three activities of daily living (dressing, eating, bathing, and the like) or constant supervision because of cognitive impairment or because of dangerous, disruptive, or difficult to manage behaviors. As needed, benefits would include personal care, homemaker/chore services, shopping and other support services, day care, respite care, and training for family caregivers.

The total annual cost to the government of the Pepper Commission proposals: an estimated $66.5 billion. In their final report, members outlined six possibilities for raising the necessary funds. Those included increases in the Social Security payroll tax, a 4 percent value-added sales tax, and additional personal taxes for those in top income brackets. Commission Chairman Senator John D. (Jay) Rockefeller IV was expected to introduce a bill based on the group's proposals in mid-1991.

The Advisory Commission on Social Security, charged by the president with addressing healthcare issues, issued an interim report in summer 1990. A final report, with recommendations for restructuring the system, was to be delivered mid-1991.

The advisory commission was contemplating a number of possible structural changes for the healthcare system. One was a plan to cover all Americans with private insurance for basic medical care, with government subsidies for premiums and out-of-pocket costs for those who cannot afford them. The government would then pick up all "catastrophic" costs above some preset level. Other options under review included expanding Medicare to cover all Americans and requiring states to set up universal coverage health programs, with costs paid by both federal and state governments.

A third group, a Department of Health and Human Services task force under the direction of Secretary Sullivan, was working on a proposal expected to address not only costs and the structure of current public and private insurance programs but also the effectiveness of medical practices and the matter of personal responsibility for health. Items for possible study included the tax-free status of employer-provided insurance, which costs the government nearly $60 billion a year, and state-mandated benefits, which drive up costs to the point that many small firms are discouraged from offering health benefits.

Medicare's Silver Anniversary

Medicare celebrated its 25th anniversary to mixed reviews. Despite the dramatic improvements in healthcare for the elderly over the last quarter century, Medicare remains an attractive target for budget cutters because of its sheer size, an estimated $108 billion in 1990, and its growth, about 10 percent a year.

As budget cutters scrambled to reduce the projected deficit in the federal budget, Medicare seemed destined for a major hit. Early efforts to impose large increases on premiums and deductibles ran into powerful opposition from seniors' groups. In the end, lawmakers trimmed about $31 billion from the program's growth from 1991 through 1995 by cutting payments to doctors and hospitals and another $10.7 billion by raising the out-of-pocket costs to beneficiaries. (At the last minute, Congress accepted one significant Medicare expansion by agreeing to coverage for mammograms to detect breast cancer.)

Under the terms of the budget package, the one-time $75 deductible for physicians' services increased to $100 in January 1991. Between 1991 and 1995, monthly Medicare premiums for Part B insurance, which covers physicians' bills, will rise from $29.90 to $46.10.

In January 1991, as mandated by a law passed in 1989, limits went into effect on the amount doctors can charge Medicare patients above what Medicare reimburses. The limit of 25 percent introduced in 1991 will decrease to 15 percent by 1993. A new fee schedule will go into effect in 1992, as will a performance-based standard that suggests how much payments to physicians should grow with respect to overall increases and to volume of services provided and technological advances. This is intended to slow both the rise in physicians' fees and the growth in the volume of services provided.

25 Years for Medicaid

The Medicaid program for the poor celebrated its 25th anniversary in even shakier condition than Medicare. According to a study by the congressional General Accounting Office, the joint federal-state program leaves millions of poor and near poor without healthcare and, at the same time, has imposed significant fiscal hardships on some states. Changes proposed by the GAO would increase federal reimbursement to poorer states like Georgia, Arkansas, and Florida, and decrease it to such states as Alaska, Massachusetts, and Connecticut.

In the final federal budget, $2.9 billion was cut from Medicaid. A provision that pharmaceutical companies give discounts on sales of drugs to Medicaid was expected to trim federal spending by $1.9 billion between 1991 and 1995 and another requirement that states purchase private insurance, if available, for the families of Medicaid beneficiaries was expected to save another $1 billion.

But at the same time, Congress continued to broaden coverage, extending it to cover, by the year 2001, all poor children through the age of 18. The previous age limit was 6. Other expansions include home care for frail elderly people and home and community-based services for those with developmental disabilities.

About half of the total Medicaid budget pays for long-term nursing home care. Through the National Governors Association, fiscally strapped states have objected to the gradual expansion of mandated benefits. To pay for the expanded coverage, many states have had to set tougher eligibility standards. An analysis by the Urban Institute suggests that only half of the nation's poor under age 65 are covered because of state eligibility requirements.

Medigap Laws Tightened

Though failing to address the overall issue of reform, Congress nibbled at other nagging health problems. One of the most significant changes tightened government regulation of so-called Medigap insurance, purchased by about 18 million elderly Americans to pay bills not covered by Medicare. Many found the policies confusing and purchased unnecessary insurance coverage.

The new rules will require standardization of policies, so consumers can compare benefits and prices. Policies that duplicate each other or Medicare coverage will be subject to civil penalties up to $25,000. Insurers will also be required to pay rebates if policies fail to return in benefits at least 65 cents of every premium dollar for individual benefits and 75 cents for group policies. Companies are no longer able to refuse to sell Medigap policies to seniors with preexisting health conditions or chronic illnesses.

Private Insurers Struggle

Employers and insurers increasingly questioned whether they were paying too much for care and whether the enormous costs of some procedures might actually outweigh any potential benefits. Economists calculate that high technology medical advances account for about 20 percent each year in the growth of health costs. The limitations placed by insurers on autologous bone marrow transplantation coverage were a highly visible example of strategies designed to control costs. This treatment involves taking bone marrow from a patient, subjecting the patient to near lethal doses of chemotherapy, then reimplanting the marrow to restore the patient's immune system. Despite the chance that 5 to 10 percent of patients will die from complications related to the procedure, the treatment is commonly used for some forms of leukemia and lymphoma, and it is a choice of growing numbers of women with metastatic breast cancer.

Unfortunately, autologous bone marrow transplants cost over $100,000. The costs are covered for the other cancers, but because the treatment is considered experimental for breast cancer, many insurers refused to pay. After patients began turning to the courts to gain coverage, Blue Cross-Blue Shield took the unprecedented step of agreeing to fund a study by the National Cancer Institute to determine the effectiveness of the treatment.

At the same time, many insurance carriers have quietly denied or limited coverage to high risk categories of workers, such as loggers and miners, to workers in occupations and cities where the AIDS virus is prevalent, or to individuals with chronic or preexisting health conditions. Several states have established risk pools to provide coverage, but in most areas, such individuals fall in the growing ranks of the uninsured.

A study by GAO confirmed that growing numbers of employers are restricting coverage available to employees. More frequently, large firms are turning to part-time workers who receive no benefits, imposing waiting periods for new employees, and requiring medical testing to identify potential employees likely to develop costly medical conditions.

On the plus side, a small number of employers are emphasizing "wellness" and rewarding fit employees with discounts, rebates, and other incentives.

Increases in costs led to a number of changes in employer-sponsored health plans. Most striking was the continued growth in managed care, either through prepaid health maintenance organizations (HMOs), designation of "preferred providers" (doctors and hospitals), and closer scrutiny of services. By the end of 1989, all but 18 percent of plans provided by employers had some managed care features.

Whether efforts by insurers to control costs will succeed remains to be seen. According to a survey by the Health Insurance Association of America, premiums rose by an average of 18 percent from the spring of 1988 to the spring of 1989, with the largest increases hitting conventional plans. Based on a number of indicators, HIAA predicted that premium inflation had peaked and increases in the next few years would be more modest.

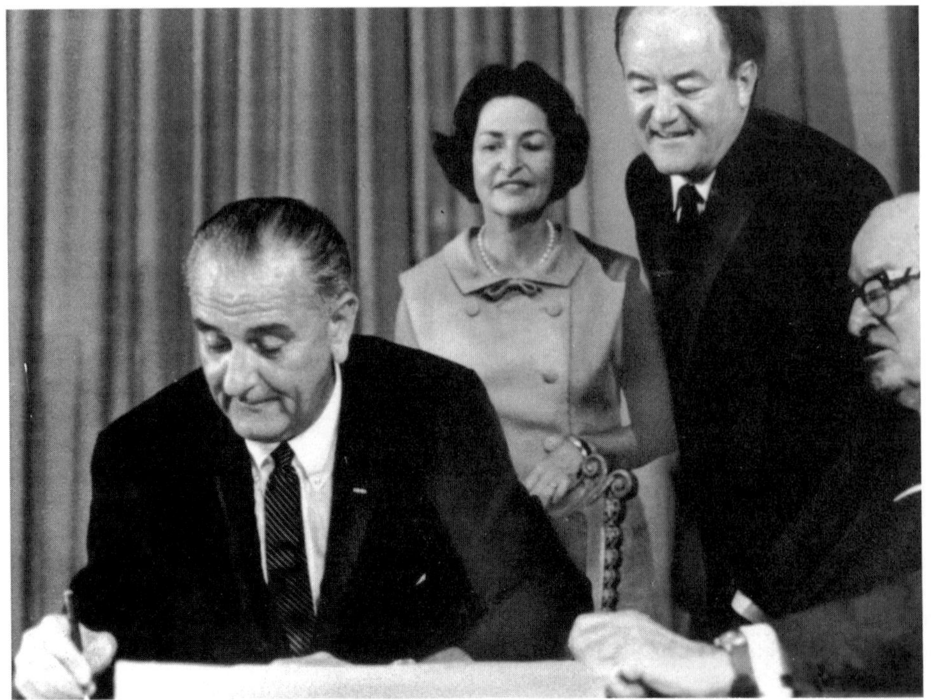

Medicare celebrated its silver anniversary in 1990. Photo shows President Lyndon Johnson signing the legislation that established the Medicare program on July 30, 1965; looking on are, from left, his wife, Lady Bird, Vice President Hubert Humphrey, and former President Harry S. Truman.

More Talk of Rationing

A survey conducted by the Northwestern National Life Insurance Company showed that a surprising 85 percent of Americans would support some form of rationing to keep healthcare both affordable and available. The support seemed tied to the fear shared by two-thirds of those surveyed that they would not be able to afford care because of rising costs.

Respondents did not agree, however, on how care should be rationed. Strongest support was given for the idea that rich and poor should abide by the same rationing rules, that publicly funded healthcare should be rationed with respect to the probability of success for a treatment, that smokers should be denied public funds to cover costs of illness caused by smoking, and that children should have priority for care at the expense of the elderly.

One notion that received little support was the Medicaid rationing initiative being designed in Oregon. Under the Oregon plan Medicaid coverage would be expanded to include all residents earning less than 100 percent of the poverty level, but only for a limited list of services. Members of the Oregon Health Services Commission completed priority rankings of some 800 medical services by early 1991, and the full program was expected to be in place by 1992.

Many medical experts think the real issue is not rationing but waste and unnecessary care. According to some studies, up to 30 percent of medical procedures performed in the United States are unnecessary. Several large-scale studies are underway to identify those procedures which are the most—and least—effective, with the eventual aim of developing practice guidelines for physicians. Beyond improving overall quality of care, one objective, of course, is to trim costs by eliminating unnecessary and ineffective treatment.

MARY HAGER

HEART AND CIRCULATORY SYSTEM

Sound Wave Technology • Heart Assist Device Approved • Enlarged Heart Poses Risk • Drugs That Dissolve Blood Clots • Surgery for Arrhythmias

Sound Wave Imaging

Recent technical improvements in the equipment used for sound wave imaging of the heart, or echocardiography, has allowed the technique to be used in increasingly novel ways. Echocardiography has long been a preferred method for evaluating many forms of heart disease because it is noninvasive, safe, and relatively inexpensive. In the past, however, the images produced were not always of the best quality, especially in patients who were elderly, obese, or had lung disease. Frequently physicians were not fully confident about echocardiographic information and ordered invasive tests such as cardiac catheterization to confirm the findings.

One important advance that has markedly improved diagnostic capabilities is the development of transesophageal echocardiography. This procedure is performed using a sonographic probe mounted on a long, flexible tube similar to an endoscope. The tube is inserted into the esophagus and then positioned at different levels in the esophagus and stomach to produce images of the heart and the large blood vessels. Because the esophagus lies just behind the heart, unobstructed by lung tissue (air hinders the passage of the sound waves), the quality of transesophageal echocardiographic images is usually superior to those obtained by conventional echocardiography.

Transesophageal echocardiography is now used at many medical centers to detect blood clots or infections in the heart and to evaluate tears in the aorta (the largest artery in the body), which can be fatal if untreated. The technique is also being used to improve the results of heart operations. The probe can monitor the heart at critical points during coronary artery bypass surgery or valve replacement without interfering with the operation.

Another sonographic technology being developed is intravascular ultrasound, which works by inserting an ultrasound catheter into the blood vessels to be imaged. Prior to the development of this technology, the only practical way to image the inside of a blood vessel was to inject a harmless dye and take an X ray, a technique called angiography. Although angiography is a powerful tool, it is limited because it creates only a lengthwise silhouette of blood vessels. Intravascular ultrasound shows a cross section through a blood vessel and can demonstrate the composition as well as the size of plaques that obstruct arteries.

A technological innovation called color flow Doppler enables physicians to immediately recognize patterns of blood flow in the heart by producing an image that is color-coded according to the direction of flow. Another technique, contrast echocardiography, provides information about blood flow by reflecting sound waves off miniscule air bubbles suspended in a harmless material that is injected intravenously.

In addition, standard echocardiography has been expanded to new clinical settings. Many emergency rooms and intensive care units now have portable ultrasound machines to immediately evaluate heart damage after trauma to the chest or during heart attacks. Echocardiography is also being used to screen patients for coronary artery obstructions by observing the heart's response to exercise or (in people who cannot exercise) to drugs that stress the heart.

Heart Device Approved

The U.S. Food and Drug Administration in January 1991 approved the experimental use of a battery-powered mechanical device to help a failing heart pump blood until a donor heart can be found. Called a left ventricular assist device, the artificial pump is implanted in the abdominal cavity just below the diaphragm and is connected to the heart's main pumping chamber, the left ventricle. Oxygenated blood drains from the left ventricle into the mechanical pumping chamber where a miniature motor propels it into the aorta to be circulated to the body.

Unlike previous heart assist devices, the battery-powered pump does not need to be connected to an external energy source and allows patients to move about freely. The batteries are worn in a shoulder holster, and power is transmitted through a wire that pierces the skin and is connected to the implanted device. An older version of the device—which requires tethering patients to an external air compressor but is otherwise identical—has been used in 33 patients in the United States.

The Heavy Heart

Several studies published in 1990 provide strong evidence that a "heavy heart" is not only a colloquialism for an emotional burden but an indication of an important health problem. It has been known for years that an enlargement of the heart is associated with a high risk of cardiac illness and death, but the scope of the problem was not recognized until improvements in echocardiography enabled physicians to accurately estimate the heart's size and weight. A May 1990 report showed that increased left ventricular mass (a thickening or enlargement of the main pumping

NEW BATTERY-POWERED PUMP TO AID A FAILING HEART

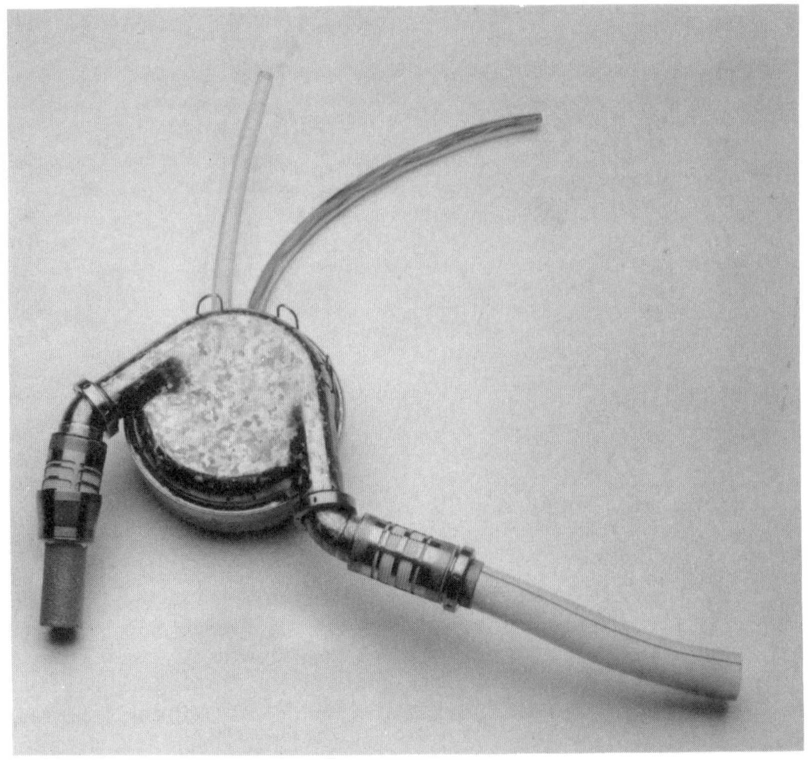

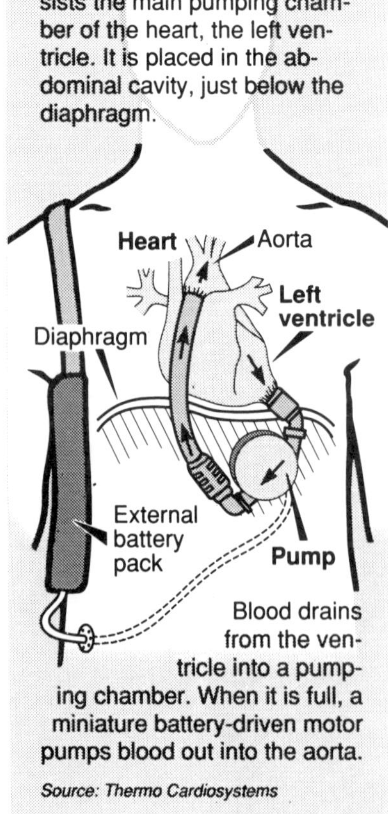

The New York Times

chamber of the heart) occurred in nearly 20 percent of apparently healthy adults and was associated with the development of heart disease and cardiac death. This increased risk of heart disease persisted even after other determinants of cardiac health such as cholesterol level, smoking, and blood pressure were accounted for.

The measurement of heart size and weight may be particularly important in patients with hypertension (high blood pressure). In a study of 253 patients, investigators showed that patients with increased left ventricular mass developed hypertensive complications ten times more frequently than those with normal heart size and no other cardiac risk factors. The study also suggested that the measurement of left ventricular mass may help determine which patients with borderline or mild hypertension can be safely treated without medication. A follow-up study of 166 patients showed that a decrease in left ventricular mass during treatment also helps reduce the likelihood of complications of hypertension.

Hypertension and Exercise

Regular aerobic exercise is an effective way to lower blood pressure without medication in patients with borderline or mild hypertension, according to a study published in May 1990. Although exercise has long been recommended as a healthful activity that seems to control blood pressure, the report is the first to show the treatment effect of exercise in a carefully controlled scientific study. The investigators studied 27 previously sedentary men, 10 of whom completed a ten-week training program consisting of fast walking, jogging, or bicycling at least four times each week for 30 minutes or more. Patients in a control group did exercise limited to stretching and easy calisthenics. At the completion of the trial, patients in the aerobic exercise group reduced their diastolic blood pressure (the bottom, or second, number of a blood pressure reading), an average of 10 mm Hg, from 95 to 85 mm Hg, whereas the control group had no change in blood pressure. Later, patients initially assigned to the control group were allowed to participate in a ten-week aerobic exercise program after which they too were found to have lower blood pressure.

Controlling Atherosclerosis

New evidence suggests that drastic lifestyle changes can stem the progression of, and perhaps reverse, atherosclerosis (hardening of the arteries) in patients with known coronary artery disease. In a study published in July 1990, 28 patients were asked to eat a very low-fat, vegetarian diet without caffeine or excessive alcohol, exercise at least three hours per week, participate in stress management techniques one hour each day, and attend a support group twice weekly for at least a year. A control group of patients, also with coronary artery disease, was not asked to make lifestyle changes, although some members did make moderate changes. Coronary angiograms were obtained at the beginning of the study and after one year to measure the severity of atherosclerosis. After a year, the group that had made drastic changes benefited, on average, in having fewer and less severe episodes of chest pain than the control patients and in having a small, but significant, reduction in size of coronary atherosclerotic plaques. The control patients' plaques had become, on average, larger.

For those at highest risk of heart disease related to atherosclerosis, an operation called an ileal bypass was proven to be beneficial in 1990. The operation involves removing several feet of the small intestine, where fat digestion, as well as absorption of other nutrients, takes place. When the bypass is performed, much smaller amounts of fat and nutrients reach the bloodstream. In a study of 838 patients with high cholesterol levels who had had heart attacks, subjects who had an ileal bypass lived longer than those treated by other means. However, the operation can cause side effects such as persistent diarrhea, kidney stones, and gallstones, so it should be reserved for the very few patients at highest risk who do not respond to other types of treatment.

Clot-Dissolving Drugs Compared

It is generally agreed that the introduction of thrombolytic agents (drugs that break up blood clots) was the most important advance in the treatment of heart attacks during the 1980s, but a great controversy persisted about which drug works best. An Italian study published in March 1990 showed no difference in effectiveness between the most commonly used agent in the United States, tissue plasminogen activator (TPA), and the most commonly used drug in Europe, streptokinase. However, many medical scientists criticized the Italian study because the blood-thinning drug heparin was not administered promptly after TPA, as is the practice in the United States, but rather 12 hours after hospital admission. An important study published in November 1990 found a higher rate of successful treatment (82 percent versus 52 percent) in 106 patients treated with heparin immediately and continuously after receiving TPA compared to 99 patients treated with daily aspirin as the principal blood-thinning agent following TPA.

In late 1989, the U.S. Food and Drug Administration approved a third thrombolytic agent, anistreplase (brand name, Eminase). Anistreplase has the advantage of being quick to administer; it can be given by injection in five minutes rather than the three hours required for infusion of TPA. The drug costs $1,500 to $1,700 per dose, compared with $2,200 for TPA and $76 to $186 for streptokinase.

In March 1991, British researchers announced the results of a long-awaited report comparing streptokinase, TPA, and Eminase. The study, which evaluated more than 46,000 patients in 16 countries over a period of 18 months, was believed to be the largest ever conducted to evaluate the treatment of heart attack. It found all three drugs to be equally effective in saving lives (about 90 percent of those receiving each drug survived), but there was one significant difference—streptokinase showed the smallest incidence of strokes due to cerebral bleeding, an uncommon but dangerous complication of treatment with thrombolytic agents. The researchers employed the European practice of administering heparin differently than in the United States, and this area remained controversial. Nevertheless, the results supported the March 1990 Italian study and raised speculation that U.S. doctors would begin to choose the much less expensive streptokinase more frequently.

Blood-thinning Drug

A blood-thinning drug available since the 1950s was reevaluated in 1990 and found effective at preventing strokes in patients with a certain type of irregular heartbeat. For years physicians have known that the risk of stroke is several times greater in individuals with atrial fibrillation (a condition characterized by an irregular pulse) and 17 times higher when atrial fibrillation is accompanied by disease of the heart valves. Although the blood-thinner warfarin (most often sold under the trade name Coumadin) has been prescribed routinely for years to prevent strokes in patients with atrial fibrillation and valvular disease, it was not known whether the benefit of stroke prevention in patients without disease of the heart valves outweighed the potential risk of bleeding. In a study published in November 1990 of patients with atrial fibrillation but without valve disease, the risk of having a stroke was 86 percent lower for patients treated with warfarin than for patients treated with aspirin or no blood-thinner. The risk of major bleeding episodes was no different between the groups.

Treating Arrhythmias

Several important papers in 1990 supported the feasibility of treating cardiac arrhythmias (irregular heartbeats) with surgical techniques. (Studies of drug treatments for arrhythmias have yielded generally disappointing results.) Over the past decade, highly specialized cardiologists called electrophysiologists have diagnosed and treated arrhythmias using procedures that involve electrical stimulation of the heart and tracking of electrical impulses in the heart. These procedures make it possible to determine the risk of future arrhythmia complications, such as loss of consciousness or death, as well as the underlying cause of arrhythmias. In many patients arrhythmias result when by small areas of the heart containing electrical pathways conduct electrical impulses abnormally. These areas can now be precisely located and either removed during open-heart surgery or destroyed with special catheters that deliver energy by direct current or radio waves.

Angioplasty Update

The use of angioplasty, the dilation of atherosclerotic plaques with a balloon catheter, has until recently usually been limited to patients with only one or two obstructions of the coronary arteries. But a new study shows that the procedure may have a role in treating patients with more severe coronary artery disease. The study reported the results of angioplasty in 3,186 patients with obstruction in two or three of the three major coronary arteries and showed that the procedure was safe and effective. The procedure was performed without complications in 97 percent of patients, and obstructions were successfully opened in 96 percent of cases. A five-year follow-up of 700 patients found that 88 percent were alive and only 16 percent required subsequent coronary artery bypass surgery. However, over one-third of patients required at least one other angioplasty procedure within six months because they experienced reobstruction of the arteries.

Because reobstruction remains a major limitation of angioplasty, alternatives to angioplasty are being explored. In November 1990 the results of a trial of over 2,000 patients undergoing a procedure called atherectomy were reported. Atherectomy involves the cutting or shaving away of coronary artery plaques with special catheters containing very small spinning blades. The results of the trial suggested that atherectomy can be performed effectively and safely in patients for whom angioplasty has previously failed or results are predicted to be poor. Other studies show that laser catheters successfully open coronary obstructions in over 80 percent of patients treated. The laser technique, still an investigational procedure, has at least one theoretical advantage over angioplasty in that it does not stretch the blood vessels. Additional studies of these newer techniques are needed to determine whether the likelihood of reobstruction at the original site is greater or less than in routine angioplasty.

A Bicycle Built for Two

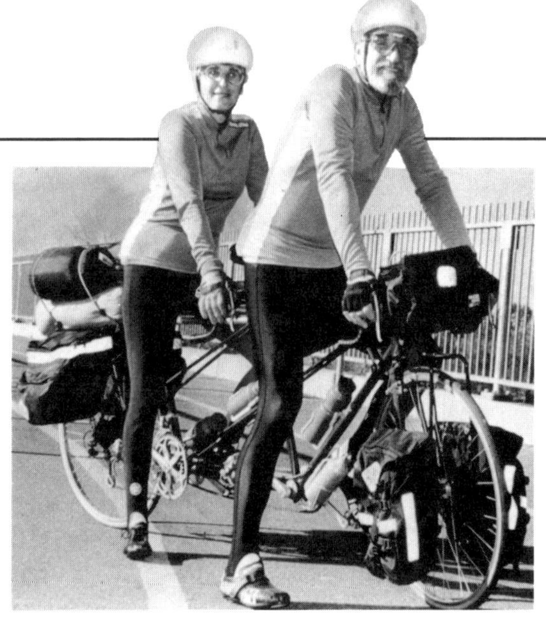

The sight of a tandem bicycle, its two riders pedaling in perfect harmony, has always conveyed a certain aura of romance. In the 1890s tandems even inspired the most popular ballad of the day, *Daisy Bell* (known to all as *A Bicycle Built for Two*). Then the two-seater bike all but disappeared for a hundred years.

But like many fads, tandem cycling has come around again, starting in the late 1980s and continuing strong into the 1990s. Tandem manufacturers say that sales have increased so rapidly they can barely keep up with the demand. The craze has been especially evident among older riders. One manufacturer says the average age of today's customer is 45, and the Tandem Club of America reports that over half its members are 50 or older. Devoted tandemers keep in touch through club newsletters, rallies, and cycling tours.

Tandem cyclists give several reasons for the appeal of their sport, among them physical fitness. Like conventional biking, tandem riding is good aerobic exercise that builds muscular strength and cardiovascular fitness. But unlike solo cycling, it allows exercise partners or couples of differing athletic abilities to ride together, rather than leaving one to watch the other disappear around the bend. The pedals of a tandem are synchronized so that both partners must pedal at the same speed, although not necessarily with the same amount of force. In this way their strengths are equalized.

Usually, the bigger and stronger member of the pair rides in front, an arrangement calling for tactful negotiation but the most aerodynamically efficient. The front rider (dubbed captain) must watch the road, steer, shift gears, and brake, and usually sets the pedal pace. The rear rider (stoker) just pedals and watches the scenery, along with perhaps some verbal back-seat driving—there are no brakes or steering controls in the rear. Both riders are advised to communicate so that the rear rider knows what's coming ahead and is not surprised by speed ups or slow downs.

Tandem cycles are expensive, costing anywhere from $1,200 to $3,700; it makes sense for a prospective tandem pair to rent one and try it out before investing in their own.

Drug Update

The FDA in 1990 approved two drugs that had received much attention when they were under investigation—morizicine (brand name, Ethmozine) and adenosine (Adenocard). Morizicine, developed in the Soviet Union in the 1970s to control arrhythmias, was one of three drugs investigated in a large, highly publicized clinical trial designed to assess the benefit of suppressing extra heart beats after a heart attack. Studies of two of the drugs, encainide and flecainide, were halted prematurely when an increased death rate was observed among patients taking them. Morizicine, however, was found to be sufficiently safe to allow ongoing study. Despite its FDA approval, physicians are now wary of all antiarrhythmic drugs.

Adenosine, which quickly became widely accepted by physicians, can help with the diagnosis and treatment of tachycardia, or abnormally rapid heartbeat. It is nearly 100 percent effective at controlling tachycardia that stems from a disorder in the conduction of electrical impulses through a structure in the heart called the atrioventricular, or AV, node. Adenosine also stresses the heart in a way that simulates exercise, allowing physicians to perform stress tests in patients who are unable to exercise adequately.

See also the feature article CHILDREN'S HEART PROBLEMS *and the Spotlight on Health article* CONGESTIVE HEART FAILURE.

MICHAEL J. KOREN, M.D.
JEFFREY FISHER, M.D.

MEDICAL TECHNOLOGY

Advances in Treating Brain Tumors and Leukemia • New Hope for Deaf Children • Device for Prenatal Screening

Shrinking Brain Tumors With Heat

Patients with certain malignant brain tumors may benefit from the VH8500 Hyperthermia Treatment System, which was approved by the U.S. Food and Drug Administration (FDA) in October 1989. With this system, manufactured by Cook Medical Products of Bloomington, Ind., heat-emitting catheters that are capable of killing tumor cells are implanted directly into the tumor. The dosage is monitored by a group of smaller independent catheters that are also implanted into the tumor to measure tissue temperature.

Malignant gliomas, which account for more than 25 percent of all brain cancers, are highly invasive and difficult to treat with conventional methods such as radiation, chemotherapy, and surgery. Moreover, as the tumor grows and normal brain tissue is compressed, patients often suffer great pain. The prognosis is poor; half of all patients with the kind of glioma called glioblastoma multiforme live only 43 weeks after diagnosis.

Forty four patients with gliomas that had not responded to conventional therapy were treated with the VH8500 Hyperthermia Treatment System. The study included 31 men and 13 women.

The catheters were surgically implanted with the aid of a computed tomography (CT) guidance system that allowed surgeons to precisely locate the tumor. Patients were anesthetized during this procedure but they were awake during the actual treatment, when the heat-delivering catheters were alternately activated and deactivated. Most reported minimal pain, usually related to the scalp penetration for insertion of the catheter.

The heat treatment not only caused the tumors to shrink, making patients more comfortable, it helped patients to survive longer than people with similar tumors who were not treated with the VH8500 system. The control group (patients with brain tumors treated conventionally) had a two-year survival rate of 4.3 percent, whereas patients treated with heat-emitting catheters had a two-year survival rate of 35 percent, with a median survival of 17 months.

The treatment itself is not without risk. There was one confirmed case of meningitis and two additional suspected cases. One patient died of hemorrhage when the catheters were removed and another experienced nonfatal hemorrhage. One of the investigators said the incidence of hemorrhage and infection "is not desirable, but it is considered acceptable given the advanced stage of the disease and poor prognosis for patients with recurrent intracranial malignancies."

Diagnosing and Treating Leukemia

A new device to detect chronic myelogenous leukemia (CML), one of a number of cancers of the white blood cells, is so sensitive that as few as 1 percent leukemic cells can be identified in a specimen. Manufactured by Oncogene Science of Manhasset, N.Y., and approved by the FDA in October 1989, the Oncogene Science (OSI) Transprobe-1 works by identifying a chromosomal abnormality called the Philadelphia chromosome that is found in the leukemic cells of more than 95 percent of patients with chronic myelogenous leukemia.

Besides serving as a diagnostic marker, the presence of the Philadelphia chromosome can be used to predict patient outcome. Patients with chronic myelogenous leukemia who have the marker survive longer than patients who do not. However, the presence of this altered chromosome in patients with another kind of leukemia, acute lymphocytic leukemia, is usually associated with decreased survival.

Another new diagnostic tool, which detects both leukemias and lymphomas (cancers of the lymphoid tissue), is the Oncor B-T Cell Gene Rearrangement Test, developed by Oncor, Inc., of Gaithersburg, Md., and approved by the FDA for marketing in October 1989. This test can help distinguish acute and chronic leukemia and non-Hodgkin's lymphomas from other cancers. It also indicates the type of cell in which the cancer originated, which helps physicians select the appropriate therapy for the patient.

Many human cancers originate in a malignant transformation of, or gene rearrangement in, a single cell. The cancer grows in size as the abnormal cell divides again and again, reproducing itself by a process called mitosis. Many leukemias and lymphomas result from malignant transformations of lymphocytes, white blood cells that fall into three categories: B cells, T cells, and null, or non-B, non-T, cells. The new test picks up any rearranged genes in T cells and in B cells. The rearranged genes thus serve as specific tumor markers.

Lymphoid cancers often show characteristics of normal cells at various stages of development, making early diagnosis difficult. A physician may sometimes see abnormal cell formation, yet be unable to identify the precise nature of the problem. Because genetic rearrangement occurs before a cancer is clinically detectable, the B-T Cell Gene Rearrangement Test can be a helpful diagnostic tool.

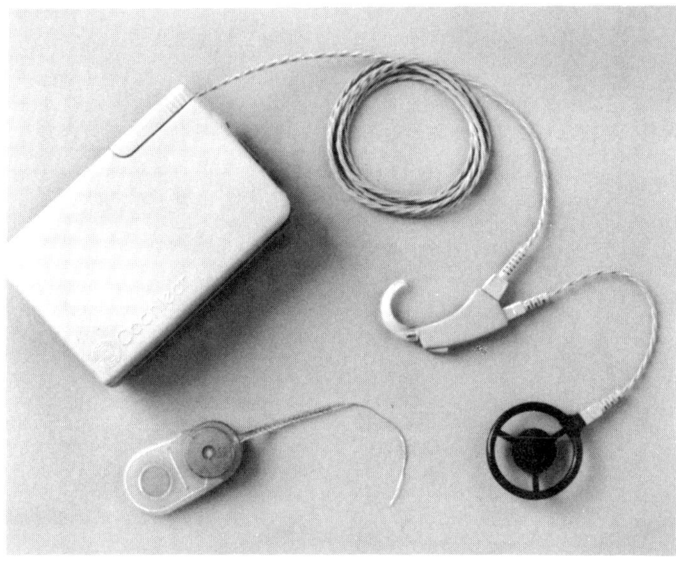

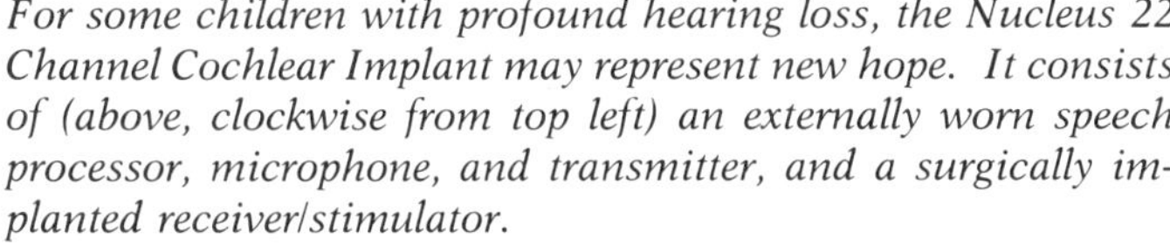

For some children with profound hearing loss, the Nucleus 22 Channel Cochlear Implant may represent new hope. It consists of (above, clockwise from top left) an externally worn speech processor, microphone, and transmitter, and a surgically implanted receiver/stimulator.

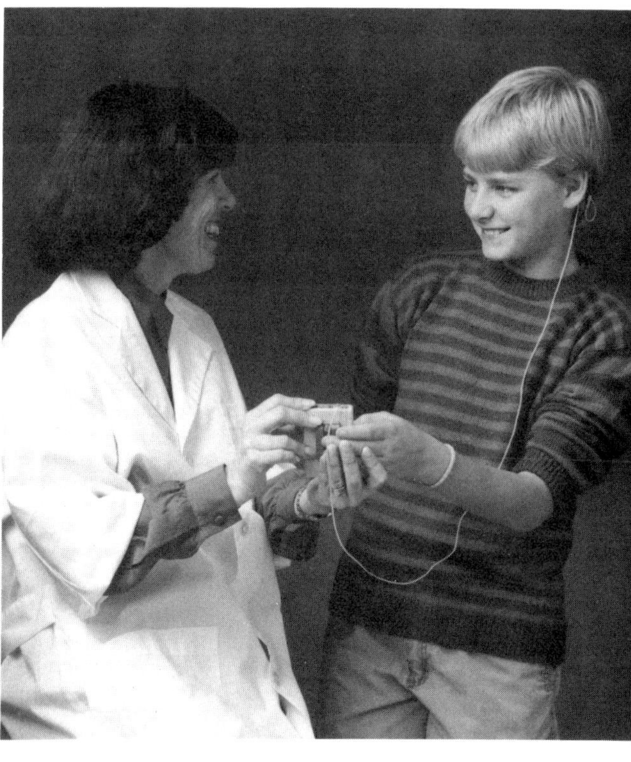

For example, a 48-year-old man who had a painless ¾ inch lump in his neck underwent a biopsy, which found a poorly differentiated malignancy that could have been metastatic cancer or lymphoma. Because these conditions require different treatments, physicians did a B-T Cell Gene Rearrangement Test, which showed genetic rearrangement consistent with a B-cell type of malignant lymphoma. Appropriate therapy could thus be started sooner than if traditional diagnostic tools had been used.

In another instance, a 71-year-old woman with lymphocytic lymphoma thought to be in remission experienced fluid buildup in her lungs and shortness of breath. A sample of the fluid showed only normal-appearing lymphocytes, and other tests were inconclusive. However, the B-T gene rearrangement analysis of the lung fluid showed B-cell markers identical to those in the original lymph-node biopsy, which meant that there had been a relapse of the lymphoma.

The Cellfree Interleukin-2 Receptor Bead Assay Kit, manufactured by T Cell Sciences in Cambridge, Mass., was approved in October 1989. It is expected to aid physicians in evaluating and monitoring the treatment of patients with hairy-cell leukemia, a rare form of chronic leukemia in which malignant cells are predominantly of B-lymphocyte origin.

Evaluating the extent of abnormal blood cells and the response to treatment in hairy-cell leukemia patients has been hindered by the lack of a reliable, noninvasive procedure. Changes in blood components were often used to gauge treatment response, but these components can return to normal even when there is an only partial remission. A biopsy of bone marrow can reveal the presence of hairy cells, but extracting marrow is an often costly and painful procedure that puts the patient at risk of infection. Bone-marrow aspiration has similar limitations and is difficult to perform successfully.

Researchers have demonstrated that hairy-cell leukemia patients who are responding well to certain treatments—specifically alpha-interferon therapy—have in their blood an increased number of interleukin-2 receptors. (Interleukin-2 is a form of protein that is secreted by T-lymphocytes as an immune response and serves as a natural "killer" cell.) The Cellfree Interleukin-2 Receptor Bead Assay Kit, by measuring the blood's interleukin-2 content, offers clinicians a means of appraising a patient's progress, while presenting none of the disadvantages of traditional means of evaluating hairy-cell leukemia patients.

An Internal Hearing Aid

Adults with profound sensorineural hearing loss (that is, hearing loss caused by damage to the parts of the inner ear called the auditory nerve and the cochlea)

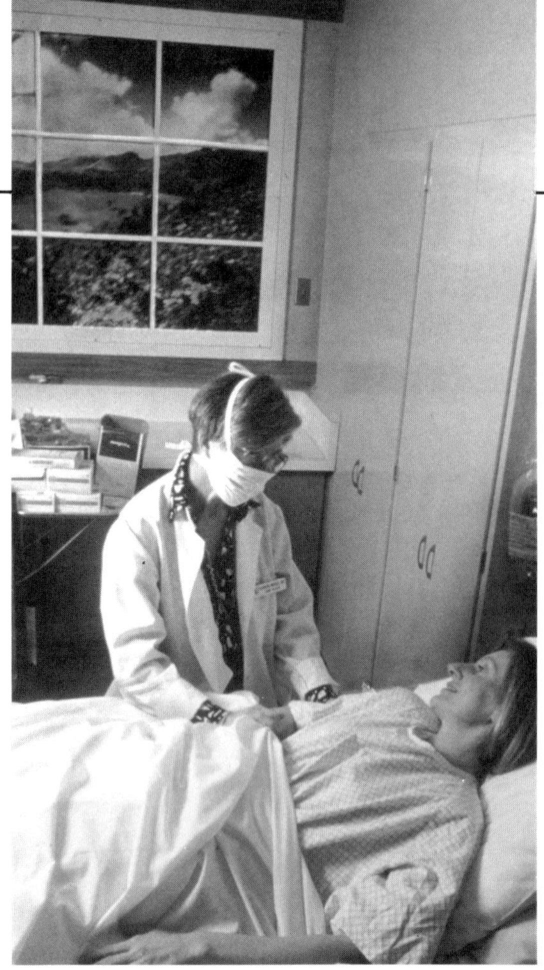

Seen From a Sickroom

Going into a hospital is no picnic for anyone. For seriously ill patients, who tend to lose track of time and place, the experience can be particularly disorienting if they find themselves in a room without a window.

California photographer Joey Fischer recently came up with an offbeat solution to the problem of the windowless hospital room; an artificial window with a "view," actually a blown-up color slide of a scene from nature, lit from behind by a computer-controlled light box. The light is programmed to change hundreds of times a day, mimicking natural changes from sunrise to sunset, thereby giving patients a sense of the passage of time. The light box can also be programmed to reflect the changing light patterns of the seasons of the year.

The idea for the windows was developed by Fischer in response to a problem encountered by Stanford University Medical Center when it renovated its cardiac intensive care unit. The renovation had left the unit with three windowless rooms, contravening a federal law that requires all inpatient hospital rooms constructed or renovated after 1977 to have windows. The center installed three of the fake windows—which come with panes, blinds, and sills—in March 1990 at a hefty cost of $20,000 apiece. California state authorities were sufficiently impressed by Fischer's creations to grant the medical center a temporary exemption, pending a follow-up of patient reactions.

The computerized windows are about to go beyond hospital walls. The U.S. Navy has ordered some of them for its submarines, while the Air Force plans to use a couple of dozen in an underground base in Turkey. Earlier, less expensive, stationary versions—essentially, giant transparencies of nature photographs—have been bought by hospitals all over the United States and used as wall and ceiling murals. Patients in these facilities, who once had nothing to look at but blank walls, may now find themselves staring at a view of snow-capped mountains, sunlit autumn foliage, or a garden massed with bright flowers.

Research has indicated that what patients see through a window may have therapeutic as well as aesthetic value. A study reported in *Science* magazine found that surgical patients whose windows looked out on a stand of trees had more positive attitudes after surgery and shorter postoperative stays than patients whose view was of a brick wall.

have been helped by cochlear implants, devices placed in the inner ear to stimulate auditory nerves and provide sound information. Those devices became available to children when the Nucleus 22 Channel Cochlear Implant, made by the Cochlear Corporation of Englewood, Colo., was approved by the FDA in June 1990. It has been tested in more than 450 children and can be used in patients aged 2 through 17.

Most hearing aids simply amplify sound. This may not be enough for people with sensorineural hearing loss. Because a cochlear implant bypasses some of the damaged parts of the inner ear, some patients who get no help from traditional hearing aids can benefit from a cochlear implant.

In order to be considered for the Nucleus Cochlear Implant, children must (1) suffer from profound sensorineural hearing loss in both ears; (2) be unable to benefit from conventional hearing aids; (3) be enrolled in an educational program that emphasizes development of auditory skills; and (4) be highly motivated and have appropriate expectations of what cochlear implants can and cannot do.

The cochlea is the snail-shaped inner ear that receives the vibrations caused by sound waves moving through the outer and middle ear. Thousands of tiny hair cells in the cochlea change these vibration into electrical energy. The electrical energy then stimulates the auditory nerve to send sound signals to the brain for interpretation.

The Nucleus Cochlear Implant system for children consists of three parts: miniaturized components that are surgically implanted; a speech processor; and a directional microphone, cables, and transmitter. The miniaturized components include a magnet, a receiver/stimulator, and a banded array of 22 electrodes that extend from the receiver/stimulator into the cochlea. Because the 22 electrodes can stimulate the nerve fibers at 22 different places, the patients can "hear" many different pitches. The speech processor, which looks like a pocket calculator and weighs about 3.5 ounces, selects and codes the elements of sound that are the most useful for understanding speech. It can be programmed to suit the sound and comfort needs of each user, and the program can be revised as the child's needs change. The microphone looks like a behind-the-ear hearing aid and is connected to the speech processor and transmitter by two cables.

Sounds are picked up by the directional microphone and routed to the speech processor. The sounds are amplified, filtered, and digitized in the speech processor; the digitized signal is sent to the receiver/stimulator by way of the transmitter, which delivers the electrical impulses to the appropriate electrodes in the cochlea. The stimulated electrodes activate the auditory nerves in the inner ear, creating the sensation of sound. This complicated process occurs in milliseconds, so that the child "hears" sounds almost as they occur.

The surgery required for the implant takes from two to three hours. An incision is made behind the ear and a small depression is formed in the mastoid bone to hold the receiver/stimulator. The electrode array is inserted through an opening in the cochlea called the round window. Once the skin heals, the only visible evidence of the surgery is a slight scar and bump. The number of electrodes that can be implanted in the cochlea is limited by the size of the inner ear, which is about 1¼ inch in length and about 1/10 inch in diameter in both children and adults.

The first child to receive a cochlear implant was a boy who lost his hearing at the age of 16 months after a bout with meningitis. He received his implant at age 9, after having spent seven years trying to learn to communicate orally. With the implant, he was able to participate in three different sports and run his own snow-cone business, which meant taking orders from customers.

Although cochlear implants do not provide normal hearing, some children with implants are able to identify everyday sounds, understand some human speech, and lip-read better. A few (about 5 percent) can even communicate without lip reading. However, not every child benefits, and it is difficult to predict success because many factors, including the number of surviving auditory nerve fibers, can affect the level of performance. In most instances, the implant must be supplemented with rehabilitation and educational programs to help people interpret what they are hearing.

Prenatal Screening

The Trophocan Chorionic Villus Sampling (CVS) Catheter, manufactured by the Concord Portex Company of Keene, N.H., was approved by the FDA in August 1990. It was the first device officially endorsed for this use, although CVS has been practiced for more than a decade. (Previously, clinicians who did CVS made their own equipment or used the Trophocan catheter before it gained FDA approval.) Similar to amniocentesis in that it detects genetic abnormalities and inherited diseases in a developing fetus, CVS is preferred by many clinicians and patients because it is usually performed during the 9th or 10th week of pregnancy, whereas amniocentesis is rarely done until the 14th or 15th week.

The chorionic tissue in the womb of a pregnant woman surrounds part of the sac where the fetus grows. Because the chorion develops from the same cells as the fetus, a sample of the chorionic villi (hair-like projections that cover the chorion's surface) have the same genetic makeup as the fetus.

As with amniocentesis, CVS is recommended for women age 35 or over, who are at increased risk of having a baby with genetic problems, such as Down syndrome; parents who are carriers of genetically inherited diseases, such as Tay-Sachs disease or muscular dystrophy; or couples who have had a child with an extra chromosome (as in Down syndrome and other disorders).

The Trophocan CVS catheter is a sterile, single-use plastic tube, almost 10 inches long and with an external diameter of roughly 1/16 inch. It contains a bendable stainless steel insert that may be curved to the shape required to reach the chorion and that is visible under ultrasound, which is used to evaluate the patient prior to the CVS procedure and to monitor placement of the device. After the catheter is inserted through the cervix to where the chorionic villi are located, the metal insert is withdrawn and a syringe containing fluid for mixing with the tissue sample is attached. The sample is obtained by gentle suction as the catheter is removed.

Clearing Blocked Arteries

A device for treating atherosclerosis, the Simpson Coronary AtheroCath, manufactured by Devices for Vascular Intervention, Inc., of Redwood City, Calif., was approved by the FDA in September 1990.

Atherosclerosis is characterized by blockages of the arteries, the vessels that carry blood from the heart to all parts of the body. Although the precise cause of atherosclerosis is unknown, most researchers believe that it begins when the endothelium, or innermost layer of the artery, becomes damaged (possibly due to high blood pressure, high levels of cholesterol, or cigarette smoking). Fatty substances, cholesterol, cellular waste products, calcium, and fibrin accumulate in the damaged area, allowing the formation of a lesion called plaque. Plaque may partially or totally block the flow of blood through the vessel. When plaque builds up in the coronary arteries—the arteries that nourish the heart itself—the result can be a heart attack.

Taming the MRI

Lots of people dread getting shots, cringe at the sight of a speculum, or make every excuse to put off visiting the dentist. But how could a noninvasive, painless diagnostic test with no known harmful effects inspire fear? Yet every day among the 21,000 Americans undergoing a magnetic resonance imaging (MRI) scan, at least 10 percent become so terrified they demand the test be stopped before it is completed. Many of these patients, who would not be considered claustrophobic in other situations, say they feel as if they've been buried alive.

MRI machines are sophisticated devices that use magnets to produce detailed images of internal organs and structures. The patient must lie on a table inside a narrow tunnel that is within a massive piece of machinery. Patients who are having a knee examined can lie with their feet sticking into the tunnel and their heads outside, but most often MRI is used on patients with brain or spinal cord problems, and they must enter the machine head first. The walls of the tunnel are about four to six inches from the patient's face, and the patient must lie completely still for 30 to 60 minutes while the scan is being done. As images are taken, the magnets make loud banging noises that vary in pitch and frequency.

Radiologists say the aborted scans are becoming so numerous and costly—a single test costs about $1,000—that they have begun searching for ways to make the test more bearable. Occasionally patients are given mild sedatives, but generally doctors prefer that they remain alert, especially if they need to follow instructions. Some medical centers have tried to teach patients relaxation techniques or they play music during the procedure. Since a radio or cassette player would interfere with the magnets, the scanners are equipped with sound systems similar to those used in airplanes, with the music piped through air hoses. Doctors report that patients who listen to music tend to remain calmer; chamber music and classical guitar are popular selections. There is one small problem, however: some patients can't help trying to "dance" in place in time to the music.

The herculean task of training such natural fidgeters as children to lie still was tackled by one team of doctors. To create a friendly atmosphere, they painted a discarded MRI machine to look like a spaceship on one side and Christopher Robin's backyard on the other; then they equipped it with a television screen connected to a device that measures the slightest body movements of the child in the machine. As long as the child lies still, cartoons play on the television, but at the slightest wiggle the picture is wiped off. After several practice sessions in the mock machine, most children learn to lie still. Unfortunately, they cannot watch the cartoons during the actual MRI test, but they do hear a replay of the sound track.

The Simpson AtheroCath is the first device that allows removal of atherosclerotic plaque from coronary arteries without open surgery. Using special kinds of X rays called angiograms to guide the catheter's movement, the physician threads it through a blood vessel to the heart and into the artery that needs treatment. The physician then positions a guidewire across the lesion or blocked area of the artery, and advances the AtheroCath over the guidewire to the lesion. A low-pressure support balloon is inflated to position the side window of the catheter in the lesion. Then a motorized unit is activated and a cutter in the side window, spinning at 2,000 revolutions per minute, removes the plaque. Next, the balloon is deflated, the catheter repositioned, and the procedure repeated until the desired result is achieved.

One advantage of the Simpson AtheroCath, it is hoped, is that the smooth surface created by the spinning cutter will make for a sturdier blood vessel and decrease the likelihood that plaque will reform.

VIRGINIA S. COWART

MEDICATIONS AND DRUGS

Combating Infections • New Drugs for Heart Disorders and Cancer • A Five-Year Contraceptive Goes on the Market

Infection Fighters

Meningitis. In late 1990, the U.S. Food and Drug Administration (FDA) approved a vaccine for preventing infections caused by *Haemophilus influenzae* type B (Hib) bacteria in infants as young as two months old. The product, Haemophilus B conjugate vaccine (brand name HibTITER), protects children against serious Hib infection, including bacterial meningitis, an inflammation of brain and spinal cord membranes that can cause death or leave survivors blind, deaf, mentally retarded, or paralyzed. Earlier versions of the vaccine had at first been recommended only for children over two years old, an age later lowered to 18 months and then to 15 months. However, because most Hib infections occur in infants between six months and one year of age this newest vaccine is expected to prevent 5,000 additional cases annually and about 800 infant deaths a year. *(See also the Health and Medical News article* PEDIATRICS.)

Shingles and Other Viral Illnesses. Two drugs that were previously approved for other purposes became available in 1990 for treating serious viral diseases. One of these, the antiviral drug acyclovir (brand name, Zovirax), which has been in use for several years to treat genital herpes, received FDA approval for treatment of shingles (herpes zoster), a painful condition caused by the same virus that is responsible for chicken pox (varicella). Shingles develops in 10 to 20 percent of people who had chicken pox as children. It occurs in adults many years later when the varicella-zoster virus emerges from its hiding place in nerve cells. As the reactivated virus reproduces and travels down nerve fibers, it produces a line of blistery sores across the body and face.

When acyclovir is taken in high oral doses as soon as possible after shingles symptoms first appear, the sores become crusty, dry up, and disappear, the virus stops spreading to new areas, and, often, the acute pain ceases. However, shingles patients who suffer chronic pain long after an acute attack that went untreated are not helped by later treatment.

Interferon alfa-2b (Intron A), a natural antiviral and antitumor substance that has been used to treat genital warts and two rare forms of cancer, was reported to be the first effective treatment for liver disease caused by hepatitis virus C. Given in a course of injections, interferon stops further viral damage to the liver in about half the patients treated. However, when high long-term dosage is needed, interferon often sets off side effects, such as fatigue and irritability, that force some patients to discontinue treatment. In such cases, patients who were improving may suffer relapses.

Bacterial Infections. Cefmetazole (Zefazone), an antibiotic in the cephalosporin family which has long been used in other parts of the world, was introduced in the United States for treating and preventing infections by a broad spectrum of bacteria. Injected into a vein every 6 to 12 hours for 5 to 14 days, it is often effective in treating abdominal infections that develop in patients who have undergone gallbladder surgery or who suffer from perforated ulcers, appendicitis, or penetrating wounds. Infected skin sores, diabetic foot ulcers, and abscesses caused by strains of *Staphylococcus aureus* resistant to other antibiotics often respond to treatment with cefmetazole. This drug, which penetrates into lung tissues, kills several kinds of bacteria responsible for pneumonia and chronic bronchitis. Excellent results have been obtained in combating urinary tract infections. In addition, a single dose of intravenous cefmetazole protects women against infections that may follow removal of the uterus (hysterectomy) and after childbirth by cesarean section. Serious toxicity has rarely been reported with this antibiotic, although diarrhea, nausea and vomiting, and stomach pain sometimes occur.

Invasive Fungi. Fluconazole (Diflucan), the first of a new chemical class of antifungal agents, was reported in 1990 to be effective against a broad spectrum of fungal microbes that cause mild to life-threatening infections. It is especially useful for people with diabetes, burn victims, and patients with impaired immune defenses, such as those with AIDS or with acute leukemia and other cancers. A single daily dose exerts long-lasting antifungal effects—a convenience for both the patient and hospital personnel.

Fluconazole is claimed to be as effective as, but much safer than, previously available antifungal agents used to treat acute cryptococcal meningitis—and for long-term maintenance therapy to prevent recurrences of this potentially dangerous infection of the central nervous system. It is also useful for treating infections caused by the yeastlike fungus *Candida albicans*, which causes mild infections of the mucous membranes of the mouth, throat, and esophagus (thrush) and severe infections of the lungs (pneumonia), the urinary tract (nephritis and cystitis), and the peritoneum (peritonitis, an inflammation of the membrane lining the abdominal cavity).

Fluconazole is very well tolerated; its most common side effects are gastrointestinal disturbances such as nausea, vomiting, abdominal pain, and diarrhea. Headaches are skin rashes may also occur.

Malaria. Mefloquine (Lariam), a new drug for preventing and treating malaria, became available in 1990 in the United States. Taken by mouth, it accumulates in the red blood cells that are the main target of malaria parasites such as *Plasmodium falciparum* and *Plasmodium vivax*. The U.S. Centers for Disease Control (CDC) recommended mefloquine for people traveling to areas where strains of *P. falciparum* have become resistant to the standard antimalarial drug, chloroquine (Aralen).

Mefloquine's preventive regimen requires travelers to take the drug at varying intervals (every one or two weeks) until up to four weeks after returning home from a malarious area. Patients diagnosed as having developed a mild to moderately acute infection swallow a single one-time dose of five tablets of mefloquine followed by at least eight ounces of water. Serious life-threatening *P. falciparum* infection is first treated intravenously with another antimalarial drug, then with oral doses of mefloquine.

Mefloquine is relatively safe. When taken in small preventative doses at weekly intervals, side effects, if they occur, are usually minor and short-lasting. The much larger dosage used for treatment of an acute infection can cause dizziness. Fever, chills, headache, muscle pain, and malaise have also been reported, but these are also malaria symptoms and thus may not have been caused by mefloquine. Signs of nervous-system disturbance may develop that may require discontinuing the drug, but such occurrences are rare.

Cardiovascular Drugs

Three drugs for normalizing irregular heart rhythms and two medications for reducing high blood pressure were introduced in 1990.

Heart Rhythm Regulators. Adenosine, a biochemical substance found in all body cells, became available in 1990 as an emergency heart drug (brand name Adenocard). It is especially effective in treating one type of arrhythmia, a heart rhythm disorder that develops when abnormal electrical impulses arise suddenly in the atria, the heart's upper chambers, and make the ventricles, the heart's main pumping chambers, beat at a very rapid rate. Injected into an arm vein, adenosine rapidly reaches the tissue at the junction of the atria and ventricles and slows conduction of the abnormally rapid impulses within one minute. In over 90 percent of cases, this terminates the attack and restores a normal heart rate.

Adenosine's short duration of action and lack of adverse interactions with other heart drugs gives it a greater safety margin than previously available antiarrhythmic drugs. The most common side effects of an adenosine injection are facial flushing, shortness of breath, and drug-induced heart rhythm irregularities, including excessive slowing of the heart. But because the injected drug is in the bloodstream for only a short time, any adverse effects that develop last only a few seconds. Still, adenosine should not be given to patients known to have underlying disorders that make them prone to heart-rate slowing unless they have been fitted with a pacemaker.

Two other antiarrhythmic drugs, morizicine (Ethmozine) and propafenone (Rhythmol), received FDA approval in 1990 for treating heartbeat irregularities originating in the ventricles. Both are reserved for use in patients whose heart rhythm abnormalities are considered to be so serious that they are in danger of sudden death from cardiac arrest. The FDA imposed this restriction on all new drugs aimed at control of ventricular arrhythmias because of the unexpected results of a recent government-sponsored trial with two other drugs of this type. Patients who took those drugs to control minor ventricular irregularities after having survived a heart attack were found to have a higher death rate than a similar group of patients who were given a dummy pill (placebo). Despite this risk, however, both morizicine and propafenone have proved effective in eliminating ventricular irregularities in some patients for a year or more.

Morizicine seems safer than propafenone for patients with a history of congestive heart failure because it is less likely to reduce the pumping power of their weakened ventricles. Both drugs can cause discomforting side effects that may prompt patients to

Birth Control Breakthrough

Norplant, a contraceptive method consisting of six soft, hormone-filled tubes implanted beneath the skin of a woman's upper arm, was approved by the U.S. Food and Drug Administration. Already used successfully in several other countries, it can prevent pregnancy for up to five years.

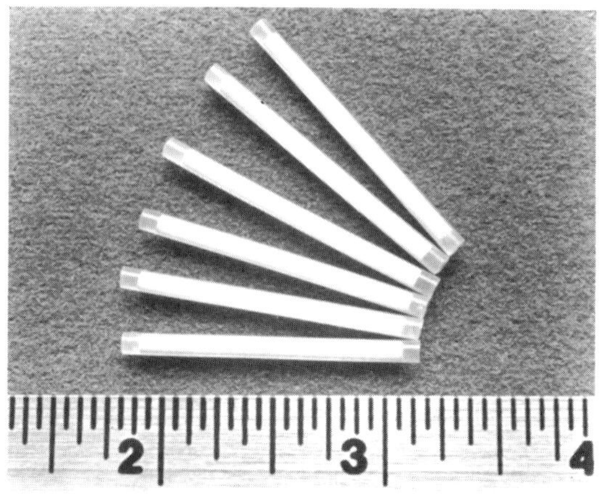

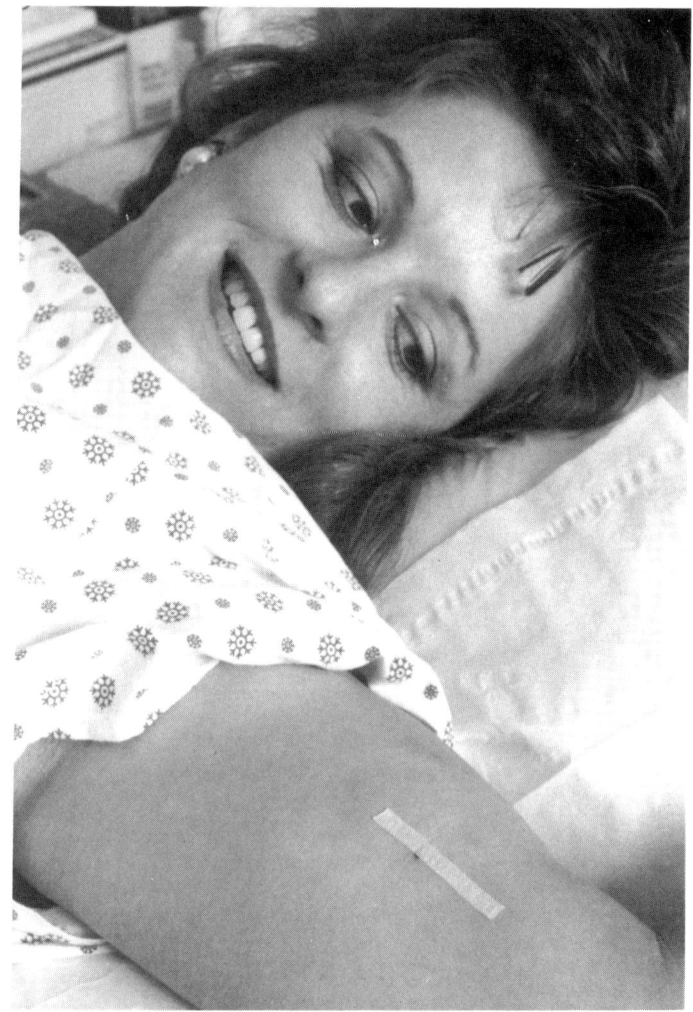

discontinue use. The most common noncardiac complaints of patients on propafenone are dizziness, blurred vision, an unusual taste in the mouth, and nausea and vomiting; morizicine can cause dizziness, nausea, and headaches. However, in one clinical trial, most patients with these complaints were taking the placebo rather than morizicine.

Blood Pressure. Doxazosin (Cardura), a drug that keeps nerve impulses from narrowing blood vessels, was approved by the FDA in 1990 for treating high blood pressure. By widening the patient's arterioles, or smallest arteries, doxazosin reduces resistance to blood flowing through these vessels. This, in turn, leads to a drop in pressure, especially when the patient is standing up. The pressure-reducing effect of doxazosin reaches a peak in 2 to 6 hours and continues for 24 hours, so the patient need take only one dose a day—a schedule that is convenient and easy to follow. Doxazosin is said to be safer than diuretics or beta blockers in treating hypertensive patients who also have diabetes, coronary heart disease, or other disorders that can worsen when they take diuretics or beta blockers.

Betaxolol (Kerlone), a new beta adrenergic blocker (a drug that blocks the effects of adrenaline and adrenaline-like substances on the heart), has been shown to have a long-lasting effect on the circulatory system. In patients with mild to moderate high blood pressure, only one oral dose daily reduces blood pressure and heart rate for at least 24 hours. Up to 80 percent of patients attain normal pressure after one month of treatment with betaxolol. In some of the remaining 20 percent, doubling the dosage or giving betaxolol together with a diuretic attains the desired degree of blood pressure reduction.

Since its side effects are usually both mild and transient, betaxolol is well-tolerated by most patients. The drug acts mainly on the heart and has fewer effects on the lungs and central nervous systems than most other beta blockers. However, a small proportion of patients who took betaxolol during clinical trials discontinued treatment because their heart rate slowed or they complained of headache, drowsiness, dizziness, and fatigue. While this drug is relatively safe for patients with bronchial asthma, it can cause spasm of the bronchial tubes in such patients if given in higher than usual doses.

Cancer Treatments

Colon Cancer. Levamisole (Ergamisol), a drug used primarily in the Third World to treat worm infestations in animals and humans, received FDA approval for use in controlling advanced colon cancer where cancer cells were found to have spread to nearby lymph nodes. Levamisole itself has not been shown to kill cancer cells, but when combined with the well-established chemotherapy drug fluorouracil (Adrucil, 5-FU) following surgical removal of colon tumors, levamisole, according to one study released in 1990, reduced deaths by 33 percent and prevented recurrences of the colon cancer in 41 percent of patients. The beneficial effects of levamisole may stem from its ability to restore the activity of white blood cells and other immune system components that had been suppressed by the cancer and by some of the measures used to treat it.

Levamisole alone causes few side effects. However, when it is used in conjunction with the standard anticancer drug 5-FU, many patients suffer the typical side effects of that therapeutic agent: loss of appetite, nausea, vomiting, and diarrhea. Because 5-FU tends also to depress the body's production of white blood cells, thereby compromising the immune system, patients receiving combination therapy must have their white blood cell counts monitored to prevent serious infections.

Bladder Cancer. BCG (Bacillus Calmette Guérin) has long been used outside the United States to confer some immunity against tuberculosis. Now a new form of this product, called BCG Live (Intravesical), marketed as TheraCys and as TICE BG, has been approved by the FDA for an entirely different purpose—treatment of a type of urinary bladder cancer called carcinoma in situ (CIS). BCG Live, when inserted directly into the patient's bladder through a catheter, has proved effective in removing cancer cells left over from diagnostic or surgical treatment procedures. The rate of new tumor development is also reduced. The benefits of BCG Live are believed to derive from the inflammatory effects it has on the lining of the bladder, but treatment-induced bladder inflammation also commonly causes painful urination and bleeding. Rarely, BCG organisms can spread into the patient's system. Because this can prove fatal, patients are watched closely for signs of infection.

Prostate Cancer. Goserelin (Zoladex), a new drug for treating men with advanced prostate cancer, has advantages over previously available medications for this disease. Like leuprolide (Lupron), a drug in use for several years, it works by reducing secretions of the main male sex hormone, testosterone, which stimulates growth of prostate tumor tissue.

Goserelin is as effective as other treatments for relief of patients' symptoms and for delaying progress of prostate cancer, but it is apparently better tolerated than procedures such as surgical castration and drugs such as diethylstilbestrol (DES), a synthetic female sex hormone that can cause blood clots and fluid retention. The main long-term side effects of goserelin are those that occur with all treatments that decrease serum testosterone to castration levels—for example, hot flashes, reduced sex drive, and impotence.

Because the first dose of goserelin tends to cause an increase in testosterone levels, some patients with advanced prostate cancer may develop a transient worsening of their condition marked by a temporary increase in bone pain, urinary obstruction, and neurological complications. Recent trials in which goserelin was given together with flutamide (Eulexin), a drug for prostate cancer that acts in a different way, suggest that the frequency of disease flare-ups following goserelin administration can be markedly reduced.

Leukemia. Idarubicin (Idamycin) has been approved for treating a type of blood cancer called acute myeloid leukemia. Given by vein either alone or combined with cytarabine, another antileukemic chemotherapeutic agent, idarubicin has brought about complete but temporary remissions in most patients with this disease. Patients also survive longer than when treated with daunorubicin, a close chemical relative of idarubicin that had previously been considered the most useful drug against acute myeloid leukemia. Damage to bone marrow, the source of both normal and leukemic blood cells, is the most serious toxic effect of idarubicin, so doctors must monitor patients closely and be ready to protect them against life-threatening infections and bleeding.

Drugs for Eye Disorders

Botulinum toxin type A (brand name Oculinum) was approved for treating two disorders that interfere with vision. In one of these conditions, blepharospasm, patients suffer eyelid contractions that often progress from brief episodes of blinking to long periods of complete eyelid closure. The other disorder, strabismus, which is characterized by excessive contractions of muscles that control eye movements can cause cross-eye, in which the eyes turn toward the nose, or walleye, in which the eyes turn away from the nose. In both disorders, injecting tiny amounts of botulinum toxin into the hyperactive muscles around the eyes makes them relax. About 85 to 90 percent of patients with blepharospasm severe enough to be incapacitating respond to injections into the upper and lower eyelids. The effects of toxin treatment last for about three months, and repeated injections can control abnormal lid contractions indefinitely. Side effects, which occur in about one out of ten patients, include transient drooping of the upper lid and eye dryness caused by impaired blinking. To avoid damage to the cornea, patients use artificial tear eye drops, soft contact lenses, or other protective measures.

Strabismus is treated with toxin injections when surgery is judged undesirable or in patients whose condition has not been entirely corrected by surgery. Side effects include temporary eyelid drooping, double vision, and undesired changes in eye position.

Metipranolol, a beta-adrenergic blocking drug, became available in eye-drop form with the brand name OptiPranolol Sterile Ophthalmic Solution. In most patients with chronic open-angle glaucoma, a condition that can cause blindness by damaging the optic nerve, a single drop applied to the surface of the eye begins to bring down excessively high pressure within the eye in less than half an hour.

Potent Pain Relievers

Two potent painkillers, dezocine (Dalgan) and ketorolac (Toredol), were marketed for treating patients suffering moderate to severe pain following major surgery, including abdominal surgery, orthopedic procedures, or removal of the uterus. Administered by injection, both drugs are claimed to be as effective as the traditional narcotic analgesics morphine and meperidine (Demerol). However, the two differ in the ways they work and in their side effects.

Injected into a vein or muscle, dezocine reaches the central nervous system where it acts to relieve pain. Like morphine, dezocine can slow a patient's breathing, but ordinary doses rarely reduce the rate and depth of respiration significantly. Dezocine also induces drowsiness—an action that is desirable for keeping patients calm and comfortable—but it does not leave patients feeling so drugged that they cannot be readily aroused when it is time to leave the recovery room. Dezocine does not cause serious adverse reactions; nausea, vomiting, and dizziness are the most commonly reported side effects.

Ketorolac, classed as a nonsteroidal antiinflammatory drug (NSAID), is the first drug of that class available in the United States in a form suitable for intramuscular injection. It relieves pain not by depressing the central nervous system, but by inhibiting production of pain-provoking prostaglandin hormones at the sites of surgery. Because of this, ketorolac does not depress respiration and causes less drowsiness than dezocine and other morphine-type drugs.

New Contraceptive Implant

In December 1990 the FDA approved a contraceptive that can prevent pregnancy for up to five years. The new product, called Norplant, contains levonorgestrel, a progestin-type synthetic female hormone used in combination with estrogen in birth-control pills. In Norplant, levonorgestrel is released slowly and steadily through matchstick-sized tubes that are implanted under a woman's skin. The doctor trained to perform the short, simple surgical procedure makes a small incision in the skin on the inside of a woman's upper arm after injecting a local anesthetic. The tubes containing the drug are then slipped through the opening and arranged in a fan-shaped pattern. Once in place, the tiny tubes stay there, releasing the contraceptive hormone until they are removed, perhaps to be replaced by a fresh set. A Norplant user who wants to discontinue the method can have the tubes removed at any time.

Norplant has proved effective in preventing pregnancy in more than 99 percent of the thousands of women in whom it has been tested worldwide. Success is somewhat lower in women weighing over 155 pounds. A small proportion of women discontinued the method during the first year mainly because they were disturbed by its most common side effect—changes in menstrual patterns and irregular spotting between menstrual periods.

Lungs of Premature Infants

A product containing synthetic chemicals called surfactants received approval for use in treating respiratory distress syndrome (RDS), a breathing disorder that is the main cause of death in premature infants. Marketed as Exosurf Neonatal, it is used both to prevent RDS and to treat the disorder when it develops during a baby's first day of life. It serves as a replacement for the natural surfactant that is lacking in the lungs of babies born too soon.

An Exosurf solution is pumped through a tube inserted into the trachea (windpipe) of infants whose lungs are being ventilated by a mechanical respirator. The foamy liquid acts like a detergent to reduce the pressure on the lining of the lungs' tiny air sacs. This keeps them from collapsing when the infant exhales. As a result, the baby's lungs inflate more readily, less energy is used up in trying to breathe, and the danger of respiratory failure is reduced.

When used immediately to treat babies diagnosed with RDS, two doses given at twelve-hour intervals produce improvement in most cases. In clinical trials, Exosurf reduced the RDS death rate in very low birth-weight infants by two thirds, and because fewer long-term complications occured, deaths from any cause during the first year of life were 44 percent less. When used to prevent RDS in infants judged to be at high risk, Exosurf cut deaths from the disorder in half and also reduced the one-year death rate from all causes.

Exosurf seems to be safe; the overall rate of adverse effects was no different in clinical trial groups treated with it than in a control group that received only ordinary room air into their airways. In one study the rate of lung bleeding reported in infants weighing under two pounds was higher in the Exosurf-treated group, but no increase in lung bleeding occurred in five other trials in infants who weighed more than two pounds at birth.

Muscle Relaxation During Surgery

Pipercuronium bromide (Arduan), a new skeletal muscle relaxant, was approved for use with general anesthetics during surgical procedures expected to last 90 minutes or longer. It can also be used before surgery to relax the patient's jaw muscles in order to make it easier for the anesthesiologist to insert a breathing tube into the windpipe. The main difficulty with pipercuronium is that some patients' muscles remain paralyzed long after surgery is completed. This can require artificial ventilation of the lungs for quite some time before the drug's effects wear off. Dosage has to be carefully adjusted for each individual based on his or her physical condition. Patients with poor kidney function receive lower doses of pipercuronium because the drug is eliminated from the body by the kidneys.

An advantage of pipercuronium is that compared to other muscle relaxants, it has few effects on the cardiovascular system. It does not, for example, elevate the heart rate or blood pressure as the muscle relaxant pancuronium sometimes does.

Congenital Immune Deficiency

Pegadamase bovine (Adagen Injection) is the first drug approved by the FDA for direct treatment of severe combined immunodeficiency, a rare genetic disorder in which infants are unable to produce sufficient amounts of adenosine deaminase (ADA), an enzyme essential for normal immune system development and function. A synthetic form of ADA, pegadamase helps to prevent the frequent infections that usually prove fatal to affected infants before they reach two years of age.

Unlike natural ADA, pegadamase rarely stimulates production of antibodies. This keeps the drug from being destroyed as rapidly as the natural enzyme and reduces the risk of allergic reactions. The long-lasting drug needs to be injected into a muscle only once a week, and it is not known to cause adverse reactions. All of the children treated in clinical trials showed gradual improvement in their immune function, and some may eventually be able to resist infection as readily as children with normal immuune systems. However, pegadamase does not cure the underlying disorder and has to be taken for life. (*See also the Health and Medical News article* GENETICS AND GENETIC ENGINEERING.)

Parkinson's Disease

Patients with Parkinson's disease, a nervous system disorder marked by muscular tremors and rigidity, may benefit from a new drug called pergolide (Permax). It is added to the treatment programs of patients whose symptoms are no longer well-controlled by the standard drug levodopa or who suffer severe side effects from high doses of levodopa. Adding pergolide permits as much as a 30 percent reduction in levodopa dosage and thus reduces some of its adverse effects.

Pergolide acts by substituting for dopamine, a nerve impulse-transmitting substance that is in short supply in the brains of Parkinson's disease patients. Combining pergolide with levodopa results in a two-pronged attack against the disease. The combination, however, tends to cause hallucinations in some patients, while others experience drops in blood pressure.

Ulcerative Colitis

Olsalazine (Dipentum) was approved for use in treating ulcerative colitis, the most common kind of chronic inflammatory bowel disease. Taken orally, this drug passes through the stomach and small intestine without being absorbed into the bloodstream. When it reaches the colon, bacteria break the compound down to an active component that exerts an antiinflammatory effect on the inflamed bowel lining. Olsalazine is said to cause fewer side effects than sulfasalazine (Azulfidine), the standard drug for ulcerative colitis. Olsalazine is not used to begin treatment of acute colitis, but once other therapy has brought the inflammatory reaction under control, colitis patients can be kept in remission for at least two years, or even indefinitely, by taking two olsalazine capsules daily.

MORTON J. RODMAN, PH.D.

MENTAL HEALTH

New Psychiatric Drugs • More Effective Treatments for Depression • Serotonin and Mental Illness • Abnormalities in the Schizophrenic Brain

New Psychiatric Drugs

In 1990 two new psychiatric medications moved from the research laboratory into general clinical practice in the United States. While many psychiatric medicines have been introduced over the years, most are simply revised new forms of already existing drugs. The medications introduced this year, clozapine (Clozaril), for schizophrenia, and clomipramine (Anafranil), for obsessive-compulsive disorder, both represent significant new additions to the therapeutic arsenal.

Clozapine has been found an effective treatment for many cases of schizophrenia that do not respond to conventional medication. Schizophrenia is a chronic psychiatric illness that seriously impairs a person's capacity to relate to others and to function at work or leisure. It affects about one in a hundred people and is a major public health concern with untold costs to the victims and their families. The social costs of schizophrenia in the United States are estimated at $10 to $20 billion yearly. Symptoms of schizophrenia include hallucinations, delusions, or false beliefs, and disorganized thinking, as well as a group of so-called negative symptoms, which include the tendency to withdraw from people, to lose motivation for work or play, and to have a blunted ability to experience emotion. Until now, all medications for schizophrenia targeted the same neurochemical systems in the brain. They primarily relieved symptoms of hallucinations, delusions, and thinking disturbance but had little effect on negative symptoms. In addition, they affected areas of the brain that control muscle function and were prone to cause tremors or involuntary movements as side effects. Approximately 10 to 20 percent of schizophrenic patients could not be helped by the existing antischizophrenia drugs.

Clozapine appears to work on different brain systems than the older drugs. One of the most dramatic features of clozapine is its ability to help chronically ill schizophrenic patients who had not benefited from any other treatments. In addition, it may reduce the negative symptoms, which have great impact upon the patient's overall quality of life. Finally, clozapine is less apt to produce neuromuscular side effects, such as tremors and involuntary movements. Unfortunately, clozapine has one important drawback: it can suppress the bone marrow's ability to produce white blood cells in 1 to 2 percent of patients. This can place the patient at risk for developing life-threatening infections. For this reason, patients receiving clozapine must have weekly blood counts taken so that the drug can be stopped if the number of white cells falls below a safe level.

Clomipramine is the first medication shown to be consistently effective in treating obsessive-compulsive disorder. The disorder, which affects 2 to 3 percent of the U.S. population sometime during their lives, is a condition in which people cannot resist an inner urge to perform some action over and over again or cannot clear their minds of intrusive repeating thoughts, even though they know that these actions and thoughts serve no real purpose. Handwashing compulsions and rituals of rechecking are typical. The syndrome can be extremely debilitating, consuming so much time, for example, that a normal work and family life is impossible. Depression often then sets in.

The paralyzing effects of depression were powerfully chronicled in the book Darkness Visible *by writer William Styron, who, despite his fame and wealth, plunged in 1985 into a despair so deep it pushed him to the brink of suicide.*

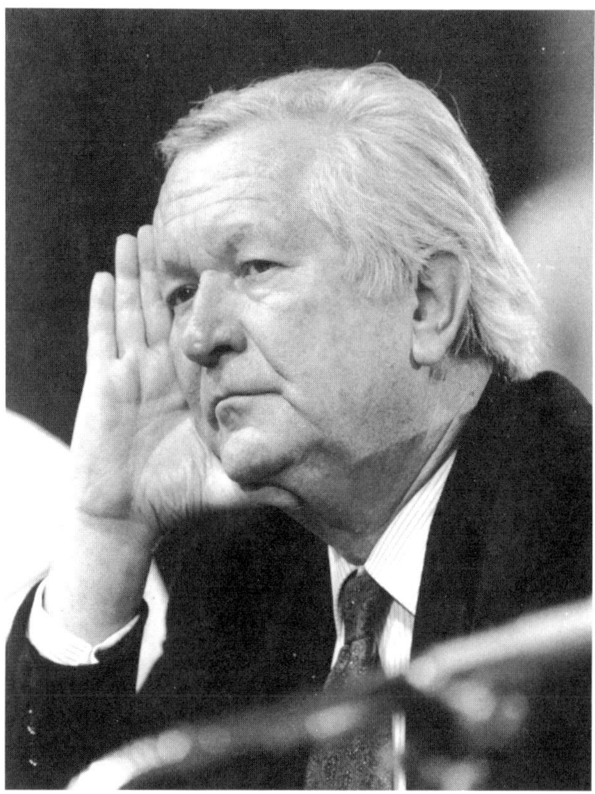

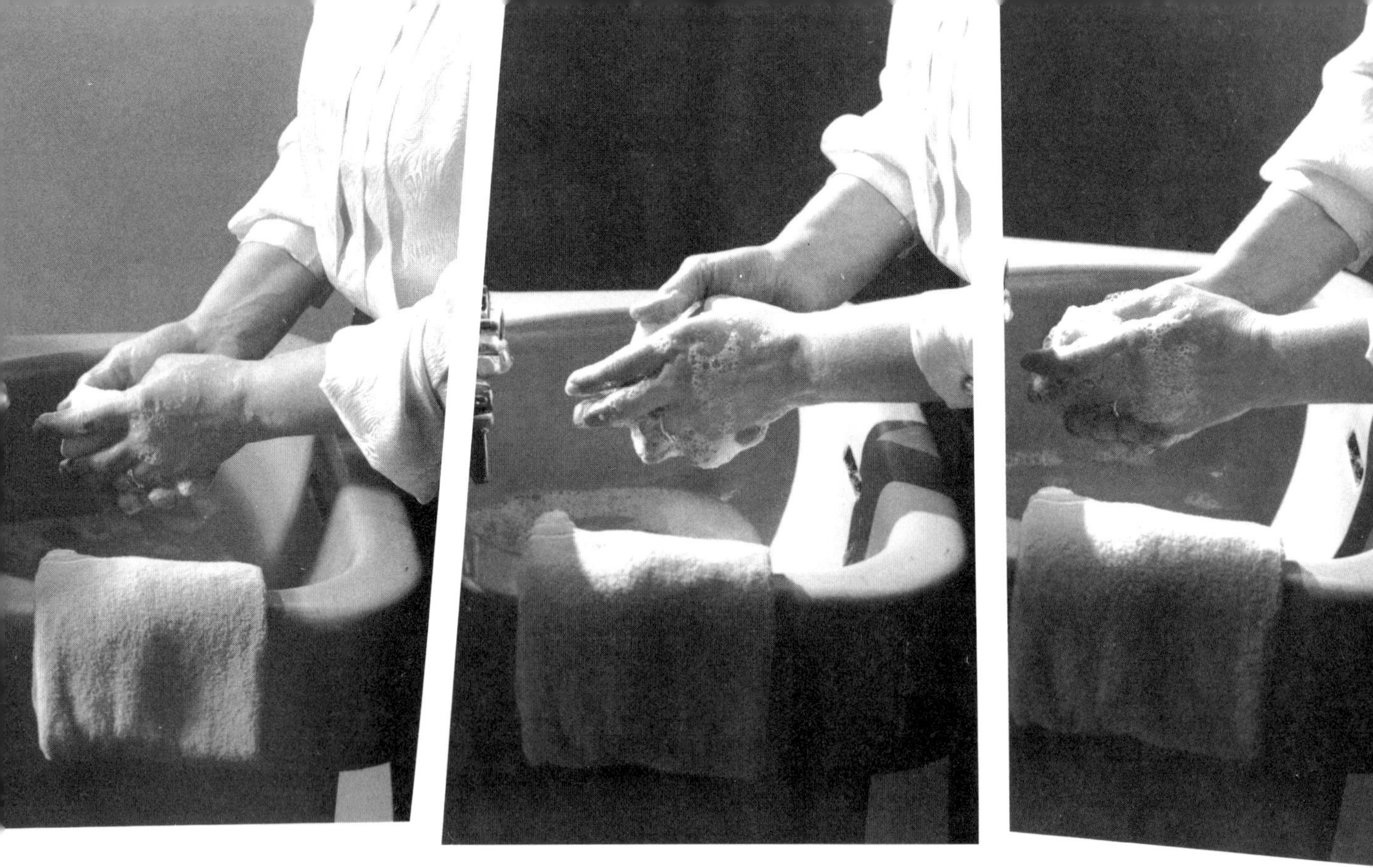

Constantly repeated hand washing is a common manifestation of what is known as obsessive-compulsive disorder, or OCD. Recently, three new drugs have proven to be effective in treating this puzzling affliction.

New Treatments for Recurrent Depression

A major study published in December 1990 suggests a new approach to treating recurrent depression and challenges some traditional ideas. Depression is a common psychiatric problem, with 13 to 20 percent of the U.S. population suffering from significant depressive symptoms at any given time and 3 to 8 percent actually meeting the criteria for a depressive illness. Fortunately, most depressions respond well to treatment with psychotherapy, antidepressant medication, or the combination. In fact, depression is one of the most treatable psychiatric illnesses. However, more than half of patients who experience a major depressive episode can be expected to have a subsequent episode months or years later. When these episodes are widely spaced apart, patients are able to lead full and satisfying lives with minimal disruption to their interpersonal relationships and careers. But when episodes occur every few years or every few months, the individual's life is severely disrupted and there is little opportunity for the patient to regain a sense of normalcy before the next episode strikes. For this reason, relapse prevention in patients with recurrent depression is a central concern.

Traditionally, treatment has included high doses of antidepressant medication throughout the depressive episode, continuation of the drug at this therapeutic level for about six months after the patient has recovered, and maintenance on a lower dose of the medication indefinitely. Some patients also continue to be seen in psychotherapy. The new study examined the effect of maintaining patients for three years on the same high dose of antidepressant medication that lifted them from their depression and the effect of three years of monthly psychotherapy sessions. It found that patients maintained on a high dose of medication appeared to improve substantially their odds of avoiding a recurrence of depression. Patients who received monthly psychotherapy sessions without medication did twice as well as those who received no follow-up treatment. Those who received both monthly psychotherapy and full-dose medication did the best: they achieved a recurrence-free interval three times longer than that achieved by those who received no follow-up treatment.

Serotonin, Compulsions, and Violence

The neurotransmitter serotonin was the focus of great interest in psychiatry in 1990. Serotonin is one of well over a dozen substances that carry nerve impulses from one nerve cell in the brain to the next across the minute gap, or synapse, between them. These neurotransmitters are released by one nerve cell and then travel across the synaptic gap to specific receptor sites on the next nerve cell. Most attach themselves to these receptor cells but some, in a normal process called reuptake, are reabsorbed by the nerve cell that released them.

New technologies that have made it possible to count the number of serotonin receptor sites in brain tissue and the availability of drugs that activate the serotonin system without affecting other neurotransmitter systems have led to a number of important findings related to obsessive-compulsive disorder and to violent behavior.

A number of drugs block the reabsorption of neurotransmitters, thus increasing the amounts that are present in the synapses at any given time. Drugs that increase the synaptic accumulation of serotonin and another neurotransmitter, norepinephrine, have been tried as treatments for obsessive-compulsive disorder. The first drugs tested worked on either the norepinephrine system alone or on the norepinephrine and serotonin systems together, but were found to be ineffective in treating obsessive-compulsive disorder. Three new drugs, fluoxetine, clomipramine (see above), and fluvoxamine, which differ from the others in that they almost exclusively block serotonin reuptakes, have been shown to be effective treatments for obsessive-compulsive disorder. Their anti-obsessional effect can be increased by adding tryptophan, which is a building block of serotonin. These findings strongly suggest that abnormal serotonin functioning results in obsessive-compulsive disorder.

An additional study using a substance called MK-212, which is known to mimic serotonin in stimulating serotonin's receptor sites on nerve cells, has added further support to the theory. Equal doses of MK-212 were given to people with obsessive-compulsive disorder and normal subjects, and the rise of two hormones (prolactin and cortisol) known to be stimulated by serotonin's action at specific receptor sites in the brain was observed. Obsessive-compulsive patients had a smaller reaction to MK-212 than did normal subjects, suggesting that in obsessive-compulsive disorder the receptors to serotonin may be less sensitive than is usually the case.

Serotonin activity in the brain may also predict a tendency toward violence. A series of recent studies suggests that low brain levels of serotonin are associated with choosing violent, as opposed to nonviolent, methods of suicide. Suicide attempters with a variety of underlying psychiatric diseases (schizophrenia, depression, and personality disorders) all had lower levels of a product of serotonin breakdown product in their spinal fluid than patients with the same psychiatric conditions who did not attempt suicide. Autopsy studies comparing the brains of patients who died of violent methods of suicide with those of persons dying of natural causes have found lower levels of serotonin and its breakdown product in the brainstems (the part of the brain that connects to the spinal cord) of suicide victims. The reduced levels occurred regardless of the psychiatric diagnosis, suggesting that it was the tendency to act violently, rather than any specific psychiatric diagnosis, that was associated with the low serotonin levels in the suicide victims.

A recent study using a radioactive tracer that selectively attached to serotonin-specific receptor sites on nerve cells allowed researchers to map out the number of these receptor sites in the brains of people who had died of violent suicide and people who had died of natural causes. This study revealed that the brains of people who complete violent suicides have more of one type of serotonin receptor (the 5-HT_2 receptor) in the prefrontal cortex, a region in the front of the brain believed to be involved in planning activities. Since nerve cells respond to low levels of neurotransmitters by increasing the number of receptors, the greater number of serotonin receptors in the violent suicides suggests that they had a lower level of serotonin in their brains.

These findings are particularly important because they link a specific type of behavior, independent of psychiatric diagnosis, to a specific neurotransmitter in the brain. In addition they may lead eventually to the development of a biochemical test that may help psychiatrists to better predict the risk of suicide in their patients.

Brain Abnormalities in Schizophrenics

The development in recent years of new techniques for looking at the brain has made it possible to identify certain structural abnormalities in the brains of schizophrenic patients. Older efforts to study brain structure relied on examination of the brain at autopsy or special X-ray procedures in which air had to be injected into the brain. In a newer, more accurate, technique called computed tomography, or CT scanning, a pencil-thin X-ray beam is directed at the brain from a number of angles within a single plane to produce an image of a single slice of the brain. Studies using CT scanning to compare the brains of schizophrenics to those of normal individuals have consistently found that on average the brains of male schizophrenics have larger natural internal cavities (called ventricles) than the brains of normal men. These findings were confirmed in 1990 in a large-scale CT scan study covering a wide age range of subjects.

A similar comparison study, also reported in 1990, using an even more precise imaging technique, magnetic resonance imaging (MRI), supported the CT scan conclusions and additionally found that patients with the most severe negative symptoms seem to have the largest ventricles. MRI uses powerful magnetic fields to produce images of the brain. It is superior to CT scanning because it distinguishes between the brain structures composed of nerve cells (the grey matter) and those composed of connecting nerve bundles (the white matter). This allows better measurement of the size of individual brain structures.

Researchers have questioned the association between large ventricles and schizophrenia, however. They have done so on the grounds that ventricle size varies widely in the general population, not all schizophrenics have large ventricles, and some actually have smaller ventricles than many normal study subjects. It is also unclear whether individuals who develop schizophrenia necessarily have larger ventricles than they would have had if they had not become schizophrenic.

An intriguing study designed to answer both of these questions was published in March 1990. The study compared MRI scans of the brains of pairs of identical twins who differed only in that one twin of each pair had schizophrenia, while the other was normal. Since identical twins have the same genes, it was expected that their brain structures would be identical except for any effect associated with schizophrenia. In almost every twin pair examined in this study, the schizophrenic twin had the larger ventricles.

This study is important not only because it confirms that ventricular enlargement is characteristic of schizophrenia, but also because it shows that the difference in brain structure is not inherited. Thus some other factor must cause the change in brain structure. Researchers say such a factor might be an injury to brain tissue occurring during pregnancy, delivery, or after birth, or it could involve a virus, toxin, or physical trauma. On the other hand, it is possible that something associated with the life experience of a schizophrenic might alter brain structure. Since there is evidence for some genetic component in the development of schizophrenia, it seems most likely that in schizophrenia there is a genetic predisposition that makes a person vulnerable to one or more nongenetic factors that in turn lead to the disease and to the abnormalities in brain structure.

See also the feature articles MIND AND BODY *and* TRAUMA: THE EMOTIONAL AFTERMATH.

HAROLD W. KOENIGSBERG, M.D.

NUTRITION AND DIET

New Diet and Weight Guidelines • Legislation on Food Labeling and Health Claims • Eating for Two Reevaluated • Fat-Free and Lower-Fat Foods

New Dietary Recommendations

The third edition of *Dietary Guidelines for Americans* was published jointly in November 1990 by the U.S. Departments of Agriculture and of Health and Human Services. It reinforces conclusions about what constitutes a healthful diet made in the previous editions and in the 1989 report *Diet and Health*, published by the National Academy of Sciences. Though the new guidelines (see the accompanying box for highlights) are similar to earlier versions, some changes were made. The two previous editions (in 1980 and 1985) had no specific guidance on fat consumption; the new edition agrees with *Diet and Health* that no more than 30 percent of a person's total intake of calories should

DIETARY GUIDELINES

- **Eat a Variety of Foods**
  Number of daily servings: 3–5 of vegetables; 2–4 of fruit; 6–11 of breads, cereals, rice, and pasta; 2–3 of milk, yogurt, and cheese; 2–3 of meats, fish, poultry, dry beans and peas, eggs, and nuts.
- **Maintain Healthy Weight**
- **Choose a Diet Low in Fat, Saturated Fat, and Cholesterol**
  Take in 30 percent or less of calories as fat, including less than 10 percent of calories as saturated fat.
- **Choose a Diet With Plenty of Vegetables, Fruits, and Grain Products**
  See Eat a Variety of Foods, above.
- **Use Sugar Only in Moderation**
- **Use Salt Only in Moderation**
- **If You Drink Alcoholic Beverages, Do So in Moderation**
  For women, no more than one drink a day; for men, no more than two drinks a day. One drink is defined as 12 ounces of beer, 6 ounces of wine, or 1½ ounces of distilled spirits.

Source: *Dietary Guidelines for Americans*, Third Edition

come from fat, with saturated fat contributing no more than 10 percent of calories. (Found in red meats and dairy products, among other sources, saturated fat is the type most closely associated with high cholesterol levels and increased risk of heart disease.) In addition, the new edition provides more specific guidance than did earlier versions on selecting foods to meet the guidelines. However, whereas *Diet and Health* recommends that people take in, on average, less than 300 milligrams of cholesterol and 6 grams or less of salt daily, the new bulletin gives no specific limits for these substances. It recommends a diet low in cholesterol, and moderation in salt consumption.

Revised Weight Guidelines. A major difference between the 1990 guidelines and earlier versions is that the weight recommendations in the 1990 edition are not based on the Metropolitan Life Insurance Company's height-weight tables, for decades a standard for "ideal" weight (for good health). The new recommendations for "healthy" weight (see the accompanying table) give suggested weight ranges according to height for adults up to age 34 and those 35 and over. The ranges are based on research suggesting that people can safely be a little heavier as they grow older. They apply to both men and women, with the proviso that the lower end of each range more often applies to women—who have less bone and muscle—while the upper end is more appropriate for men.

Finding Your Healthy Weight. The 1990 bulletin advocates a three-step method for determining "healthy" weight. First, check to see whether your body weight is within the range given in the table for your age and height. Second, since excess fat in the abdomen increases the risks of high blood pressure, heart disease, diabetes, and gallbladder disease, determine whether body fat is concentrated in the abdomen or hips. Do this by measuring waist and hip circumferences and dividing the waist by the hip measurement. The resulting figure is called the waist-to-hip ratio. The distribution of body fat is healthier if the ratio is less than 0.80 for women and 0.95 for men, according to some experts; the guidelines warn that increased health risks are associated with ratios close to or greater than one. The third step in determining healthy weight is to check with your physician to be sure you have no medical problem for which weight gain or loss is recommended.

If your weight is within the range for someone of your height and age, body fat is not overly concentrated in the abdomen, and your physician sees no special weight problem, you do not need to change your weight. The purpose of the three criteria is to identify only those people who need to gain or lose weight for reasons of health (as opposed to fashion) and thus to discourage the national obsession with thinness and off-again, on-again dieting in the United States.

SUGGESTED WEIGHTS FOR ADULTS

Height[1]	Weight in pounds[2]	
	Age 19–34	35 and Over
5′0″	97–128	108–138
5′1″	101–132	111–143
5′2″	104–137	115–148
5′3″	107–141	119–152
5′4″	111–146	122–157
5′5″	114–150	126–162
5′6″	118–155	130–167
5′7″	121–160	134–172
5′8″	125–164	138–178
5′9″	129–169	142–183
5′10″	132–174	146–188
5′11″	136–179	151–194
6′0″	140–184	155–199
6′1″	144–189	159–205
6′2″	148–195	164–210
6′3″	152–200	168–216
6′4″	156–205	173–222
6′5″	160–211	177–228
6′6″	164–216	182–234

[1] without shoes [2] without clothes
Source: *Dietary Guidelines for Americans,* Third Edition

Not all scientists agree that it is healthy for adults to gain weight as they get older. Moreover, there are practical difficulties in using the new weight table. For example, does a woman of 5′4″ who weighs, say, 112 pounds at age 20 become "unhealthy" if she maintains that weight beyond age 35 (when her suggested weight range changes from 111-146 to 122-157)? On the other hand, is she at a "healthy" weight if she gains 30 pounds to weigh 143 at age 40? Scientists will doubtless continue to debate the usefulness of this new table for the public.

Single copies of *Dietary Guidelines for Americans* are available free from the Consumer Information Center, Dept. 514-x, Pueblo, Colo. 81009.

Food Labeling Legislation

Passage of a new federal law in late 1990 should result in improved nutrition labeling of foods sold in the

United States. A publication released in September by a committee of the Institute of Medicine and the National Academy of Sciences, *Nutrition Labeling—Issues and Directions for the 1990s*, greatly influenced provisions of this law, which primarily affects packaged and processed foods.

Nutrition Information. Nutrition labeling for most food products has been voluntary. Only manufacturers who make nutritional claims (such as "low in fat") or who fortify food with vitamins or minerals have been required to list on labels the amounts of certain nutrients in the product, and even then they have not had to list saturated fat, sugar, cholesterol, or percentage of calories from fat. The new law requires that labels for most packaged foods give the product's total number of calories and number of calories from fat; specify how much protein, total fat, saturated fat, cholesterol, sodium, total carbohydrates, complex carbohydrates, sugars, and dietary fiber the product contains; and give the quantities of some vitamins and minerals. The Food and Drug Administration (FDA) is to formulate detailed regulations to implement the new law and designate which vitamins and minerals must be listed.

Foods exempted from the law's labeling requirements include meat and poultry products, restaurant and take-out foods, infant formulas, and products sold by companies with sales of less than $500,000. The law gives the FDA authority to require displays of nutrition information about the most popular fresh produce and seafoods if this is not done voluntarily.

Controlling Health Claims. The new law will restrict health claims that can be made on labels regarding cholesterol, saturated fat, and fiber. The FDA is to decide what specific claims manufacturers will be allowed to make about relationships between diet and disease. For example, if the FDA concluded that consumption of dietary fiber decreased the risk of colon cancer, manufacturers would be allowed to claim their product lowered that risk if the item met FDA specifications as to fiber content.

The FDA is also to establish standard definitions for terms often used by manufacturers in making nutritional claims, such as "free," "low," "light," "reduced," "less," and "high." For example, the FDA will specify how little fat a product must contain to be labeled "low-fat" or "fat-free"; how few calories to be labeled "light"; or how much calcium to be labeled "high in calcium."

The new labels will enable motivated consumers to find out more than they currently can about the nutritional content of most foods on the market. However, the FDA will need time to finalize the regulations, and changes based on the new law are not expected to show up on labels until 1993.

Nutrition Guidelines for Pregnancy

Increased Weight Gain. New guidelines from the Institute of Medicine and National Academy of Sciences for weight gain during pregnancy were released in mid-1990. For the previous 30 years, physicians had been warning women not to gain more than 25 pounds during pregnancy. This admonition provoked such anxiety that some women would starve themselves before prenatal checkups. The new publication, *Nutrition During Pregnancy*, sanctions weight gains of 25-35 pounds for women who are of normal weight at conception. Young adolescents and blacks should aim for the top of this range, since these women tend to have smaller babies than others of normal weight at conception if they gain the same amount of weight during pregnancy. Women who are underweight prior to pregnancy should gain 28-40 pounds, with young adolescent and black women aiming for the upper end of this range. Women who are overweight at conception should gain 15-25 pounds, with obese women aiming for a 15-pound gain. (Obesity is generally defined as 20 percent or more above normal weight.) The new recommendations are based on research indicating that inadequate weight gain during pregnancy is associated with babies of low birth weight. Low birth weight greatly increases the infant's risk of serious health problems.

Vitamin and Mineral Supplements. A great many American women take vitamin and mineral supplements in the course of normal pregnancies. According to *Nutrition During Pregnancy*, however, supplements generally are not necessary unless a woman is carrying more than one fetus, is a heavy cigarette smoker, abuses drugs or alcohol, or has a poor diet. The publication recommends that health professionals evaluate the diets of all pregnant women at the first prenatal visit. The only supplement that healthy women with adequate diets need during pregnancy is 30 milligrams a day of iron during the last six months.

Healthier Fast Food

Lower-Fat Burgers. Fast food restaurants responded to consumer pressure by making available wider choices of foods lower in total fat or in saturated fat. McDonald's made news in March 1991 by announcing plans for a "McLean" burger, a quarter-pound burger with only half the fat of the chain's regular quarter-pounder. The patty is made by grinding lean beef with water and a small amount of carrageenan, a carbohydrate extracted from seaweed. Carrageenan and water are needed to make the new meat patty approach the juiciness and flavor of a higher-fat patty, since low-fat beef alone tends to become dry with cooking. The McLean, served on a bun with lettuce, tomato, onion, pickles, mustard, and ketchup, contains 310 calories and 10 grams of fat (29 percent of calories). The new burger is not likely to replace McDonald's standard one, for many people prefer the taste of fattier meat, but it will provide a welcome alternative for those who are trying to follow a lower-fat diet.

Nutritionists generally applauded McDonald's for its new burger, and some have urged the firm to go further by offering a vegetarian (meatless) burger, a product already selling well in the United Kingdom.

Less Saturated Fat, More Information. A number of fast food chains—including Wendy's, Burger King, Jack in the Box, and McDonald's—have recently reduced the saturated fat in their French fries by switching from beef tallow to vegetable oil for cooking the fries. (Some chains—Hardee's, for example—have always used vegetable oil.) It should be noted that the new French fries are just as high in calories and total fat as the old.

McDonald's has increased the variety of its offerings, making it easier for customers to choose foods that fit into lower-fat diets. These include lower-fat breakfast cereals, a bran muffin containing no fat, and low-fat frozen yogurt and milk shakes. In addition, McDonald's now posts nutrition information, so that customers can find out the number of calories and the amount of fat, sodium, and other nutrients in all its menu items. McDonald's had for many years resisted making such information available. Since it is the

Red Meat Revisited

Red meat—beef, pork, lamb—has been firmly branded public enemy number one in the perennial battle against heart disease, with ground beef the single greatest source of fat in the American diet. High in both cholesterol and saturated fat, which raise blood cholesterol levels, red meat is the focus of a barrage of health warnings. Experts caution that overconsumption can increase the risk of heart attack and stroke, and they advise limiting one's intake or, perhaps, even cutting it out altogether.

So *adding* a large quantity of fat to meat in cooking would make it even more lethal, right? Wrong, at least according to biophysicist Donald Small of Boston University School of Medicine. An enthusiastic cook, himself plagued by high cholesterol levels, Small had a large stake in discovering a way to eat red meat without exceeding American Heart Association guidelines for fat and cholesterol consumption. He came up with a solution in his own kitchen—and promptly patented it for commercial use.

As unlikely as it sounds, Small's method involves cooking ground meat in a large quantity of vegetable oil (which is high in *un*saturated fat). Any ground meat and any vegetable oil can be used, with two to four cups of oil for every two pounds of meat. The oil and meat are heated to just below boiling point and stirred for five minutes to mix them as thoroughly as possible. The mixture is then heated to boiling point and cooked for five more minutes, browning the meat and boiling off excess juices, or broth. The meat is next strained, and the oil—which now contains animal fats that have leached into it from the meat—and any remaining broth are collected in a bowl. Then boiling water is poured over the meat and drained off into the same bowl. The fat and oil are now separated from the broth, either with a gravy skimmer or through refrigeration for perhaps an hour, which causes the fat to float to the top and solidify. Finally, the broth is added back to the meat.

In a paper published in January 1991 in the *New England Journal of Medicine*, Small and two colleagues reported that this extraction process reduced the fat content of meat by an average of 68 percent and its cholesterol content by 39 percent. In addition, the meat's proportion of unsaturated to saturated fat increased, as some of its original fat was replaced by vegetable oil. The result was a meat comparable in fat content to skinless chicken breast—frequently recommended for healthy eating.

Ground meat prepared by Small's method can be used in many different dishes: soups, chili, sauces, lasagna, casseroles, and stuffed peppers or cabbage, to name a few. Small is experimenting with possible binders, such as egg whites and oatmeal, to beef up the repertoire.

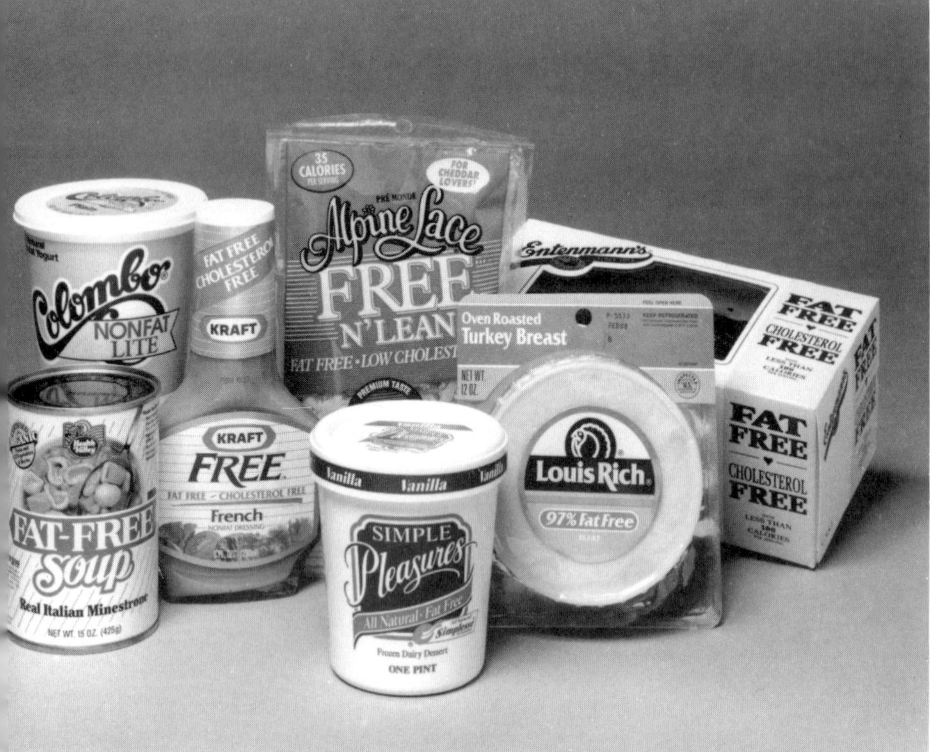

Because of increased consumer interest in healthful eating, supermarket shelves boast an ever broader selection of fat-free and low-fat foods. Careful reading of the labels is necessary to determine which products are genuinely healthful choices.

pacesetter in the fast food industry, other companies are likely to follow suit.

Lower-Fat Foods in Supermarkets

In response to consumer demand, food processors and manufacturers are offering supermarket shoppers an ever-increasing choice of lower-fat substitutes for standard foods. Since the presence of fat in a food strongly affects its flavor, texture, and "mouth feel" (the sensation on the tongue of richness), individuals must decide for themselves whether a given food is an acceptable substitute for a traditional item. All lower-fat substitutes must carry nutrition labels; these should be read carefully.

Many lower-fat foods still derive most of their calories from fat. The important information in this regard is the percentage of calories from fat, but this is not always given on the label. To calculate it, find the grams of fat in one serving, multiply by 9 to obtain the number of calories from fat, divide the result by the number of calories in one serving, and multiply by 100. Foods with 30-35 percent or more of their calories coming from fat are high in fat. Note the serving size on the label to prevent mistaken estimates of the amount of fat in the portion you plan to eat. (Some suggested serving sizes are rather small.)

Companies now offer lower-fat cheeses, yogurt, margarine, salad dressings, cakes, cookies, and frozen desserts, among other foods. Substitutes for cheddar and Swiss cheeses are made with low-fat milk and are lower in calories, fat, and cholesterol than their traditional counterparts. Nonetheless, 35-70 percent of their calories come from fat. Plain skim-milk yogurt provides fewer calories, with only 4 percent of them coming from fat, than does whole-milk yogurt, which furnishes 48 percent of its calories as fat.

So-called light margarine is made by replacing half the fat with water—thus, both calories and fat are lower than in regular margarine. While this product spreads well, it spatters when used for sautéing. If it is used in place of regular margarine or shortening in baked products, the amount of liquid in the recipe must be decreased.

A large number of low-fat or non-fat salad dressings are now available, but many are higher in sugar than their regular counterparts, and they vary tremendously in taste. Reduced-calorie mayonnaise contains half the calories and fat of regular mayonnaise, due to the use of starch and gums as thickeners and increased amounts of water; still, 90 percent of its calories come from fat. Among traditional substitutes for mayonnaise, Miracle Whip is also available in a "light" form, which provides 80 percent of its calories from fat compared with 90 percent in the regular product. The "light" version contains starch, microcrystalline cellulose, and gum, giving it a thicker, stickier texture than the original.

Lower-fat cakes and other baked products are also becoming widely available. Among cake mixes advertised as low in fat, some brands are markedly lower in fat than others. For example, according to the labels, one brand of spice cake mix provides 5 grams of fat per slice while another provides 11. Among already baked products, one nationally known brand (Entenmann's) offers cakes, cookies, and muffins that contain no fat or cholesterol. They are made with flour, sugar, skim milk, egg whites, and baking powder; a high sugar content makes them sweeter than their regular counterparts. Some supermarkets offer their own brands of similar products.

Lower-fat or "light" alternatives to ice cream can be found in supermarket freezer cases next to the real thing, but they cannot be labeled "ice cream" because they do not contain the legally required amount of fat. Some so-called light frozen desserts provide 110-120 calories per half-cup serving, with 3-4 grams of fat (representing 25-30 percent of calories). This compares with 135-150 calories and 7-8 grams of fat (providing nearly 50 percent of calories) for regular ice cream, and 175 calories with 12 grams of fat (62 percent of calories) for rich ice cream. The lowered fat content in the light desserts is due to the use of milk in place of cream.

Some fat-free frozen desserts are made with skim milk, sugar, and gums and provide 100 calories per half-cup with no fat. Many sherbets (sometimes called sorbets) contain no fat because they are made with fruit juice, but others contain milk and can derive as much as 20 percent of their calories from fat.

Fat Substitutes

New fat-free frozen desserts made with a fat substitute called Simplesse went on the market in the United States in 1990. Simplesse is a blend of egg white and milk protein treated so as to form tiny, spherical particles that slide over one another, creating the feel on the tongue of smoothness and creaminess usually associated with fat. It was approved by the FDA in February 1990 for use in frozen desserts.

As of early 1991, two frozen desserts contained Simplesse. The first, Simple Pleasures, has no fat (because Simplesse replaces cream) and about 10 percent fewer calories than regular ice cream. The other Simplesse product, Fat Freedom Eskimo Pie, consists of a center resembling vanilla ice cream (but made with Simplesse) held between two fat-free chocolate wafers; it contains no fat and provides 130 calories.

The manufacturer of Simplesse has applied to the FDA for approval of its use in mayonnaise, salad dressings, sour cream, cheese spreads, dips, and margarine. However, Simplesse can be used only in foods that do not require cooking because high heat destroys the properties that allow it to masquerade as fat. Other fat substitutes to be used in unheated food have also been submitted for FDA approval, including one called Oatrim, made from oat bran, and Trailblazer, another egg-white, milk-protein product.

One fat substitute that can be used in cooking and frying, Olestra, has been submitted to the FDA. Olestra consists of sucrose (table sugar) molecules and fatty acids linked together to form a substance the body cannot absorb. The manufacturer proposes to replace with Olestra 35-75 percent of the calories from fat in oils, shortenings, and prepared foods.

Whether consumption of foods containing fat substitutes will result in lower fat intake by the general public is questionable, since people may well rationalize that by eating some nonfat products they can eat more fat in other foods. This seems to have been the case with sugar substitutes, which became popular in the 1970s and 1980s. During that time, U.S. consumption of caloric sweeteners (sugars and corn sweeteners) increased rather than decreased. It should also be noted that fat substitutes cannot make foods that supply nothing but calories more nutritious, and nutritionists will continue to emphasize the benefits to be gained from a diet high in whole grains, fresh fruits, and vegetables, even should fat substitutes come into widespread use.

See also the feature articles PEAS, BEANS, AND OTHER LEGUMES *and* THIRST QUENCHERS *and the Spotlight on Health articles* EATING OUT WISELY, SAFE COOKWARE, *and* THE VIRTUES OF OLIVE OIL.

ELEANOR R. WILLIAMS, PH.D.

OBSTETRICS AND GYNECOLOGY

Dangers of AIDS • Hormone Replacement Therapy Evaluated • Genetic Testing Update • Fetal Surgery Success

AIDS and Women

A report from the U.S. Centers for Disease Control published in 1990 predicted that AIDS (acquired immune deficiency syndrome) would probably become one of the five leading causes of death in American women of reproductive age by 1991.

Most recent evidence indicates that the human immunodeficiency virus (HIV), which causes AIDS, is communicated like any other microorganism that is sexually transmitted or present in bodily fluids. Women can be infected with HIV through sexual contact with infected partners, by injecting drugs with needles that have previously been used by an infected person and not sterilized, through blood transfusions, or through direct contact with the blood or other bodily fluids of an infected individual. Fetuses and infants may contract HIV infection from their mothers through the placenta, during passage through the birth canal, or through breast milk. Fortunately, since HIV tests became available in 1985, routine testing of blood products has resulted in a very sharp drop in the number of cases of HIV infection from transfusions.

Women accounted for 7 percent of AIDS cases reported in the United States before 1985 but an estimated 12 percent of those reported in 1990—when there were some 5,000 new cases in women. Unfortunately, many women continue to believe that they are not at risk for HIV infection. Women at most risk are those with bisexual partners (26 percent of cases) or those who use intravenous drugs themselves or are sexual partners of intravenous drug users (53 percent of cases). HIV-infected women who have babies often pass on to the newborn the double problem of HIV and drug exposure, and the mothers are often themselves too sick to care for the infants, leading to a growing crisis in providing healthcare and social services for these needy children. About 30 percent of children born to HIV-infected mothers develop AIDS.

The number of American babies born with AIDS continues to rise. Because the mothers are often too ill to care for their children, great demands have been placed on healthcare providers, such as these staff members at Boston's Children's Hospital.

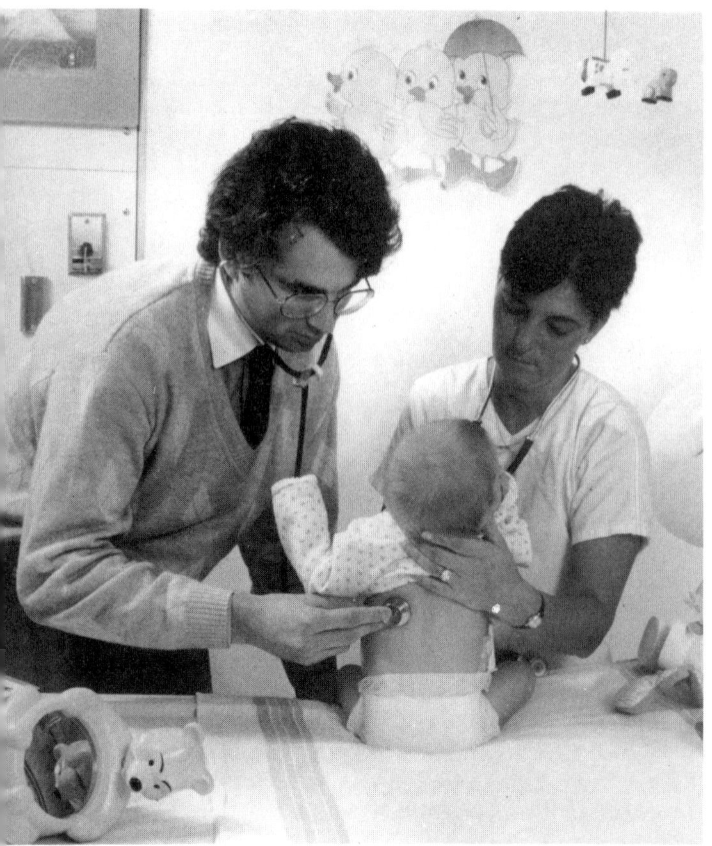

An estimated 1 million persons in the United States have been infected with HIV—that is, up to one in every 250. A 1990 study of college students, a group in which intravenous drug use or transfusion-acquired HIV infection would probably be quite rare, found that one in every 500 tested positive for HIV. Although knowledge about AIDS is fairly widespread on campuses, most studies have shown that only a minority of young adults are systematically using condoms or practicing other forms of "safe" sex (sexual activity with no exchange of bodily fluids).

Hormone Replacement Therapy

During 1990 information about the benefits to menopausal and postmenopausal women of hormone replacement therapy continued to accumulate, along with some possible causes for concern. Few issues are as controversial for women going through menopause—the years immediately before and after the ovaries stop releasing eggs and menstruation ceases—as the issue of whether or not to go on hormone replacement therapy (HRT). At menopause the ovaries decrease production of estrogen and progesterone, two hormones that build up the uterine lining each menstrual cycle to prepare it to receive a fertilized egg. As a result, many women experience hot flashes, mood swings, or depressive episodes, and HRT can alleviate these symptoms.

HRT usually consists of a combination of estrogen and a progesterone equivalent. Besides relieving the immediate symptoms of menopause, it can also protect against two serious possible long-term complications of decreased estrogen production: osteoporosis (thinning of the bones) and coronary heart disease. Women on HRT gain a 50-60 percent reduction in the risk of fractures due to osteoporosis and, for women on low doses, a 50 percent reduction in the death rate from heart disease.

Unfortunately, the news is not all good. The bone

and heart benefits come only with long-term HRT, and many women are reluctant to take the hormones for long periods, for a variety of reasons. For up to 90 percent of women, the most common HRT dosages result in monthly bleeding similar to menstrual periods, which most women have little desire for after menopause has freed them from that particular nuisance. Side effects such as bloating, nausea, and breast tenderness are common, although these can usually be avoided by reducing the dose. Any bleeding except for the pseudoperiods mentioned above necessitates a biopsy of the endometrium (uterine lining), since the wrong balance of estrogen and progesterone in HRT may increase the risk of endometrial cancer.

Moreover, several recently published studies have raised the possibility that HRT may slightly increase the risk of breast cancer. Although many other studies are reassuring on this issue, many women resist taking HRT out of concern about its long-term safety. Yet only a minority of women over 50 have ever had a mammogram (breast X ray), one of the most important tools in early detection of breast cancer. (The American Cancer Society recommends that women age 50 and over have annual mammograms.) Aggressive breast cancer screening programs in Sweden and England seem to be decreasing death rates from breast cancer dramatically. Furthermore, the U.S. death rate from heart disease in women over the age of 50 is more than five times the death rate from breast cancer. Does this suggest that the protection against death from heart disease conferred by HRT may outweigh any added risk of breast cancer? Women continue to face a very real dilemma in evaluating the pros and cons of HRT.

Advances in Prenatal Testing

The availability of prenatal genetic testing for relatively common conditions such as Down syndrome (a developmental disorder characterized by mental retardation and physical abnormalities) has helped couples to feel more comfortable planning pregnancies at later ages. The tendency to produce a fetus with a chromosomal abnormality such as the one responsible for Down syndrome increases with maternal age. At age 30 a woman has a 1 in 900 chance of bearing a baby with Down syndrome; at age 40 her risk is almost 1 in 100.

Unfortunately, the two most common tests for chromosomal abnormalities, though highly accurate, increase the risk of miscarriage: amniocentesis, in which a small amount of the amniotic fluid that surrounds the fetus in the uterus is removed; and chorionic villus sampling (CVS), in which a small sample of cells is taken from the placenta. Therefore, these tests are usually recommended only to women who will be 35 or over at the time of childbirth—in whom the risk of a Down child exceeds the risk of miscarriage from the test. The majority of Down syndrome infants, however, are born to women under 35, and physicians have long sought and patients long desired a test that would not involve any increased risk to the pregnancy and that could be used to screen younger women.

If the results of work by several different researchers are used in combination, blood tests can now be used to help detect before birth approximately 70 percent of Down syndrome babies, regardless of the mother's age. The blood tests indicate the mother's blood levels of alpha-fetoprotein (AFP), a protein produced by the fetus as it develops, and human chorionic gonadotropin (hCG), a hormone whose levels rise through the first 12 weeks of a healthy pregnancy. Women with abnormal levels are then offered standard genetic testing (amniocentesis or CVS). Some women in their middle and late 30s may even feel comfortable forgoing the more invasive tests if blood tests for AFP and hCG reveal that the risk of their baby having Down syndrome is quite low.

Tests on blood can also identify a gene defect responsible for most cases of cystic fibrosis (CF), an inherited abnormality that causes severe lung disease, poor growth, and, ultimately, early death. The defect was first identified in 1989. Screening of all potential parents has not been recommended, however, because of the cost involved and because the defect that has been identified occurs in only 75 percent or fewer of the people who are CF carriers. The blood test is recommended only for those with a family history of CF. A child of two carriers has a one in four chance of developing the disease, and either CVS or amniocentesis can be used to screen pregnancies in cases where both parents are found to be carriers.

All of these prenatal screening techniques involve simply testing for particular potential genetic defects and offering the parents involved the option of terminating the pregnancy if a defect is found. Many couples are uncomfortable with this choice and forgo genetic screening altogether. There is hope that research in progress may soon allow physicians to splice healthy genes into fetuses with genetic abnormalities, so that they can actually cure defects rather than simply detecting them.

See also the feature article PRENATAL SCREENING.

Breakthrough in Prenatal Surgery

The first successful major surgery on a fetus was reported in May 1990—by which time the patient was a thriving boy of nine months named Blake Schultz. A sonogram had shown that the fetus suffered from a diaphragmatic hernia, a congenital defect that is fatal in about 75 percent of cases. It occurs when the diaphragm (the wall of muscle that separates the chest cavity from the abdominal cavity) fails to close as the fetus develops. This allows the abdominal organs to migrate into the chest cavity, stunting the growth of the fetal lungs. Without surgery, Blake would probably have died soon after birth, unable to breathe. But when the fetus was about 25 weeks old, surgery was performed by doctors at the University of California at San Francisco. In a 54-minute procedure, with mother and fetus under general anesthesia, the doctors opened the uterus and the fetus's left side and returned the abdominal organs to their proper place. They patched the diaphragm closed and enlarged the abdomen to hold the repositioned organs. The mother was unharmed by the procedure, and the baby was born seven weeks later. Such operations, however, carry a high level of risk for the fetus (several previous attempts to repair diaphragmatic hernias were unsuccessful), and they are still considered highly experimental. They are unlikely to be widely performed in the immediate future.

See also the feature article WHAT IS ENDOMETRIOSIS? *and the Spotlight on Health article* COPING WITH MORNING SICKNESS. LINDA HUGHEY HOLT, M.D.

OCCUPATIONAL HEALTH

Repetitive Motion Disorders • Fetal Safety or Sex Discrimination? • Protecting Workers From Chemicals

Ergonomics

Ergonomics, or human engineering, an applied science that studies the safe interaction of people and things in the home, office, and the factory, received increased attention in 1990. On December 27, San Francisco Mayor Art Agnos signed into law an ordinance regulating the equipment used at computerized work stations. The law requires ergonomic workstations (equipped with adjustable chairs, adequate lighting, and adjustable computers with detachable keyboards) and worker safety training at firms having more than 15 employees who work at least four hours a day at video display terminals (VDTs). The law also mandates that employees who routinely perform "repetitive keyboard motions" for four hours or more per shift be given 15 minutes of alternate work every two hours.

During 1990 the U.S. National Institute for Occupational Safety and Health (NIOSH) released a series of health hazard evaluation reports stating that workers who were required to repeat the same motions with hands and arms throughout the day suffered a wide range of health problems known as cumulative trauma disorders. In January 1990, a preliminary NIOSH study conducted at Newsday Inc., a daily newspaper published in New York City and neighboring Long Island, to assess the ergonomic hazards of computer keyboards found that 331 of 834 reporters and other workers surveyed reported cumulative trauma disorders of the hand, wrist, elbow, shoulder, and neck.

In a study of 119 checkers and 56 other grocery workers at supermarkets in New Jersey and New York, NIOSH found that 30 percent of the checkers and nearly 20 percent of the other workers had cumulative trauma disorders of the wrist, hands, or both. Compared to other grocery workers, the checkers had three times as many cases of carpal tunnel syndrome, in which the nerves going through a narrow space at the base of the hand (the carpal tunnel) become painfully compressed.

During 1990 the U.S. Occupational Safety and Health Administration (OSHA) continued a series of high-profile plant inspections focusing on ergonomic problems. In July, Ford Motor Company agreed to pay $1.2 million in fines and expand a model ergonomics program to cover 81 facilities. Four months later, OSHA announced that General Motors Corporation would establish a comprehensive ergonomics program for its 302,000 employees in 138 plants. The agreement stemmed from OSHA inspections of two GM plants early in the year, one of which resulted in a citation for 27 willful violations of OSHA's general regulations concerning ergonomic hazards.

Fetal Protection

In an important sex-discrimination suit, the U.S. Supreme Court in March 1991 ruled in the case of *United Automobile Workers* v. *Johnson Controls*. In 1982, Johnson Controls, an automobile battery manufacturer based in Milwaukee, adopted a policy barring women "who are pregnant or who are capable of bearing children" from jobs where they might be exposed to lead. The company said it took the step to protect unborn children. Fetal exposure to lead can result in stillbirth, low birthweight, premature delivery, and birth defects. However, the United Automobile Workers argued that the policy violated Title VII of the Civil Rights Act of 1964, which bars employment practices that discriminate on the basis of sex. The Supreme Court agreed, ruling that "decisions about the welfare of future children must be left to the parents . . . rather than to the employers."

Occupational Stress

Computer monitoring, in which a computer records every keystroke made by a VDT worker, can be used to measure an employee's ability to complete a task in a set amount of time. In October 1990 the Communications Workers of America released a study, conducted by the Department of Industrial Engineering at the University of Wisconsin, which found that telephone company VDT workers who are monitored by computers suffer more health problems than VDT workers who are supervised solely by human managers. Monitored workers reported "more boredom, high tension, extreme anxiety, depression, anger, and severe fatigue than non-monitored workers," researchers observed, as well as more neck pain and twice the number of sore wrists.

In April 1990, Dr. Peter L. Schnall of the New York Hospital-Cornell Medical College and a team of nine coauthors published the results of a study in which they found a relationship between occupational stress and elevated blood pressure. The researchers reported that employees who had jobs characterised by low decision-making latitude (i.e., inability to develop new skills, be creative, and choose how to perform tasks) and high psychological demands (i.e., a heavy workload, insufficient time to complete work) were three times more likely to suffer from high blood pressure as workers with less stressful jobs.

Asbestos

Asbestos continued to be the deadliest occupational health hazard in the United States. In June 1990 the Collegium Ramazzini, an international society of environmental and occupational health scientists, sponsored a conference in New York City on asbestos-related lung disease and cancer caused by exposure to asbestos fibers in pipe insulation, fireproofing, and floor and ceiling tiles in industrial settings, public and commercial buildings, and homes. At the meeting, physicians Irving Selikoff and Stephen Levin reported that asbestos-related lung scarring was found in 28 percent of the 660 New York City public school custodians that they screened. The percentage of custodians with lung abnormalities increased with the length of time on the job.

At an asbestos conference in September, Selikoff discussed a study of insulation workers exposed to asbestos. After examining death certificates covering a 20-year period, he found that 375 members in the Western States Conference of the asbestos workers' union had died of cancer, as compared to an expected 112 cancer deaths in the same number of other Ameri-

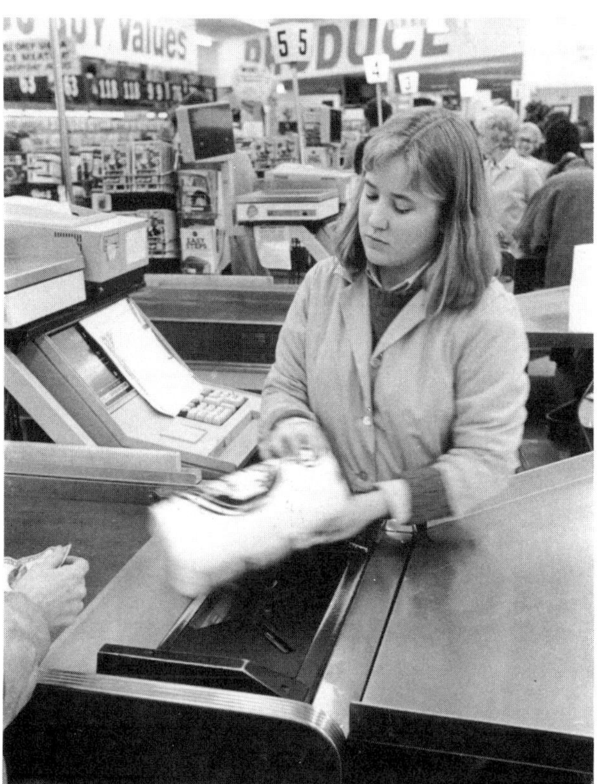

Workers who perform repetitive motions, such as checking out groceries or keyboarding, suffer a variety of health problems, according to reports released by the U.S. National Institute for Occupational Safety and Health. Among the complications are disorders of the hand, wrist, elbow, shoulder, and neck.

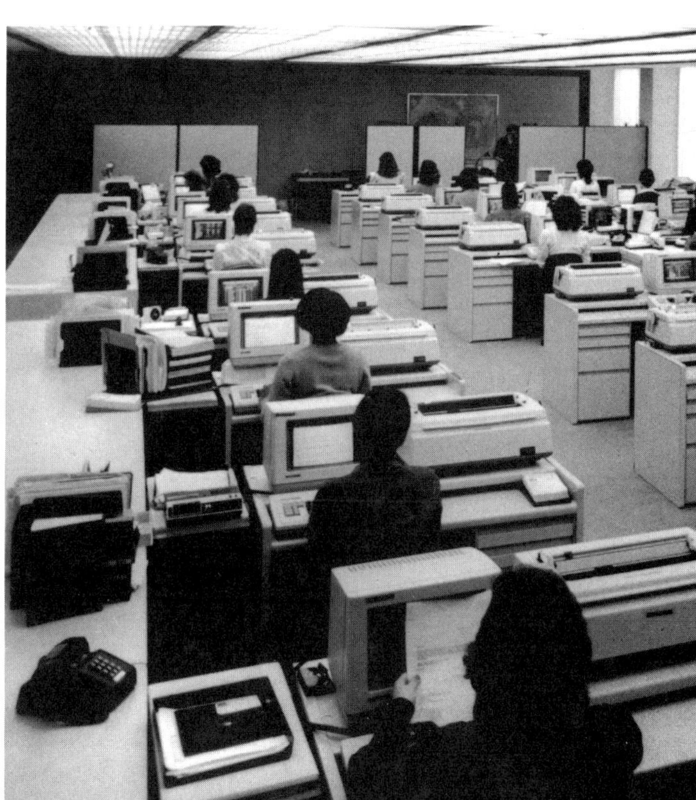

can white males. Selikoff also found 70 deaths from asbestosis, a progressive and potentially fatal disease characterized by scarring of the lung tissue. He noted that nearly two-thirds of the asbestos-related deaths occurred before the age of 65.

Neurotoxins

On May 16, 1990, the Office of Technology Assessment of the U.S. Congress issued a report, "Neurotoxicity: Identifying and Controlling Poisons of the Nervous System," which warned that while toxicological testing focuses on the threat of cancer from toxic chemicals, the adverse effects of these substances (i.e., their neurotoxicity) on the central nervous system "may pose an equal or greater threat to public health." The study concluded that the government's response to neurotoxicity was "fragmented" and that an improved federal response will require more testing, improved monitoring programs, and more aggressive regulation.

In an article in the *American Journal of Industrial Medicine* in the spring of 1990, University of Pittsburgh researchers who studied 567 female employees at a semiconductor manufacturing plant found that increased exposure to industrial solvents was significantly related to depression, severe headaches, lightheadedness, and other neurologic disorders. The study also found that solvent exposures were associated with major appetite changes, unusual taste in the mouth, weakness or fatigue, rashes, and abdominal pain.

Non-Ionizing Radiation

In December 1990 the U.S. Environmental Protection Agency (EPA) noted in a draft report that studies of children and adults exposed to electromagnetic fields (EMFs) in residential and occupational settings "suggest a causal link" between these exposures and elevated levels of cancer and other health problems. (EMFs, which exert force on surrounding objects, are generated when electric currents pass through power lines, VDTs, and household wiring and appliances.) The EPA said that while the strongest evidence of a health effect from EMF exposure came from studies of cancer in children, occupational studies provided additional but weaker evidence of elevated risks of leukemia and other malignancies due to EMF. However, the EPA cautioned that few measurements of occupational EMF exposure had been taken and that job classifications had come "generally from sources that could be characterized as sketchy."

See also the Health and Medical News article PUBLIC HEALTH.

STEPHEN G. MINTER

PEDIATRICS

Infant Meningitis Vaccine • Progress Against Cystic Fibrosis • Treating Epilepsy • Passive Smoking and Respiratory Diseases • New Asthma Treatment • Improving Access to Healthcare

Meningitis Vaccine

In October 1990 the U.S. Food and Drug Administration (FDA) approved a new vaccine, Haemophilus b conjugate vaccine, for use in infants. Given as a series of injections beginning at two months of age, the vaccine is effective against the bacterium called *Haemophilus influenzae* type b (Hib), a major cause of meningitis in American children under five years of age and especially those between 6 and 18 months old. Meningitis is an inflammation of the lining of the brain and spinal cord that can sometimes be fatal and often results in complications such as blindness, deafness, mental retardation, and paralysis.

The Hib bacterium can also cause other diseases, including serious infections of the skin, lungs, heart, and bloodstream. One of the most threatening is inflammation and swelling of the epiglottis, a small structure that guards the opening of the trachea (windpipe), preventing food from entering it during swallowing. The inflammation can progress rapidly and, if not promptly diagnosed and treated, can result in obstruction of the trachea and death. The new vaccine promises to be effective in preventing this life-threatening condition.

The risk of developing a serious Hib infection before age five is about one in 200. The mortality rate is as high as 5 percent, and the proportion of nervous system complications in meningitis survivors may be as high as 38 percent.

Haemophilus b conjugate vaccine is manufactured by Praxis Biologics, Inc., and marketed as HibTITER. The only vaccine previously available for Hib was effective only in children aged 15 months or older, leaving some of the most vulnerable infants without protection. A large-scale clinical trial of the new vaccine in infants less than six months old found that its effectiveness approached 100 percent, with no serious side effects.

Current U.S. recommendations are that all children be immunized against Hib beginning at two months of age or as soon as possible thereafter, rather than at 15 months of age as was previously done. The new vaccine should be administered in three doses given at two-month intervals. A booster dose should be administered at 15 months or later.

Gene Therapy for Cystic Fibrosis?

Two different research teams reported in 1990 that they had successfully used gene replacement therapy in laboratory experiments to correct a gene defect responsible for cystic fibrosis (CF). In CF thick, sticky mucus builds up in the lungs and elsewhere, impairing breathing and other functions and leading to chronic lung infections with destruction of lung tissue. Among Caucasians, CF is the most common fatal inherited disease, occurring once in every 2,000 live births. Some 30,000 Americans have cystic fibrosis. A large proportion are children; most people with the disease do not survive beyond their early 30s.

The identification in 1989 of the gene defect that causes about 70 percent of CF cases paved the way for the most recent advances and has already led to development of a prenatal screening test for use in cases where there is a family history of the disease. The defective gene produces an abnormal version of a protein that is responsible for the transport of chloride, a component of salt, across cell membranes. The protein is known as the cystic fibrosis transmembrane conductance regulator (CFTR). The abnormal CFTR is thought to impede the movement of chloride ions into and out of cells, pulling water into cells and leading to the buildup of the thick mucus.

A team of researchers at the University of Iowa, Tufts University, and the Genzyme Corporation reported in September 1990 that insertion of a gene for normal CFTR into abnormal cells taken from the airways of CF patients corrected the defect in chloride transport. At the same time, another team led by scientists from the University of Michigan announced similar results from inserting the normal gene into pancreatic cells with the CF gene defect. Both groups of researchers worked in the laboratory with cells that had been removed from CF patients; scientists have not yet tried to actually insert the normal gene into a patient. Though it will probably be several years at least before CF patients see any direct benefits from 1990's experimental successes, the potential is now increased for more effective treatment of CF.

Advances in Treating Epilepsy

It is now clear that two newer drugs for epilepsy, carbamazepine (brand name, Tegretol) and valproic acid (Depakene), are the drugs of choice for a majority of children and adolescents with epilepsy. Epilepsy is a brain disorder characterized by sudden attacks of altered or lost consciousness. Its victims experience seizures, often called convulsions or spells, in which abnormal electrical discharges from the brain result in uncontrolled movements, lapses in consciousness, strange feelings, or unusual behavior. The goal of drug treatment is to achieve maximum seizure control with minimum side effects. The newer drugs are at least as effective as older drugs, such as phenobarbital and phenytoin, with fewer side effects. They can minimize problems such as sedation and difficulties with balance and walking and may allow improved fine muscle control (important, for example, in writing). Equally important, carbamazepine and valproic acid are less likely than the earlier drugs to interfere with mental functioning, allowing improved concentration, memory, and learning.

A National Institutes of Health consensus conference held in 1990 focused on the question of how soon to recommend surgery when a patient's epileptic seizures prove unresponsive to treatment with drugs. Surgical removal of abnormal brain tissue can sometimes stop certain types of seizures. The consensus panel recommended that surgery be considered earlier in the course of the disorder, especially for patients whose seizures have proved difficult to control, and not be used as a last resort. If two years of drug therapy have failed to control the patient's seizures, surgery may be considered, the panel concluded. The longer a patient's seizures go uncontrolled, the greater the risk that they will worsen and impair the sufferer's ability to function in society. One effect of the suggested change in treatment procedure favoring earlier surgery would be that more children and adolescents would have the surgery.

Obsessive-Compulsive Disorder

A 1990 study from the Yale Child Study Center supports the hypothesis of a genetic, or hereditary, basis for obsessive-compulsive disorder (OCD). This condition, which afflicts up to a million American children and adolescents, is characterized by persistent ideas or fears that are unfounded and the irrational compulsion to repeat ritualized actions (for example, repetitive hand washing because of an exaggerated fear of germs). Of 21 children and adolescents with OCD studied by the Yale researchers, 15 (71 percent) had a parent with OCD or obsessive-compulsive symptoms.

An antidepressant drug approved by the FDA in 1989 to treat OCD was first marketed in 1990. The drug, clomipramine (brand name, Anafranil), can be used to treat OCD in children and adolescents. Although Anafranil was approved by the FDA only for use in people over ten years of age, the severity of the illness in younger children may dictate its use at an earlier age, with the full consent of the parents and, if appropriate, the child.

Parental Smoking and Children's Health

University of Arizona researchers reported a relationship between parental smoking and illnesses of the lower respiratory system in young children. They studied a large number of babies and found that the likelihood of an infant's having a lower respiratory illness, such as pneumonia or asthma-like wheezing, was significantly higher if the mother smoked cigarettes, particularly a pack or more a day.

The importance of parents not smoking in the presence of their children was further underscored by a report published in September 1990 in the *New England Journal of Medicine*. Researchers from Yale University and the National Cancer Institute, among other institutions, reported a link between inhalation of cigarette smoke in household air (passive smoking) and the development of lung cancer decades later. The researchers studied 191 nonsmokers with lung cancer and an equal number of healthy nonsmokers. They concluded that household exposure to 25 or more "smoker years"—the equivalent of two parents smoking for 12½ years each—during childhood and adolescence doubled a person's risk of developing cancer of the lung. They estimated that about one in six cases, or about 17 percent, of lung cancer in nonsmokers appear to be caused by long-term exposure to cigarette smoke in the home during childhood and adolescence.

Asthma Education Program

With the number of new asthma cases increasing steadily in the United States, particularly among children, the National Heart, Lung, and Blood Institute in early 1990 released a report containing new guidelines for doctors on the diagnosis and management of the disorder. Asthma is a chronic respiratory disease characterized by attacks of wheezing and breathing difficulties. An acute attack can be fatal, but the disorder is treatable, and with appropriate care most asthma patients can lead normal, active lives.

The new treatment guidelines emphasized that inflammation of the airways has been found by recent research to be a prominent feature of the disease—and one that should be more aggressively treated. It is now recommended that anti-inflammatory medication be a part of daily treatment for moderate to severe asthma cases, while bronchodilators, currently the most commonly used drugs for asthma, continue to be used for relief during acute asthma attacks.

The guidelines also focused on the importance of patient education, of controlling allergies, and of physicians' using a spirometer—an instrument that measures the amount of air breathed in and out of the lungs—to assess asthma severity and monitor treatment.

Access to Healthcare

The American Academy of Pediatrics (AAP) announced in October 1990 a specific proposal to provide health insurance to all American children and pregnant women. The proposal, outlined in a special report in the *New England Journal of Medicine*, was in response to the growing numbers of uninsured children and the relative decline in health status of some groups of American children compared to children in other developed countries.

Too many infants, children, and adolescents in the United States are not sharing the benefits of the remarkable advances in pediatrics because of financial limitations on their access to healthcare. The technology now exists for sustaining life in very low birth weight babies—even those weighing less than 2 pounds at birth—and the FDA's 1990 approval of a new type of drug (known as a pulmonary surfactant) for babies with respiratory distress syndrome has greatly improved the prospects for babies on breathing machines (ventilators). Yet infant mortality in the United States remains embarrassingly high, at 10.1 deaths per thousand live births. Infants born to substance-abusing mothers are at risk for central nervous system damage, and rising numbers are infected at or before birth with the human immunodeficiency virus, which causes AIDS. There has also been a resurgence of congenital syphilis (syphilis contracted at or before birth from an infected mother).

Probably the most alarming fact, which has sparked widespread concern both within and outside the medical community, is that at least 10 million children and perhaps 14 million women of childbearing age in the United States have no health insurance. In 1990 the Pepper Commission, a bipartisan U.S. congressional commission on healthcare, in recommending a universal insurance plan that included preventive care, identified the needs of children and pregnant women as the first to be addressed.

The plan proposed by the AAP would provide guaranteed access to healthcare for all persons up to 22 years of age and all pregnant women. This would include preventive care, primary and major medical care, and coordination of medical and other types of care (such as mental health services) where appropriate. Employers would be expected either to provide a basic package of benefits for employees and their dependents or to pay a payroll tax on all employees' wages. State-funded insurance, to cover those not insured by employers, would be financed from employer payroll taxes, premiums, and federal and state Medicaid funds currently allocated to children and pregnant women.

See also the feature articles HOW TO CHOOSE CHILD CARE *and* CHILDREN'S HEART PROBLEMS *and the Spotlight on Health articles* STEROIDS AND TEENAGERS *and* CIRCUMCISION: PROS AND CONS.

GEORGE D. COMERCI, M.D.

PUBLIC HEALTH

U.S. Health Objectives Set • Rise in Streptococcal Infections • Measles Resurgence

New Health Objectives

In September 1990 the U.S. Department of Health and Human Services, in cooperation with several other agencies, brought out the report *Healthy People 2000*, detailing national public health objectives for the 1990s. These objectives are expected to help guide public health priorities and practice over the next decade.

The report defined three broad goals: to increase the span of healthy life for Americans, to reduce the health disparities among different groups of Americans, and to achieve access to preventive services for all Americans. To achieve these goals, three main groupings of specific objectives were developed: health promotion, health protection, and preventive services.

Within the category of health promotion, there are objectives in the areas of physical activity and fitness, nutrition, tobacco use, use of alcohol and other drugs, use of family planning, improved mental health, decreased violent and abusive behavior, and improved educational and community-based programs. In the area of health protection there are objectives for unintentional injuries, occupational safety and health, environmental health, food and drug safety, and oral health. Under preventive services there are objectives regarding maternal and infant health, heart disease and stroke, cancer, diabetes and chronic disabling conditions, human immunodeficiency virus (HIV, the virus that causes AIDS) infection; sexually transmitted diseases, and clinical preventive services. In addition, there is a specific objective to improve health data systems and the surveillance of disease and there are age-related objectives for children, adolescents and young adults, adults, and older adults.

Streptococcal Infections

When Jim Henson, creator of the Muppets, died from streptococcal pneumonia in May 1990 at the relatively young age of 53, the world was shocked, but epidemiologists were not especially surprised. Serious streptococcal infections, particularly rheumatic fever, had been increasing for the past few years. In addition, an unusually toxic form of the streptococcus bacterium was becoming more prominent, especially in persons in their 40s and 50s. This form causes a rapidly progressive illness, called toxic streptococcal syndrome, which is similar to toxic shock syndrome but much more lethal. The best hope for overcoming this toxic form is early treatment with massive amounts of antibiotics; indeed, Henson's physicians said that he

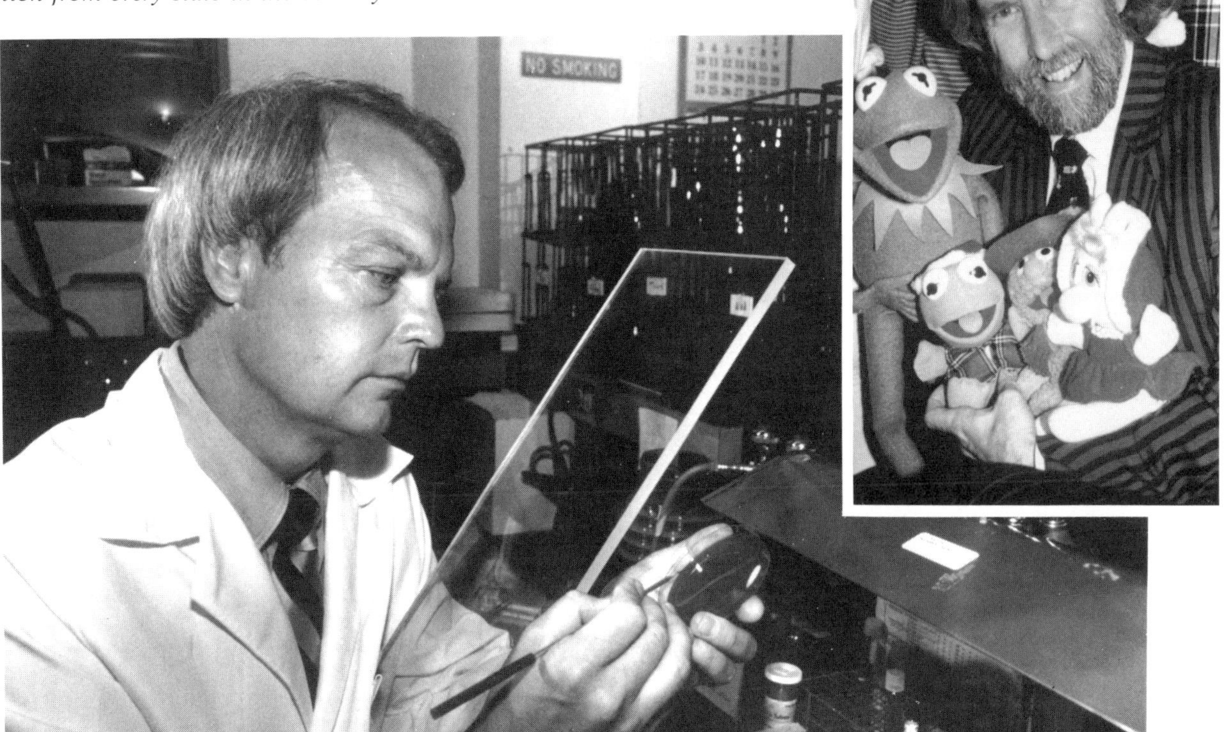

Muppet creator Jim Henson (right), who died in May 1990, was the victim of an unusually toxic form of streptococcus bacteria whose spread has caused considerable worry among health officials. Dr. Dennis Stevens, below, a leading U.S. strep researcher, reported that he had received accounts of the infection from every state in the country.

might have been saved if treatment had been started only a few hours earlier. Signs of advanced streptococcal infection include high fever, chills, dizziness when standing, and, in the case of pneumonia, coughing up of sputum and shortness of breath.

Head Injuries and Motorcycles

A study published in November 1990 reported that over a seven-year period, more than 15,000 deaths occurred in the United States from head injuries associated with motorcycle crashes. The states without comprehensive laws requiring helmet use by motorcycle riders had almost twice the rate of head injury deaths as states with comprehensive helmet-use laws. Also, two states that weakened their helmet-use laws during this period saw significant increases in the death rates from motorcycle-crash head injuries.

Nuclear Power Plants and Leukemia

A recent study conducted in Massachusetts suggested that persons who lived near the Pilgrim nuclear power plant in Plymouth for a long time experienced a leukemia rate four times as high as did those who lived farthest from the plant for the shortest time periods. The study was begun after a British study found an increase in childhood leukemia near some British nuclear plants. On the other hand, two other studies, one in the United States and one in France, found no overall increase in leukemia risk in counties or regions near nuclear power plants. More studies are needed to clarify the situation.

Electromagnetic Fields and Cancer

Although it has long been known that nuclear radiation can cause some types of cancer, until recently it was not suspected that electromagnetic radiation, which is much more prevalent, could do so as well. Data are increasing, however, that suggest that electromagnetic fields also pose a cancer risk, although it is probably a small one. One 1990 report by the U.S. Environmental Protection Agency, for example, linked electromagnetic fields to leukemia and brain cancer in children.

Electromagnetic fields are produced by such structures as electricity distribution lines along streets (especially if they are high-power transmission lines or from local power substations), as well as common household items such as electric blankets, hair dryers, shavers, and electric appliances. Because an electromagnetic field is most intense nearest its source, the best protection is distance. Whenever possible, it is best to say a foot or two away from electromagnetic field sources in the home.

Rise in Salmonellosis

In recent years, Americans have been eating more poultry and less beef and pork. The annual per capita consumption of chicken in the United States has gone up from about 40 pounds in 1970 to more than 70 pounds in 1990. With the increased production and consumption of poultry, however, has come a rise in a type of food poisoning caused by the *Salmonella* bacterium, which is often found in chickens and their eggs. The number of reported cases of *Salmonella* infection increased from about 33,700 in 1980 to about 47,800 in 1989, and this is considered a mere fraction of the total number of infections, which some experts put at 2 to 3 million a year in the United States. Salmonellosis is usually not fatal, except in debilitated persons, but even a healthy person can become seriously ill and require hospitalization. An estimated 2,000 Americans die from *Salmonella* infection every year. One strain of the bacterium, *Salmonella enteritidis*, has caused numerous outbreaks of food poisoning in the northeastern United States in recent years.

There is no reason, however, to be afraid of poultry if it is adequately cooked and if proper food handling practices are followed, including thorough cleaning in hot water of any utensils or containers that come in contact with uncooked poultry and keeping poultry refrigerated when not being prepared or served.

Influenza Epidemic

In the winter of 1989-1990 the United States was hit hard by one of the so-called A strains of influenza, resulting in an estimated 60 million cases of the disease. Of the two major strains of influenza, A and B, the A group is usually the more serious because the virus mutates so frequently that past exposure and even current vaccines may not protect against it. The strain that swept through the United States in 1989-1990 was called A-Shanghai because it was first identified there. Many new influenza A strains appear to originate in Asia, probably because high population densities there promote new genetic variations in the virus. The primary prevention is influenza vaccine, which may or may not be of much help, depending on whether or not the virus has changed since the vaccine was developed.

The winter flu season of 1990-1991 was milder, with a type B influenza accounting for most cases. The vaccine available was similar enough to the virus strain to protect those who had been immunized.

Viruses in Drinking Water

Viruses are increasingly being identified in U.S. drinking water. Better detection methods may partly account for this, but there are other explanations. The current methods of sewage and water treatment in the United States cannot rid drinking water of all of the viruses and parasites in it, even though the water may pass all required safety tests after being filtered and chlorinated. In addition, U.S. sewage treatment is inadequate in many areas, and intestinal organisms that enter the water upriver are taken into water intake systems lower downstream. There is no quick or inexpensive test that can detect these organisms; even a partial solution would require a major overhaul and upgrade of American sewage treatment systems, as well as more research to find better methods of treating sewage.

L-tryptophan Update

In 1989 it was discovered that a rare blood disorder called eosinophilia-myalgia syndrome (EMS) was associated with taking large doses of the amino acid L-tryptophan, a supplement believed to relieve insomnia, premenstrual syndrome, and depression, among other conditions. At first it was thought that this was merely another case of taking too much of a good thing. In 1990, however, it was discovered that most of the cases of EMS occurred in people who took pills produced by just one supplier, the Showa Denko chemical company in Japan. Special analyses identified an unknown substance (called "peak E") in three-quarters of the pill samples taken by EMS patients; these pills had been made by using a new strain of bacteria in the fermentation process that produces L-tryptophan. Yet only 1 percent of the people taking these pills actually got EMS, and some researchers theorized that the new bacteria introduced small amounts of a new substance that was capable of producing EMS only in a small number of people with certain genetic patterns.

Measles

The winter of 1989-1990 brought more than 80 local outbreaks of measles across the United States, and by the end of 1990 more than 26,000 cases and some 90 deaths had been reported. These figures were in contrast to the lowest frequency ever, in 1983, when 1,497 cases and no deaths were reported. A federal advisory panel blamed the measles epidemic on a breakdown in the national vaccination system.

Compounding the problem, in May 1990 the U.S. federal government announced that it had used all of the $10 million of emergency money set aside to buy measles vaccine to be distributed to poor people through local and state health departments.

JAMES F. JEKEL, M.D., M.P.H.

SEXUALLY TRANSMITTED DISEASES

Sexual Behavior Found Largely Unaffected by Awareness of Disease Risks • New Data on Gonorrhea Resistance • Improvements in Diagnosis

Sexual Behavior of College Women

A study of college women published in March 1990 showed that awareness of sexually transmitted diseases (STDs) does not always result in intelligent sexual behavior. This group of well-educated young adults was surveyed over a 14-year period that saw major public health campaigns involving STDs.

The researchers surveyed the sexual practices of women at a university in the northeastern United States in 1975, 1986, and again in 1989—that is, before and after the start of the current epidemics of genital herpes, genital chlamydia infection, and AIDS. Among other things, the women were questioned about aspects of sexual behavior potentially affecting the spread of STDs, such as frequency of condom use, number of sexual partners, and anal intercourse. Among sexually active women, the proportion whose partners regularly used condoms increased between 1975 and 1989, but the majority of women surveyed in 1989 said their partners did not use condoms regularly, despite the women's knowledge of sexually transmitted diseases and fear of AIDS. From 1975 to 1989, no significant differences were found in the number of male sexual partners in a given year or in the percentage of women who engaged in anal intercourse.

Syphilis Rates

The incidence of syphilis in the United States has continued steadily upward since 1985, reaching the level of approximately 18 cases of primary and secondary syphilis for every 100,000 persons in 1989. This reflects a widening gap between blacks and whites, with blacks having more cases than whites. (The overall incidence among black men and women was about 122 cases per 100,000 in 1989.) Congenital syphilis (syphilis contracted by the fetus during pregnancy or birth) is also on the rise. However, from 1982 to 1989, the number of cases of primary and secondary syphilis among white men decreased 69 percent, to about 3 per 100,000, and the number of cases among white women remained low, about 2 per 100,000. (*See also the Spotlight on Health article* THE RESURGENCE OF SYPHILIS.)

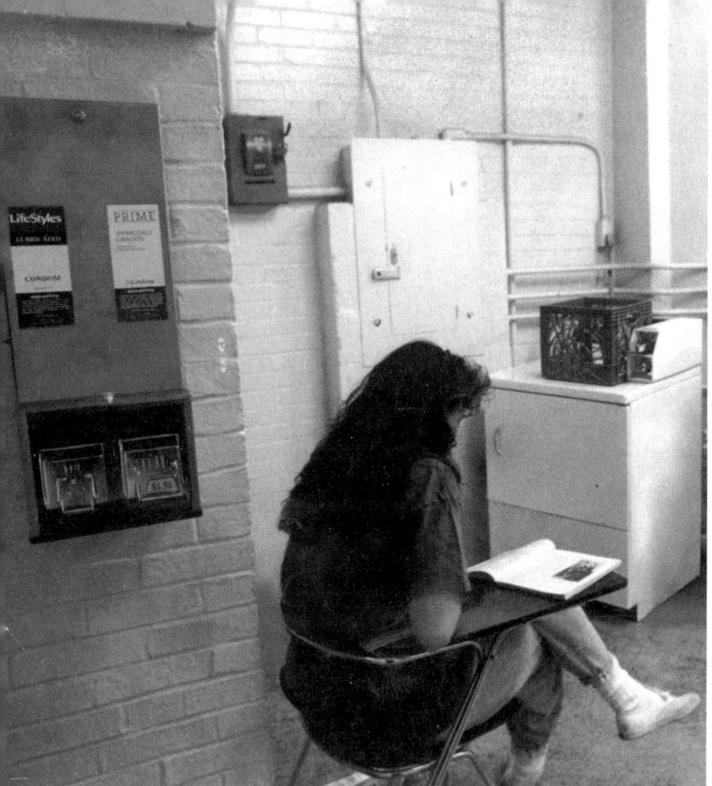

Despite colleges' efforts to protect students from sexually transmitted diseases—such as condom dispensers like the one in this University of Massachusetts dormitory—a survey has found that a majority of sexually active college women did not have their partners use condoms regularly, even though they were well aware of the risk.

Gonorrhea Resistance

A study published in September 1990 substantiated the 1989 decision by the U.S. Centers for Disease Control (CDC) to no longer recommend the antibiotics penicillin or tetracycline as the preferred treatment for gonorrhea. In recent years gonorrhea has become more difficult to treat because of its increased resistance to these older antibiotics.

In September 1987 the CDC began a program in selected clinics throughout the country to observe resistance to antibiotics by the bacterium that causes gonorrhea. Among the strains of the bacterium studied up to the end of 1988, 21 percent were found to be resistant to one or more antibiotics. However, none were resistant to the antibiotic ceftriaxone. The treatment most commonly used now is an injection of ceftriaxone followed by tetracycline, taken orally. (The tetracycline is given because a chlamydia infection may be present.)

Diagnostic Advances

Researchers at the University of Washington have introduced a promising new option—a combination of two tests—for diagnosing chlamydia. Genital chlamydia infections are believed to strike 4 million people yearly in the United States. Women in their childbearing years are particularly vulnerable because infection with chlamydia can result in pelvic inflammatory disease, with subsequent infertility and ectopic pregnancy (pregnancy outside the uterus). The rate of ectopic pregnancy in the United States has been on an upward trend since 1970. Many women with chlamydia have no symptoms, and so screening tests that can detect this infection are particularly important.

The gold standard among tests for diagnosing chlamydia uses tissue cultures, but even this method is not 100 percent effective; between 10 and 30 percent of infected patients receive negative, rather than positive, results. Moreover, the test is expensive and requires highly trained personnel. In the two-step Washington method, by contrast, all specimens undergo a simple laboratory test called an enzyme immunoassay, whereby specially treated beads are used to detect chlamydia antigens. Specimens for which this test gives positive results are then checked by means of a more complex test called a direct fluorescent antibody assay, in which the bacterium causing chlamydia is identified with an antibody specific to it that is labeled with a fluorescent dye. Although this test is highly accurate, it requires considerable expertise. Researchers are experimenting with other methods that they hope will yield accurate tests for diagnosing chlamydia in laboratories that lack tissue culture techniques.

Finnish researchers have developed an improved technique for diagnosing the human papilloma virus (HPV), which causes infections of the genital tract that may not be visible to the naked eye or may show up as flat condylomas (wartlike growths) or warts. There are many varieties of HPV, and types 16 and 18 have been found to be closely associated with cervical cancer in women. A test approved by the U.S. Food and Drug Administration (FDA) in 1988 detects the genetic material, or DNA, of specific types of the virus and can pinpoint the more risky types, yielding results in four to fourteen days. The new Finnish method, now undergoing testing, provides more rapid detection of the virus DNA, with results in only one day.

Hepatitis B Transmission

A Pittsburgh study found that the hepatitis B virus is transmitted more readily among homosexual men than is the virus that causes AIDS—the human immunodeficiency virus (HIV). Both viruses are major health problems in homosexual men. Hepatitis B virus, ordinarily transmitted by intimate contact or by contaminated blood, causes "serum" hepatitis.

There are an estimated 300,000 new cases of hepatitis B yearly in the United States, and anywhere from 50 to 70 percent of urban homosexual men are infected. Usually, rest is all that is needed for recovery, but about 6 to 10 percent of infected patients develop chronic hepatitis B. This can result in chronic liver disease, cirrhosis, liver cancer, and death.

The Pittsburgh study showed that insertive, rather than receptive, anal intercourse with an infected partner presented the major risk for hepatitis B virus infection among homosexuals, suggesting that the male urethra may be an important route for entry of the virus. The hepatitis B virus was discovered to be almost nine times more effective than HIV in infecting homosexual men—a finding that emphasizes the importance of hepatitis B immunization and the use of condoms during intercourse.

Unfortunately, Americans have been slow to be vaccinated against hepatitis B. For this reason, vaccination of children was recommended in February 1991 by the Immunization Practices Advisory Committee of the U.S. Public Health Service. It was the first time that the federal panel had advised vaccinating children against a disease that usually strikes adults.

Condoms and STDs

A new FDA pamphlet entitled *Condoms and Sexually Transmitted Diseases . . . Especially AIDS* explains different types of STDs and provides practical information on condoms, lubricants, and spermicides. Up to 100 copies may be obtained by educators without cost by calling the National AIDS Information Clearinghouse at 1-800-458-5231. Others can receive a free copy by calling the National AIDS Hotline at 1-800-342-2437.

See also the Health and Medical News article AIDS.

ROBERT C. NOBLE, M.D.

SKIN

Better Sunscreens • New Drug to Combat Fungal Infections • Why Hair Grows • Improved Anesthetic for Skin Surgery

Sunscreens With Melanin

Researchers are testing a sunscreen that contains melanin, a natural chemical produced by the skin that helps protect us against the damaging effects of ultraviolet light. As the public becomes increasingly aware of the effects on the skin of sunlight, which includes ultraviolet light, the demand for better sunscreens increases. Scientists have been relatively successful in formulating sunscreens that offer highly effective protection against the short wavelengths of ultraviolet light, which are the most likely to cause sunburn and skin cancer. However, less progress has been made in developing sunscreens with improved protection against the long wavelengths. These longer wavelengths are largely responsible for photoaging—physical changes in the skin that cause it to become wrinkled and leathery, with unsightly spots and growths that may become cancerous.

In their attempts to develop a sunscreen that will yield substantial protection against both the short and the long wavelengths of ultraviolet light, researchers are now taking a lesson from nature and trying melanin. Melanin is produced by specialized skin cells called melanocytes. In response to stimulation by sunlight, melanocytes are capable of producing increased quantities of melanin. They then supply this melanin to the other cells of the epidermis, or outer layer of the skin. When the skin is reexposed to sunlight, the melanin dispersed through the epidermis absorbs both short wavelength and long wavelength ultraviolet light. By doing so, melanin greatly protects us against the cancer-producing and cosmetically damaging effects of sunlight.

Chemists are now capable of biosynthesizing large quantities of melanin in the laboratory. The melanin, processed further to give it a powdery consistency, can then be incorporated into existing sunscreens. Preliminary studies indicate that melanin-containing suncreens do safely provide increased protection against the longer wavelengths of ultraviolet light. The melanin is absorbed into the skin surface, but it does not penetrate through the skin or get absorbed into the blood.

New Antifungal Drug

Preliminary studies of an antifungal agent called terbinafine have shown it to be highly effective in curing common superficial fungal infections. Fungal infections account for approximately 2.5 percent of new visits to dermatologists each year. Although most fungal infections are merely nuisances, disturbing new evidence suggests that more virulent fungal organisms are evolving. Even more upsetting is the evidence that some of these new organisms display resistance to existing antifungal medications. Thus, there is an increasing need to develop new systemic antifungal drugs. (Systemic drugs are taken into and circulate throughout the body—oral medications, for example—as opposed to topical medications, which are applied directly on the skin.)

Presently there are only two systemic antifungal agents that have been approved by the United States Food and Drug Administration: griseofulvin and ketoconazole. Fortunately, numerous other promising antifungals are on the horizon, with terbinafine being one of the most promising.

The most impressive results of the preliminary studies of terbinafine are its effects on fungal infections of the nails. Fingernail and toenail fungal infections, called onychomycoses by dermatologists, are notoriously resistant to treatment. Antifungal creams and lotions applied to the surface of the nails are uniformly ineffective. The existing systemic antifungals are only sometimes effective. In the limited number of cases in which they are, they must be taken for 6 to 12 months—they work by being incorporated into the growing nails and thus must be taken until a complete new nail is formed, 6 months for a fingernail, 12 months for a toenail.

Terbinafine has been shown to be effective in treating onychomycosis when it is taken for 6 to 12 months. However, most exciting is the preliminary evidence that a twice-daily dose of the drug taken for only two weeks proved effective in clearing up onychomycosis in four out of five cases. Terbinafine apparently diffuses from the nail bed through the old nail, thus combating the fungus in both the old and the new nails within a few weeks. Studies of terbinafine have shown it to be safe and relatively free of side effects whether taken long-term or short-term.

How Hair Grows

The recent discovery of the location of the stem cells, or parent cells, that regulate hair growth promises future advances in the understanding of normal and abnormal hair growth.

Scientists have long been baffled by the question of what controls the normal hair cycle. They have known that the cells that produce a hair are located in the very base of the hair, in the hair bulb. These cells, called matrix cells, are known to go through phases of prolonged rapid replication, resulting in growth of a hair. However, they periodically stop replicating, and the hair's growth then stops. After a few months the matrix cells again begin replicating; they form a new hair, and the old hair is shed.

Until recently, researchers investigating hair growth have focused their attention on the matrix cells but have failed to uncover the mechanism that controls their replication. For example, it has been unclear how a new hair develops even after plucking has destroyed the old hair bulb and matrix cells. Recent research has yielded new insight into these questions, with the discovery of a population of stem cells located in a site separate from the hair bulb. This site is called the hair bulge region. Unlike the hair bulb and matrix cells, the hair bulge and its stem cells remain undamaged by hair plucking. The stem cells normally replicate very slowly; however, in response to a yet unidentified stimulus, they give rise to the matrix cells that can produce a new hair. The discovery of the existence and location of the stem cells in the bulge area, researchers believe, should lead to new approaches to treating hair problems and hair loss.

Topical Anesthetic Cream

Recent studies have documented the effectiveness of a new anesthetic cream in partially numbing normal skin. The most unpleasant part of most simple skin surgery is the pain associated with the injection of local anesthetics, such as lidocaine. Because normal skin is an effective barrier to chemical penetration, topical anesthetics generally have little impact. But the new product, EMLA (eutectic mixture of local anesthetics), has been shown to produce significant reduction in the pain associated with needles when applied to the skin and then kept covered with a dressing for 60 minutes.

EMLA contains lidocaine and prilocaine. Although the 60 minute wait for EMLA to work is an inconvenience, it is certainly worthwhile when, for example, skin surgery in children is necessary.

Even more promising is evidence that the anesthetic effect obtained with the application of EMLA cream may be sufficient to permit simple skin surgery without the injection of any additional local anesthetic. For example, the curettage (scraping) of viral lesions associated with the skin disease molluscum contagiosum was painlessly completed on children after EMLA cream was applied.

See also the Spotlight on Health article ATHLETE'S FOOT.

EDWARD E. BONDI, M.D.

SMOKING

New Surgeon General's Report • Gene Linking Smoking and Lung Cancer • Sales to Minors • Tobacco Stocks Targeted

Benefits of Quitting

In September 1990 the U.S. Surgeon General issued the first comprehensive report focused on the health benefits of quitting smoking. The major benefits include: decreased risk of lung cancer and of cancers of the larynx, esophagus, pancreas, bladder, and cervix; decreased risk of heart attack, stroke, and chronic lung disease; higher birthweight babies for women who quit anytime up to the 30th week of pregnancy; and decreased chance of early death.

The report said that quitting smoking also reduces the risk of developing duodenal and gastric ulcers, influenza and pneumonia, and peripheral artery occlusive disease, that is, blockages in the arteries of the extremities, especially the legs and feet. (*See also the Spotlight on Health article* LEG CRAMPS.) It also noted that quitting smoking reduces the risk of a recurrent heart attack. The report concluded that "the health benefits of smoking cessation far exceed any risks from the average five-pound weight gain that may follow quitting."

Help for Quitters

According to the Surgeon General's report, more than 38 million Americans have quit smoking cigarettes, but more than 50 million continue to smoke. A Gallup poll conducted in July 1990, however, concluded that 74 percent of these smokers want to quit. One group that began getting some extra encouragement to stop is the 13 million American smokers over the age of 50. The U.S. Public Health Service launched a $100,000 media campaign aimed at helping this group to stop smoking.

Smokers in Seattle who are covered by King County Medical Blue Shield can now count on help from their health insurer in quitting cigarettes. The plan announced that it would pay 75 percent of the cost of services from a physician or psychologist who helps a person quit or for participation in an approved smoking-cessation program, with a lifetime cap on reimbursement of $500.

An experimental self-help smoking-cessation program for pregnant women at a Maxicare HMO in Texas found that mailing eight brochures with advice on quitting smoking was an effective way to encourage these women to stop smoking for the majority of their pregnancy. Those women who quit gave birth to infants who weighed more at birth than those who did not and were less likely to give birth prematurely. Maxicare investigators said that preventing just one premature birth saved enough money to pay for smoking-cessation programs for 500 women.

Smokers who use nicotine gum to help kick the smoking habit will find it more effective if they avoid mixing acidic drinks—including coffee, beer, colas, and fruit juices—with the gum, according to a study by the National Institute on Drug Abuse. These beverages neutralize the nicotine in the gum, a reaction which can be avoided by waiting 15 minutes before drinking them.

Research

In 1990 researchers achieved some understanding of how cigarette smoke may trigger the gene that causes lung cancer in the cells of susceptible people. According to a study published in August 1990, a gene known as CYP1A1 is more likely to be switched on by cigarette smoke in some people than in others, perhaps explaining why not all smokers develop lung cancer. Once activated, the gene produces a protein of a type capable of turning the chemicals found in cigarette smoke into powerful cancer-causing substances. The gene may be useful as a marker to identify people who are at highest risk for developing lung cancer.

Leukemia and childhood asthma were added during 1990 to the growing list of medical problems known to be caused by smoking. A study published in December in the *Journal of the National Cancer Institute* found the incidence of leukemia in people who smoke 25 or more cigarettes per day to be three times higher than in people who never smoked. The study also showed a fivefold risk of myeloma, a cancer of the bone marrow's plasma cells. The risk for both diseases rises with the number of cigarettes smoked daily as well as with the number of years a person smokes.

According to research from the Harvard School of Public Health, published in *Pediatrics* in April 1990, mothers who smoke have children with higher rates of asthma, increased use of asthma medications, and an earlier onset of the disease.

Evidence that exposure during childhood to secondhand smoke can lead to lung cancer appeared in the *New England Journal of Medicine*. The study found that the risk of lung cancer was about double for nonsmokers who had grown up in households with

A 1990 U.S. Surgeon General's report which listed the impressive health benefits from giving up cigarettes provided strong incentives to smokers to kick the habit (in photo, a Smokenders seminar in Toronto).

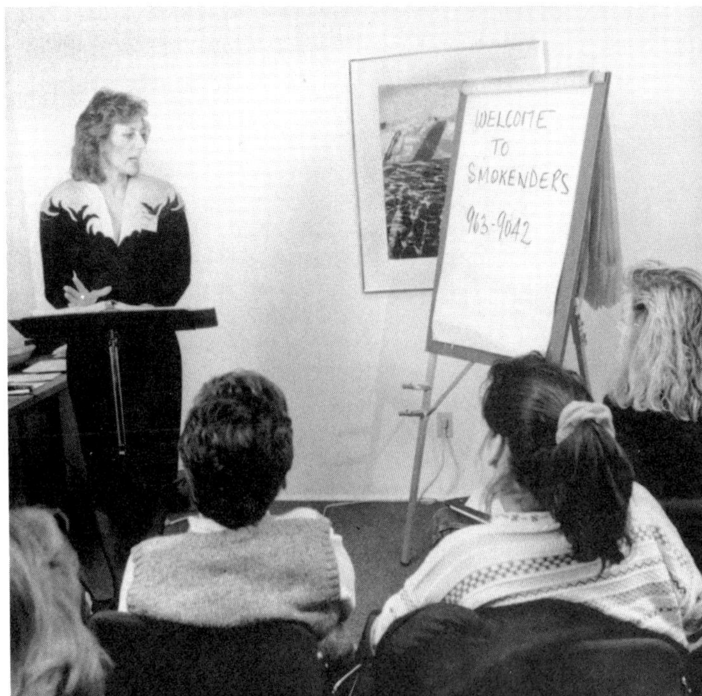

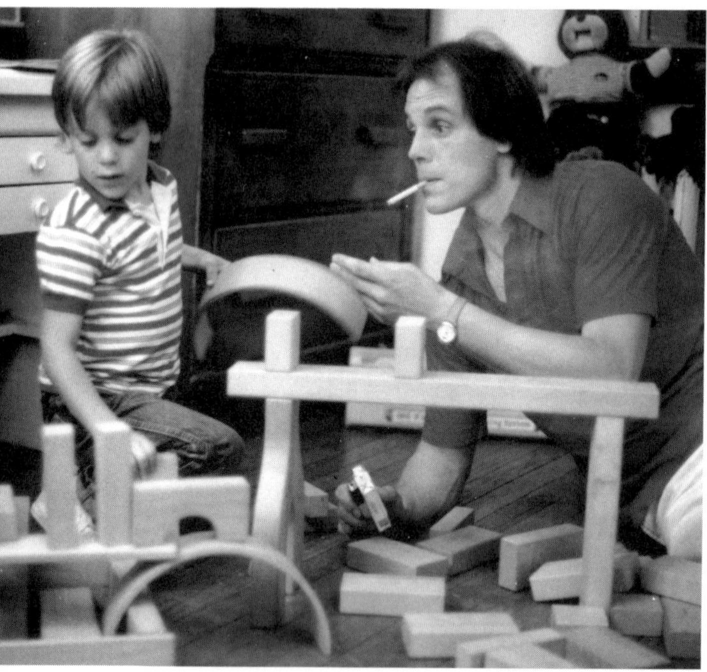

The dangers of secondhand smoke were underlined by a new study which reported that children who grow up in smokers' homes face a lung cancer risk about double that of children raised in a smoke-free environment.

smokers as for those who had been raised in a smoke-free environment, and that about 17 percent of lung cancer cases in nonsmokers can be attributed to this cause.

A comprehensive report from the U.S. Environmental Protection Agency (EPA), released in draft form in June 1990, tentatively concluded that passive smoking, the breathing of ambient cigarette smoke by nonsmokers, causes an estimated 3,800 adult lung cancer deaths a year, as well as increased childhood respiratory illness. The document was accompanied by a guide to workplace smoking policies recommending that government and private employers reduce or eliminate involuntary exposure to secondhand smoke.

Tobacco Exports

As the market for cigarettes in the United States continued to decline, tobacco companies looked for markets abroad. Politicians and health officials attacked U.S. tobacco companies' efforts to market cigarettes overseas. In particular, there was praise for a decision by a General Agreement on Tariffs and Trade panel, which, in considering the controversy over the export of tobacco products from the United States to Thailand, concluded that the export of tobacco products is an international health issue, not simply an issue of international trade. While the panel held that under GATT Thailand could not ban the import of tobacco, neither could the United States accuse Thailand of unfair trade practices because it bans all cigarette advertising. This finding followed the breaking down in recent years of barriers to sales of American tobacco to South Korea, Taiwan, and Japan.

In September 1990, Philip Morris and RJR Nabisco, the United States' two biggest tobacco companies, announced they would sell about 34 billion cigarettes to the Soviet Union, increasing the producers' profits and helping to ease the shortage of cigarettes in that country.

Sales to Minors

As of May 1990 there were laws prohibiting the sale of tobacco to minors in 44 states and the District of Columbia, but they were rarely being enforced, according to the inspector general of the U.S. Department of Health and Human Services. In addition, the tobacco industry was being accused of spending large annual sums to advertise and promote its products to young people.

As a result of concern about access to cigarettes by young people despite the legal prohibitions, cigarette vending machines were targeted by antismoking groups during 1990. The state of Indiana banned the sale of tobacco products through vending machines, as did the township of East Brunswick, N.J. A New York City law restricted the machines to bars.

In order to counter criticism that its advertising is designed to appeal to children and young teenagers, the tobacco industry announced in December that it would begin an ad campaign to discourage smoking by anyone under the age of 18.

Tobacco as an Investment

While the tobacco business continued to be highly profitable, ownership of stock in the companies became unpopular in some quarters, while other stockholders have decided they'd rather fight than switch. In late 1989, Harvard University decided to sell its stock in tobacco corporations, and the City University of New York followed suit in May 1990. Other universities were said to have sold their tobacco stocks quietly in order to avoid losing research contracts supported by tobacco companies.

One coalition of stockholders—the Interfaith Center on Corporate Responsibility—decided to include antitobacco measures among its efforts to influence corporate policies. The group coordinated the introduction of stockholder resolutions to amend the bylaws of three cigarette manufacturers and a maker of cigarette papers to prohibit them from producing or marketing tobacco products by the year 2000. Target companies were Philip Morris, Loews Corporation, American Brands Inc., and Kimberly-Clark. In all cases the corporate boards of directors recommended against the resolutions, but the resolutions received some support at the annual meetings of stockholders.

Advertising and Promotion

The year brought continuing protests against tobacco advertising, especially billboards, aimed at blacks and women. After a group of protesters in New York City's Harlem area whitewashed billboards containing cigarette and liquor advertisements aimed at blacks, billboard owners began replacing some of the ads with public service announcements. As a further response to protests against the use of billboards for tobacco and alcohol advertisements, the Outdoor Advertising Association of America announced in August 1990 that it would place a decal of a child on all billboards within 500 feet of schools, churches, or hospitals to indicate that these locations are off limits to ads for those products, including tobacco, that are illegal to sell to minors. In addition, the Tobacco Institute announced in December that its industry would not advertise cigarettes within 500 feet of schools.

The American College of Obstetricians and Gynecologists also criticized tobacco companies' advertising policies, charging that the companies aim ads at young women with little education—the only group in which the rate of smoking is increasing.

While tobacco companies continued to claim that ads encourage people to switch brands, not to start smoking, critics countered that a ban on tobacco advertising in Canada had contributed to a 10 percent decrease in sales in the first four months of 1990. All print advertising for tobacco products has been banned since January 1990. Tobacco companies argued that the decrease in sales resulted from the high price of smoking, caused by a tax increase of $1 per pack of cigarettes that was instituted at the same time as the advertising ban.

BARBARA SCHERR TRENK

TEETH AND GUMS

High-Tech Dentistry • Implants Become More Common • Antianxiety Pill • Tooth Whiteners

Using New Technology

High tech, so prevalent today in medical procedures, has been slow to make an impact on dental practice. But that seems to be changing, with lasers, ultrasound, and a new imaging technique called radiovisiography increasingly finding their way into dental offices.

Dental Laser. In May 1990 the U.S. Food and Drug Administration (FDA) approved the first laser designed specifically for dental use. The laser energy is delivered through a slender handpiece with a flexible, hair-thin optical fiber at its end, providing the dentist access to virtually all areas of the mouth. The instrument, which delivers short bursts of thermal energy, was initially approved only for treatments involving the soft tissues of the mouth, such as surgical procedures and therapy for periodontal (gum) disease. In minor oral surgery the thermal laser energy seals tiny blood vessels as it vaporizes diseased gum tissue, resulting in minimal bleeding and little pain. Periodontists hope that in patients with deep periodontal pockets (gaps that form below the gum line between the tooth roots and surrounding gum and other tissue) the thermal energy will not only remove the diseased tissue lining the pocket but sterilize the bacteria-laden pocket as well. The American Academy of Periodontology cautioned, however, that there were not yet published studies that "support the effectiveness and relative utility of lasers as compared to conventional forms of instrumentation during periodontal therapy." That is, the laser may be no better than standard scaling (scraping) to clean out periodontal pockets.

The FDA was asked by the laser's manufacturer to also approve it for use on hard tissue—bone or teeth. There was hope that with further research lasers might eventually be used for removing tooth decay and for desensitizing overly sensitive tooth areas, as well as in root canal treatment.

Ultrasound. High-frequency sound waves have been in use for many years in dentistry, in a device designed to remove tartar during tooth cleaning. Now there is a modified ultrasound device approved by the FDA for use in root canal treatment. In the traditional procedure the infected canals are cleaned, widened, and shaped (in preparation for filling them) using a series of manually manipulated files and reamers. Supporters of the new ultrasonic device claim that it is faster and more effective in removing infected tissue from and killing bacteria in the canals. Other specialists counter, however, that further research is needed to determine whether the ultrasound procedure is indeed superior to the conventional method or merely an alternative.

Radiovisiography. In a completely new FDA-approved system for X-raying the teeth and jaws, called radiovisiography, an electronic X ray sensor placed within the mouth replaces the conventional X

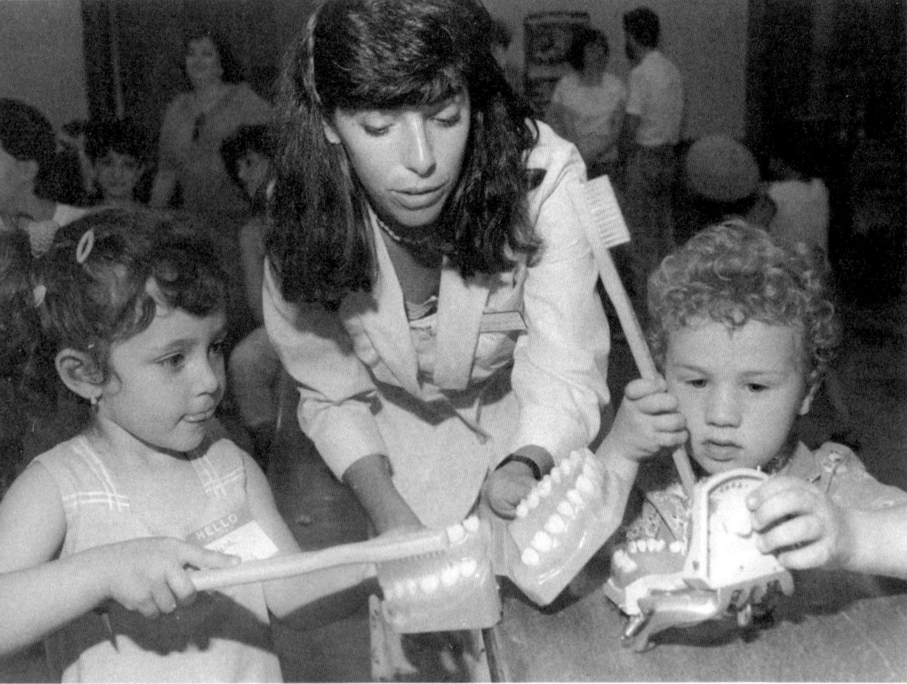

In Boston a Tufts dental student instructs two young Soviet émigrés in toddler toothbrush technique. Four-year-old Svetlana (left) has the right idea; Aleksandr (right) has a little trouble figuring out which end is up.

ray film. The sensitivity of the sensor is so great that the X ray dosage required is reduced by 80 percent. Once exposed, the sensor instantly transmits a video image to a TV monitor—no darkroom or chemicals are required. The high-resolution image can be enlarged fourfold, the contrast can be altered for more precise viewing, images can be viewed in color, and multiple images can be viewed simultaneously for purposes of comparison. After the image has been studied, a special printer can produce in about ten seconds a hard copy for the patient's record. The image itself can be stored in the database of the office computer for comparative study at a later time or transmitted to other offices for consultation purposes.

Implants

Implants, for many years considered to be experimental, are fast becoming part of mainstream dentistry. Implants are anchoring devices permanently inserted into the jawbone (in a surgical procedure usually performed by an oral surgeon or periodontist who has had special training). Crowns, bridges, or dentures are then attached to the implants. A recent survey of specialists in oral and facial surgery showed that from 1986 to 1989 there was a threefold increase in the number of implants inserted per year.

In 1990 the American Dental Association announced a formal acceptance program and guidelines for manufacturers of the various implant devices. Full acceptance of a device by the ADA requires five-year studies showing safety and effectiveness; provisional acceptance is given based on three-year studies. By the end of 1990 one device had achieved full acceptance, and four others had provisional acceptance.

As confidence in implants grows, researchers have even used them in patients with severely atrophied (shrunken) jawbones—people who are virtually dental cripples because they have great difficulty wearing dentures. The researchers reported in March 1990 that at the end of 33 months there was a success rate of 94 percent for the 130 implants placed in 28 such patients, who ranged in age from 30 to 78.

Alleviating Anxiety

Investigators reported in July 1990 that the drug triazolam (brand name, Halcion) given in pill form, was just as effective as intravenous sedation in alleviating the anxiety that accompanies oral surgery. Triazolam is a derivative of diazepam (commonly sold as Valium). A group of 75 patients undergoing extraction of wisdom teeth were the test subjects. Although all of the patients still experienced some anxiety during the extractions (performed under local anesthesia), anxiety was markedly reduced both by the triazolam pill and by intravenous Valium. Not only is an oral medication more easily administered, but the pill takers also experienced faster mental and physical recovery from the drug after the extractions.

Bleaching Agents

In the relatively short time since a new generation of tooth whiteners and brighteners was introduced early in 1989, a large number of these bleaching agents have become available. Most of the products are used under the supervision of a dentist; some, however, have been added to toothpastes sold over-the-counter and by mail order (and widely advertised). All of these new products do not rely on traditional abrasives or detergents to remove "unsightly stains," but on various kinds of oxygenating agents, chemicals that whiten or bleach teeth by a process similar in principle to bleaching hair or clothes. A few products use hydrogen peroxide as the bleaching agent, but most rely on carbamide peroxide—a more stable, slow-release form of hydrogen peroxide.

The new whiteners that are supervised by dentists go beyond the removal or bleaching of surface stains from food, beverages, or tobacco; they actually penetrate the teeth and alter their intrinsic color. Natural tooth color is quite variable, but as teeth age they generally tend to take on a yellower appearance as the enamel wears away. Fillings also cause teeth to darken in time. Some teeth may be markedly discolored from use of tetracycline. If taken during pregnancy, this antibiotic can react with the fetus's developing teeth and cause them to become permanently stained. The same result can occur if a child takes tetracycline during tooth development, a process which is ongoing up to about age eight. Consumption of excessive levels of fluoride while teeth are being formed in early childhood can also cause them to become discolored.

Bleaching such discolored teeth in the dental office by applying high concentrations of bleaching agent is an old procedure. With the new generation of whiteners, however, tooth lightening may be achievable by home application of bleaching gels. The gels are put into custom-made plastic trays (mouthpieces similar to those used by football players and boxers) and kept in place over the teeth for several hours a day for periods ranging from 3 to 12 weeks. The degree of whitening reported in formal studies was variable, with yellow color responding best to the treatment and gray-blue and dark brown stains proving much more resistant. It was not determined in the studies how often the whole series of applications might have to be repeated, although most experts maintained that the process would almost certainly have to be done more than once and perhaps as often as one or two times a year.

The American Dental Association cautioned that oxygenating agents can be irritating to oral tissue and may produce tooth sensitivity and that long-term use may enhance the effect of carcinogens. While manufacturers of both the over-the-counter and the dentist-supervised oxygenating agents argued that their products, being cosmetics, did not require approval by the FDA, the agency was reported to be investigating the whiteners, holding out the possibility that they could be classified as drugs and hence held to stricter safety standards than cosmetics.

See also the Spotlight on Health article PREVENTING GUM DISEASE.

IRWIN D. MANDEL, D.D.S.

WORLD HEALTH NEWS

AIDS Update • Famine in Africa • Mad Cow Disease • Vitamin A Helps Measles • Cholera Outbreak in Peru

AIDS Continues to Spread

In 1990 the number of AIDS cases continued to rise in areas already hard hit by the disease, such as Africa and the United States, and it appeared as a serious problem in Asia, especially in Thailand among intravenous drug users and prostitutes. In addition, China was stunned in 1990 by an outbreak of AIDS among intravenous drug users in the southwest province of Yunnan, which is close to the heroin-producing nations of Myanmar (formerly Burma), Thailand, and Vietnam. This outbreak forced Chinese authorities to relinquish their previously adamantly held position that neither intravenous drug use nor AIDS were problems in their country.

Authorities in India said that the AIDS threat was growing in that country because risk factors such as intravenous drug use and prostitution were common and HIV, the human immunodeficiency virus, which causes AIDS, had already appeared among drug users and prostitutes. Moreover, there had been little education about AIDS to help prevent its spread. Whereas less than one percent of prostitutes in India tested in 1987 were HIV positive, studies suggested that up to 20 percent of prostitutes in major Indian cities were infected by 1990. About 70 percent of one group of prostitutes was reported positive for the HIV virus.

When HIV was first discovered, at least half of the known infected persons were in industrialized nations. Now about two-thirds of the infections are in the developing world, and projections are that by 2000 about three-fourths will be in the Third World. Childhood mortality rates, which had been decreasing in some developing countries, began rising again because of AIDS. The disease, which often kills people in their most productive years, may devastate the economies of some of these countries. Previous estimates of the numbers of people infected with HIV led scientists to predict that from 15 million to 20 million people would be infected by the virus worldwide by the year 2000, with from 5 million to 6 million actual AIDS cases by that date. But the rapid introduction of the virus into the Third World, coupled with the AIDS epidemic in Central Africa, make it likely that these figures will be revised upward.

The most severely stricken area of the world is Africa south of the Sahara. The number of infected people there has apparently doubled in just three years, from 2.5 million in 1987 to 5 million in 1990. In Africa, as in most of the developing world, HIV is spread mainly by heterosexual activity, and whole families have been devastated by the disease, as infected men pass the virus to their wives who, in turn, pass it to their newborn children. Without adequate medical resources, little can be done for those who come down with AIDS symptoms. And, as one American traveler involved in a bus accident in Rwanda discovered, contact with the blood of others may be all it takes to become infected with HIV. He suffered cuts and was covered with the blood of other victims of the accident in an area with a high HIV infection rate. He had no other likely exposures.

Finally, the AIDS epidemic has complicated an already difficult economic situation in Africa. As one AIDS specialist said, "AIDS is just one more reason for those with capital to look elsewhere when they are investing, traveling, or contemplating starting new industries."

Famine

Famine and war combined to hit Ethiopia and Sudan severely in 1990. In Ethiopia at various times during 1990 both sides in the civil war refused to allow emergency food shipments to reach starving people in the north of the country. When the rains failed for the second year in a row, the food situation was even more seriously aggravated. In Sudan, also split by civil war, refugees forced to flee south from Khartoum, the capital, suffered increasing malnutrition and starvation. When the government blocked food supplies sent by the United States from being distributed to the refugees, the United States threatened to withhold any further food aid.

In 1990 the United Nations Children's Fund reported that in the African nation of Malawi malnutrition and stunted growth among children was high, despite the lack of war or rebellion. Malawi, also cited by many outside observers for severe civil rights violations in 1990, maintained that all was well, despite the malnutrition and extremely high infant mortality rates. Ironically, the president of the country, Ngwazi Hastings Kamuzu Banda, is a physician.

Africa was not the only area threatened by famine. In 1990, for the third year in a row, the world produced less grain than it consumed, and world grain reserves dwindled. This, in turn, threatened to increase the price of grain, making it more difficult for poor countries to buy it or for relief organizations to buy grain for them.

Part of the pressure on food supplies was the result of the expanding world population, which was estimated to be about 5.3 billion in early 1991 and expected to reach more than 6 billion by 2000. Control of the world's population must be given high priority if famines are to be prevented in the future. Improvements in agriculture, including storage and transportation, control of pollution, and prevention of war will also be necessary.

Cattle Disease in Britain

Great Britain was devastated in 1990 by fear of what the British press dubbed "mad cow disease." This is a disease of cattle (and possibly other animals) that causes them to suffer brain damage and death. The public showed concern that it might be possible to get the disease by eating beef, although there is no evidence that this can happen. British beef sales plummeted at home, and many nations, including the United States, outlawed the importation of British beef and beef products, causing severe damage to this vital British industry.

The technical name for the disease is bovine spongiform encephalopathy, or BSE. The name comes from the fact that the disease produces many small holes in the brain (making it appear sponge-like) before it kills the animal. By late 1990, the disease had killed or forced the slaughter of almost 14,000 cattle in Britain, and the pace of slaughter was continuing at more than 1,000 head per month. The cattle become aggressive, unsteady, and froth at the mouth before they die, symptoms similar to those of rabies, although the diseases are quite different.

The causative agent of mad cow disease has not been identified, but the disease is clearly infectious. It appears to be in the same category as scrapie in sheep and two human diseases, kuru and Creutzfeldt-Jakob disease, which also produce gradual death through brain damage. Although these sometimes are called slow virus diseases, no viruses have been found for them or for mad cow disease. Some researchers have suggested the improbable idea that the disease is caused by the small protein-containing threads in the cells which lack any genetic material (DNA or RNA).

Investigators call these threads prions, for proteinaceous infectious particles. If this theory is proved, currently held theories of infection and of larger biological processes would be challenged.

As of early 1991, the British government was calming the public and its trading partners, the beef industry was trying to recover, and scientists were attempting to learn more about this mysterious disease.

Vitamin A and Measles

In 1990, South African doctors reported that children suffering from measles who are treated with vitamin A, even if they give no indication of a vitamin A deficiency, recover more quickly than children who are not given the vitamin supplement. Children who have not been vaccinated against measles and come down with the disease are at risk of severe illness, brain damage, and death. The children in the study had been hospitalized with measles complicated by pneumonia, diarrhea, or croup. There were no adverse effects observed from the vitamin A treatment. In their article in the *New England Journal of Medicine*, the doctors recommended that all children with severe measles be given vitamin A supplements.

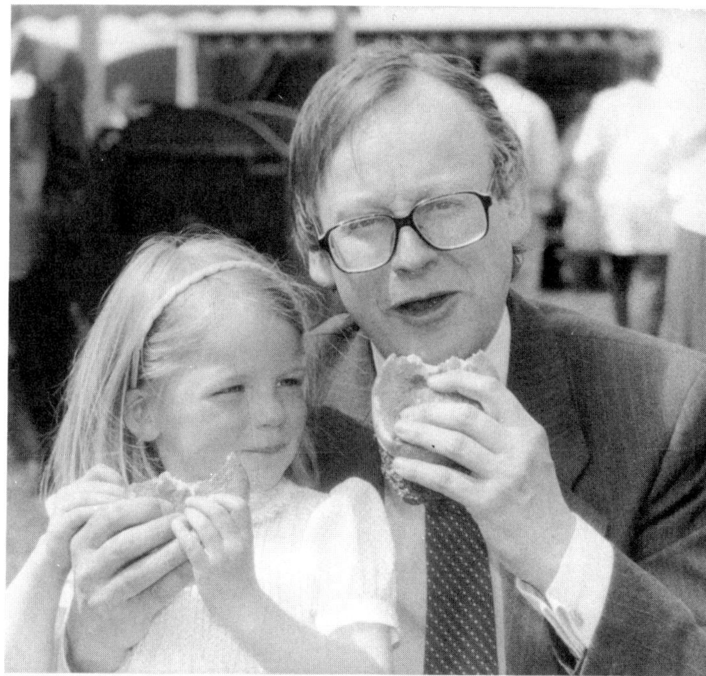

"I have no worries about eating the beefburgers at all," said British agriculture minister John Selwyn Gummer, as he and his four-year-old daughter, Cordelia, enjoyed lunch at an Ipswich boat show. The gesture was designed to allay fears of what the British press called "mad cow disease," an extensive illness of British cattle which, despite medical evidence to the contrary, consumers feared might be transmissible to humans.

Guinea Worm

In 1986 the World Health Assembly of the World Health Organization gave Guinea worm top priority for an attempt at worldwide eradication similar to the successful effort against smallpox in the 1970s. In 1990 India and Pakistan noted marked progress in eliminating Guinea worm, a parasite ingested from contaminated water and which grows under the skin of human beings, causing abscesses and pain. Health officials expect that Guinea worm will be eradicated from India and Pakistan soon, leaving only sub-Saharan Africa still infected. The United States government offered both financial and technical support for Third World Guinea worm eradication programs in 1990. U.S. corporations have also participated in the Guinea worm eradication program by making donations to local programs. American Cyanamid provides free of charge the chemical Abate, which kills the copepods (a kind of crustacean) that transmit the disease, and Du Pont has donated small-mesh nylon gauze that can be used to filter the copepods from infested water before drinking.

Fake Medications

While the developing nations may be more likely to be targeted by makers of false medications who operate from a large international black market, even the developed nations are subject to fake medicines, as was discovered again in 1990, when a drug ring selling bogus Zantac (an antiulcer drug) was uncovered. The false drug had been made in Singapore and Turkey, put into pill form in Greece, and sold for handsome profits in Switzerland and the Netherlands.

Peruvian Cholera Outbreak

In early 1991 the first major outbreak of cholera in the Western hemisphere in the 20th century occurred in Peru. Cholera, an acute infectious disease, is caused by a bacterium that lodges in the intestines and is characterized by severe diarrhea, vomiting, muscle cramps, and collapse. If body fluids are not replced within hours of the first symptoms, the disease can be fatal. The cholera bacterium is usually transmitted through infected water, directly or by contaminating raw or lightly cooked food. The Peruvian government urged people to cook all foods—especially vegetables and fish (often eaten raw in Peru)—thoroughly before eating and to boil water before drinking.

JAMES F. JEKEL, M.D., M.P.H.

Index

Page number in *italics* indicates the reference is to an illustration.

B

C

F

N

O

P

Q

R

S

T

U

V

W

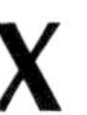

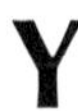

Z

Photo/Art Credits

1: top left, H.M. Lambert/Superstock; top right, John Launois/Black Star; center, Rick Kopstein/Monkmeyer Press; bottom right, George Goodwin/Monkmeyer Press; **2:** Dennis Kendrick; **3:** top left, David Frazier; top right, Don Renner; center, Dennis Oda/Sipa Press; right, Suzanne Szasz/Photo Researchers; **4-5:** Martin Rogers/TSW-Click/Chicago Ltd.; **7:** David Madison; **8:** David Stoecklein/The Stock Market; **10:** H.M. Lambert/Superstock; **11:** David Madison; **12:** Derek Berwin/The Image Bank; **13:** bottom, Whitney Lane/The Image Bank; inset, Trevor, Inc./Monkmeyer Press; **16:** Robert Winslow; **19:** Bob Daemmrich; **21:** top, Stewart D. Halperin; bottom, Lawrence Migdale; **22-23:** Miriam Schaer; **24:** Robert Winslow; **25:** top, Bob Daemmrich; center & bottom, Bob Daemmrich/The Image Works; **26:** Bob Daemmrich; **27:** Focus On Sports Inc.; **29:** Julie Houck/TSW-Click/Chicago Ltd.; **30:** John Neubauer; **31:** Steven LaBadessa; **33:** art by Corinne Hekker Graphics; **35:** Bob Brown; **36:** top, Leonard Lessin/Photo Researchers; bottom, Mark D. Phillips/Photo Researchers; **38-39:** George Rose/Gamma-Liaison; **40:** top, John Launois/Black Star; bottom, Eric Sander/Gamma-Liaison; **42:** David Madison; **43:** John Launois/Black Star; **44:** James Sugar/Black Star; **47:** UPI/Bettmann Newsphotos; **48:** Ford Environmental & Safety Communications; **50-51:** Brown Brothers; **52-53:** The Bettmann Archive; **54:** top, Brown Brothers; bottom, The Bettmann Archive; **55:** The Bettmann Archive; **56:** left to right, Culver Pictures, Inc.; Brown Brothers; **57:** left to right, Culver Pictures, Inc.; The Bettmann Archive; **58:** left & right, UPI/Bettmann Newsphotos; bottom, Culver Pictures, Inc.; **60:** Culver Pictures, Inc.; **61:** Brown Brothers; **65-67:** art by Dennis McArthur; **71:** illustration by Kye Carbone; **72:** art by Corinne Hekker Graphics; **73:** Jeffrey Reed/Stock Shop; **74:** Michael L. Abrahamson; **77:** Renaud Thomas/FPG; **80-81:** art by Robert Romagnoli; **82:** Ann Sager/Photo Researchers; **83:** Day Williams/Photo Researchers; **84:** Don Renner; **85:** Grant DeDuc/Monkmeyer Press; **86-87:** art by Robert Romagnoli; **88:** David Conklin/Monkmeyer Press; **89:** David Stoecklein/Stock Market; **90:** Rick Kopstein/Monkmeyer Press; **92:** Alexander Tslaras/Science Source/Photo Researchers; **93:** Sybil Shackman/Monkmeyer Press; **95:** Kenneth Jarecke/Contact Press Images; **96:** left to right, David Grossman; Erika Stone/Peter Arnold, Inc.; **98:** top, Charlie Archambault/U.S. News & World Report; bottom, Kevin Horan/U.S. News & World Report; **99:** both, Kevin Horan/U.S. News & World Report; **100:** Doug Menuez/Reportage; **102-103:** illustration by Robert Pasternak; **104:** Eric Carle/Shostal/Superstock; **105:** Barbara Burnes/Photo Researchers; **106:** Larry Smith/Leo de Wys, Inc.; **107:** Joe Munroe/Photo Researchers; **108:** Dr. Nigel Smith/Superstock; **109:** Porterfield/Chickering/Photo Researchers; **110:** Don Renner; **114-115:** Martin Gershen/Photo Researchers; **116-117:** Lynne Buschman; **119:** Will & Demi McIntyre/Photo Researchers; **120:** Reuters/Bettmann Newsphotos; **121:** Nancy Pierce/Photo Researchers; **123:** Rob Nelson/Picture Group; **125:** Linda L. Creighton/U.S. News & World Report; **127:** Howard Friedman; **128:** Deborah Heart & Lung Center; **129:** Jim Olive/Peter Arnold, Inc.; **132:** AP/Wide World Photos; **133:** James Caccavo/Picture Group; **134:** Don Renner; **135:** AP/Wide World Photos; **137:** Lynne Buschman; **139:** left & center, Science Photo Library/Photo Researchers; right, St. Mary's Hospital Medical School/Science Photo Library/Photo Researchers; **142-143:** illustration by Stephen Sweny; **144:** Dick Luria/Photo Researchers; **146:** Phil Huber/Black Star; **147:** New England Deaconess Hospital; **150:** George Goodwin/Monkmeyer Press; **152-153:** Steve Lowry; **157-159:** Ruth Soffer; **161:** Joseph Lynch/Medical Images, Inc.; **162-163:** Paul Fusco/Magnum Photo, Inc.; **164:** left to right, Marc Cohen/Visible Ink; Department of Health & Human Services; **165-166:** American Cancer Society; **167:** both, The University of Texas MD Anderson Cancer Center; **168:** American Cancer Society; **170:** J. Wilson/Woodfin Camp; **171:** top, Tom DeWall; inset, Victoria Cavalier; **172:** both, St. Vincent's Hospital; **173:** UPI/Bettmann Newsphotos; **175:** Jerry Berndt; **177:** Doug Jamieson; **180:** Ruth Soffer; **182:** Dennis Kendrick; **184:** art by Dennis McArthur; **187:** Giraudon/Art Resource; **190:** Dennis Kendrick; **193-194:** Lynne Buschman; **196:** both, United Cerebral Palsy Association; **200:** Lynne Buschman; **202:** The Bettmann Archive; **203-204:** Ruth Soffer; **205:** Brian Drake/Viesti Associates; **208:** Ruth Soffer; **211:** art by Corinne Hekker Graphics; **213:** Dennis Kendrick; **216:** art by Corinne Hekker Graphics; **218:** Jerry Berndt; **220-222:** Dennis Kendrick; **223:** Alon Reininger/Contact Press; **226-229:** Dennis Kendrick; **233:** AP/Wide World Photos; **235:** Ruth Soffer; **237-238:** Doug Jamieson; **239:** Jon Chase/NYT Pictures; **241:** Barney Taxel/NYT Pictures; **243-245:** AP/Wide World Photos; **247:** Alon Reininger/Contact Press Images; **248:** John S. Stewart; **250:** left to right, Orange County Register; Sam Mircovich; **252-253:** Kim Komenich/People Weekly/© 1990 The Time Inc. Magazine Company; **255:** both, Tass/Sovfoto; **257:** Robert Goldstein/Medi Chrome; **259:** Lisa Beane; **260:** Mark Hinojosa/© 1990 New York Newsday; **263:** Suzanne Szasz/Photo Researchers; **267:** Rick McCawley/Miami Herald; **268:** Dennis Oda/Sipa Press; **273:** Chris Sheridan/Monkmeyer Press; **274:** National Cancer Institute; **276:** AP/Wide World Photos; **278:** Steve Goldberg/Monkmeyer Press; **283:** Canapress Photo Service; **284:** Mimi Forsyth/Monkmeyer Press; **286:** Health & Human Services; **288:** left to right, courtesy Thermo Cardio-Systems, Inc.; NYT Pictures; **291:** Jeanne Maewong/NYT Pictures; **293:** left to right, Cochlear Corporation; Nicholas De Sciose; **294:** Rick Browne/Photoreporters; **299:** left to right, Wyeth-Ayerst Laboratories; John Storey/People Weekly/© 1990 The Time Inc. Magazine Company; **303:** AP/Wide World Photos; **304-310:** Don Renner; **312:** Ira Wyman/Sygma; **315:** left to right, Ray Ellis/Photo Researchers; Tom Hollyman/Photo Researchers; **319:** left to right, David R. Frazier; Adam Scull/Globe Photos; **322:** Steve Miller/NYT Pictures; **325:** Brian Willer; **326:** Richard Hutchings/Photo Researchers; **328:** Jon Chase/NYT Pictures; **331:** Jim James/The Press Association Ltd.